Pancreatic Disease

Springer
London
Berlin
Heidelberg
New York
Hong Kong
Milan
Paris
Tokyo

C.D. Johnson and C.W. Imrie

Pancreatic Disease

Basic Science and Clinical Management

With 82 Figures

Springer

C.D. Johnson, MChir, FRCS
University Surgical Unit
Southampton General Hospital
Southampton, UK

C.W. Imrie, BSc, MB, FRCS
Royal Infirmary
Glasgow, UK

British Library Cataloguing in Publication Data
Pancreatic disease: basic science and clinical management
1. Pancreas – Diseases 2. Pancreas – Cancer 3. Pancreatitis
I. Johnson, C.D. (Colin David), 1952- II. Imrie, C.W.
(Clement William)
616.3'7
ISBN 978-1-4471-3491-6 ISBN 978-1-85233-904-3 (eBook)
DOI 10.1007/978-1-85233-904-3

Library of Congress Cataloging-in-Publication Data
Pancreatic disease: basic science and clinical management/ C.D. Johnson and C.W. Imrie (eds).
p. ; cm.
Includes bibliographical references.

1. Pancreas–Diseases. I. Title: Pancreatic disease in the twenty-first century. II. Johnson, C. D. (Colin David), 1952- III. Imrie, C. W.
[DNLM: 1. Pancreatic Diseases–diagnosis. 2. Pancreatic Diseases–etiology. 3. Pancreatic Diseases–therapy. 4. Therapies, Investigational. WI 800 P1892 2004]
RC857.P3225 2004
616.3'7–dc21 2003054423

springeronline.com

Originally published by Springer-Verlag London Limited in 2004
Softcover reprint of the hardcover 1st edition 2004

Typeset by EXPO Holdings, Malaysia
28/3830-543210 Printed on acid-free paper SPIN 10900925

Preface

This volume continues our series dealing with current areas of progress and controversy in our understanding of pancreatic disease, its mechanisms, and its treatments.

The contributors met in Southampton to discuss the advances in this field as we look forward to practice in the 21st century. We are fortunate to have world leading experts in several areas, which enables us to present a rounded view of topics such as the diagnosis and management of cystic lesions of the pancreas, the role of stellate cells in the pathogenesis of chronic pancreatitis, and the rapidly developing insights into the genetic basis of pancreatic disease.

A new feature in this volume is the inclusion of a symposium on the management of neuroendocrine tumours of the pancreas. These tumours may produce hormonal symptoms which require the skills of endocrinologists, or other physicians with specialist expertise not normally part of the pancreatologist's range. We are grateful to our authors, who show what can and should be achieved in the management of these sometimes difficult tumours.

Of course, no review of pancreatic disease would be complete without consideration of the current status of pancreatic cancer, and acute pancreatitis. Although we are surgeons, we recognise that progress in the treatment of pancreatic cancer will come through collaboration with our colleagues in oncology, by the use of adjuvant therapy after resection, by the development of more effective chemotherapy, and by application of novel treatments for the majority of patients with irresectable disease. Acute pancreatitis continues to pose problems for clinicians. This book contains useful contributions on the themes of detection of severe pancreatitis, the management of infected necrosis, and the role of enteral nutrition. Finally, we have taken a step back from considering how to manage pancreatic disease, to look at ways in which we can help patients with severe symptoms, when the underlying cause, be it chronic pancreatitis or cancer, cannot be cured.

As editors we have had the pleasure of reading all the chapters in this book. We hope that you, the reader, will enjoy it as much as we have. If you are involved in the management of patients with pancreatic disease, this book will bring your practice up to date; the insights it offers may well underpin developments in treatment that will shape your practice over the next 20 years.

C.D. Johnson
C.W. Imrie
Editors

Contents

Diabetes and Chronic Pancreatitis

3 Hereditary Pancreatitis and Genetic Predispositions

4 Acute Pancreatitis

Selecting Severe Acute Pancreatitis for Trials and for Treatment

Management of Necrosis in Acute Pancreatitis

Enteral Nutrition in Acute Pancreatitis

5 Symptom Relief in Pancreatic Disease

Contributors

Basil J. Ammori
Department of Surgery
Manchester Royal Infirmary
Manchester
UK

Minoti Apte
The University of New South Wales
Pancreatic Research Group
Liverpool Hospital
Liverpool, NSW
Australia

Max G. Bachem
Department of Clinical Chemistry and Pathobiochemistry
University Hospital
Ulm
Germany

Nick Bansback
University of Sheffield
Sheffield
UK

Claudio Bassi
Surgical and Gastroenterological Department
Endocrine and Pancreatic Unit
G.B. Rossi Hospital
University of Verona
Verona
Italy

Adrian C. Bateman
Department of Cellular Pathology
Southampton General Hospital
Southampton
UK

Hans G. Beger
Department of General Surgery
University of Ulm
University Hospital of Surgery
Ulm
Germany

F. Berger
Department of Pathology and Cytology
Lyon Sud Hospital
Lyon
France

F.P. Bernard
Department of Digestive Diseases
Edouard Herriot Hospital
Lyon
France

R.P. Bleichrodt
Department of Surgery
University Medial Center Nijmegen
Nijmegen
The Netherlands

Dale E. Bockman
Department of Cellular Biology and Anatomy
Medical College of Georgia
Augusta, Georgia
USA

Markus W. Büchler
Department of General Surgery
University of Heidelberg
Heidelberg
Germany

John Buckels
Queen Elizabeth Hospital
Birmingham
UK

H.C.J.L. Buscher
Department of Surgery
University Medical Center Nijmegen
Nijmegen
The Netherlands

Anton Buter
University Department of Surgery
Glasgow Royal Infirmary
Glasgow
UK

Martyn Caplin
Centre for Gastroenterology
Royal Free Hospital
London
UK

Ross Carter
Lister Department of Surgery
West of Scotland Pancreatico-biliary Unit
Glasgow Royal Infirmary
Glasgow
UK

Mark Cartmell
Plymouth Postgraduate Medical School
University of Plymouth
Derriford Hospital
Plymouth
UK

Luca Casetti
Surgical and Gastroenterological Department
Endocrine and Pancreatic Unit
G.B. Rossi Hospital
University of Verona
Verona
Italy

Richard M. Charnley
Consultant in Hepato-Pancreato-Biliary Surgery
Freeman Hospital
Newcastle-upon-Tyne
UK

Eithne Costello
Department of Surgery
Royal Liverpool University Hospital
Liverpool
UK

Jane E. Creighton
Department of Surgery
Wansbeck Hospital
Ashington
UK

Mark Deakin
North Staffordshire Hospital
Stoke-on-Trent
UK

Peter de Porre
Johnson & Johnson Pharmaceutical Research & Development
Beerse
Belgium

Christos Dervenis
1st Department of Surgery
Konstantopoulion "Agia Olga" Hospital
Athens
Greece

Pierluigi Di Sebastiano
Department of General Surgery
University of Heidelberg
Heidelberg
Germany

Fabio F. di Mola
Department of General and Laparoscopic Surgery
G. D' Annunzio University
Chieti
Italy

Helen Doran
Departments of Public Health and Surgery
University of Liverpool
Liverpool
UK

J. Dumortier
Department of Digestive Diseases
Edouard Herriot Hospital
Lyon
France

Janet A. Dunn
Cancer Research UK Clinical Trials Unit
University of Birmingham
Birmingham
UK

Massimo Falconi
Surgical and Gastroenterological Department
Endocrine and Pancreatic Unit
G.B. Rossi Hospital
University of Verona
Verona
Italy

David R. Fine
Division of Infection Inflammation and Repair
University of Southampton
Department of Gastroenterology
Southampton University Hospitals NHS Trust
Southampton
UK

Deborah Fitzsimmons
School of Nursing & Midwifery
University of Southampton
Southampton
UK

Helmut M. Friess
Department of General Surgery
University of Heidelberg
Heidelberg
Germany

Paula Ghaneh
Department of Surgery
Royal Liverpool University Hospital
Liverpool
UK

Bernhard Glasbrenner
Department of Internal Medicine II
St. Franziskus-Hospital
Münster
Germany

Thomas Gress
Department of Internal Medicine I
University Hospital
Ulm
Germany

Adolf Grünert
Department of Clinical Chemistry and Pathobiochemistry
University Hospital
Ulm
Germany

Amor Hajri
IRCAD/INSERM
Department of Tumor Biology and Gene Therapy
Strasbourg
France

Christopher M. Halloran
Department of Surgery
Royal Liverpool University Hospital
Liverpool
UK

Pascal Hammel
Service de Gastroentérologie
Fédération Médico-chirurgicale d' Hépato-Gastroentérologie
Hôpital Beaujon
Clichy
France

Helen Hickey
Cancer Research UK Trials Unit
Royal Liverpool University Hospital
Liverpool
UK

Verena Hlouschek
Department of Medicine B
Westfälische Wilhelms-Universität
Münster
Germany

W. Martin Howell
Histocompatibility & Immunogenetics Laboratory
Southampton General Hospital
Southampton
UK

Clement W. Imrie
Lister Department of Surgery
Upper Gastrointestinal Unit
Glasgow Royal Infirmary
Glasgow
UK

Rainer Isenman
Department of General Surgery
University Hospital of Surgery
University of Ulm
Ulm
Germany

Jan B.M.J. Jansen
Department of Gastroenterology
University Medical Centre
Nijmegen
The Netherlands

Colin D. Johnson
University Surgical Unit
Southampton General Hospital
Southampton
UK

Stefan Kahl
Department of Gastroenterology, Hepatology and Infectious Diseases
Otto-von-Guericke University
Magdeburg
Germany

Jutta Keller
Department of Medicine
Israelitic Hospital
Hamburg
Germany

Andrew Kingsnorth
Plymouth Postgraduate Medical School
University of Plymouth
Derriford Hospital
Plymouth
UK

Günter Klöppel
Department of Pathology
University of Kiel
Kiel
Germany

Markus Kosmahl
Department of Pathology
University of Kiel
Kiel
Germany

Paul Georg Lankisch
Department of Internal Medicine
Municipal Clinic of Lüneburg
Lüneburg
Germany

Mike Larvin
Academic Division of GI Surgery
Derby City General Hospital
Derby
UK

Peter Layer
Department of Internal Medicine
Israelitic Hospital
Hamburg
Germany

Markus M. Lerch
Division of Gastroenterology, Endocrinology and Nutrition
Ernst-Moritz-Arndt Universität
Greifswald
Germany

Philippe Lévy
Fédération Médico-Chirurgicale d'Hépato-Gastroentérologie
Hôpital Beaujon
Clichy
France

Matthias Löhr
Department of Medicine II
Medical Faculty Mannheim
University of Heidelberg
Heidelberg
Germany

Daniel Longnecker
Department of Pathology
Dartmouth-Hitchcock Medical Center
Lebanon, New Hampshire
USA

Peter Malfertheiner
Department of Gastroenterology, Hepatology and Infectious Diseases
Otto-von-Guericke University
Magdeburg
Germany

David Malka
Fédération Médico-Chirurgicale d'Hépato-Gastroentérologie
Hôpital Beaujon
Clichy
France

Stefano Marcucci
Surgical and Gastroenterological Department
Endocrine and Pancreatic Unit
G.B. Rossi Hospital
University of Verona
Verona
Italy

Julia Mayerle
Division of Gastroenterology, Endocrinology and Nutrition
Ernst-Moritz-Arndt Universität
Greifswald
Germany

Colin J. McKay
University Department of Surgery
Glasgow Royal Infirmary
Glasgow
UK

Mary McStay
Centre for Gastroenterology
Royal Free Hospital
London
UK

Frank C. Mooren
Department of Sport Medicine
Westfälische Wilhelms-Universität
Münster
Germany

Eva Morris
University of Sheffield
Sheffield
UK

Irina Mountian
Johnson & Johnson Pharmaceutical Research & Development
Beerse
Belgium

B. Napoléon
Department of Digestive Diseases
Edouard Herriot Hospital
Lyon
France

John P. Neoptolemos
Department of Surgery
University of Liverpool
Liverpool
UK

K. Palmer
University Surgical Unit
Southampton General Hospital
Southampton
UK

Christian Partensky
Fédération Digestive
Service de Chirurgie Digestive
Hôpital Edouard Herriot
Lyon
France

Paolo Pederzoli
Surgical and Gastroenterological Department
Endocrine and Pancreatic Unit
G.B. Rossi Hospital
University of Verona
Verona
Italy

Vanina Popova
Johnson & Johnson Pharmaceutical Research & Development
Beerse
Belgium

James Powell
Department of Clinical and Surgical Sciences
Royal Infirmary of Edinburgh
Edinburgh
UK

Catherine Price
Pain Clinic
Southampton University Hospitals NHS Trust
Southampton
UK

Pauli A. Puolakkainen
The Hope Heart Institute
Seattle, Washington
USA

John K. Ramage
Department of Gastroenterology
North Hampshire Hospital
Aldermaston Road
Basingstoke
UK

Michael G.T. Raraty
University of Liverpool
Liverpool
UK

Stéphane Richard
Service de Néphrologie
Hôpital Necker Paris
Laboratoire de Génétique Oncologique
Faculté de Médecine
le Kremlin-Bicêtre
France

Philippe Ruszniewski
Fédération Médico-chirurgicale d'Hépato-Gastroentérologie
Hôpital Beaujon
Clichy
France

Manuel Ruthenbürger
Division of Gastroenterology, Endocrinology and Nutrition
Ernst-Moritz-Arndt Universität
Greifswald
Germany

Roberto Salvia
Surgical and Gastroenterological Department
Endocrine and Pancreatic Unit
G.B. Rossi Hospital
University of Verona
Verona
Italy

D. Sandeman
Endocrinology/Diabetes
Southampton General Hospital
Southampton
UK

Jan Schmidt
Department of General Surgery
University of Heidelberg
Heidelberg
Germany

Alexandra Schmid-Kotsas
Department of Clinical Chemistry and Pathobiochemistry
University Hospital
Ulm
Germany

J.Y. Scoazec
Department of Pathology and Cytology
Edouard Herriot Hospital
Lyon
France

Fanny Shek
Amelie Waring Fellow of the Digestive Disorders Foundation
Tissue Remodelling and Repair Division
University of Southampton
Southampton
UK

Shailesh Shrikhande
Department of General Surgery
University of Heidelberg
Heidelberg
Germany

Marco Siech
Department of General Surgery
University Hospital
Ulm
Germany

Peter Simon
Division of Gastroenterology, Endocrinology and Nutrition
Ernst-Moritz-Arndt Universität
Greifswald
Germany

Ajith Siriwardena
Hepatobiliary Unit
Department of Surgery
Manchester Royal Infirmary
Manchester
UK

Deborah D. Stocken
Cancer Research UK Clinical Trials Unit
University of Birmingham
Birmingham
UK

Robert Sutton
Department of Surgery
University of Liverpool
Liverpool
UK

Helena Tabry
University Surgical Unit
Southampton General Hospital
Southampton
UK

Benoît Terris
Service d'Anatomie Pathologique
Hôpital Beaujon
Clichy
France

Waldemar Uhl
Department of General Surgery
University of Heidelberg
Heidelberg
Germany

Helgi van de Velde
Clinical R&D Oncology
Johnson & Johnson Pharmaceutical Research & Development
Beerse
Belgium

R. van Dongen
Department of Anaesthesiology
University Medical Center Nijmegen
Nijmegen
The Netherlands

H. van Goor
Department of Surgery
University Medical Center Nijmegen
Nijmegen
The Netherlands

Valérie Vilgrain
Service de Radiologie
Hôpital Beaujon
Clichy
France

Susan E. Ward
ScHARR
University of Sheffield
Sheffield
UK

F. Ulrich Weiss
Division of Gastroenterology, Endocrinology and Nutrition
Ernst-Moritz-Arndt Universität
Greifswald
Germany

Jens Werner
Department of General Surgery
University of Heidelberg
Heidelberg
Germany

Evelyn M.I. Williams
Department of Public Health
University of Liverpool
Liverpool
UK

Jeremy Wilson
The University of New South Wales
Director of Medicine and Gastroenterology
Bankstown-Lindcombe Hospital
Bankstown, NSW
Australia

Part 1
Pancreatic Tumours

Neuroendocrine Tumours

1 Epidemiology of Pancreatic Neuroendocrine Tumours

Helen Doran, John P. Neoptolemos, Evelyn M.I. Williams and Robert Sutton

Pancreatic neuroendocrine tumours are rare neoplastic growths of endocrine pancreatic tissue with both neural and endocrine features, frequently causing clinical syndromes from uncontrolled hormone secretion.[1,2] Those tumours that cause such syndromes have been classified as 'functional' whilst those without obvious hypersecretion have been classified as 'non-functional'.[1-3] However, 'non-functional' tumours secrete various peptides and proteins, including chromogranins, plasma levels of which can be used as tumour markers.[1,3,4] There are a number of well recognised syndromic tumours, the commonest being insulinoma and gastrinoma, although many gastrinomas arise in the duodenum (see Table 1.1). A minority of patients presenting with pancreatic neuroendocrine tumours have one of four inherited disorders producing tumours at many sites: multiple endocrine neoplasia type 1 (MEN-1)[5], von Hippel-Lindau disease[6] (see Ch. 12), neurofibromatosis[7] and tuberous sclerosis.[8]

Incidence and Prevalence

Autopsy Series

Pancreatic neuroendocrine tumours have been found in 0.1–1.6% of autopsies in unselected series.[10] This wide variation is likely to be attributable to varying methods of identification; systematic sectioning of the pancreas in transverse blocks 0.3–0.5 cm thick, with subsequent thorough examination of all slides made from each block, will give higher figures. In one autopsy series using meticulous identification the percentage with pancreatic neuroendocrine tumours was 10%.[16] However, as in other endocrine glands, many tumours are small adenomas that are slow growing and without significant hormonal effects, and so do not present during life. In a 25 year study of 11 472 autopsies conducted in Hong Kong, pancreatic neuroendocrine tumours were identified in only 10 cases, only one of which had presented during life.[10] Another study suggests that tumours not presenting in life are more likely to occur in the body and tail of the gland, and contain more pancreatic polypeptide than any other hormone.[18] Such studies have helped to develop our understanding of natural history, but provide limited insight into clinical features.

Table 1.1. Principal clinical features of less rare types of pancreatic neuroendocrine tumours

Tumour	Symptoms	Diagnosis	Malignancy	Survival
Insulinoma	Confusion, sweating, dizziness, weakness, unconsciousness, relief with eating	Inappropriate insulin secretion during hypoglycaemia from up to 72 h fasting	10% of patients develop metastases	Complete resection cures most patients
Gastrinoma	Zollinger–Ellison syndrome of severe peptic ulceration and diarrhoea	Elevated serum gastrin when patient off all acid suppression treatment	Metastases develop in 60% of patients; likelihood correlated with size of primary	Complete resection results in 10 year survival of 90%; less likely if large primary
Glucagonoma	Necrolytic migratory erythema, weight loss, diabetes mellitus, stomatitis, diarrhoea	Elevated serum glucagon. Other hormones can be elevated	Metastases develop in 60% or more patients	More favourable with complete resection; prolonged even with liver metastases
Vipoma	Verner–Morrison syndrome of profuse watery diarrhoea with marked hypokalaemia	Hypochlorhydria, + hypercalcaemia; elevated serum VIP	Metastases develop in up to 70% of patients; majority found at presentation.	Complete resection: five year survival of 95%; with metastases: 60%
Somatostatinoma	Symptomatic cholelithiasis; weight loss; diarrhoea and steatorrhoea	Elevated serum somatostatin	Metastases likely in about 50% of patients	Complete resection associated with five year survival of 95%; with metastases, 60%
Non-syndromic pancreatic neuroendocrine tumour	Symptoms from pancreatic mass and/or liver metastases	A variety of hormones may be elevated, including chromogranins	Metastases develop in up to 50% of patients	Complete resection associated with five year survival of at least 50%

Clinical and Surgical Series

Clinical series have been compiled from collections of cases that include tumours identified incidentally on radiological imaging or pathological examination of a pancreatic specimen performed for another reason. In surgical series functioning tumours have more often been reported.[17,19] Without assessment of the population base from which each series was drawn, no proper epidemiological picture can be drawn.

Prevalence

For indolent neoplastic lesions such as pancreatic neuroendocrine tumours, prevalence is an important measure of population disease burden. Prevalence estimates are reported at 1.0 per 100 000,[20,21] but these estimates were made over three decades ago using older histological techniques. More recent data from the SEER project identified 401 islet cell tumours amongst 22 747 pancreatic cancers (< 2%).[21] However, these data are also limited, because only malignant tumours were included, and more importantly, most pancreatic cancers are associated with a survival of less than six months, quite different from most pancreatic neuroendocrine tumours.

Incidence

All Pancreatic Neuroendocrine Tumours

There are two population-based studies that have assessed the overall incidence of pancreatic neuroendocrine tumours identified during life,[6,7] but in neither was the autopsy rate reported. Watson and co-workers used cases identified in Northern Ireland that had been entered into a neuroendocrine tumour database compiled in conjunction with a specialist reference laboratory conducting hormone assays.[22] From these data they estimated the incidence to be 2.0 per million per year. Eriksson and co-workers took all cases treated in Uppsala over a 20 year period and assumed a local population base, despite an international referral practice; they calculated 4.0 cases per million per year.[23]

Insulinoma

Estimates for this tumour have ranged from 0.67–4.0 cases per million per year, varying widely despite the use of reference populations.[6,8,9,23,24]

Gastrinoma

The reported incidence of this tumour has ranged from 0.1–4.0 cases per million per year,[23,25] with that for the defined Northern Ireland population the incidence reported by Watson and colleagues was 0.5 per million per year.[22] Historically, insulinoma was considered the most common pancreatic neuroendocrine tumour but more recent reports suggest that gastrinoma is more common.[22,26] However, the terms Zollinger–Ellison syndrome and gastrinoma have been used interchangeably, without specification as to tumour location, and most studies have given combined pancreatic and extra-pancreatic gastrinoma rates. Earlier studies cited the pancreas as the organ most frequently harbouring a gastrinoma (40–53%).[27,28] However these reports contained a significant number of cases where tumour was not detected (27–34%). Small, occult duodenal gastrinomas account for a significant number of such cases.[1,3]

Glucagonoma

The Northern Ireland study of Watson and colleagues estimated the annual incidence of glucagonoma at 0.05 per million (1 per 20 000 000) per year,[22] accounting for 2.5% of all their pancreatic neuroendocrine tumours. Other estimates suggest that glucagonoma accounts for 8% of all syndromic pancreatic neuroendocrine tumours and for 5% of all pancreatic endocrine tumours presenting during life.[29,30] A more recent report suggests that glucagonoma is an underdiagnosed condition, because it is asymptomatic for long periods, and produces non-specific symptoms; this report suggests that the true incidence may approach that of insulinoma and gastrinoma,[31] although this has not been confirmed.

Vipoma

VIPomas, which are usually located in the pancreas, produce the Verner–Morrison or WDHA (watery diarrhoea, hypokalaemia and achlorhydria) syndrome from an excess of vasoactive intestinal polypeptide.[1,3,22] Their incidence has been estimated at 0.12–2.0 per million per year,[6,23] comprising 3–5% of all pancreatic neuroendocrine tumours.[32]

Ppoma

Marked differences in the reported incidence of pancreatic polypeptide producing tumours (PPoma) have arisen because historically, many non-syndromic tumours were not tested for pancreatic polypeptide. The principal documented physiological action of pancreatic polypeptide is inhibition of biliary and pancreatic exocrine secretion.[37] The incidence of pancreatic polypeptide hypersecretion is variable depending on the type of endocrine cell tumour; all pure PPomas present with elevated pancreatic polypeptide levels.[37,38] Thus, although 50–75% of patients with non-syndromic tumours have increased basal levels of pancreatic polypeptide,[18] and cells producing pancreatic polypeptide are found in 28–74% of other syndromic tumours, pure or dominant PPoma have been estimated to comprise only 1–2% of all pancreatic neuroendocrine tumours.[38]

Rarer Syndromic Tumours

The more infrequent pancreatic neuroendocrine tumours are reported primarily as case series; incidence is difficult to estimate. Somatostatinomas, like gastrinomas, occur in both pancreatic and extra-pancreatic sites, although the distinction between sites has rarely been made.[40,41] Somatostatinomas have been estimated to account for about 1% of all active neuroendocrine tumours of the gut and pancreas.[42] Other very occasional tumours include those producing growth factor releasing hormone or growth hormone, parathyroid hormone or parathyroid related hormone, or adrenocorticotrophic hormone.[1–3] Some of these tumours may be misclassified as non-syndromic if a full screen of potential ectopic hormones is not performed.

Carcinoid

Carcinoid tumours of the pancreas are rare, and reports must include at least immunohistochemical analysis or appropriate hormone assays to avoid confusion from vague terminology. A detailed report is that of thirty cases collected up to 1995,[43] which found the most frequent symptom to be pain, followed by diarrhoea and weight loss. An atypical carcinoid syndrome characterised by skin flushing was found in 10 cases (33%). Elevated urinary 5-hydroxyindole acetic acid levels were found in 25 (83%).

Small Cell Carcinoma

Small cell carcinoma is a poorly differentiated pancreatic tumour composed of small to intermediate sized cells with neuroendocrine features. It is extremely rare and estimated to account for less than 1% of all (exocrine and endocrine) pancreatic malignancy.[44]

Non-syndromic Pancreatic Neuroendocrine Tumours

The reported incidence of non-syndromic tumours has varied from 15–40%,[18,33,34] depending on assay and classification procedures.[36] Earlier reports included glucagonoma and somatostatinoma as non-syndromic tumours, as these do not produce obvious hormone-specific symptoms when serum hormone levels are low.[30] However, more recent reports suggest higher numbers of non-syndromic tumours, because of increased accuracy in their detection[1,3,16,22] (see Table 1.2).

Incidence Trends Over Time

In the past 20 years more accurate identification of pancreatic neuroendocrine tumours has resulted from heightened awareness, supported by improved diagnostic technology as well as development of specialist tertiary referral units. Specific reports detailing changes in the incidence of these tumours over time suggest that the percentage of non-syndromic tumours has increased during the last two to three decades.[26,32] A study from the Mayo Clinic examining insulinomas diagnosed in Olmstead County between 1927–1986 demonstrated a significant increase in incidence over time, with no detectable change in age or gender distribution,[26] However, clinical practice has changed so dramatically it is not possible to conclude whether such an increase is real or artefactual.

Table 1.2. Location, association with MEN-1 and incidence of less rare types of pancreatic neuroendocrine tumours

Tumour	Location	Metastases	% MEN-1	Incidence
Insulinoma	Pancreas	10%	5%	1–2 per million
Gastrinoma	50% pancreas	60%	25–40%	1–2 per million
Glucagonoma	Pancreas	50–80%	10%	0.1 per million
Vipoma	Pancreas	40–70%	5%	0.1 per million
Somatostatinoma	50% pancreas	70%	45%	< 0.1 per million
Non-syndromic tumour	Pancreas	60%	20%	1–2 per million

Sex Distribution

The overall sex distribution for all pancreatic neuroendocrine tumours appears to be approximately equal, with variations between syndromic types. For insulinoma most series have reported a higher incidence in women;[8,18,31,45,46] for gastrinoma the male to female ratio has been reported at 3:2;[47,48] whilst for glucagonoma it is 1:2.[31] Somatostatinoma has been reported to be commoner in women[42,49] as has VIPoma,[18,50] whereas small cell carcinoma has been found predominantly in men.[44,51]

Age Distribution

The crude median age for all pancreatic neuroendocrine tumours has been reported to be 52 years, with children below 15 years of age rarely affected.[23,44] Insulinoma has a very wide age range but the crude peak incidence occurs between 40–50 years.[8,29,45,46] Gastrinomas can occur at any age and in one series children formed almost one in 10 of those affected.[47] The peak incidence of sporadic gastrinoma occurs between 40–60 years, whereas in association with multiple endocrine neoplasia, the peak age is between 20–40 years.[25] The reported median age for glucagonoma is between 40–70 years,[1,52] for somatostatinoma between 30–60 years[42,49] and small cell carcinoma between 40–75;[44,51] as the numbers are few, the ranges are wide.

Geographical and Ethnic Variation

There are no studies examining geographical variation in a meaningful way, although there are reported series from both east and west.[6,10]

Risk Factors for Pancreatic Neuroendocrine Tumours

Inherited Diseases

Multiple Endocrine Neoplasia Type 1(MEN-1)

This syndrome is characterised by pituitary, parathyroid and pancreatic islet cell tumours, produced by mutation of the MEN-1 gene encoding menin,[5,55] a nuclear protein that suppresses cell proliferation.[56] Numerous microscopic neuroendocrine tumours (0.3–5 mm in diameter) occur throughout the pancreas, occassionally associated with one or more larger tumours. In individuals with an established diagnosis of MEN-1, between 30–85% have clinical evidence of pancreatic neuroendocrine tumours.[30,58] Autopsies of patients with MEN-1 have shown pancreatic neuroendocrine tumours to be invariably present,[58] but most are non-syndromic and clinically silent. Thus in one surgical series of 132 patients with pancreatic neuroendocrine tumours, non-syndromic tumours were identified in only eight of 36 (22%) patients with MEN-1, the other 28 having syndromic tumours.[59] Of these, gastrinoma is the commonest; up to 50% of MEN-1 patients display typical symptoms.[60] Of all patients with gastrinomas, MEN-1 is present in one of every four.[31]

Von Hippel–Lindau Disease (VHL)

This disease is inherited as an autosomal dominant disorder with high penetrance, this produces brain and spinal cord haemangioblastomas, retinal angiomas, renal cell carcinomas, pancreatic neuroendocrine tumours, phaeochromocytomas, endolymphatic sac tumours and also papillary cystadenomas of the epididymis and broad ligament.[6] It results from mutation of the tumour suppressor VHL gene, and may rise de novo through somatic mutation.[3,6]. (See Ch. 12.)

Neurofibromatosis

Type 1 neurofibromatosis (NF1) affects about 1 in 4000 individuals, and is inherited as an autosomal dominant condition with variable penetrance of mutations in the tumour suppressor NF1 gene encoding the protein neurofibromin; 50% of affected individuals have new mutations.[7] It is characterised by multiple pigmented and thickened patches of skin, neurofibromata of nerves and occasionally, phaeochromocytomas. Pancreatic neuroendocrine tumours occur in a small minority of affected individuals.[1,3]

Tuberous Sclerosis

This rare disorder arises from mutation in the tumour suppressor TSC1 or TSC2 genes, producing focal hyperplasia of neuroglia and neuronal tissue of the brain, astrocytoma, rhabdomyoma of the heart, adenoma sebaceum, and uncommonly, pancreatic neuroendocrine tumours.[8]

Sporadic Pancreatic Neuroendocrine Tumours:

Allelic loss of chromosome 11Q, which includes the MEN-1 gene, is the most frequent chromosomal alteration in these tumours.[61] Somatic mutations of the MEN-1 gene have been found in 25–50% of sporadic pancreatic neuroendocrine tumours, excepting insulinoma, in which somatic MEN-1 mutations are uncommon.[62,63] Somatic mutations of VHL have been found occasionally. It appears that many of the commoner oncogenes and tumour suppressor genes (p53, DPC4/SMAD4, PTEN, K-ras, c-myc, c-erb2, c-fos) are of little importance in pancreatic neuroendocrine tumour development, although p16/MTS1 may have a role in gastrinoma.[61,64]

Risk of Malignancy

Traditional histopathological criteria of malignancy have limited application in the assessment of primary pancreatic neuroendocrine tumours. Thus uniformity of tumour cell appearance can be deceptively reassuring, whilst vascular and/or perineural invasion are unusual. Only the presence of local invasion and/or metastases are definitive in determining malignancy.[34,63,64] Metastases are most commonly found in the liver (up to 80% of cases), less frequently in regional lymph nodes, whilst dissemination to other distant sites is unusual.[65] Generally, tumours composed of cells producing eutopic hormones (that are normally produced by pancreatic islets) have a much lower malignancy risk that tumours producing ectopic hormones (gastrin, VIP, neurotensin, ACTH), which is useful in prognostic evaluation.[64] Overt malignancy has been found in 4–16% of patients with insulinoma,[33,46,46,64–67] with a large series of 951 patients reporting overt metastatases in 5%.[46] In contrast, malignant features have been reported in 23–90% of patients with gastrinomas, with a consensus of around 60%.[33,47,64,68–70] Over 60% of patients with glucagonoma have invasive or metastatic disease,[33] as do 50–75% of those with somatostatinomas[33,49] and 50–90% of those with VIPomas.[33,50] Between 45–90% of patients with non-syndromic tumours have been reported to have invasive or metastatic disease, a wide range that is probably a reflection of selection factors such as referral patterns, as well as methods of classification and management.[7,33,35] The vast majority of tumours secreting hormones such as ACTH, PTH and vasopressin are malignant.[64]

Management and Prognosis

Staging

Until recently (see Table 1.3[74]), there has been no relevant staging system, and only now are randomised controlled trials underway to test alternative strategies in therapy. Furthermore, gastrointestinal carcinoids and pancreatic neuroendocrine tumours have often been considered together as gastroenteropancreatic endocrine tumours, so that figures for survival are imprecise.

Survival

Overall Survival

The Uppsala group reported a median survival from diagnosis of 8.7 years for all pancreatic neuroendocrine tumours, reduced to 6.7 years for those with malignant tumours; 80% of those with benign tumours were alive at 10 years.[2,23] Most malig-

Table 1.3. Consensus classification of pancreatic neuroendocrine tumours developed under the auspices of the World Health Organisation [74]

Well differentiated:			
	Confined to pancreas:		
		Benign behaviour:	
			Nonangioinvasive
			< 2 cm in size
			Ki-67 proliferation index < 2%
			< 2 mitoses per10 high power fields
		Uncertain behaviour:	
			Angioinvasion
			> 2 cm in size
			Ki-67 proliferation index >2%
	Gross local invasion or metastasis:		
		Low grade malignant:	
			Often have angioinvasion and/or perineural invasion
			Metastases
Poorly differentiated:			
	High grade malignant:		
		Highly atypical cells	
		Metastases	

nant pancreatic neuroendocrine tumours grow slowly and are generally associated with far longer survivals than other solid tumours. For patients with regional and/or distant metastases, overall 5-year survivals of between 30 and 40% have been reported.[29,66,73,74] In patients with untreated or unresponsive metastatic disease, a median survival of 3–4 years has been observed from the time of diagnosis,[73] approximately 8 years from the onset of symptoms.[75] Whilst curative resections are rarely possible for metastatic disease, combinations of therapies including surgical debulking and hormonal inhibition can achieve effective palliation for prolonged periods.[76] Now that the effects of life-threatening hypersecretion can usually be controlled, the commonest cause of death is liver failure from slow tumour progression.[36,64,76] However, pharmacological suppression of hormonal hypersecretion is not always effective, and the debilitating effects of liver metastases may still warrant hepatic resection or other ablative therapies.[77]

Comparison of Syndromic and Non-syndromic Tumours

The overall survival for syndromic tumours, especially those producing eutopic hormones, has been consistently longer than for non-syndromic tumours. These latter tend to present at a later stage; the rate of liver metastasis amongst patients with non-syndromic tumours has been estimated at 60–90% of cases.[64] Eriksson and coworkers reported a 5 year survival rate of 42% for non-syndromic tumours compared to 80% for syndromic tumours.[7,17] Most series confirm non-syndromic tumours to have a poorer survival[7,19] but some authors contradict this.[35,64,80]

Insulinoma

All series report insulinoma to have an excellent prognosis because of the high incidence of benign disease, and surgical excision is curative for most patients.[78] In earlier reports, peri-operative mortality was attributed to pancreatic fistulas, pseudocysts and pancreatitis; more often after enucleation than after distal pancreatectomy,[19,46] but with increasing specialisation the complications of pancreatic surgery have fallen. Even limited metastatic disease can be cured by surgery: 5-year survival rates for metastatic insulinoma have been reported at 30–46%.[8,34]

Gastrinoma

Zollinger reported an overall survival of 50% at 10 years for malignant gastrinoma.[68] Even with liver metastasis the overall 5-year survival has been reported at 20–38%.[66,68] Gastrinoma is associated with lymph node involvement in 60–80% of cases.[23] Interestingly, lymph node involvement without hepatic or distant metastasis does not appear to exert a major influence on survival from gastrinoma.[48] This finding suggests that the presence of lymph node metastases should not necessarily discourage an aggressive surgical approach.

Other Syndromic Tumours

The majority of patients with glucagonoma have metastatic disease at the time of presentation. However, this tumour tends to progress slowly and patients may survive for years without treatment.[66] VIPomas, often metastatic at the time of diagnosis, may be associated with extended survivals, with a median of 3.6 years.[27] Patients with pancreatic carcinoids have fared less well, the median survival being 7 months in a series of 30 patients, 21 of whom had metastases.[79]

Summary

Pancreatic neuroendocrine tumours are a rare group of neoplasms with complex patterns of behaviour requiring detailed specialist management. Interpretation of the current literature is limited by difficulties in classification, diagnosis and staging, with no randomised controlled trials that compare alternative treatments. Descriptive epidemiological studies are based on clinical or autopsy series with poorly defined reference populations. Only two population-based studies provide estimates of the incidence in life, one at 2.0 per million per year, the other at 4.0 per million per year, whilst autopsy series suggest a more frequent occurrence. The course of these tumours is often indolent, and although ectopic hormone production can be life threatening, crude survival rates of 50% or more at 5 years have been recorded, even for more malignant forms. There is a need for further population-based studies with accurate ascertainment to evaluate the epidemiology of these tumours.

References

1. Jensen RT. Pancreatic endocrine tumors: recent advances. Ann Oncol 1999; 10 (Suppl 4):S170–6.
2. Eriksson B, Oberg K. Neuroendocrine tumours of the pancreas. British Journal of Surgery 2000; 87:129–31.

3. Gumbs AA, Moore PS, Falconi M, et al. Review of the clinical, histological, and molecular aspects of pancreatic endocrine neoplasms. J Surg Oncol 2002; 81:45–53.
4. Stridsberg M, Oberg K, Li Q, et al. Measurements of chromogranin A, chromogranin B (sectretogranin I), chromogranin C (secretogranin II) and pancreastatin in plasma and urine from patients with carcinoid tumours and endocrine pancreatic tumours. J Endocrinol 1995; 144:49–59.
5. Thakker RV. Multiple endocrine neoplasia. Horm Res 2001; 56 (Suppl 1):67–72.
6. Lubensky IA, Pack S, Ault D, et al. Multiple neuroendocrine tumors of the pancreas in von Hippel-Lindau disease patients. Am J Pathol 1998; 153:223–31.
7. Ballester R, Marchuk D, Boguski M, et al. The NF1 locus encodes a protein functionally related to mammalian GAP and yeast IRA proteins. Cell 1990; 63:851–9.
8. Van Slegtenhorst M, Nellist M, Nagelkerken B, et al. Interaction between hamartin and tuberin, the TSC1 and TSC2 gene products. Hum Mol Genet 1998; 7:1053–7.
9. Lopez-Kruger R, Dockerty MB. Tumors of the islet of Langerhans. Surg Gynecol Obstet 1947; 85:495–504.
10. Creutzfeldt W, Arnold R, Creutzfeld C, et al. Pathomorphologic, biochemical and diagnostic aspects of gastrinomas (Zollinger-Ellison syndrome). Hum Pathol 1975; 6:47–62.
11. Grimelius L, Hulquist GT, Stenkvist B. Cytological differentiation of asymptomatic pancreatic islet cell tumours in autopsy material. Virch Arch Pathol Anat Histo 1975; 365:275–88.
12. Creutzfeld W. Endocrine tumours of the pancreas, clinical, chemical and morphological findings. Monograph Pathol 1985; 21:208.
13. Weil C. Gastro-enteropancreatic endocrine tumours. Klinic 1985; 63:433–59.
14. Lam KY, Lo CY. Pancreatic endocrine tumours: a 22 year clinico-pathological experience with morphological, immunohistochemical observation and a review of the literature. Eur J Surg Oncol 1997; 23:36–42.
15. Kimura W, Kuroda A, Morioka Y. Clinical pathology of endocrine tumours of the pancreas: analysis of autopsy cases. Digestive Diseases and Sciences 1991; 36:933–42.
16. Delcore R, Friesen SR. Gastrointestinal neuroendocrine tumours. J Am Coll Surg 1994; 178:187–211.
17. Kent RB, van Heerden JA, Weiland LH. Nonfunctioning islet cell tumours. Ann Surg 1981; 198:185–90.
18. Broughan TA, Leslie JD, Soto JM, et al. Pancreatic islet cell tumours. Surgery 1986; 99:671–8.
19. Shein PhS, De Lellis RA, Kahn CR, et al. Islet cell tumours. Current concepts and management. Ann Int Med 1973; 79:239–57.
20. Moldow RE, Connelly RR. Epidemiology of pancreatic cancer in Connecticut. Gastroenterology 1968; 55:677–86.
21. Carriaga MT, Henson DE. Liver, gallbladder, extraheptic bile ducts, and pancreas. Cancer 1995; 75:171–90.
22. Watson RG, Johnston CF, O'Hare MM, et al. The frequency of gastrointestinal endocrine tumours in a well defined population – Northern Ireland 1970–1985. Quart J Med 1989; 267:647–57.
23. Eriksson B, Oberg K, Skogseid B. Neuroendocrine pancreatic tumours: clinical findings in a prospective study of 84 patients. Acta Oncol 1989; 28:373–7.
24. Kavlie H, White TT. Pancreatic islet beta cell tumors and hyperplasiā: experience in 14 Seattle hospitals. Ann Surg 1972; 175:326–35.
25. Cullen RM, Ong CE. Insulinoma in Auckland 1970–85. New Zealand Med J 1987; 100:560–2.
26. Service FJ, McMahon MM, O'Brien PC, et al. Functioning insulinoma – incidence, recurrence and long survival of patients: a 60 year study. Mayo Clin Proc 1991; 66:711–9.
27. Peplinski G, Norton J. Gastointestinal endocrine cancers and nodal metastasis Biological significance and therapeutic implications. Surg Oncol Clin North Am 1996; 5:159–71.
28. Stamm B, Hacki WH, Kloppel G, et al. Gastrin producing tumours and the Zollinger Ellison syndrome. In: Dayal Y, ed. Endocrine pathology of the gut and pancreas. Boston: CRC Press 1991; 155–94.
29. Mozell E, Woltering E, Stenzel P, et al. Functional endocrine tumours of the pancreas: clinical presentation, diagnosis and treatment. Curr Prob Surg 1990; 303–86.
30. Fox PS, Hoffman JW, Wilson SD, et al. Surgical Management of Zollinger Ellison Syndrome. Surg Clin North Am 1974; 54:395–407.
31. Jensen RT, Doppman JL, Gardener JD. Gastrinoma. In: Go VLW, DiMagno EP, Gardner JD, et al, eds. The exocrine pancreas: biology, pathobiology and disease. New York: Raven Press 1986; 727–44.
32. Thompson GB, van Heerden JA, Grant CS, et al. Islet cell carcinomas of the pancreas: a twenty year experience. Surgery 1988; 104:1011–7.
33. Frantz VK. Tumours of the endocine pancreas. In: Armed Forces Institute of Pathology, ed. Atlas of Tumour Pathology. Washington DC 1997; 145–209.

34. Edney JA, Hormann S, Thompson JS, et al. Glucagonoma Syndrome is an Underdiagnosed Clinical Entity. Am J Surg 1990; 160:625–9.
35. Heitz PU. Pancreatic endocrine tumours. In: Kloppel G, Heitz P, eds. Pancreatic Pathology. Edinburgh: Churchill Livingstone 1984; 206–32.
36. Greenberg GR, McCloy RF, Adrian TE, et al. Inhibition of pancreas and gallbladder by pancreatic polypeptide. Lancet 1978; 2:1280–2.
37. Drian TE, Uttenthal LO, Williams SJ, et al. Secretion of pancreatic polypeptide in patients with endocrine tumours. New Eng J Med 1986; 315:287–91.
38. Tomita T, Friesen SR, Pollock GH. PP-producing tumours. In: Dayal Y, ed. Endocrine pathology of the gut and pancreas. Boca Raton: CRC Press 1991; 280–304.
39. Ganda OP, Soeldner JN. "Somatostatinoma": a somatostatin containing tumour of the endocrine pancreas. New Engl J Med 1977; 296:963–7.
40. Larsson LI, Hirsch MA, Holst JJ, et al. Pancreatic somatostatinoma: clinical features and physical implications. Lancet 1977; 1:677.
41. Dayal Y, Ganda Om P. Somatostatin producing tumours. In: Dayal Y, ed. Endocrine Pathology of the Gut and Pancreas.: Boca Raton: CRC Press 1991; 241–77.
42. Maurer CA, Baer HU, Dyong TH, et al. Carcinoid of the pancreas: clinical characteristics and morphological features. Eur J Cancer 1996; 32:1109–16.
43. Reyes CV, Wang T. Undifferentiated small cell carcinoma of the pancreas: a report of 5 cases. Cancer 1981; 47:2500–2.
44. Broder LE, Carter SK. Pancreatic islet cell carcinomas. Clinical features of 52 patients. Ann Intern Med 1973; 79:101–7.
45. Thompson NW, Eckhauser PE. Malignant islet cell tumours of the pancreas. World J Surg 1984; 8:940–51.
46. White TJ, Edney JA, Thompson JS, et al. Is There a Prognostic Difference Between Functional and Nonfunctional Islet Cell Tumours? Am J Surg 1994; 168:627–30.
47. Galbut DL, Markowitz AM. Insulinoma: diagnosis, surgical management and long-term follow-up. Review of 41 cases. Am J Surg 1980; 139:682–90.
48. Stefanini P, Carboni M, Patrassi N, et al. Beta-islet cell tumours of the pancreas: results of a study on 1067 cases . Surgery 1974; 75:597–609.
49. Ellison EH, Wilson SD. The Zollinger Ellison Syndrome:Re-appraisal and Evaluation of 260 Registered Cases. Ann Surg 1964; 160:512–8.
50. Ellison EC. Forty year appraisal of gastrinoma: back to the future. Ann Surg 1995; 222:512–24.
51. Konomi K, Chijiiwa K, Katsuta T, et al. Pancreatic somatostatinoma: a case report and review of the literature. Int Surg Oncol 1990; 43:259–6.
52. Capella C, Polak J, Buffa R, et al. Morphological patterns and diagnostic criteriaof VIP producing endocrine tumours. A histological,histochemical, ultrastructural and biochemical study of 32 cases. Cancer 1983; 52:1860–74.
53. O'Connor TP, Wade TP, Sunwoo YC, et al. Small cell undifferentiated carcinoma of the pancreas. Report of a patient with tumour marker studies. Cancer 1992; 70:1514–9.
54. Norton JA. Somatostatinoma and rare pancreatic endocrine tumours. In: Clark OH, Duh Quang-Yang, eds. Textbook of Endocrine Surgery. Philadelphia: W.B.Saunders company 1997; 626–34.
55. Chandrasekaharappa SC, Guru SC, Manickam P, et al. Positional cloning of the gene for multiple endocrine neoplasia-type 1. Science 1997; 276:404–7.
56. Guru SC, Goldsmith PK, Burns AL, et al. Menin, the product of the MEN1 gene, is a nuclear protein. Proc Natl Acad Sci USA 1998; 95:1630–4.
57. Calender A, Giraud S, Cougard P. Multiple endocrine neoplasia type 1 in France: clinical and genetic studies. J Intern Med 1995; 238:263–8.
58. Majewski JT, Wilson SD. The MEN-1 syndrome: an all or non phenomenon. Surgery 1979; 86:475–84.
59. Solcia E, Sessa F, Rindi G, et al. Pancreatic endocrine tumours: general concepts; non functioning tumours and tumours with uncommon function. In: Dayal Y, ed. Endocrine Pathology of the Gut and Pancreas. Boston: CRC Press 1991; 105–32.
60. Pipeleers-Marichal M, Somers G, Willems G, et al. Gastrinomas in the duodenums of patients with multiple endocrine neoplasia type 1 and the Zollinger Elllison syndrome. New Engl J Med 1990; 1990:723–7.
61. Jensen RT. Carcinoid and pancreatic endocrine tumours: recent advances in molecular pathologenesis, localisation, and treatment. Curr Opin Oncol 2000; 12:368–77.
62. Zhuang Z, Vortmeyer AO, Pack S, et al. Somatic mutations of the MEN1 tumor suppressor gene in sporadic gastrinomas and insulinomas. Cancer Res 1997; 57:4682–6.

63. Bergman L et al. Identification of somatic mutations of the MEN-1 gene in sporadic endocrine tumours. Br J Cancer 2000; 83:1003–8.
64. Muscarella P, Melvin WS, Fisher WE, et al. Genetic alterations in gastrinomas and nonfunctioning pancreatic neuroendocrine tumors: an analysis of p16/MTS1 tumor suppressor gene inactivation. Cancer Res 1998; 58:237–40.
65. Heitz PU, Kasper M, Polak JM, et al. Pancreatic Endocrine Tumours. Immunohistochemical Analysis of 125 Tumours. Hum Pathol 1982; 13:271.
66. Legaspi A, Brennan M. Management of islet cell carcinoma. Surgery 1988; 104:1018–23.
67. Madeira I, Terris B, Voss M, et al. Prognostic factors in patients with endocrine tumours of the duodenopancreatic area. Gut 1998; 43:422–7.
68. Danforth DN Jr, Gorden P, Brennan MF. Metastatic insulin secreting carcinoma of the pancreas: clinical course and the role of surgery. Surgery 1984; 96:1027–37.
69. Carty S, Jensen RT, Norton JA. Prospective study of aggressive resection of metastatic pancreatic endocrine tumours. Surgery 1992; 112:1024–32.
70. Solcia E et al. Classification and histiogenesis of gastroenteropacreatic endocrine tumours. Eur J Clin Invest 1990; 20:S72–S81.
71. Zollinger RM. Gastrinoma:factors influencing prognosis. Surgery 1984; 97:49–54.
72. Stabile BE, Morrow DJ, Passaro EJ. The gastrinoma triangle:operative implications. Am J Surg 1984; 147:25–31.
73. Stabile BE, Passaro E. Benign and malignant gastrinoma. Am J Surg 1964; 149:144–9.
74. Solcia E, Kloppel G, Sobin LH (eds). Histological Typing of Endocrine Tumours. New York: Springer-Verlag, 2001.
75. Que FG, Nagorney DM, Batts KP, et al. Hepatic Resection for Metastatic Neuroendocrine Carcinomas. Am J Surg 1995; 169:36–41.
76. Modlin IM, Sandor A. An analysis of 8305 cases of carcinoid tumours. Cancer 1997; 79:813–29.
77. Modlin IM, Lewis JJ, Ahlman H, et al. Management of unresectable malignant endocrine tumours of the pancreas. Surg Gynecol Obstet 1994; 176:507.
78. Moertal CG. An odyssey in the land of small tumours. J Clin Oncol 1987; 5:1503–22.
79. Strodel WE et al. Pancreatic polypeptide producing tumours. Silent lesion of the pancreas? Arch Surg 1984; 119:508.
80. Rothmund M, Angelini L, Brunt M, et al. Surgery for benign insulinoma: an international review. World J Surg 1990; 14:393–9.

2 Quality of Life Issues Identified by Healthcare Workers and Patients with Metastatic Carcinoid/Neuroendocrine Tumours

J.K. Ramage

The symptom complexes produced by carcinoid tumours and neuroendocrine tumours (NET) and the quality of life issues associated with the various syndromes and their treatments are unique, setting them apart from gastrointestinal malignancy in general.[1] The patients are often young, with dependent families and have a long course of disease while undergoing therapies. These therapies are often very expensive and many do not have conclusive supporting evidence of an effect of prolonging life. In addition to the cost in human terms, the economic costs of treatments of this condition are considerable (see Table 2.1).

It is clear that both quality and quality of life are important factors when deciding on funding expensive treatments and adequate assessment of the former are needed to justify the huge expense of these therapies.

Patients are being encouraged to have a greater say in the care and treatment they receive and are being empowered in this by patient support groups and 'physican–patient partnerships'. It is hard for patients to make up their minds about treatment on the basis of survival figures alone- a 10% improvement in 5-year survival is not a helpful statistic for an individual case. Patients will want to know how they will actually feel in the later stages of the disease and how the treatment will affect their quality of life. Currently studies of therapies do not address this systematically. It is important to develop a quality of life score that is representative of the patients' (and relatives or carers) feelings to empower them in decision making about their care.

Measurement of quality of life should therefore be used as an endpoint in studies of the various therapies, and this has not been standardized in clinical

Table 2.1. Costs of treatments used for carcinoid/NET

Treatment	Per patient
Octreotide injections	£700–1100/month
Interferon injections	£500/month
Hepatic artery embolisation	£2000/treatment
Chemo-embolisation	£3000/treatment
Chemotherapy (usually 5FU based)	£4000/3 months care
Surgical resection of liver tumours	£7000/treatment
Targeted nuclear medicine therapy	£10 000/treatment
Liver transplantation	£50 000/transplant

trials to date.[2;3] There is a clear need to develop a disease-specific quality of life questionnaire for carcinoid tumours to supplement the already validated European Organisation for the Research and Treatment of Cancers core questionnaire (QLQ-C30).

Previous studies[4;5] have shown initial reduction in quality of life scores following diagnosis, with recovery to acceptable levels some months afterwards. QLQ C-30 scores showed good quality of life but it was clear that many issues were not covered by this core questionnaire. No significant differences were found in quality of life between carcinoid and pancreatic endocrine tumours. We have administered the QLQ-C30 in 60 carcinoid/ NET patients and found similar results to those of the Swedish group. The functional scales were virtually identical and symptom scores showed minor differences. (see Fig. 2.1)

We have set out to develop a disease specific quality of life questionnaire module to supplement the QLQ-C30 in patients with carcinoid and neuroendocrine tumours. This project is proceeding in conjunction with the EORTC Quality of Life Study Group.

Methods

Likely issues were raised from an in-depth literature search, followed by semi-structured interviews with 15 healthcare professionals of different specialities

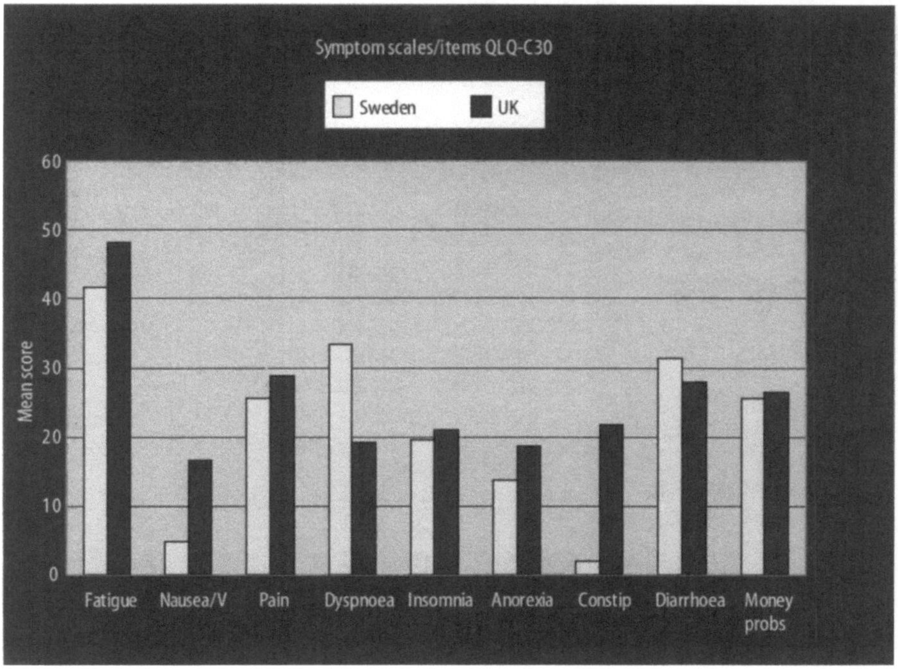

Figure 2.1. Symptom scales of QLQ C-30 in patients in UK compared to Sweden (Larsson et al).

involved with patients with carcinoid tumours and 23 patients with these tumours. Respondents were asked to rank importance of issues not covered by the QLQ C-30. Issues were developed in 2 languages (English and Swedish). In addition 60 patients were given QLQ-C30 to assess general symptoms of malignancy.

Results

In general healthcare professionals scored individual symptoms highest whereas patients reported emotional and anxiety issues highest. The highest average score from the health care workers was for flushing (3.73), whereas the highest total from the patients is for concern for family members (2.82). Fig. 2.2 shows the top five issues scored from 60 patients with carcinoid/neuroendocrine tumours. The least important issue for the healthcare workers was multiple infections with a mean at 1.8 and for patients it was fever, with a mean of 1.21. The greatest difference between the two groups was for wheezing where the healthcare workers scored 2.8 and the patients scored 1.3 (see Fig. 2.3).

QLQ-C30 values in the 60 patients revealed good functional scales, indicating that patients' perception is that they function relatively normally in everyday life, and certainly better than for many cancer patients (see Fig. 2.4).

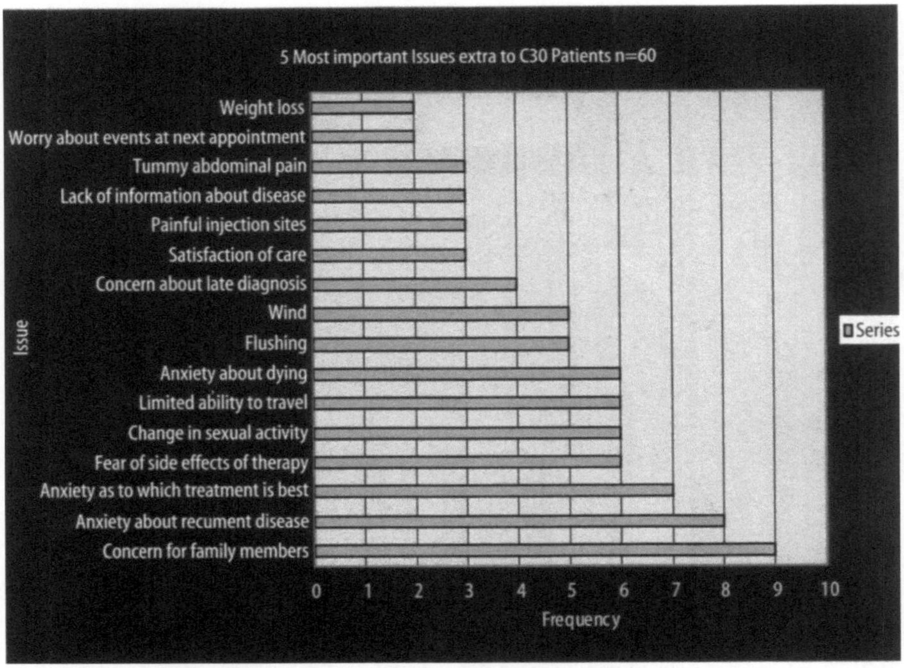

Figure 2.2. Frequency of the five most important additional issues to C-30 standard questionnaire in 60 patients with carcinoid/NET.

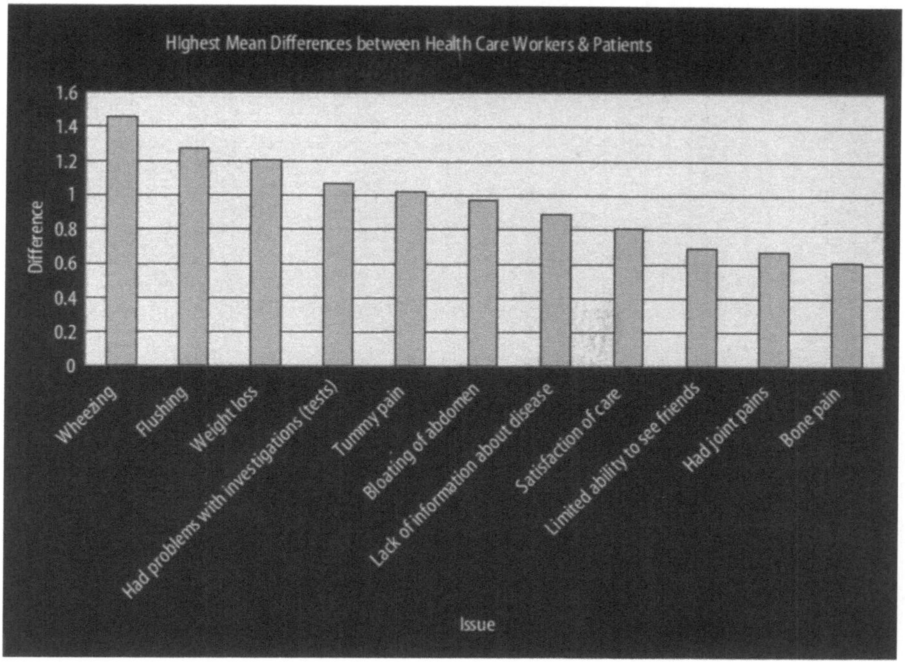

Figure 2.3. Mean differences between patients and healthcare professionals perception of most important symptoms extra to those covered in QLQ C-30.

Conclusions

There is a difference between the healthcare professional's perceptions of the importance of an issue in terms of quality of life compared with the patient with carcinoid tumours:

1. Healthcare workers are more pessimistic than the patients and therefore tend to score the issues higher than the patients.
2. Healthcare workers attribute more importance to individual symptoms whereas patients attribute much more importance to issues of emotion and satisfaction with care than to symptoms

Further work is needed to develop a list of questions from these issues followed by implementation as part of the process of developing a new EORTC module. This will subsequently need validating in multinational clinical trials.

Acknowledgements

Dr Albert Davies, SRN's Nikie Jervis (KCH) and Barbara King (NHH), members of the EORTC quality of life study group.

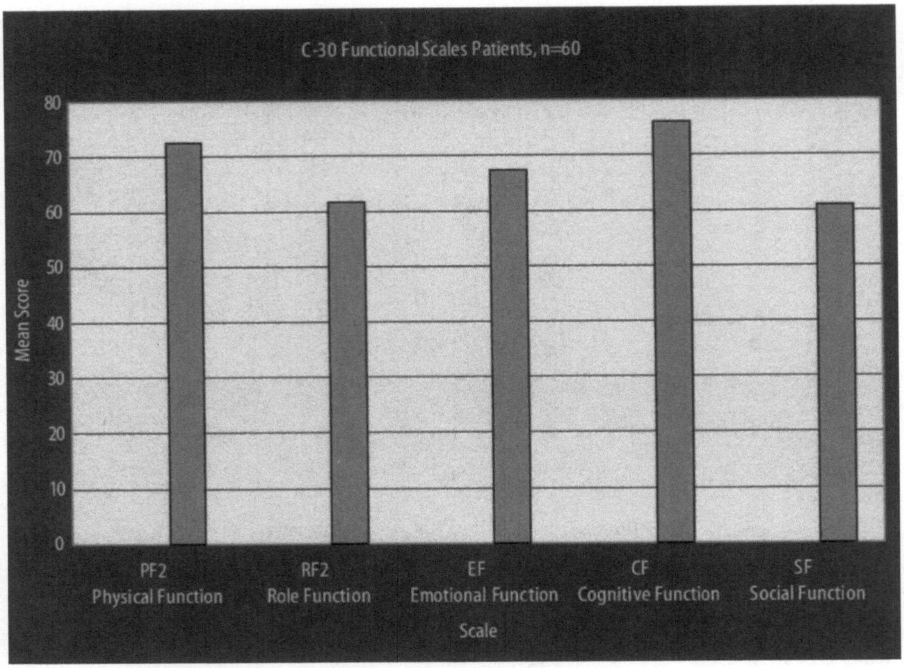

Figure 2.4. QLQ C30 functional scales in patients with carcinoid/NET tumours showing good overall quality of life with this tool.

References

1. Buchanan KD, Johnston CF, O'Hare MM, et al. Neuroendocrine tumors. A European view. Am J Med 1986; 81:14–22.
2. O'Toole D, Ducreux M, Bommelaer G, et al. Treatment of carcinoid syndrome: a prospective crossover evaluation of lanreotide versus octreotide in terms of efficacy, patient acceptability, and tolerance. Cancer 2000; 88:770–6.
3. Wymenga AN, Eriksson B, Salmela PI, et al. Efficacy and safety of prolonged-release lanreotide in patients with gastrointestinal neuroendocrine tumors and hormone-related symptoms. J Clin Oncol 1999; 17:1111.
4. Larsson G, Sjoden PO, Oberg K, et al. Health-related quality of life, anxiety and depression in patients with midgut carcinoid tumours. Acta Oncol 2001; 40:825–31.
5. Larsson G, Sjoden PO, Oberg K, et al. Importance-satisfaction discrepancies are associated with health-related quality of life in five-year survivors of endocrine gastrointestinal tumours. Ann Oncol 1999; 10:1321–7.

3 Diagnosis and Localisation of Insulinoma

D. Sandeman

Insulinoma is a rare but usually rewarding condition to manage. A recent estimate of incidence from Olmsted County, USA is four per million.[1] Insulinoma presents with symptoms of hypoglycaemia; patients are often referred to the endocrinologist with 'turns'. Whilst insulinoma is rare, 'turns' are common, and it often seems that one has to see all of the million to pick up the four insulinomas!

Insulinoma is almost always pancreatic in origin (although ectopic tumours have been reported in the porta hepatis and duodenum). They are however usually small (less than 1 cm) and can be difficult to locate. Ideally they should be located prior to surgery to facilitate a successful outcome.

This chapter reviews the diagnosis of hypoglycaemia and the localisation of insulinoma.

Symptoms of Hypoglycaemia

The classic neuroglycopenic symptoms of hypoglycaemia (sweating, hunger, tremor, palpitations and anxiety) are seldom present in true spontaneous hypoglycaemia, probably due to the preservation of brain glucose uptake in the face of low blood sugars.[2] Presentation with dramatic symptoms will result in an early diagnosis, however this usually suggests that the symptoms are due to stress and panic attacks rather than hypoglycaemia. For this reason when a patient presents with strong symptoms of hypoglycaemia with a background history suggestive of anxiety/depression it may be helpful to prescribe an antidepressant rather than undergoing investigation. Usually the symptoms of 'hypoglycaemia' are the first to resolve well before those of anxiety depression.

The classical hypoglycaemic symptoms are listed and in Table 3.1. Most patients present with mild symptoms such as episodes of altered concentration or behaviour. They seldom complain of weight gain or spontaneously become aware of the precipitation of hypoglycaemia by fasting or exercise although these are usually present when prompted.[3] Patients are usually well between episodes and again persistent symptoms should suggest an alternative diagnosis or the presence of an underlying chronic cause of hypoglycaemia. The elderly however may present with symptoms suggestive of fatigue or dementia as the only mode of presentation.

Table 3.1. Symptoms of hypoglycaemia

Neurogenic Symptoms
• Cholinergic (Parasympathetic mediated)
Sweating
Hunger
Paraesthesia
• Adrenergic (Adrenal & Sympathetic mediated)
Tremor
Palpitations, tachycardia
Anxiety
Systolic hypertension
Neuroglycopaenic Symptoms
Impairment of consciousness, change in behaviour
Seizures
Weakness, warmth
Confusion, poor concentration
Drowsiness
Faintness
Blurred vision

Post-prandial Hypoglycaemia

This is a controversial area. Many people have been diagnosed with post-prandial hypoglycaemia on the basis of symptoms (usually autonomic) occurring 1–2 hours after a meal and a confirmatory blood glucose of 2.8 mmol/l or less during an oral glucose tolerance test.

However careful analysis of the investigation suggests that the diagnosis does not satisfy Whipple's Triad (suggestive symptoms, biochemical confirmation of hypoglycaemia and a response to glucose). Although such patients present with hypoglycaemic symptoms there is a poor correlation of the blood glucose levels and symptoms.[4] Healthy individuals will often have symptoms of hypoglycaemia at a blood glucose concentration of less than 2.8 mmol/l, however 10% of normal subjects will reach such a nadir during a prolonged glucose tolerance test without symptoms.

Post-prandial hypoglycaemia certainly occurs but is rare. It may result from ingestion of unripened ackee fruit, following insulin therapy or sulphonylurea use, ingestion of large quantities of alcohol and simple sugars, or in hereditary disorders of carbohydrate metabolism or noninsulinoma pancreatogenous hypoglycaemia.

Symptoms commonly occur both in the general population and the pre-diabetic stage of Type II diabetes and following upper GI surgery (bariatric or vagotomy or partial gastrectomy). It is again not clear how consistently these symptoms relate to a low glucose in these circumstances.[5,6]

The management is probably pragmatic suggesting a low carbohydrate, high fibre diet or frequent snacks. In the absence of the suggestion of a specific diagnosis a pragmatic approach to management is probably of more use than pursuing the diagnosis of hypoglycaemia in most patients.

Diagnosis of Hypoglycaemia

Whipple's Triad must be fulfilled. Patients must be shown to have symptoms of hypoglycaemia at the time of the low blood glucose and these should be relieved by ingestion of glucose.

Capillary Glucose Measurement

In view of the frequency of suggestive symptoms, which are often not due to hypoglycaemia it is useful to ask the patient to perform a capillary or filter paper blood glucose estimation during the times of symptoms (diabetic home blood glucose testing is not sensitive at low blood sugar levels). The principal purpose of this approach is to exclude hypoglycaemia as the cause of symptoms. If hypoglycaemia is confirmed further investigation will be necessary, usually by prolonged fast.[6] A capillary or filter paper test of less than 2.5 mmol/l is diagnostic of hypoglycaemia and greater than 4 mmol/l excludes hypoglycaemia as the cause.[7]

Prolonged Fasting

Prolonged supervised fasting allows the confirmation of hypoglycaemia and the observation of symptoms in response to glucose. It also allows the measurement of insulin, C peptide and sulphonylurea concentration, allowing the differential diagnosis of hypoglycaemia.

The standard accepted test is a 72 h fast. The duration of the test can be reduced if symptoms occur early. The majority of patients will be diagnosed after 48 h fasting, however 14% of patients were not hypoglycaemic in this period and required a further 24 hours to make a confident diagnosis.[8] The test is simple in its conception however it is often poorly done. The principal problems relate to documentation of symptoms and correlation with blood samples. A suggested protocol is shown in Table 3.2.

Interpretation of Prolonged Fast

The combination of hypoglycaemic symptoms with a blood glucose of less than 2.2 mmol/l confirms hypoglycaemia as the cause of the symptoms.

The presence of hyperinsulinaemia (greater than 30 pmol/l) confirms hyperinsulinaemia as the cause. C peptide should be present (greater than 300 pmol/l). If C peptide is absent and insulin present it would suggest facticious insulin administration. Blood or urine should be tested for the presence of sulphonylurea. Sulphonylureas will cause inappropriate insulin secretion and in every way mimic an insulinoma. If these criteria are fulfilled a confident diagnosis of insulin mediated hypoglycaemia is made.

Table 3.2. Prolonged fasting

- the patient is admitted in the morning of the test and the time of the last food intake documented.
- the patient can drink calorie free and caffeine free beverages. The patient is active during waking hours, blood is taken for measurement of plasma glucose, insulin and C peptide every six hours until the blood glucose is less than 3.3 mmol/l and then hourly. Insulin and C peptide are only measured in those samples in which the blood glucose is less than 3.3 mmol/l.
- the fast is ended when the blood sugar is less than 2.2 mmols and when the patient has symptoms or signs of hypoglycaemia or 72 hours have elapsed.
- at the end of the fast plasma B hydroxybutarate, sulphonylurea are measured. The patient is then fed.
- The decision to end the fast early should be made on the basis of a low blood sugar accompanied by symptoms rather than a low blood glucose alone (Adapted from Ref 9).

C-peptide Suppression Test

The prolonged fast is probably the most reliable way of diagnosing an insulinoma and has the advantage of allowing Whipple's Triad to be tested. The principal utility of a C-peptide test is when a suspicion remains of persistent symptoms either following surgery or following a failed three day fast.

The principle of this test is that the production of insulin by the tumour is not sensitive to hypoglycaemia. The patient is therefore given an infusion of insulin (0.1 units per kg over 60 minutes) in order to produce hypoglycaemia (less than 2.2 mmol/l). If the C-peptide remains above 400 pmol/l the test is positive suggesting persistent insulinoma.

Differential Diagnosis of Hypoglycaemia

It is not the purpose of this chapter to review all causes of hypoglycaemia. (Table 3.3). Hypoglycaemia can clearly result from the use of drugs such as insulin and sulphonylureas or also following alcohol ingestion. Alcohol usually only causes hypoglycaemia if ingested in large quantities and is associated with little food. Hypoglycaemia usually occurs 6–24 hours after the alcohol intake.

Hypoglycaemia is a feature of cortisol deficiency usually presenting at a time of increased glucose use. Severe liver disease, cardiac failure, renal failure and sepsis are associated with hypoglycaemia, but usually only during acute severe episodes.

Hypoglycaemia also occurs with non-islet cell tumours. Principally these are mesenchymal tumours, fibrosarcomas, mesotheliomas and leiomyosarcomas. They are usually large, located in the thorax or abdomen. They produce

Table 3.3. Causes of hypoglycaemia

Post prandial hypoglycaemia	
Noninsulinoma pancreogenic hypoglycaemia (Nesidioblastosis)	
Pre-diabetic stage of Type II diabetes	
Bariatric Surgery	
Vagotomy	
Partial gastrectomy	
Fasting Hypoglycaemia	
Insulinoma	
Drugs:	Insulin
	Sulphonylurea
	Alcohol
	Haloperidol
	Quinine
Organ Failure (usually critical)	
	Liver
	Renal
	Sepsis
	Prolonged Starvation
Non-Islet cell tumours	
	Mesenchymal
	Haematopoietic
	Epithelial (Hepatomas)
Congenital deficiencies in carbohydrate metabolism	

hypoglycaemia by the production of insulin like growth factor II which stimulates the insulin receptor.[9] Hypoglycaemia is seen with hepatomas, gastric and lung carcinoma, adrenacortical carcinoma and exocrine pancreatic tumours.

Insulin receptor antibodies have been suggested to cause hypoglycaemia in patients with lymphoma.[10]

Nesidioblastosis and Noninsulinoma Pancreatogenous Hypoglycaemia

These conditions require special mention.

Nesidioblastosis is due to primary islet cell hyperplasia. This is a disease of infancy but can persist into adulthood. There are two forms, the commoner form is diffuse with islet cell hyperplasia throughout the pancreas. This is difficult to treat, a near total pancreatectomy will result in failure to cure many and impaired glucose tolerance or diabetes.[11] The focal form occurs in about 40% of cases and can be diagnosed by pancreatic venous sampling following selective intra-arterial calcium injection. The importance of differentiating between the two is that the focal form can be treated with partial rather than total pancreatectomy.[11]

Noninsulinoma pancreatogenous hypoglycaemia is a very rare disorder that needs to be differentiated from an insulinoma. This condition presents in adults and is characterised by islet cell hypertrophy and nesidioblastosis. The diagnosis should be made biochemically. Patients with this condition exhibit only postprandial hypoglycaemia, in contrast to patients with insulinomas who have predominantly fasting hypoglycaemia. None exhibit hypoglycaemia during fasting including a prolonged 72 h fast.[12]

Localisation studies in these patients fail to reveal a tumour, including intraoperative ultrasonography. The selective arterial calcium stimulation test when performed is positive, as defined by a doubling of the basal hepatic venous serum insulin concentration in a series of five patients. This was positive either in one or all three arteries. The patients were treated by debulking surgery, the degree of surgery was determined by the result of the selective arterial calcium stimulation test. The pancreas to the left of the superior mesenteric vein was resected when the test was positive only after splenic artery injection, but extended to the right of the superior mesenteric artery vein when the test is positive in an additional artery. In all patients symptomatic hypoglycaemia was cured.[12]

Localisation of Insulinoma

Octreotide Scanning

Usually octreotide scanning is a good first port of call for diagnosing neuroendocrine tumours. The advantage is that whole body scintigraphy localises the tumour wherever it lies, allowing a later targeted approach of other modalities. Most pancreatic endocrine tumours have a high concentration of somastatin receptors and can be imaged reliably with the octreoScan. This technique is particularly useful for gastrinomas, glucagonomas, non-functioning pancreatic tumours, and carcinoid tumours, where the advantage of instantaneous whole body scanning allows the detection of metastases.[13] However Octreotide scintigraphy is less useful in the localisation of insulinomas. Sensitivity rates for insulinomas depend on the size of the tumour. If the tumour can be located by conventional imaging up to 53% of tumours are seen by scintigraphy. However if the tumour is difficult to find the sensitivity has been reported as low as 14%.[14]

CT Scanning

CT is usually performed in order to image in the upper abdomen of all patients. The primary lesion is usually only visualised with enhanced scan. Lesions as small as 0.7 cm can be seen, but not consistently, and the sensitivity overall for CT is between 31% and 59%.[15,16]

Hepatic metastases are hypodense lesions, that become isodense with contrast scanning. Both a contrast and non-contrast scan should therefore be performed in order to visualise the primary tumour and hepatic secondaries. Spiral CT sanning improves sensitivity, up to 92%, and multislice CT should be more reliable.[17]

Ultrasonography

Trans-abdominal ultrasonography will fail to localise all but the largest tumours. It has the distinct advantage of being non-invasive. Endoscopic ultrasonography can be useful in those who have tumours not located by CT scanning. Unfortunately it is not widely available and is very operator dependent but in the best hands can locate up to 95% of tumours.[18] Intra-operative ultrasonography is more sensitive than gentle palpation of the pancreas as occasionally insulinomas can be of a similar consistency to the pancreas and difficult to palpate. It should perhaps be used in all cases allowing visualisation of an adenoma that is missed by other modalities particularly reducing the risk of missing multiple tumours.

Angiography

Angiography when performed alone is not adequate to diagnose islet cell tumours as false positives occur.

The combination of angiography with selective intra arterial calcium stimulation and hepatic venous sampling allows a localisation of most cases of insulinoma.

In this technique the right hepatic vein is cannulated to sample venous blood, selective visceral arteriography is performed by cannulation of the proximal gastroduodenal, proximal splenic, hepatic and superior mesenteric arteries. The test is performed by injecting calcium into each artery and a positive test will be indicated by a doubling of the hepatic venous insulin levels within two minutes of this injection. Each artery is injected with a bolus of 10% calcium gluconate (0.0025 mmol/kg). Blood is sampled from the hepatic vein at 0, 30, 60, 90, 120 and 180 seconds. Each artery is cannulated in turn after an interval of 30 minutes. If on the angiography prior to the procedure a suggestive lesion is seen on arteriography then this artery should be studied last as it may provoke hypoglycaemia which may terminate the study.[19,20] In a study of seven patients in whom other techniques have failed to demonstrate an insulinoma, six solitary insulinomas and one nodular hyperplasia were diagnosed after surgery. In all cases the use of the selective arterial calcium infusion allowed accurate localisation of the insulin secreting lesion.[20]

Conclusion

The diagnosis of hypoglycaemia can be difficult. Many patients present with supposedly hypoglycaemic symptoms which are just a manifestation of hyper-adrenergic symptoms due to anxiety. These patients are most easily excluded by the discovery of a normal blood glucose in the presence of symptoms either during a prolonged fast or with a capillary glucose testing. In the presence of confirmed hypoglycaemia the diagnosis of insulinoma is simple as long as Whipple's Triad is tested. This requires biochemical hypoglycaemia to be associated with symptoms and respond to treatment. If genuine hypoglycaemia associated with hyperinsulinaemia is confirmed during a prolonged fast and facticious insulin administration excluded by the measurement of C peptide, the diagnosis of insulin mediated hypoglycaemia is confirmed. Noninsulin pancreatogenic hyperglycaemia does not produce fasting hypoglycaemia but post-prandial hypoglycaemia. Sulphonylurea use should be excluded as it will mimic insulinoma.

Having confirmed the diagnosis of insulinoma biochemically and clinically these tumours can be difficult to locate. Regrettably scintigraphy fails to identify most insulinomas and therefore is not a primary test. For most patients investigation will start with CT which should be helical or multislice. If this is negative an attempt at localisation should be made by angiography with selective intra-arterial calcium infusion and hepatic venous insulin sampling. This will localise the tumour in most cases.

It is strongly recommended that most patients have intra-operative ultrasonography. This will confirm the presence of a tumour often missed by other modalities and reduce the risk of missing a secondary tumour.

Identification of spontaneous hypoglycaemia, confirmation of the cause and tumour site in patients with insulinomas is challenging, but surgery is usually curative and the benefits to the patients often dramatic making this one of the most satisfying conditions to manage.

References

1. Service FJ, McMahon MM, O'Brien PC, et al. Functioning Insulinoma – Incidence, recurrence and long-term survival of patients: A 60 year study. Mayo Clin Proc 1991; 66 (7):711–9.
2. Boyle PJ, Kempers SF, O'Connor Am & Nagy RJ. Brain glucose uptake and unawareness of hypoglycaemia in patients with Insulin-dependent diabetes mellitus. N Eng J Med 1995; 333:1726–31.
3. Service FJ, Dale AJD, Elveback LR, et al. Insulinoma – clinical and diagnostic features of 60 consecutive cases. Mayo Clin Proc 1976; 51:417–29.
4. Lev-Ran A, Anderson RW. The diagnosis of post-prandial hypoglycaemia. Diabetes 1981; 30:996–9.
5. Wellbourn RB, Butler TJ, Capper WM. Discussion on postgastrectomy hypoglycaemia. Diabetes 1975; 24:1005–10.
6. Faludi G, Beresky G, Gerber P. Functional hypoglycaemia in early latent diabetes. Ann N Y Acad Sci 1968; 148:868.

7. Snorgaard O, Binder C. Monitoring of blood glucose concentrations in subjects with hypoglycaemic. Symptoms during everyday life. Br Med J 1990; 300:16–18.
8. Service FJ and Natt N. The Prolonged Fast. J Clin Endocrinol Metab 2000; 85 (11):3973–4.
9. Service FJ. Hypoglycaemic Disorders. N Eng J Med 1995; 332:1144–52.
10. Marks V, Teale JD. Tumours producing Hypoglycaemia. In James V, ed Hypoglycaemia: Endocrine Related Cancer 1988; 5:111–29.
11. Saudubray JM, Robert JJ, Nichoul-Fekete C, et al. Clinical features of 52 neonates with hyperinsulinism. N Eng J Med 1999; 340 (15):1169–75.
12. Service FJ, Natt, Thompson GB, et al. Noninsulinoma pancreatogenous hypoglycaemia: a novel syndrome of hyperinsulinaemic hypoglycaemia in adults independent of mutations in Kir 6.2, and SUR1 genes.J Clin Endocrinol Metab 1999; 84 (5):1582–9.
13. Modlin IM, Tong LH. Approaches to thee diagnosis of Gut Neuroendocrine Tumours: The Last. Word (today). Gastroenterology 1997; 112:583–90.
14. Zimmer T, Stolzel U, Bader Me et al. Endoscopic Ultasonography and Somatostatin Seintigraphy in the Pre-operative localisation of Insulinomas and Gastrinomas. Gut 1996; 39:562–8.
15. King CM, Reznek RH, Dacie JE, et al. Imaging Islet Cell Tumours. Clin Radiology 1994; 49 (5):295–30.
16. Galiber AK, Reading CC, Charboneau JW, et al. Localisation of pancreatic insulinoma: comparison of pre- and intra. Operative US with CT and angiography. Radiology 1988; 166 (2):405–8.
17. Legman P, Vignaux O, Dousset B, et al. Pancreatic Tumours: Comparison of dual-phase medical CT and endoscopic. Sonography. Am J Roetgenol 1988; 170 (5):1315–22.
18. Boukham Mp, Karam JM, Shaver J, et al. Localisation of Insulinomas. Archives of Surgery 1999; 134:818–23.
19. Doppman JL, Miller DL, Chang R, et al. Insulinomas: Localisation with Selective Intra arterial injection of calcium. Radiology 1991; 178 (1):237–41.
20. Pereira PL, Roche AJ, Maier GW, et al. Insulinoma and Islet cell hyperplasia in value of the calcium intra arterial. Stimulation test when findings of other preoperative studies are negative. Radiology 1988; 206 (3):703–9.

4 GI Hormone Producing Tumours: Syndromes and Treatment Options

Mary McStay and Martyn E. Caplin

Neuroendocrine tumours of the pancreas (also called pancreatic endocrine tumours or islet cell tumours) may be *functioning* or *non-functioning*. Functioning tumours are those associated with a clinical syndrome that is caused by hormone release, and are named according to the hormone that they secrete (Table 4.1). Non-functioning neuroendocrine tumours of the pancreas include those that have all the histological characteristics of a neuroendocrine pancreatic tumour (NPT), but no associated clinical syndrome related to hormone hypersecretion. NPTs are rare tumours, with an incidence of less than 1/100 000 population/year. Non-functioning tumours form the biggest group (30–40%), followed by gastrinomas and insulinomas, which have approximately the same incidence. With the exception of insulinomas, the majority of NPTs are malignant.

Eight of the NPTs are well established and are included in most classifications. These are gastrinomas, insulinomas, VIPomas, glucagonomas, somatostatinomas, growth-hormone releasing factor secreting tumours (GRFomas), ACTH secreting tumours of the pancreas (ACTHomas), and 'non-functioning' tumours, which may in fact be pancreatic polypeptide-secreting tumours (PPomas). Other rarer NPTs have recently been considered as causing syndromes, including NPTs causing hypercalcaemia (producing parathyroid hormone and parathyroid hormone-related protein), NPTs secreting calcitonin and NPTs causing the carcinoid syndrome.

Pathophysiology and Pathology of Neuroendocrine Tumours

The histological diagnosis of neuroendocrine tumours relies first on the identification of general markers of neuroendocrine differentiation, and then cell-specific characterisation. Neuroendocrine differentiation is evaluated by immunohistochemistry using antibodies against secretory granule proteins (chromogranin A, synaptophysin) and cytosolic proteins (neuron-specific enolase, protein gene product 9.5). The cell-specific characterization of neuroendocrine tumours requires hormone immunohistochemistry. According to the World Health Organisation (WHO) classification, neuroendocrine tumours of the gastroenteropancreatic tract are classified as well-differentiated and poorly differentiated depending on their histological and functional features.

Table 4.1. The different types of pancreatic neuroendocrine tumours and their associated hyperfunctional syndromes

Tumour	Cell type	Predominant hormone	Major clinical symptoms	Tumour location	Percent malignant
Gastrinomas	G	Gastrin	Recurrent peptic ulcer	Pancreas 50% Duodenum 50%	90
Insulinoma	B	Insulin	Hypoglycaemia (fasting or nocturnal)	Pancreas	10
VIPoma	?	Vasoactive intestinal polypeptide (VIP)	Watery diarrhoea, hypokalaemia, achlorhydria	Pancreas 90%	60
Glucagonoma	A	Glucagon	Diabetes mellitus, necrolytic migratory erythema	Pancreas	90
Somatostatinoma	D	Somatostatin	Diabetes mellitus	Pancreas 55% Duodenum 45%	80
GRFoma	?	Growth-hormone releasing-hormone	Acromegaly	Pancreas 30% Lung 50% Jejunum 15%	60
ACTHoma	?	ACTH	Cushing's syndrome	Pancreas 90%	95
PPoma	PP/F	Pancreatic polypeptide (PP)	Hepatomegaly, abdominal pain	Pancreas 100%	80

Well-differentiated tumours are positive for most markers of neuroendocrine differentiation in the vast majority of tumour cells. Poorly differentiated tumours do not express chromogranin A, but retain cytosolic markers together with synaptophysin. Other helpful features used to classify these tumours, and therefore to attempt to gauge their behaviour, include general morphologic description; mitotic rate (two or more mitoses per 10 high power [×400] microscopic fields); proliferative index (as assessed by nuclear Ki67 expression); tumour size; evidence of invasion of blood vessels, nerves, or adjacent organs by the neoplasm; predominant tumour synthesis of a specific hormone; or complete non-functionality of the tumour at an immunohistological level. Well-differentiated tumours are then named according to the specific endocrine cell of which they are composed (usually the cell types normally observed in the anatomical site of the tumour). Tumours falling into the two major categories of well-differentiated and poorly differentiated exhibit significant differences in phenotype and behaviour. The behaviour of well-differentiated tumours can be unpredictable, varying from benign to low-grade malignant;[1] according to the several clinicopathological parameters mentioned above, a tentative risk class is assigned to the tumour. Poorly differentiated (small cell) endocrine carcinomas are highly aggressive and are associated with a poor prognosis.

MEN-1 Syndrome

The MEN-1 syndrome is most commonly associated with primary hyperparathyroidism, and tumours of the endocrine pancreas and anterior pituitary.

This autosomal dominant inherited syndrome is associated with a germline genetic mutation in the MEN1 gene, on chromosome 11.[1] Genetic mapping studies show somatic loss of heterozygosity (LOH) suggesting that development of MEN1 associated tumours is a two-step process: firstly, a germline mutation affecting the first MEN1 allele; and then a somatic inactivation of the unaffected allele by LOH.[1,2] The MEN1 gene was cloned in 1997[3,4] and encodes a 610 amino acid protein called menin. Menin is a putative growth-suppressor protein, which specifically binds JunD, a transcription factor acting through the activator protein-1 (AP1 complex).[5] AP1 is a regulatory system within the cell, which is involved in a plethora of functions including apoptosis, mitosis and response to endogenous or exogenous growth factors.

Characteristically, hyperparathyroidism is the initial manisfestation of MEN-1, usually presenting in the third decade of life, and followed by the development of an NPT between the ages of 35 and 50 years. Recognition of MEN-1 is an important first step in the management of NPTs, because patients with and without MEN-1 differ in clinical presentation, clinical management approaches, and also prognosis. The presence of additional endocrinopathies may need specific management and may have an influence on the main tumour management. For example, in patients with gastrinoma and hyperparathyroidism, the presence of hypercalcaemia resulting from hyperparathyroidism often stimulates the release of gastrin from the tumour, and parathyroidectomy has to be performed before gastrinoma surgery. Patients with MEN-1 may develop multiple tumours simultaneously, and more than one type of NPT over time, thus the chances of surgical cure and the approach to long-term follow-up will differ from patients without

MEN-1. Additionally, screening of other family members of MEN-1 patients is indicated. Systematic biological screening performed on these patients includes: measurement of parathyroid hormone, serum calcium, prolactin, luteinising hormone, follicle stimulating hormone, growth hormone, adrenocorticotrophic hormone (ACTH), morning cortisol and 24 h urinary cortisol.

Other hereditary neoplasia syndromes associated with NPTs include neurofibromatosis type 1 and von Hippel-Lindau disease. Neurofibromatosis type 1 (NF1) is inherited in an autosomal dominant manner, arising from mutation of the NF1 gene. The NF1 gene is a tumor suppressor gene encoding a large protein (neurofibromin) that functions primarily as a RAS negative regulator.[6] The hallmark feature of NF1 is the presence of neurofibromas arising either in the dermis or in peripheral nerve. However, patients also have an increased incidence of other tumours, including phaeochromocytomas and duodenal tumours, including somatostatinomas. Clinically von Hippel-Lindau(VHL) disease displays an autosomal dominant pattern of inheritance. Germline mutation of the VHL tumour suppressor gene on chromosome 3 causes a hereditary cancer syndrome characterised by the development of retinal and central nervous system haemangioblastomas. Other tumours associated with VHL disease include clear cell renal carcinomas, phaechromocytomas, and neuroendocrine tumours of the pancreas.[7]

Clinical Syndromes of Neuroendocrine Tumours

Gastrinomas

Gastrinomas have an annual incidence of 0.5–1.5 per 10^6 persons,[8] the majority of the tumours are located either in the pancreas or the duodenum. Less frequent sites are the small intestine and the stomach.[9] Approximately 20% of patients have a family history of neuroendocrine tumours, and 20–25% of patients (particularly those with duodenal tumours) have the MEN1 syndrome. MEN-1-associated gastrinomas usually present at an earlier age, and most MEN-1 patients have coexisting hyperparathyroidism or pituitary disease at the time of presentation. As gastrin is trophic for the enterochromaffin cells in the fundus of the stomach (ECL cells), prolonged hypergastrinaemia may lead to the development of so-called ECLomas, which are also mostly benign neuroendocrine tumours.[10] ECLomas are more frequent in patients with MEN1-associated gastrinoma (15–30%) than in those with sporadic gastrinoma (<5%).

Gastrinomas manifest with the characteristic Zollinger–Ellison syndrome (ZES), which is caused by hypergastrinaemia associated with hypersecretion of gastric acid. The most common symptom is abdominal pain caused by *peptic ulceration.*[11] Ulcers are most commonly found in the first part of the duodenum (approximately 75%), and are usually single, but can be multiple. Ulcers are found much less often in the stomach, and in contrast to the common peptic ulcer, which is associated with *Helicobacter pylori* or ingestion of non-steroidal inflammatory drugs, may also by found in the second, third and fourth parts of the duodenum (14%), and in the jejunum (11%).[12] Ulcers are often recurrent and/or resistant to medical or surgical treatment.

Gastroesophageal reflux disease is also common. Approximately 60% of patients with Zollinger-Ellison Syndrome have dysphagia, or endoscopic evidence of erosive oesphagitis, including its complications of stricture formation, Barrett's epithelium, and perforation.[13,14] A recently appreciated, important endoscopic sign is the presence of prominent endoscopic folds, which was present in 94% of patients in a large prospective series of patients.[11]

The other characteristic component of the syndrome is *diarrhoea*, which occurs in the majority of patients.[11] This is of the secretory or motor variety, and is always associated with hypersecretion of gastric acid, making it easily distinguishable from the diarrhoea associated with VIPomas, which is associated with hypochlorhydria.[15] The diarrhoea may accompany, precede or follow the peptic ulcer disease, or in some cases it may be the only manifestation. The large amounts of hydrochloric acid in the upper GI tract lowers the intraluminal pH, producing other effects: steatorrhoea, through the inactivation of pancreatic lipase, and the insolubilisation of some primary bile acids; vitamin B malabsorption, by interference with intrinsic factor-mediated vitamin B12 absorption by the distal ileum.[12]

An estimated 60% of gastrinomas run a malignant course. Approximately 50% of patients with pancreatic or duodenal gastrinomas have lymph node and/or liver metastases at presentation. For many years, the main causes of death among gastrinoma patients were the complications of peptic ulcer disease: perforation, haemorrhage and pyloric stenosis. However, with the advent of effective acid-reducing pharmacological agents, in particular proton pump inhibitors, the primary morbidity has changed to that of tumour growth and spread.

Insulinoma

Insulinomas have an annual incidence of $1–2/10^6$ persons/year, and usually occur in patients between 30 and 60 years of age. Insulinomas are small (81% measure 20 mm or less),[16] usually solitary, and are almost always confined to the pancreas. They are evenly distributed within the head, body and tail of the pancreas. Approximately 10% of the tumours are malignant tumours, these are usually larger than benign lesions, and can lead to widespread metastases. Multiple tumours occur in up to 10% of patients and should raise the possibility of MEN-I syndrome.

The tumour is characterised by hypersecretion of insulin and hypoglycaemia. Symptoms occur as the result of hypoglycaemia and characteristically occur when a meal is delayed or missed, with fasting, or during exercise.[17] Most patients present with neurological symptoms of hypoglycaemia, such as visual disturbances, altered mood/confusion, weakness, transient motor defects, fatigue, dizziness, and even coma. Hypoglycaemia can also cause symptoms of adrenergic hyperactivation, such as hunger, palpitations, sweating and tremor. When the diagnosis is made late, hypoglycaemia may even cause permanent cerebral damage. The symptoms can be partially masked by a tendency to over-eat in order to compensate for the hypoglycaemia. For this reason, insulinoma patients are often overweight.[18]

VIPoma

Vasoactive intestinal polypeptide (VIP)-secreting tumours (VIPomas) account for less than 10% of pancreatic neuroendocrine tumours. They are much more common in women (with a female:male ratio of 3:1), and most frequently occur at around the fourth decade of life.[9] Up to 90% of VIPomas originate from the pancreas, and are usually solitary tumours. The remaining 10% are tumours of the nervous system, such as ganglioneuromas, neuroblastomas and phaeochromocytomas. Approximately 5% of VIPomas are MEN-1-associated. Over 60% of pancreatic VIPomas are malignant, and by the time of diagnosis up to 60% have metastasized to lymph nodes, liver, kidneys, or bone.[8,19]

The hypersecretion of VIP produces a syndrome characterised by severe secretory diarrhoea, associated with hypokalaemia and dehydration, and is commonly called the *Verner-Morrison Syndrome*. The diarrhoea is intermittent in 53% of patients, and continuous in 47%. The volume of diarrhoea is large, with the majority of patients having more than 3 l/day.[20] The pathogenesis of the severe hypokalaemia is probably primarily caused by faecal loss, and if left uncorrected may be severe enough to cause life-threatening cardiac arrthymias. Other electrolyte abnormalities include: hypochlorhydria, hypercalcaemia, hyperglycaemia, and hypomagnesaemia.[17] A less frequent symptom is cutaneous flushing, which is characteristically erythematous, and occurs in 20% of patients.

Glucagonomas

Glucagonomas are less than half as common as VIPomas, with an annual incidence of 0.01–0.1 new cases per million. They are slightly more common in women (55%), and usually occur after 45 years of age.[21] Most glucogonomas are large solitary tumours, which are almost exclusively found in the pancreas. They generally exhibit highly malignant behaviour: approximately 90% of patients already have lymph node and/or liver metastases at presentation.[8] Glucagonoma is rarely associated with MEN-1.

Glucagonomas secrete excessive amounts of glucagon and cause a distinct syndrome that is characterized by a specific dermatitis (*necrolytic migratory erythema*), weight loss, diabetes mellitus, and anaemia. The cutaneous lesions are one of the most common manifestations of the disease, being present in about 90% of patients. Characteristically, the skin lesion starts as an erythematous area that subsequently becomes papular, with superficial blistering that frequently erodes and crusts. Healing is associated with hyperpigmentation of the area involved. The eruption is usually localized to the buttocks, groin, perineum, elbows, hands, feet and perioral area. The glucagon-induced hypoaminoacidaemia that develops in the majority of patients is implicated in the pathogenesis of the rash.

Glucose intolerance, with or without frank diabetes mellitus, develops in 85%, principally due to the hyperglycaemia that results from glucagon-stimulated hepatic glycogenolysis and gluconeogenesis. Weight loss is almost universal, and probably reflects the known catabolic actions of glucagon. Weight loss may be as severe as 20–30kg, and may occur even with small non-metastatic tumours. Normochromic, normocytic anaemia develops in 60% of patients, and is probably caused by an inhibitory effect of prolonged hyperglucagonaemia on erythropoiesis.[22] Other abnormal laboratory findings commonly found include hypoalbuminaemia (in 80% of patients), and hypocholesterolaemia (reduced VLDL in 80% of patients), which both reflect reduced hepatic synthesis.

Less common symptoms include; deep venous thrombosis (20%), pulmonary emboli (10%), diarrhoea (15%), and psychiatric disturbance.

Somatostatinoma

Somatostatinomas are usually solitary tumours, which originate in the pancreas or small intestine. They are rare tumours, and account for less than 5% of pancreatic neuroendocrine tumours. Somatostatinomas of the pancreas and small intestine differ in several respects: a clinical syndrome is encountered more frequently (18.5% versus 2.5%), the large size of the tumour (>20 mm)(85.5% versus 41.4%), the association with neurofibromatosis type 1 (von Recklinghausen's disease)(1.2% versus 43.2%), and the presence of psammoma bodies (2.5% versus 49.4%).[23] The majority of somatostatinomas are overtly malignant at presentation, and have evidence of metastatic spread to the liver and/or lymph nodes.[24]

Somatostatinomas release large amounts of somatostatin and cause a distinct clinical syndrome characterized by diabetes mellitus, gallbladder disease, and diarrhoea with steatorrhoea. Approximately 40% of patients with somatostatinomas remain asymptomatic, and the tumour is discovered incidentally. The development of diabetes mellitus, which is usually mild, is likely to be secondary to the inhibitory action of somatostatin on insulin, glucagon and growth hormone release, as well as the replacement of functional pancreatic tissue. Gallbladder disease may be a result of somatostatin inhibition of gallbladder emptying. Diarrhoea and steatorrhoea probably reflect inhibition by somatostatin of pancreatic secretion of enzymes and bicarbonate, gallbladder motility, and intestinal absorption of lipids.[17] All of these symptoms may also occur in patients treated with somatostatin analogues, such as octreotide. Other symptoms include weight loss, which may be secondary to malabsorption, and hypochlohydria, which is probably secondary to inhibition of gastric acid secretion.[17]

GRFomas

GRFomas are defined as extracranial tumours that are predominantly or exclusively composed of cells that synthesize and release growth hormone-releasing factor (GRF) (also known as GHRH), which leads to growth hormone (GH) hypersecretion and acromegaly. The average age of GRFoma patients at presentation is 40years, and at variance with pituitary adenoma, GRFoma is 3 times more common in women than in men. Differentiation of GRF-driven acromegaly from GH hypersecretion from a pituitary adenoma can be difficult. Radiological imaging of the sella turcica is often unhelpful, since 40–45% of patients with GRFomas show a hypophyseal mass resembling an adenoma, usually due to hyperplasia of somatotrophs. Detection of an extrahypophyseal tumour, together with an elevated plasma GRF level, is the most useful aid to diagnosis.

GRFomas have been reported in the pancreas (30% of cases), bronchus (50% of cases, where they can be associated with bronchial carcinoid tumours), and in the jejunum (15% of cases). Approximately 30% of tumours are overtly malignant at the time of diagnosis. About 40% of patients with GRFomas have other associated secretory syndromes, especially through the expression of the MEN-1 syndrome. Co-existing endocrinopathies include hyperparathyroidism, Zollinger-Ellsion syndrome, hypoglycaemia, Cushing's syndrome and phaeochromocytoma.[24]

ACTHomas

These tumours are very rare, and are usually located in the pancreas (90% of cases). They produce ACTH and ectopic Cushing's syndrome. The tumours often co-secrete, and so the syndrome is often associated with another syndrome. Approximately 95% have metastasised at the time of diagnosis.

NPTs Causing Carcinoid Syndrome

Tumours secreting 5-hydroxytryptamine (5HT) or pancreatic 'carcinoids' account for 1–2 % of NPTs. These tumours also produce other peptides such as histamine, kinins, substance P and prostaglandins. Unless these secretory peptides are released directly from metastases into the systemic circulation (intestinal drainage is into the portal system), they do not usually cause any signs or symptoms. Paracrine secretion in the intestine may however cause diarrhoea. Therefore, systemic features of the carcinoid syndrome only usually become apparent when liver metastases are present. This syndrome is characterised by flushing and diarrhoea, and less commonly by wheezing, abdominal pain and heart disease. Pancreatic carcinoids with excess production of histamine may cause an atypical carcinoid syndrome (generalised flushing, lacrimation, hypotension, cutaneous oedema, bronchoconstriction). Approximately 10% of carcinoid tumours are associated with MEN1.[25]

NPTs Causing Hypercalcaemia

Hypercalcaemia has been reported with NPTs secreting parathyroid hormone-related protein that mimics the actions of parathyroid hormone. The tumours are usually large and have metastased to the liver by the time of diagnosis.[17,26]

Nonfunctioning Tumours

The incidence of non-functioning pancreatic endocrine tumours is $1–2/10^6$ persons/year, and these tumours represent about 60% of the total number of pancreatic neuroendocrine tumours. By definition, nonfunctioning endocrine tumours of the pancreas are those that have all the histological characteristics of a pancreatic neuroendocrine tumour, but no associated clinical syndrome related to hormone hypersecretion. These tumours are often producing hormones, but remain clinically 'silent' for a number of reasons. The peptides or hormones produced may not produce a known specific clinical syndrome, for example, pancreatic polypeptide (PPomas), α- and β-human chorionic gonadotrophin, calcitonin, and chromogranin A. In other cases, the tumour may produce a peptide which is well known to produce a clinical syndrome, but fails to release it, or produces it at only very low plasma concentrations. It may also be that the tumour only produces biologically inactive precursor forms of the peptide, or that it simultaneously produces an inhibitory peptide, such as somatostatin.[27]

The tumours are usually unifocal, and are predominantly situated in the head of the pancreas. Between 20 and 40% of non-functioning pancreatic neuroendocrine tumours are MEN-1-associated, and in this situation may be multifocal. Patients present with symptoms related to expanding tumour mass, most commonly jaundice and epigastric pain, but also with weight loss, steatorrhoea, upper gastrointestinal bleeding, recurrent pancreatitis, fatigue and malaise. An increasing number are being detected incidentally. Reported malignancy rates at presentation are 60–90%.[29,30]

It should be noted that a tumour which has presented as a non-functioning tumour, can later turn into a functioning tumour, for example a gastrinoma.[27]

Diagnosis

Pancreatic neuroendocrine tumours produce specific symptoms and hormones. The diagnosis is therefore based on clinical symptoms, hormone measurement, radiological and nuclear medicine imaging and histological confirmation. The gold standard is histology and should be obtained wherever possible. The minimum diagnostic criteria for the various syndromes includes histology and the following tests:

Fasting Gut Hormones

Insulinoma

The demonstration of inappropriately high insulin levels in the presence of hypoglycaemia after prolonged fasting is used to diagnose insulin-producing tumours. Hypoglycaemia is usually defined as a blood glucose below 2.2 mmol/l (40 mg/dl). Within 24 h of fasting, most patients develop hypoglycaemia, and by 72 h, virtually all patients will be hypoglycaemic. Paired samples of insulin and glucose are taken every 3–4 h. The test is terminated, and intravenous glucose is administered, when the serum glucose drops to 2.2 mmol/l or below, and/or the patient becomes symptomatic. The test is considered positive for insulinoma if the ratio of plasma insulin (in μU/ml) to glucose (in mg/dl) is more than 0.3. A value of 20 pmol/mmol (insulin concentration [pmol/l] divided by glucose concentration [mmol/l]) can also be used to differentiate patients with and without insulinoma.[31]

Caution must be taken to exclude factitious hypoglycaemia, which may be particularly prevalent amongst medical workers or in relatives of diabetic patients. This can be done by measurement of C-peptide (endogenous flanking peptide of insulin) and pro-insulin (which is elevated in up to 90% of patients with insulinoma). Levels of these peptides will be normal or low following administration of insulin. In the case of deliberate or accidental use of sulphonyureas, elevated levels of insulin and C-peptide are found, but proinsulin levels are normal or low. In this case, serum can be screened for the presence of hypoglycaemics.[18]

Gastrinoma

The most important diagnostic test for gastrinoma is an elevated fasting serum gastrin in the presence of gastric acid secretion after discontinuation of acid reducing medications (ie. H2 receptor antagonists and proton pump inhibitors).

A level of greater than 1000 pmol/ml, is virtually diagnostic of ZES. However, hypergastrinaemia can also be present in a number of other conditions, including *Helicobacter pylori* infection, and gastric outlet obstruction. Many patients with ZES will have only a modest elevation of fasting serum gastrin (between 100 and 1000pmol/l), and in these patients a secretin stimulation test may be of some help.[25] Secretin is a potent stimulator of gastrin release from gastrinomas, but has little effect on other types of gastrinaemia.

Other Hormones

The diagnosis of glucagonoma syndrome can be made easily by measurement of fasting plasma glucagon. In the vast majority of patients with the syndrome, basal levels of glucagon exceed the normal range by six-fold.[21]

The Verner–Morrison syndrome can be diagnosed by demonstration of an elevated fasting plasma VIP level. The usual increase in plasma VIP is 50-fold above the normal mean concentration. A raised plasma pancreatic polypeptide level is frequently also seen in pancreatic VIPomas.[32]

Somatostatinoma

Plasma somatostatin levels are usually elevated in pancreatic somatostatinomas. Levels may however be inconclusive or normal in duodenal or small intestinal tumours.[17]

GRFoma

Plasma GRF (GHRH) levels are usually elevated in patients with GRFoma, and are normal in patients with pituitary acromegaly. Growth hormone (GH) and insulin-like growth factor-1 (IGF-1) are invariably elevated, and GH levels fail to suppress after an oral glucose load in all forms of acromegaly.[33]

ACTHoma

These patients usually have an elevated plasma ACTH and high cortisol levels. This does not however differentiate an extra-pituitary ACTH-producing tumour from pituitary-dependent Cushing's disease, with which it may share some clinical features. Factors favouring the diagnosis of an extra-pituitary ACTH-secreting tumour include, the presence of hypokalaemia with metabolic acidosis, the co-secretion of other gut hormones, male sex, and advanced age.[34]

Chromogranin A

The chromogranins are a unique family of water-soluble acidic glycoproteins found in the storage vesicles of neuroendocrine cells and released during exocytosis. Chromogranin A (CgA) was the first discovered chromogranin and is found throughout the diffuse neuro/endocrine system. It is an excellent immunohistochemical marker of neuroendocrine differentiation, and because it is co-released with resident peptide hormones/amines contained within the secretory granules, it can also serve as a serum marker of neuroendocrine activity. The serum concentration of CgA is elevated in patients with various neuroendocrine tumours. Nonfunctioning neuroendocrine tumours, for which no peptide marker is available, usually retain the ability to secrete CgA. CgA can therefore be used as a tumour marker for nonfunctioning neuroendocrine tumours. Elevated levels are strongly correlated with tumour volume.[35] CgA measurements are very reliable markers in the follow-up of treatment. Furthermore, increases in CgA usually precede radiological evidence of progression.[36] Independent observations that increased levels of chromogranin A correlate with a bad prognosis in different tumours might indicate that chromogranin A or its splice products act as stimulators of tumour growth. Other general markers for neuroendocrine tumours include pancreatic polypeptide and human chorionic gonadotrophin subunits.

Somatostatin and its analogues exert their effect via a family of G-protein-coupled receptors. So far, five subtypes have been cloned, somatostatin receptors 1–5 (sst1–5).[37] The natural compound, somatostatin 14, binds with high affinity to all the receptors. The only somatostatin analogues widely used clinically, octreotide and lanreotide, bind with high affinity to sst2 and sst5.[38] The somatostatin receptors have been identified on many normal cells of neuroendocrine origin, on inflammatory and immune cells, and on a large variety of human cancers. More than 90% of pancreatic endocrine tumours express two or more of the five subtypes of receptor at high density.[39, 40] Knowledge of this property of these tumours has been utilised in the development of *imaging techniques* and in novel therapeutic strategies. Radiolabelled somatostatin analogues, such as [Indium-111-diethylenetriamine pentaacetic acid (DTPA)-D-Phe^1]-octreotide (Ocreoscan), have proved to be very useful for tumour scintigraphy and internal radiotherapy of somatostatin receptor overexpressing tumours.

Assessment of Tumour – Localisation and Extent

The next key step in the management of pancreatic neuroendocrine tumours is the determination of the primary tumour location, and the tumour extent (location and extent of metastases). This information is essential both for patients whose disease is amenable to surgical resection, and for the clinical management of patients with advanced disease.

Somatostatin Receptor Scintigraphy (SRS)

Numerous studies have now established somatostatin receptor scintigraphy (SRS) using Indium-111-DTPA,D-Phe^1-octreotide as the initial imaging modality of choice in patients with any type of neuroendocrine tumour, except insulinoma. SRS has greater sensitivity in detecting both the primary tumour, hepatic metastases, and bone metastases,[41,42] than other conventional radiological techniques (computed tomography [CT], magnetic resonance imaging [MRI], ultrasound, and angiography), and also allows the whole body to be scanned in one examination (Fig. 4.1). The sensitivity of detection of somatostatin receptor-positive tissues is further increased by performing single photon emission computed tomography (SPECT), which also gives a better anatomical delineation than planar views.[43,44]

Despite the high sensitivity of SRS, there are some limitations to its use. Since numerous normal tissues, as well as benign and pathological processes (for example, thyroid disease and breast disease), can have high densities of

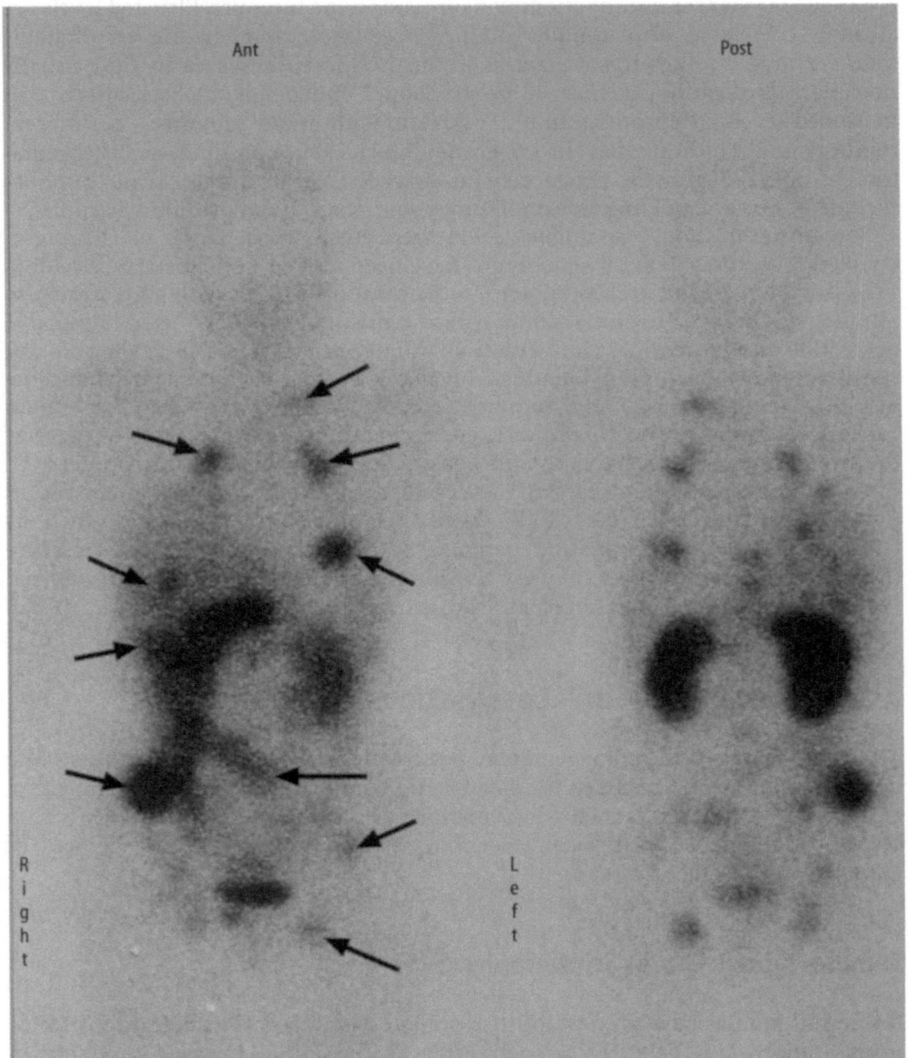

Figure 4.1. Indium-111-DTPA,D-Phe[1]–octreotide scan demonstrating avid uptake of tracer (indicated by the arrows) in a patients with multiple metastases from a PTHrP-secreting pancreatic neuroendocrine tumour.

somatostatin receptors, they can appear as focal lesions ('false-positive' localizations) in up to 15% of patients. The rate of 'false-positive' localisations can be reduced considerably if care is taken to consider the SRS with the clinical context.[45] Further, SRS detection rate is closely related to tumour size, and therefore may frequently miss small (ie. <1cm) gastroenteropancreatic tumours, most frequently at the primary site.[46] SRS fails to image insulinomas adequately for two reasons: the majority of these tumours are small (90% are <1cm in diameter), and only 50% of insulinomas express somatostatin type 2 receptors.[47] Finally, even with SPECT imaging, it may not be possible to adequately distinguish two or more closely-related images as being separate, which instead show as a single image. Given the above, SRS is not used alone, but in combination with CT and MRI in order to assess the localisation and extent of the tumour, in order to plan further treament, to monitor the effects of treatment, and to monitor the progression of disease.

Positron Emission Tomography

Positron emission tomography (PET) using the standard tracer ^{18}F-labelled deoxyglucose (FDG) is currently being assessed, but appears to have low sensitivity for well differentiated NPTs, but perhaps higher sensitivity for the more aggressive poorly differentiated tumours. The alternative tracers, ^{11}C-labeled 5-hydroxytrytophan and L-dihydroxyphenylalanine (L-DOPA) are also being assessed. ^{11}C-labeled 5-hydroxytrytophan has improved sensitivity in serotonin-producing (usually carcinoid) tumours. Currently, PET provides no advantage compared with CT and is ineffective in the detection of non-functional neuroendocrine pancreatic tumours.[48]

Control of Hormonal Symptoms

The third step in management of patients with pancreatic endocrine tumours is to control the symptoms of the hormone-excess state. Treatment with the somatostatin analogue octreotide has been shown to be clinically effective both in terms of improving the symptoms and reducing serum hormone levels in patients with VIPoma, glucagonoma, GRFoma, and 5HT-secreting pancreatic neuroendocrine tumours. Standard doses of octreotide (50–500µg 2–3 times a day subcutaneously) produce symptomatic and biochemical responses in 30–75% of patients over a mean duration of 12 months.[49] Both of these effects appear to be dose related. Since the response rate varies markedly between patients, it is important to titrate the dose of the octreotide until adequate symptom and biochemical control has been achieved.

Octreotide is well tolerated by the majority of patients. Adverse effects are generally mild and transient, lasting less than 1 week. They include diarrhoea, pain at the injection site, abdominal pain, nausea, and flatulence. Octreotide therapy is also associated with an increased risk of cholelithiasis in the long term. A significant recent advance is the development of long-acting forms of octreotide and sustained-release forms of lanreotide (Sandostatin LAR® and Somatuline® LA respectively). These depot forms are more convenient than the usual preparations of octreotide or lanreotide which usually need to be administered subcutaneously every 4 to 8 hours. Sandostatin LAR® is usually administered monthly; Somatuline® LA every 10 to 14 days.

Eventually, however, the majority of patients with neuroendocrine tumours show desensitisation to the effects of somatostatin analogues within weeks to months. The mechanism regarding this escape phenomenon is not yet clarified. Novel somatostatin receptor subtype-selective somatostatin analogues are being developed that may prevent desensitisation.[50]

The effect of long-acting somatostatin analogues in the prevention of hypoglycaemia in insulinoma patients is unpredictable. Hypoglycaemia may even be aggravated through the supression of counterregulatory hormones such as glucagon. Diazoxide inhibits the release of insulin from normal B cells and insulinoma cells, and may be effective in the prevention of hypoglycaemia patients with insulinoma. Long-acting somatostatin analogues can suppress gastric acid secretion, however its effects cannot compete with the acid-suppressing effects of agents, such as proton-pump inhibitors or histamine receptor antagonists, which should be given to Zollinger–Ellison patients.

Surgical Removal of Localised Disease/debulking

Surgery remains the only curative modality currently available for resectable neuroendocrine tumors. Complete surgical resection may be possible in those tumours that are localised at presentation (60% of gastrinomas, 90% of insulinomas, 10–20% of nonfunctioning tumours, and 10–40% of VIPomas and glucagonomas).[51] Furthermore, up to 15% of patients with a pancreatic neuroendocrine tumour and metastatic disease to the liver, have disease confined to one hepatic lobe, which may be resectable.[52]

The surgical management varies with tumour type, location and size. Benign insulinomas and gastrinomas less than 5cm in diameter may be treated with enucleation. Malignant gastrinomas more than 5cm in diameter should be managed with either a Whipple resection and periduodenal node resection or distal pancreatectomy, depending on the location of the tumour (most tumours are in the head of the pancreas). Intraoperative ultrasound should be performed during the surgical procedure. VIPomas, somatostatinomas, and nonfunctioning tumours should be treated with either excision or Whipple resection, with local lymph node resection. Most glucagonomas are malignant and located in the tail of the pancreas, therefore, distal pancreatectomy with resection of the peripancreatic lymph nodes and spleen is the recommended surgical treatment. Postoperative anticoagulation is also recommended because glucagonomas are associated with an increased risk of thromboembolic disease. Additionally, debulking of metastatic tumour can improve survival when cure cannot be achieved.

Prior to any surgery, or indeed any interventional treatment of neuroendocrine tumours, special care must be taken to assess the type of hormone production by the tumour, as large quantities of hormones may be released during the procedure. For glucagonoma, VIPoma, and 5HT-secreting pancreatic neuroendocrine tumours, preoperative treatment with octreotide is usually adequate. Patients with large insulinomas may require hypertonic glucose after tumour removal, and close glucose monitoring. Patients with gastrinoma should maintain their medication with proton pump inhibitors for a while after tumour resection, since they have elevated gastric acid secretion due to hypertrophic gastric mucosa[53]

The surgical treatment of pancreatic endocrine tumours in the setting of MEN-1 is slightly different. Tumours are frequently multiple, and patients with multiple tumours and MEN-1 may run a more indolent course.[54, 55] The surgical approach for MEN-1-associated gastrinomas remains controversial, because of their indolence, multiplicity, and reduced chance of achieving complete resection. There is no absolute clarity over whether intervention offers survival or disease-free benefit in these patients. Currently surgical intervention is advocated when the tumours exceed 2.5 cm in diameter, as tumour size is associated with a higher likelihood of liver metastases, which ultimately affects survival[56]

Antitumour Treatment in Patients with Advanced Disease

Metastatic neuroendocrine tumours of the pancreas progress at markedly different rates in individual patients. One recent study of patients with metastatic gastrinoma illustrates this observation.[57] In this series of patients who had not yet received anti-tumour treatment, 26% showed no tumour growth over a mean follow-up time of 29 months, 32% had slow growth (1–50% volume increase per month) over a 19-month period, and 42% had rapid growth (>50% volume increase per month) over an 11-month period. During a mean follow-up period of 3.1 years, 62% of the patients in the rapid-growth group died, but no patients in the no-growth or slow-growth growth group died. These results, and others, have led to the recommendation that patients with advanced tumour secondary to metastatic gastroenteropancreatic tumour should have their disease reassessed at an interval of 4–6 months after the initial staging investigations, and that only those patients with growing tumours should receive anti-tumour treatment at this stage.[52]

A number of different treatment modalities exist for patients with advanced metastatic disease. These will be discussed within two treatment categories: interventional management of liver metastases (below) and extrahepatic metastases (page 47).

Interventional Management of Liver Metastases

Liver Resection

Palliative liver resections can be considered for some patients with slow tumour growth and severe hormonal symptoms. There is a significant operative mortality for elective liver surgery and this must be taken into account. Prophylactic use of antibiotics has decreased infectious complications, but morbidity is still more frequently associated with sepsis than with bleeding during surgery.[50] Patients with bilobar or more than 75% liver parenchymal involvement are less likely to benefit from surgical resection.[58]

Hepatic Embolisation and Chemoembolisation

Hepatic artery embolisation provides an effective alternative treatment for hepatic metastases, with reduction in hormonal symptoms and pain[59] as well as reduction in tumour burden (Fig. 4.1) and increase in median survival.[58] Immediately before embolisation an arteriogram is performed to demonstrate the arterial anatomy, tumour blood flow, and the patency of the portal vein. The hepatic arteries feeding the liver segment containing the metastases are then selectively embolised by filling the arterial tree distal to the point of injection with embolisation material, eg. polyvinyl alcohol (PVA) particles, causing a temporary, but complete ischaemia.[60] Objective response rates may be further improved by combining the embolisation material with cytotoxic agents. In a recent study using a combination of 5-fluorouracil and streptozotocin, a reduction in tumour size occurred in 50% of patients, and 90% of patients had improvement in symptoms due to hormone hypersecretion. The mean duration of the response was 24 months (range 6 to >63 months).[61] There are however no controlled trials to suggest that chemoembolisation is any better than particle embolisation alone. Again, this therapy should be used with caution when more than 75% of the liver parenchyma is replaced by tumour.[58] For large volume liver metastases, our practice is to perform particle embolisation of a single lobe, and if intra-arterial chemotherapy is to be given, that is injected into both lobes. The procedure is then repeated 2–3 months later with particle embolisation being performed on the other lobe.

Peroperative Techniques

Radiofrequency ablation (RFA), causing selective thermocoagulation, is a novel method for destroying liver tumours, and may be performed percutaneously or at laparotomy or laparoscopy. The latter approaches facilitate the use of intraoperative ultrasound scanning which may demonstrate occult hepatic disease and allow isolation of the liver from adjacent structures. Initial experience using laparoscopic RFA indicates that it is effective in reducing symptoms and achieving good local tumour control, and has low associated morbidity.[62] Other novel relatively non-invasive surgical techniques include *cryosurgery*[63] and the *interstitial laser* (γ-knife).

Taking advantage of the high expression of somatostatin receptors by pancreatic neuroendocrine tumours, intraoperative tumour detection techniques are evolving, using radiolabelled octreotide and a scintillation detector (*radioguided surgery*) to help localise mainly small tumours.[64]

Liver Transplantation

In patients with advanced metastatic disease which is confined to the liver, liver transplantation may be considered. The results from retrospective single and multicentric analyses show that most liver recipients experience significant liver palliation despite a high tumour recurrence rate, although in some patients a long-term cure can be achieved.[65] These series included gastroenteropancreatic tumours of various histological types, including carcinoid tumours. At a time of organ donor shortage, there is an ethical debate about transplanting tumour patients. Total hepatectomy and liver replacement should only be considered in patients with metastatic neuroendocrine tumours confined to the liver in situations where: the tumours are not accessible to curative surgery or major tumour reduction, the tumours are causing symptoms that are not responding to medical or interventional treatment, or hormonal symptoms that are life threatening.[66] Rigorous pre-transplant work-up involving SRS with SPECT, and CT or MRI is required to exclude extra-hepatic disease.

Extrahepatic Metastases

Chemotherapy

Chemotherapy is generally only considered for advanced progressive pancreatic endocrine tumours (increase of >25% of the main tumour masses in a period of 12 months, or tumoural symptoms not treatable by other means).[67] A combination of streptozocin, 5FU and Adriamycin significantly prolongs survival, inhibits tumour progression, and produces major shrinkage of well-differentiated tumours in up to two-thirds of cases.[68] Its efficacy sometimes enables secondary surgical excisions, which were initially not possible, to be made. A similarly high response rate has also been reported using a combination of etoposide and cisplatin in undifferentiated endocrine tumours of the pancreas.[69] (Midgut and carcinoid tumours have a much lower response rate). Unfortunately, in all patients, there is a high rate of tumour recurrence or new progression at more than 12 months.

Biotherapy

Somatostatin. Recent studies have shown somatostatin analogues to have an anti-tumour-growth effect in a small proportion of patients with progressive malignant pancreatic endocrine tumours. The molecular mechanisms responsible for this effect are both direct and indirect. Direct action may result from blockade of mitogenic growth signal or induction of apoptosis following interaction with specific somatostatin receptors. Indirect effects include the reduced or inhibited secretion of bioactive peptides, that may have a growth-promoting effect on the tumour cells, inhibition of angiogenesis, and effects on the immune system.[70] Approximately 50% of patients demonstrated stabilisation of tumour progression when treated with standard or ultrahigh dose octreotide. Up to 6% of patients demonstrated a reduction in tumour size.[53,71]

Alpha-interferon. Alpha-interferon (α-IFN) is known to inhibit the cell cycle, to inhibit the production of growth factors and receptors secreted by the tumours, to have an-antiangiogenic effect, and an immuno-modulatory effect by stimulation of natural killer cells and macrophages. The biochemical response rate in pancreatic endocrine tumours treated with moderate doses of α-IFN (3–6 mega units given 3 to 7 times a week) is about 50%; tumour stabilisation occurs in approximately 80% of patients, significant tumour reduction occurs in only 15% over a mean duration of 20 months.[72] The use of polyethylene glycosylated recombinant interferons in the future will hopefully facilitate treatment and may reduce side-effects.

Combination of α-IFN and octreotide. In two recent studies on patients with progressive metastatic pancreatic endocrine tumours, the majority of patients, who were not responding to either agent previously used alone, showed an improved response with the combination of α-IFN and octreotide.[73,74]

Receptor-targeted Therapy

The common expression of somatostatin receptors on pancreatic endocrine tumours and their avid uptake of Indium-111-DTPA,D-Phe^1-octreotide for scintigraphic scanning, has led to the development of receptor-targeted radionuclide therapy. The concept of targeted therapy is to visualise the tumour with the diagnostic scan and use this to make an estimate of tumour load. Then the isotope label on the peptide is changed, preferably for a β-emitter, in order to target the radiotherapy to the tumour cell ('magic bullet'). The path length of β-particles is several cells thick, and so the cross fire of the β-particles emitted from the radiolabelled peptide bound to the tumour cell can also, in theory, kill neighbouring somatostatin receptor-negative tumour cells. This assumption led to the development of Yttrium-90-DOTA-D-Phe^1-Tyr^3-Octreotide(^{90}Y-DOTATOC), a chelated somatostatin analogue with high affinity for the somatostatin receptor which is labeled with a β-emitting radionuclide. In a recent trial, predominately in patients with therapy resistant and progressive disease, therapy with this novel agent was well tolerated and had a remarkable objective response rate (36%), an improved survival rate (76% at 2 years), and a reduction in tumour-associated pain (12%).[75]

Yttrium-90-DOTA-lanreotide has also recently been developed, the design based principly on the high affinity of Indium-111-DOTA-lanreotide for sst 2,3,4, and 5, and relatively low affinity for sst 1. Preliminary treatment results from a multicentre trial in patients with progressive disease are promising, and again show that the treatment is well tolerated.[76] The results of a large Novartis sponsored trial with their Yttrium 90-DOTA analogue performed in patients with neuroendocrine tumours is awaited. Currently other radionuclide therapies using alternative isotopes are being assessed, including Lutetion-1777-DOTA-octreotide.

Indium-131-meta-iodobenzylguanidine(MIBG) therapy, based on a positive Indium-123-MIBG scan, produces symptomatic and hormonal improvement and modest tumour regression/stabilisation in patients with metastatic carcinoid tumours.[77] It has very much less effect on pancreatic endocrine tumours, probably reflecting the very much reduced sensitivity of Indium-123-MIBG in detecting these tumours (9% of tumours detected in one series).[78]

Bony Metastases

Painful bone metastases can be treated with either radiotherapy or in a clinical trial with bisphosphonates. Disseminated bony metastases may be treated with radionuclide therapy.

Prognosis

The prognosis of NPTs is still not entirely clear. The reasons for this are multifactorial. Part of the problem is that NPTs are relatively rare tumours, often with a slow evolution, that are only diagnosed once they have widespread metastases. Another problem is that many studies have not differentiated between carcinoid tumours and NPTs, let alone between the different types of NPT. Gastrinomas are the most studied of the NPTs. Recent well-designed studies have yielded useful information about these tumours.[54,79] Firstly, that only 25% of patients with gastrinoma pursue an aggressive course, the rest pursuing a non-aggressive course. The 10-year survival was 96% in the indolent group, compared to a 10-year survival of 25% with the aggressive tumour course. The factors associated with a poor prognosis include: liver metastases (either initially or with the development of time); the extent of liver metastases; the development of bone metastases or ectopic Cushing's syndrome; a large primary tumour (>3 cm); female gender; MEN-1 absent; a short clinical course prior to diagnosis; a markedly increased gastrin prior to diagnosis; and a primary tumour that was pancreatic rather than duodenal. The development of bone metastases or ectopic Cushing's syndrome were particularly predictive of a poor prognosis, with patients only surviving 1.9 ± 0.4 and 1.7 ± 0.4 years after their diagnosis, respectively.[79]

There is much less data available on the other NPTs. The majority of insulinomas (>90%) are cured by surgical resection. The majority of patients with the remaining NPTs (particularly non-functional NPTs) have hepatic metastases at presentation. However numerous studies have shown that the presence of liver metastases, primary tumour size (>3cm) liver metastases progression, presence of other metastases, and the histological features of poor tumoral differentiation, are associated with a poor prognosis.

Developments in the Management of Neuroendocrine Pancreatic Tumours

NPTs are rare and complicated tumours, which often need complicated strategies for optimal management. The increasing number of investigative procedures and therapeutic options available to diagnose and treat NPTs requires the ability to co-ordinate specialists from a variety of disciplines including gastroenterologists, oncologists, interventional radiologists, nuclear medicine physicians, pathologists and surgeons. In order to do this, only a multidisciplinary approach in a specialist centre is appropriate. Furthermore, scientific research and controlled clinical trials are needed to determine the efficacy of the many treatment options available for these tumours. As they are rare, multicentre collaboration is very important and from this can be sought a consensus of opinion on guidelines for the management of carcinoid tumours based on the best evidence available. Organisations such as the European Neuroendocrine Tumour Group (ENET) and the UK Neuroendocrine Tumour Group (UK NETwork) and have been the first to take a lead in this multidisciplinary approach. We must also remember that patients with rare tumours need even more in the way of support, and hence the importance of developing readily available literature and patient support groups.

References

1. Larsson C, Skogseid B, Oberg K, et al. Multiple endocrine neoplasia type 1 gene maps to chromosome 11 and is lost in insulinoma. Nature 1988; 332:85–87.

2. Bystrom C, Larsson C, Blomberg C, et al. Localisation of the MEN1 gene to a small region within chromosome 11q13 by deletion mapping in tumors. Proc Natl Sci USA 1990; 87:1968–1972.
3. Chandrasekharappa SC, Guru SC, Manickam P, et al. Positional cloning of the gene for multiple endocrine neoplasia type 1. Science 1997; 276:404–407.
4. European Consortium on MEN 1: Identification of the multiple endocrine neoplasia type 1 (MEN 1) gene. Hum Mol Genet 1997; 6:1177–1183.
5. Karim M, Liu Z, Zandi E. AP1 function and regulation. Curr Opin Cell Biol 1997; 9:240–246.
6. O'Connell P, Cawthon R, Xu GF, et al. The neurofibromatosis type 1 (NF1) gene: identification and partial characterization of a putative tumor suppressor gene. J Dermatol 1992 Nov; 19 (11):881–4.
7. Kondo K, Kaelin WG. The von Hippel-Lindau tumour supressor gene. Experimental Cell Research 2001; 264:117–125.
8. de Herder WW. An algorithm for the treatment of gastroenteropancreatic neuroendocrine tumors: when to treat; how to treat. In The Expanding Role of Octreotide I: Advances in Oncology. Eds Lamberts SWJ & Dogliotti L. BioScientifica Ltd., pp. 143–54.
9. Tomassetti P, Migliori M, Lalli S, et al. Epidemiology, clinical features and diagnosis of gastroenteropancreatic endocrine tumours. Annals of Oncology 2001; 12 (Suppl 2):85–9.
10. Jensen RT. Gastrointestinal endocrine tumours. Gastrinoma. Bailliere's Clinical Gastroenterology 1996; 10:603–43.
11. Roy PK, Venzon DJ, Shojamanesh H, et al. Zollinger-Ellison syndrome. Clinical presentation in 261 patients. Medicine (Baltimore) 2000; 79 (6):379–411.
12. McGuigan JE. Zollinger-Ellison Syndrome and other hypersecretory states. In: Feldman M, Scharschmidt BF, Sleisenger MH (eds): Sleisenger & Fordtran's Gastrointestinal and Liver Disease: Pathophysiology/Diagnosis/Management. W.B.Saunders Company 1998; Vol 1:679–95.
13. Miller LS, Vinayek R, Frucht H, et al. Reflux oesophagitis in patients with Zollinger-Ellsion syndrome. Gastroenterology 1990: 98:341–6.
14. Bondeson AG, Bondeson L, Thompson NW. Stricture and perforation of the oesophagus: Overlooked threats in the Zollinger-Ellison syndrome. World J Surg 1990; 14:361.
15. Mignon M, Jais Ph, Cadoit G, et al. Clinical features and advances in biological diagnostic criteria for Zollinger-Ellison syndrome. In Mignon M, Jensen RT (eds): Endocrine Tumours of the Pancreas: Recent Advances in Research and Management. Basel: Karger 1995; 223–39.
16. Soga J, Yakuwa Y, Osaka M. Insulinoma/hypoglycaemic syndrome: a statistical evaluation of 1085 reported cases of a Japanese series. J Exp Clin Cancer Res 1998; 17 (4):379–88
17. Jensen RT, Norton JA. Endocrine tumours of the pancreas. In: Feldman M, Scharschmidt BF, Sleisenger MH (eds): Sleisenger & Fordtran's Gastrointestinal and Liver Disease: Pathophysiology/ Diagnosis/Management. W.B.Saunders Company 1998; Vol 1:871–95.
18. Creutzfeldt W. Insulinomas: Clinical presentation, diagnosis, and advances in management. In: Mignon M, Jensen RT (eds): Endocrine Tumours of the Pancreas: Recent Advances in Research and Management. Basel: Karger 1995; 148–65.
19. Soga J, Yakuwa Y. Vipoma/diarrheogenic syndrome: a statistical evaluation of 241 reported cases. J Exp Clin Cancer Res 1998; 17 (4):389–400.
20. Matuchansky C, Rambaud JC. VIPomas and endocrine cholera: Clinical presentation, diagnosis, and advances in management. In Mignon M, Jensen RT (eds), Endocrine Tumours of the Pancreas: Recent Advances in Research and Management. Frontiers of Gastrointestinal Research, Vol. 23, Basel, Switzerland, S. Karger, 1995, pp. 166–82.
21. Guillausseau PJ, Guillausseau-Scholer C. Glucogonomas: Clinical presentation, diagnosis, and advances in management. In Mignon M, Jensen RT (eds), Endocrine Tumours of the Pancreas: Recent Advances in Research and Management. Frontiers of Gastrointestinal Research, Vol. 23, Basel, Switzerland, S. Karger, 1995; pp. 183–93.
22. Naets JP, Guns M. Inhibitory effect of glucagons on erythropoesis. Blood 1980; 55:997.
23. Soga J, Yakuwa Y. Somatostatin/inhibitory syndrome: a statistical evaluation of 173 reported cases as compared to other pancreatic endocrinomas. J Exp Clin Cancer Res 18 (1):13–22.
24. Sassolas G, Chayvialle JA. GRFomas, somastatinomas: clinical presentation, diagnosis, and advances in management. In Mignon M, Jensen RT (eds), Endocrine Tumours of the Pancreas: Recent Advances in Research and Management. Frontiers of Gastrointestinal Research, Vol. 23, Basel, Switzerland, S. Karger, 1995; pp. 195–207.
25. Carcinoid tumour. Caplin ME, Buscombe JR, Hilson AJ, et al. Lancet 1998; 352:799–805.
26. Mao C, Carter P, Schaefer P, et al. Malignant islet cell tumour associated with hypercalcaemia. Surgery 1995; 117 (1):37–40.
27. Eriksson B, Őberg K. PPomas and nonfunctioning endocrine pancreatic tumours: clinical presentation, diagnosis, and advances in management. In Mignon M, Jensen RT (eds), Endocrine Tumours of

the Pancreas: Recent Advances in Research and Management. Frontiers of Gastrointestinal Research, Vol. 23, Basel, Switzerland, S. Karger, 1995; pp. 208–22.
28. Cheslyn-Curtis S, Sitaram V, Williamson RCN. Management of non-functioning neuroendocrine tumours of the pancreas. British Journal of Surgery 1993; 80:625–7.
29. Evans DB, Skibber JM, Lee JE, et al. Nonfunctioning islet cell carcinoma of the pancreas. Surgery 1993; 114:1175–82.
30. Cheslyn-Curtis S, Sitaram V, Williamson RCN. Management of non-functioning neuroendocrine tumours of the pancreas. British Journal of Surgery 1993; 80:625–7.
31. Nauck M, Creutzfeldt W. Insulin-producing tumours and the insulinoma syndrome. In Dayal Y (ed), Endocrine Pathology of the Gut and Pancreas. Boca Raton, CRC Press, 1991; pp. 197–225.
32. Long RC, Bryant MG, Mitchell SJ, et al. Clinicopathological study of pancreatic and ganglioneuroblastoma tumours secreting vasoactive intestinal polypeptide (vipomas). Br Med J 1981; 282:1767–71
33. Doga M, Bonadonna S, Burrattin A, et al. Ectopic secretion of growth hormone-releasing hormone (GHRH) in neuroendocrine tumours: relevant clinical aspects. Ann Oncol 2001; 12 (Suppl 2):89–94.
34. Terzolo M, Reimondo G, Ali A, et al. Ectopic ACTH syndrome: molecular bases and clinical heterogeneity. Ann Oncol 2001; 12 (Suppl 2):83–7.
35. Nobels FRE, Kwekkeboom DJ, Bouillon R, et al. Chromogranin A: its clinical value as marker of neuroendocrine tumours. Eur J Clin Invest 1998; 28:431–40.
36. Eriksson B, Őberg K, Stridsberg M. Tumours markers in neuroendocrine tumours. Digestion 2000; 62 (Suppl 1):33–8.
37. Patel YC, Greenwood MT, Warsynska A, et al. All five cloned somatostain receptors (hSSTR1-5) are functionally coupled to adenylate cyclase. Biochem and Biophysical Research Communications 1994; 198:605–12.
38. Lamberts SWJ, van der Lely AJ, de Herder WW, et al. Octreotide. New England Journal of Medicine. 1996; 334:245–54.
39. Reubi JC, Laissue J, Waser B, et al. Expression of somatostatin receptors in normal, inflamed, and neoplastic human gastrointestinal tissues. Annals of the New York Academy of Sciences 1994; 733:122–37.
40. Jensen RT, Norton JA. Carcinoid tumours and the carcinoid syndrome. In DeVita VT, Hellman S, Rosenberg SA (eds): cancer: Principles & Practice of Oncology, 5th edition. New York: Lippincott-Raven 1997; 1706.
41. Termanini B, Gibril F, Reynolds JC, et al. Value of somatostatin receptor scintigraphy: a prospective study in gastrinoma of its effect on clinical management. Gastroenterology 1997; 112 (2):335–47.
42. Gibril F, Doppman JL, Reynolds JC, et al. Bone metastases in patients with gastrinomas: a prospective study of bone scanning, somatostatin receptor scanning, and magnetic resonance imaging in their detection, frequency, location, and effect of their detection on management. J Clin Oncol 1998; 16 (3):1040–53.
43. Kwekkeboom D, Krenning EP, de Jong M. Peptide receptor imaging and therapy. J Nucl Medicine 2000; 41 (10):1704–13.
44. Chow A, Caplin ME, Buscombe JR, et al. Somatostatin receptor scintigraphy in neuroendocrine tumours: is single photon emission tomography (SPECT) required? Gut 2001; 48 (Suppl 1):A186.
45. Gibril F, Reynolds JC, Chen CC, et al. Specificity of somatostatin receptor scintigraphy: a prospective study and effects of false-positive localizations on management in patients with gastrinomas J Nucl Med 1999; 40 (4):539–53.
46. Alexander HR, Fraker DL, Norton JA, et al. Prospective study of somatostatin receptor scintigraphy and its effect on operative outcome in patients with Zollinger-Ellison syndrome. Ann Surg 1998; 228 (2):228–38.
47. Wulbrand U, Wied M, Zofel P, et al. Growth factor recptor expression in human gastroenteropancreatic neuroendocrine tumours. Eur J Clin Invest 1998; 28:1038–49.
48. Ahlstrőm H, Eriksson B, Bergstrőm M, et al. Pancreatic neuroendocrine tumours:diagnosis with PET. Radiology 1995; 195:333–7.
49. Gorden P, Comi RJ, Maton PN, et al. NIH conference. Somatostatin and somatostatin analogue (SMS 201-995) in treatment of hormone-secreting tumours of the pituitary and gastrointestinal tract and non-neoplastic diseases of the gut. Ann Intern Med 1989; 110:35–50.
50. Hofland LJ, de Herder WW, Lamberts SWJ. Mechanism of action of somatostatin and interferon in gastroenteropancreatic tumours. In The Expanding Role of Octreotide I: Advances in Oncology. Eds Lamberts SWJ & Dogliotti L. BioScientifica Ltd, Bristol 2002; pp. 89–102.

51. Jensen RT. Carcinoid and pancreatic endocrine tumours: recent advances in molecular pathogenesis, localization, and treatment. Curr Opin Oncol 2000; 12 (4):368–77.
52. Jensen RT. Role of somatostatin receptors in gastroenteropancreatic tumours. In The Expanding Role of Octreotide I: Advances in Oncology. Eds Lamberts SWJ, Dogliotti, pp. 45–71. BioScientifica Ltd, Bristol, 2002.
53. Ahlman H, Wängberg B, Jansson S, et al. Interventional treatment of gastrointestinal neuroendocrine tumours. Digestion 2000; 62 (Suppl 1):59–68.
54. Weber HC, Venzon DJ, Lin JT, et al. Determinants of metastatic rate and survival in patients with Zollinger-Ellison syndrome: a prospective long-term study. Gastroenterology 1995 Jun; 108 (6):1637–49.
55. Jensen RT. Management of the Zollinger-Ellsion syndrome in patients with multiple endocrine neoplasia type 1. J Int Med 1998; 243:477–88.
56. Li ML, Norton JA. Gastrinoma. Curr Treat Options Oncol 2001; 2 (4):337–46.
57. Sutcliff VE, Doppman JL, Gibril F, et al. Growth of newly diagnosed, untreated metastatic gastrinomas and predictors of growth patterns. J Clin Oncol 1997; 15 (6):2420–31.
58. Chamberlain RS, Canes D, Brown KT, et al. Hepatic neuroendocrine metastases: does intervention alter outcomes? J Am Surg 2000; 190 (4):432–45.
59. Brown KT, Koh BY, Brody LA, et al. Particle embolization of hepatic neuroendocrine metastases for control of pain and hormonal symptoms. J Vasc Interv Radiol 1999; 10 (4):397–403.
60. Chuang VP, Wallace S. Hepatic artery embolisation in the treatment of hepatic neoplasms. Radiology 1981; 140:51–8.
61. Kim YH, Ajani JA, Carrasco CH, et al. Selective hepatic arterial chemoembolisation for liver metastases in patients with carcinoid tumour or islet cell carcinoma. Cancer Invest 1999; 17 (7):474–8.
62. Berber E, Flesher N, Siperstein AE. Laparoscopic radiofrequency ablation of neuroendocrine liver metastases. World J Surg 2002; 26:985–90.
63. Seifert JK, Cozzi PJ, Morris DL. Cryotherapy for neuroendocrine liver metastases. Seminars in Surgical Oncology 1998; 14:175–183.
64. Benjegard SA, Forssell-Aronsson E, Wangberg B, et al. Intra-operative tumour detection using ^{111}In-DTPA-D-Phe^{1}-octreotide and a scintillation detector. Eur J Nucl Med 2001; 28 (10):1456–62.
65. Ringe B, Lorf T, Dőpkens K, et al. Treatment of hepatic metastases from gastroenteropancreatic neuroendocrine tumours: role of liver transplantation. World J Surg 2001; 25:697–9.
66. Olausson M, Friman S, Cahlin C, et al. Indications and results of liver transplantation in patients with neuroendocrine tumours. World J Surg 2002; 26 (8):998–1004.
67. Rougier P, Mitry E. Chemotherapy in the treatment of neuroendocrine malignant tumours. Digestion 2000; 62 (Suppl 1):73–8.
68. Moertel CG, Lefkopoulos M, Lipsitz M. Streptozocin-doxorubicin, streptozocin-fluorouracil or chlorozotocin in the treatment of advanced islet-cell carcinoma. N Engl J Med 1992; 36:519–23.
69. Moertel CG, Kvols LK, O'Connell MJ, et al. Treatment of neuroendocrine carcinomas with combined etoposide and cisplatin. Cancer 1991; 68:227–32.
70. Arnold R, Simon B, Wied M. Treatment of neuroendocrine GEP tumours with somatostatin analogues. Digestion 2000; 62 (Suppl 1):84–91.
71. Shojamanesh H, Gibril F, Louie A, et al. Prospective study of the antitumour efficacy of long-term octreotide treatment in patients with progressive metastatic gastrinoma. Cancer 2002; 15 (2):331–43.
72. Eriksson B, Őberg K. An update of the medical treatment of malignant endocrine pancreatic tumours. Acta Oncol 1993; 32:203–8.
73. Frank M, Klose K, Wied M, et al. Combination therapy with octreotide and α-interferon. Effect on tumour growth in metastatic endocrine gastroenteropancreatic tumours. Am J Gastroent 1999; 94:1381–7.
74. Fjällskog ML, Sundin A, Westlin JE, et al. Treatment of malignant endocrine pancreatic tumours with a combination of alpha-interferon and somatostatin analogs. Med Oncol 2002; 19 (1):35–42.
75. Waldherr C, Pless M, Maeke HR, et al. The clinical value of [90Y-DOTA]-D-Phe1-Tyr3-octreotide (90Y-DOTATOC) in the treatment of neuroendocrine tumours: a clinical phase II study. Ann Oncol 2001; 12:941–5.
76. Virgolini I, Britton K, Buscombe J, et al. In- and Y-DOTA-lanreotide: results and implications of the MAURITIUS trial. Semin Nucl Med 2002 Apr; 32 (2):148–55.
77. Kaltsas GA, Mukherjee JJ, Grossman AB. The value of radiolabelled MIBG and octreotide in the diagnosis and management of neuroendocrine tumours. Ann Oncol 2001; 12 (Suppl 2):S47–50.

78. Kaltsas G, Korbonits M, Heinz E, et al. Comparison of somatostatin analog and meta-iodobenzyl-guanidine radionuclides in the diagnosis and localisation of advanced neuroendoctine tumours. J Clin Endocrinol Metab 2001; 86 (2):895–902.
79. Yu F, Venzon DJ, Serrano DJ, et al. Prospective study of the clinical course, prognostic factors and survival in patients with longstanding Zollinger-Ellsion syndrome. J Clin Oncol 1999; 17:615–30.

Pancreatic Cancer

5 Progress by Collaboration: ESPAC Studies

Robert Sutton, Deborah D. Stocken, Janet A. Dunn, Helen Hickey, Michael G.T. Raraty, Paula Ghaneh, John Buckels, Mark Deakin, Clement W. Imrie, Helmut Friess, Markus W. Büchler and John P. Neoptolemos

Pancreatic cancer is amongst the top ten fatal cancers of the Western world, accounting for 57 000 deaths per year in Europe and 29 000 deaths per year in the United States.[1] It is particularly difficult to treat because of its inaccessible location, late presentation, and frequently aggressive tumour biology. Five-year survival in the 10–15% of affected patients who undergo potentially curative surgery is limited to 17–24%,[2,3] whilst overall 5-year survival in all patients is less than 0.5%.[4] Although significant improvements in surgical outcome have been obtained with increasing specialisation and case-load,[3,5] and further benefits may be anticipated with earlier investigation and referral of high risk groups,[6] the role of adjuvant and neo-adjuvant treatment accompanying surgery remains uncertain.[7–10] Interestingly, chemotherapy is the principal modality in the treatment of advanced pancreatic cancer.[11]

Adjuvant Therapy after Resection

Most resectable pancreatic cancer is identified in the head of the gland, and can be treated by pancreatoduodenectomy.[12] No survival advantage has been shown to result from more radical resections than from a standard Kausch–Whipple pancreatoduodenectomy,[13] nor from routine resection of the pylorus and antrum.[14] Determinants of outcome include the stage of disease, tumour grade and resection margin status (R0 = no tumour within 1mm of margin; R1 = microscopic tumour within 1 mm of margin; R2 = macroscopic tumour at margin of resection); most patients die within 2 years from local recurrence and/or hepatic metastases.[14–17]

Prior to the European Study Group for Pancreatic Cancer (ESPAC) studies, there had been three trials of adjuvant treatment following pancreatic cancer resection. The Gastrointestinal Tumor Study Group (GITSG) trial randomised 43 patients to either 40 Gy radiotherapy with fluorouracil then weekly fluorouracil for up to 2 years or no adjuvant treatment.[7] Median, 2-year and 5-year survivals were significantly higher in the adjuvant treatment group.[7,8] An adjuvant regimen of fluorouracil, doxorubicin and mitomycin improved median but not 5-year survival compared to no adjuvant treatment in a randomised study of 61 resected patients in Norway.[9] Using the GITSG regimen but without follow-on fluorouracil, the European Organisation for Research and Treatment of Cancer (EORTC) found no benefit in 114 patients randomised to either adjuvant or no extra treatment following resection.[10] Few conclusions can be drawn from these data, as all three trials were inadequately powered. Despite this, the GITSG trial has been highly influential in determining treatment policy in the United States, where adjuvant chemoradiotherapy has been widely recommended.[17]

Value of Randomised Clinical Trials

Experimental investigation requires manipulation of an independent (experimental) variable by an investigator or by natural means. During a cholera outbreak over 150 years ago John Snow compared the mortality rates from cholera for 300 000 London residents subscribing to two water companies, one of which drew water from the river Thames where large amounts of sewage were discharged, the other from a region free of sewage effluent.[18] Snow discovered that the mortality rate for residents supplied with water containing sewage was higher; he then removed the handle from the offending water pump, and the outbreak stopped.[18]

The value of a comparative investigation is obvious. It took a century for such a scientific approach to become sufficiently well developed and accepted so that it was adopted in clinical trials of alternative treatments for human disease.[19,20] Control of the experimental variable and random assignment between groups are essential features, used in the first randomised trials of the treatment of tuberculosis,[19] sponsored by the Medical Research Council. During the second half of the 20th Century the randomised controlled trial has assumed centre-stage in the assessment of health care interventions, and is the principal experimental method by which the effects of alternative treatments can be assessed. Thus over 90 000 references are currently indexed in Medline under the term 'controlled clinical trial'. By working and reworking this method in many different applications, critical components have been honed and become more widely recognised. These have been summarised through consensus by the CONSORT (Consolidated Standards of Reporting Trials) group (see Table 5.1).[21,22] Although improvements in the design, conduct and reporting of randomised clinical trials have been evident in recent years, considerable room for improvement remains.[22] Nevertheless, the adoption of an 'evidence-based' approach for choosing treatment is to be welcomed, nowhere less than in pancreatology.

Large Randomised Trials

It is no longer feasible for one individual to investigate the effect of an experimental intervention on hundreds of thousands of people; teams of investigators are usually required. Many of the considerations in the design and conduct of randomised clinical trials are statistical in nature, such that without statistical input, randomised clinical trials are compromised.[23] This is particularly important in the determination of sample size (number of patients recruited), the 'power' of the trial (the probability of detecting a specified effect size if it truly exists, if the trial plan is fully enacted), as well as in the planning, calculation and interpretation of the quantitative evaluation of the data. With increasing difficulty in deciding between treatments, and smaller but still significant potential margins of benefit

Table 5.1. Current items included in CONSORT recommendations for the reporting of randomised clinical trials.[21,22]

Part of paper	Item	Description
Title and abstract	1	Method of treatment allocation
Introduction	2	Rationale
Methods		
Participants	3	Eligibility criteria
Interventions	4	Detail of the alternative treatments
Objectives	5	Specific hypotheses to be tested
Outcomes	6	Primary and secondary endpoints
Sample size	7	How determined and stopping rules
Randomisation		
Sequence	8	Methods used to generate
Concealment	9	Whether hidden until allocated
Implementation	10	Who did what
Blinding	11	Patients and/or investigators
Statistics	12	Methods for analysis
Results		
Participant flow	13	Numbers at each stage of trial
Recruitment	14	Dates including follow up
Baseline data	15	Demographic and clinical features
Number analysed	16	Recruited and whether intention-to-treat
Outcomes	17	Summary of outcomes including effect size
Ancillary analyses	18	Stating what pre-specified
Adverse events	19	Broken down by group
Discussion		
Interpretation	20	Including hypotheses, bias, cautions
Generalisability	21	Applicability to whole population
Overall evidence	22	Results in the context of the field

associated with one treatment over another, it is often the case that large-scale randomised clinical trials are necessary.[23] Such trials recruit large numbers of patients (many hundreds if not thousands) to be able to detect smaller differences between treatments and achieve a greater likelihood of demonstrating a difference if one really exists. Although the first randomised clinical trials recruited fewer than one hundred patients into each arm, cardiovascular trials were the first to recruit many thousands of patients.[24] Such trials are only possible if the condition under investigation is common, if affected patients can readily be recruited and given trial treatments, and if many centres can take part. To ensure that many hundreds of patients are recruited and given trial treatment, and that requisite data are collected, a 'pragmatic' design is necessary, to minimise the workload on contributing clinicians.[23] Also, a culture shift is required among these responsible clinicians so that they are willing to contribute and gain 'ownership' of such trials, especially when large-scale trials are new to a specific area of clinical practice. Prior to ESPAC studies, there had been no large-scale trials of any treatment for resectable pancreatic cancer, nor few for any other condition in any other field of pancreatology.

Quality Assurance in Large Trials

Several of the components in the design, conduct and reporting of randomised clinical trials have been demonstrated to reduce bias and to increase the reliability of reported results. These include appropriate generation of the unbiased treatment allocation procedure for successive patients (using random allocation), allocation concealment (to avoid predictability of the next treatment allocation and so avoid selection bias), blinding (of both investigators and patients, when possible), intention-to-treat analysis (where all randomised patients are included in the analysis and are analysed according to their treatment allocated, whether received or not) and follow-up of more than 90% of patients. These components have been incorporated into the Jadad score,[25] whereby an individual trial can be graded from zero to five (from low to high quality), depending on the number of appropriate components that were present. The Jadad score has been validated as a measure of the quality of a randomised clinical trial,[25] and can be supplemented by further assessments, including the CONSORT checklist and trial flow diagrams, and other important components such as stratification (of both randomisation and analyses) to account for important prognostic factors and the importance of well-defined and reliable endpoints.

Design and Conduct of ESPAC-1

This section outlines considerations that went into the design and conduct of ESPAC-1, and progress made through multicentre, multinational collaboration. The results of ESPAC-1 have been reported in full elsewhere.[26,27]

Pragmatism

The ESPAC-1 study was designed as a simple, pragmatic trial which required the collection of a small dataset on each patient so as to encourage maximum recruitment. It set out in 1994 to recruit 280 patients into a two-by-two factorial design, to detect an excess of 20% deaths at 2 years between each main comparison, at the 5% significance level with 90% power (Fig. 5.1). This calculation assumed that approximately 80% of patients would have negative resection margins (R0) and a 2-year survival of 20–40%, and that the remaining 20% of patients with positive resection margins (R1) would have a 2-year survival of 1–20%. However, because of the wide variation in access to and attitudes towards chemoradiotherapy, clinicians could randomise additional patients between chemotherapy or no chemotherapy (without randomising to chemoradiotherapy), or to chemoradiotherapy or no chemoradiotherapy (without randomising to chemotherapy). Clinicians had to provide details on any additional therapy that they wished to give, e.g. they might randomise a patient to either chemotherapy, or no chemotherapy, and give background radiotherapy. Thus, there were three randomisation options, and although randomisation into the original two by two factorial design was encouraged, clinicians were able to exercise considerable discretion, so that the maximum recruitment of patients was ensured. Recruitment continued until the target 280 patients randomised via the two-by-two design had been reached with all patients randomised outside the two-by-two design providing additional power to each treatment comparison.

Randomisation was by phone call or fax to one of four randomisation centres (UK, Switzerland, Germany, France), where eligibility was checked (ductal adenocarcinoma of the pancreas, macroscopically resected, no local spread or

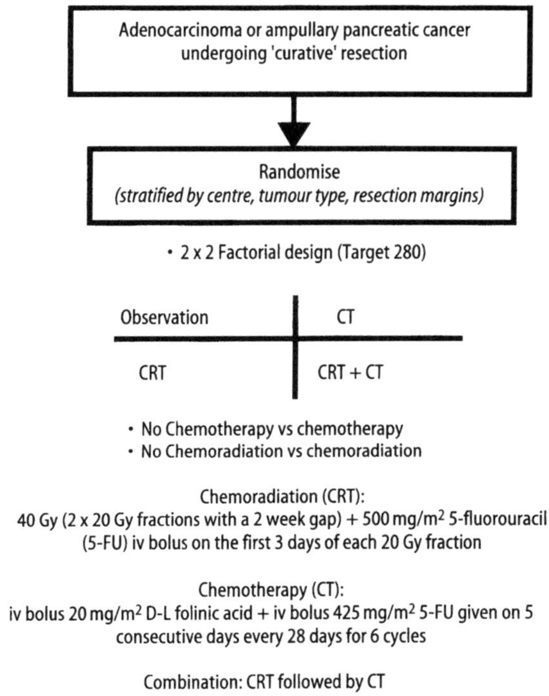

Figure 5.1. Principal components of the design of the ESPAC 1 trial.[26,27]

metastases, life expectancy of more than 3 months, fit enough for adjuvant treatment, informed consent) before treatment was allocated. Randomisation was stratified (as separate groups) by randomisation centre and resection margin status (R0 or R1). Adjuvant therapy was started as soon as possible after full recovery from resection, and all patients were followed up every 3 months until death. At each clinic visit all patients were asked to complete an ESPAC-1 quality of life form, consisting of the EORTC QLQ-C30 version 1 plus ESPAC-1 disease specific questions.

The Independent Data Monitoring Committee for the trial comprised a pancreatic surgeon (Mr RCG Russell, Consultant Surgeon at the Middlesex Hospital, London), a medical oncologist (Dr S O'Reilly, Consultant Clinical Oncologist, Clatterbridge Centre for Clinical Oncology, Wirral), and a statistician (Dr RP A'Hern, Department of Computing and Information, the Royal Marsden, London).

Recruitment

A steady increase in patient entry occurred in ESPAC-1, through planning, pragmatism, publicity and persistence (Figures 5.2 and 5.3). The recruitment phase lasted from February 1994 to June 2000 when target recruitment into the two-by-two design was reached. This was obtained without an established culture of multicentre, multinational randomised trials in the treatment of

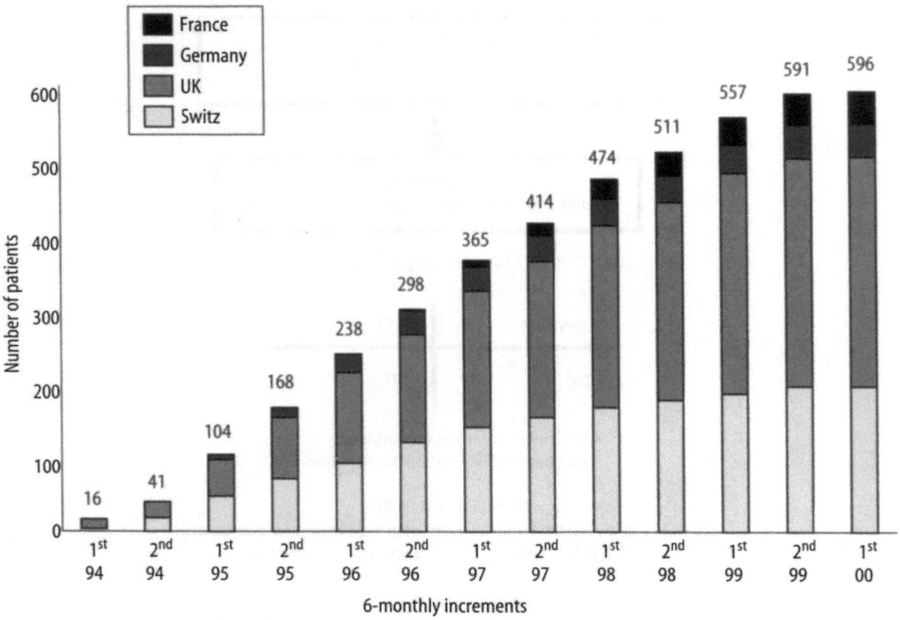

Figure 5.2. Cumulative recruitment of patients into ESPAC 1. Recruitment was halted early in 2000, accounting for the small number of patients recruited during the 1st half of 2000.

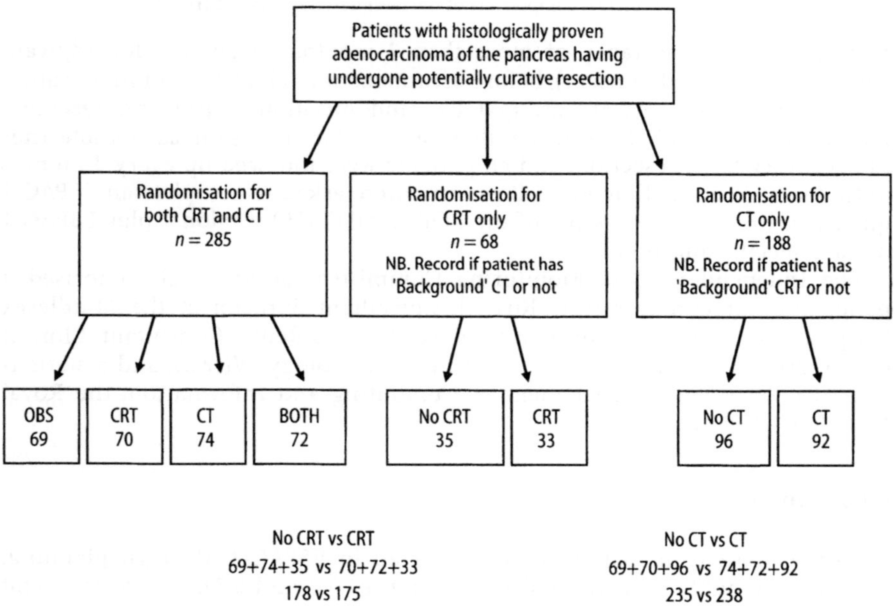

Figure 5.3. Flow chart detailing number of patients entered into the various randomisation options and their allocated treatment in ESPAC-1.

(resected) pancreatic cancer. New centres joined throughout the course of the trial, such that 83 clinicians in 61 cancer centres in 11 countries entered patients into ESPAC-1. Such widespread participation suggests that the key questions addressed were relevant and timely, and that widespread uncertainty existed as to the place of adjuvant chemoradiotherapy and/or chemotherapy following resection for pancreatic cancer. A significant step in maintaining the increase in recruitment was pragmatic expansion of the trial to include single-arm randomisation options for chemoradiation only and chemotherapy only (see above). Clinicians were thus free to administer treatment that they considered indicated (e.g. radiotherapy), whilst contributing to the trial in a manner that they considered appropriate.

Data Collection

The collection of data was the responsibility of each of the four randomisation centres, with central co-ordination initially in Birmingham, then from late 1996 onwards, in Liverpool. Each randomisation centre checked patient eligibility, and collected and translated data. Within each randomisation centre a leading clinician was responsible for national data collection and verification, as were national co-ordinators in other countries, who pursued clinicians proactively to obtain due or missing data items. As the trial was pragmatic in design, minimum details were required at each 3 monthly follow up visit, with completion of a quality of life form by each patient. Because of the large number of European centres participating in the trial, central audit of treatment practice could not be made, although each had local quality assurance measures in place. However, a sub-study was undertaken to assess toxicity data during treatment on a representative sample that underwent chemoradiotherapy, or chemotherapy, or both. Ineligibility was reported for seven patients (three patients were randomised twice in error, one patient had no pancreatic resection, one had metastases at entry and two had previous breast cancer), who were excluded from interim analysis, but all except the three duplicate randomisations will remain in the final analysis on an intention to treat basis. Protocol violations were reported for 51 patients (9% of 541 eligible, all but one of whom declined or withdrew from the treatment to which they were randomised), but these patients were kept in the relevant group to which they were randomised for the analyses.

Analysis and Interpretation of ESPAC-1

The primary endpoint was death, and the two main comparisons were of survival between those patients randomised to chemotherapy or not, and of survival between those randomised to chemoradiotherapy or not. Patients from the two by two factorial randomisation were analysed separately and then combined with the additional patients from each single arm randomisation.

Survival was calculated from the date of resection until the date of death, whatever the cause, or censored at the date of the latest follow up visit. Stratified log-rank analyses of treatment effects were undertaken with adjustment for known prognostic factors. Also, Cox's proportional-hazards modelling was used to investigate known prognostic factors, and to construct a base model to test further the effect of prognostic factors on treatment effects.

Whereas ESPAC-1 demonstrated no benefit from adjuvant chemoradiotherapy (randomisation to chemoradiotherapy only was closed early in 1999 on the advice of the Independent Data Monitoring Committee), there was a potential benefit from adjuvant chemotherapy. When data from patients entered into the two by two randomisation were combined with data from patients entered into the chemotherapy only randomisation, this benefit was highly significant. The median survival was 19.7 months (IQR 16.4–22.4) in 238 patients randomised to chemotherapy versus 14.0 months (11.9–16.5) in 235 patients randomised to no chemotherapy; the survival benefit was evident in resection margin positive (R1) as well as resection margin negative (R0) patients. However, for the subset of 285 patients randomised into the two by two factorial design, the survival benefit from adjuvant chemotherapy did not reach statistical significance at 17.4 months (13.5–21.8) for 146 patients randomised to chemotherapy versus 15.9 months (13.5–19.2) for 139 patients randomised to no chemotherapy.

Univariate significant predictors of survival were resection margin status, tumour grade, nodal involvement and tumour size. Stratification of the treatment effects by each of these factors made no difference to the results outlined above. Cox's proportional hazards model identified tumour grade, tumour size, nodal involvement and age as independent prognostic factors, which allowed calculation of overall treatment effects adjusted for these factors and background therapy. A hazard ratio of 1.18 (95% CI 0.87–1.61) for chemoradiotherapy and 0.66 (0.51–0.89) for chemotherapy was obtained from this analysis (Fig. 5.4).

Toxicity data were collected on 246 patients receiving chemoradiotherapy (74), chemotherapy (118) or both (54). Serious side effects were reported in 44 patients (27%), the most common of which were stomatitis (14), neutropenia (11) and diarrhoea (10). Despite this, the average overall quality of life scores increased similarly for all treatment groups during the first 3 months from baseline.

Several conclusions could be drawn from these interim data. First, that no benefit resulted from this adjuvant chemoradiotherapy regimen. Second, that there is overall a strong indication of benefit from adjuvant chemotherapy, a trend which was seen but which was not significant in the patients entered into the two by two randomisation, although the actual magnitude remains to be determined. Third, that chemoradiotherapy had a confounding negative effect on the benefit of chemotherapy alone, making interpretation of the chemotherapy effect more difficult. Fourth, that through collaboration, large scale trials of the adjuvant treatment after resection of pancreatic cancer can be undertaken successfully. Fifth, that the success of ESPAC-1 offers unparalleled opportunity to pursue further questions in pancreatic cancer treatment.

Problems and Solutions with ESPAC-1

ESPAC-1 scores highly on the Jadad scale and on CONSORT criteria. It would not have been feasible nor ethical to undertake double-blinding in this study, which would have fulfilled the remaining quality criterion that the trial did not

Figure 5.4. **a** Hazard ratio plot of the chemoradiation randomisation options in ESPAC-1 (CRT = chemoradiation) **b** Hazard ratio plot of the chemotherapy randomisation options in ESPAC-1 (CT = chemotherapy). ▶

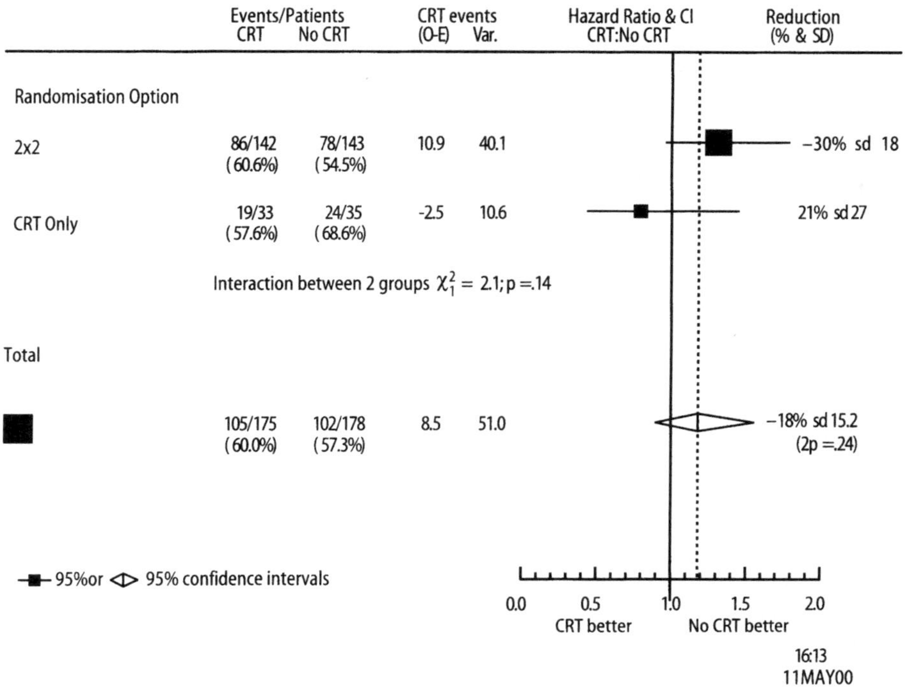
Events/Patients
CRT No CRT
CRT events
(O-E) Var.
Hazard Ratio & CI
CRT:No CRT
Reduction
(% & SD)
Randomisation Option
2x2
86/142 (60.6%)
78/143 (54.5%)
10.9
40.1
−30% sd 18
CRT Only
19/33 (57.6%)
24/35 (68.6%)
-2.5
10.6
21% sd 27
Interaction between 2 groups $\chi_1^2 = 2.1$; p =.14
Total
105/175 (60.0%)
102/178 (57.3%)
8.5
51.0
−18% sd 15.2
(2p =.24)
95%or 95% confidence intervals
0.0
0.5
1.0
1.5
2.0
CRT better
No CRT better
16:13
11MAY00

a

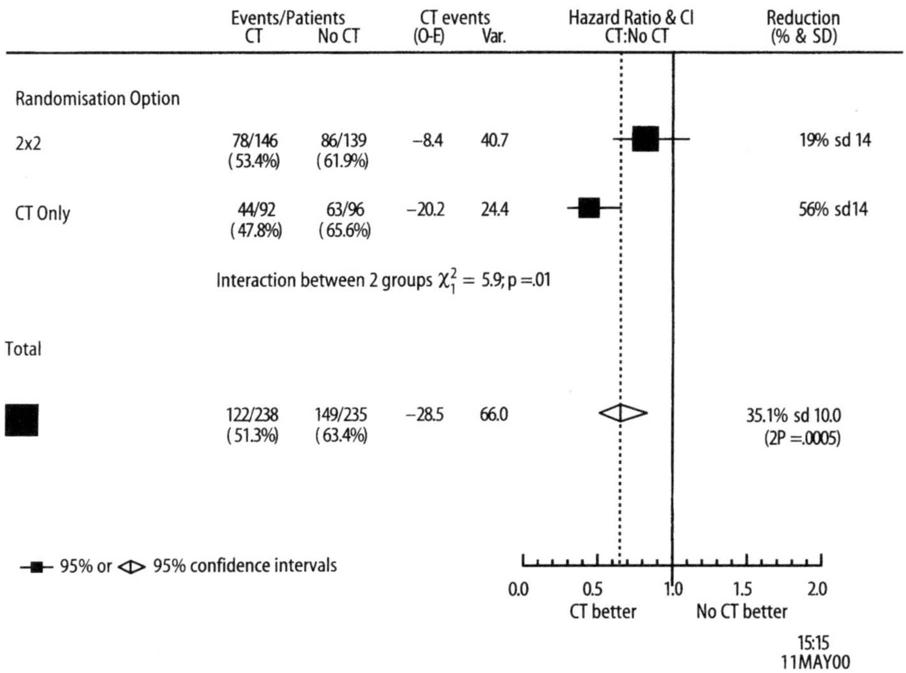
Events/Patients
CT No CT
CT events
(O-E) Var.
Hazard Ratio & CI
CT:No CT
Reduction
(% & SD)
Randomisation Option
2x2
78/146 (53.4%)
86/139 (61.9%)
−8.4
40.7
19% sd 14
CT Only
44/92 (47.8%)
63/96 (65.6%)
−20.2
24.4
56% sd14
Interaction between 2 groups $\chi_1^2 = 5.9$; p =.01
Total
122/238 (51.3%)
149/235 (63.4%)
−28.5
66.0
35.1% sd 10.0
(2P =.0005)
95% or 95% confidence intervals
0.0
0.5
1.0
1.5
2.0
CT better
No CT better
15:15
11MAY00

b

meet. The original two by two design was modified to allow clinicians to also randomise to either chemoradiotherapy or chemotherapy, in order to make the trial pragmatic hence increasing recruitment; this strategy was effective, as judged by the additional number entered into these alternatives. Thus 285 patients were randomised into the two by two design, compared to 68 into the chemoradiotherapy arm and 188 into the chemotherapy arm, doubling patient entry into the trial.

The international basis for recruitment took several years to strengthen, but has increased the ability to generalise the results, and has ensured more rapid take-off for subsequent trials. Randomisation via four separate randomisation centres was not ideal, as a single, central randomisation service is more effective and manageable. Also, data collection required streamlining, with national nominees responsible for their countries. This feature has been further refined for ESPAC-3, as outlined below.

ESPAC-2

Members of the ESPAC study group (HG Beger, Ulm and H Jeekel, Rotterdam) have pursued the hypothesis that loco-regional (intra-arterial) administration of chemotherapy together with radiotherapy may offer advantages over systemic administration, as an adjuvant to pancreatic cancer resection.[28] A comparison of this treatment against surgery alone is central to ESPAC-2. It is different from ESPAC-1, in that placement of cannulae into specific arteries is required, making the trial more specialised. ESPAC-2 also continues to explore the role of chemoradiotherapy, with a higher dose of radiotherapy. Recruitment began in 1999, prior to publication of the results of ESPAC-1; the recruitment objective is for 120 patients, with 60 in each arm. Because this will be a smaller trial than ESPAC-1, for any effect to be detected reliably, it must be more marked than that seen with adjuvant chemotherapy in ESPAC-1.

ESPAC-3

Design

ESPAC-1 showed potential benefit from adjuvant chemotherapy, but sufficient doubt remained to require any similar, further trial of adjuvant chemotherapy to require a no treatment arm. At the same time, the optimum regimen remains uncertain. From trials of gemcitabine in advanced pancreatic cancer, there appears to be a survival advantage with well maintained quality of life, more evident than with any other chemotherapeutic regime.[11,29,30] Thus ESPAC-3 was designed to determine what the optimal chemotherapeutic regime might be (either the same regimen as used in ESPAC-1 or gemcitabine), whilst also assessing the effect of adjuvant chemotherapy *per se* (Fig. 5.4).[30] Importantly, the international collaborative network that built up in ESPAC-1 presented an ideal opportunity to address the relatively simple questions posed in ESPAC-3. By continuing to pursue a pragmatic approach, it is anticipated that this large-scale trial will be undertaken with recruitment that is at least as fast as that of ESPAC-1 (and so far has been, see below). Thus it is planned to recruit 990 patients into ESPAC-3, widening collaboration to include centres in Canada, Japan and Australasia.

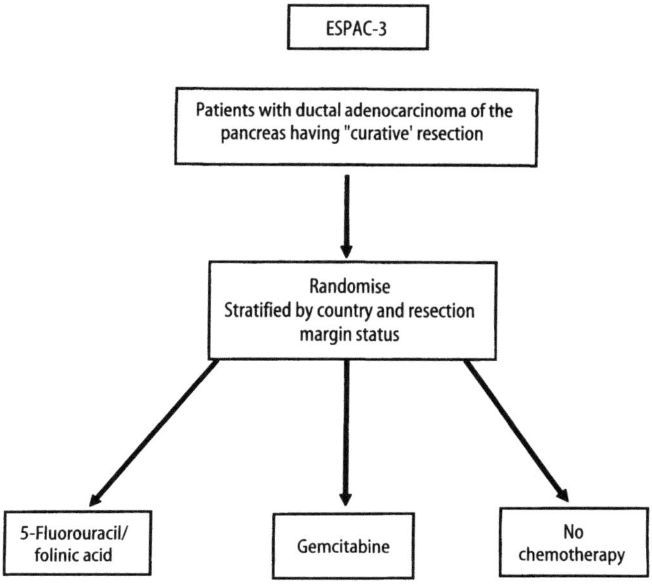

5-Fluorouracil/folinic acid: folinic acid (D-L 20 mg/m^2 iv bolus), 5-fluorouracil (425 mg/m^2 iv bolus) 5 days every 28 days, x6 cycles

Gemcitabine: gemcitabine (1000 mg/m^2 iv infusion) once weekly x3 weeks, 1 week rest, x6 cyces

Figure 5.5. Principal components of the design of the ESPAC 3 trial.

Organisation

Experience of ESPAC-1 has led to a number of modifications for ESPAC-3. First, randomisation is being undertaken by one central service (in Liverpool). However, the onus on National Coordinating Centres remains, since these must establish and maintain the link with the randomisation (and central data collection) service. The critical role of National Coordinating Centres has been formalised in the organisation of ESPAC-3, to:

- Collect ethics confirmation
- Maintain list of consultant/ hospital contacts
- Ensure completeness of randomisation data
- Provide fast/ effective/ available 'randomisation' service
- Collect patient consent forms
- Translate data collection/ patient consent forms
- Actively track, collect, chase trial data and QoL data
- Actively follow-up randomised patients
- Liase, advise and co-ordinate local hospitals
- Be the point of contact for data queries/ missing data

The trial is a large-scale randomised trial, with minimum impact on participating clinicians to ensure maximum participation. Methods of analysis will be similar to ESPAC-1, with the potential for even more data on prognostic factors. Furthermore, the continuing follow up on living patients entered into ESPAC-1, together with data fed to the Independent Data Monitoring Committee of ESPAC-3, may permit a definitive conclusion to be drawn as to the beneficial effect of adjuvant chemotherapy against surgery alone. Should this occur, the no treatment arm can be dropped, to ensure maximum recruitment to either chemotherapy arm. Despite being a European Study Group trial, other centres in other countries are encouraged to participate. Thus Australia and Canada are contributing to the recruitment, also with interest from the Japanese Pancreatic Group.

Progress

ESPAC-3 has been open to recruitment since June 2000, and in May 2003, 234 patients had been recruited in 68 centres: 34 centres in the UK, 8 in Canada, 8 in Australia, 4 in Germany, 3 in Hungary, 2 in Greece, 2 in Italy, 2 in Sweden, 1 in Czech Republic, 1 in Finland, 1 in Poland, 1 in Serbia and Montenegro. It is anticipated that recruitment will start shortly in Belgium, Ireland, Japan and New Zealand. This exemplifies the success of the collaborative approach, that has extended more widely than the original remit of ESPAC.

References

1. Parkin DM, Muir CS, Whelan SL, et al. Cancer incidence in five continents, vol VI. Lyon: International Agency for Research on Cancer, 1992 (IARC Scientific Publications number 120).
2. Nitecki SS, Sarr MG, Colby, et al. Long-term survival after resection for ductal adenocarcinoma of the pancreas: is it really improving? Ann Surg 1995; 221:59–66.
3. Birkmeyer JD, Warshaw AL, Finlayson STG, et al. Relationship between hospital volume and late survival after pancreatoduodenectomy. Surgery 1999; 126:178–183.
4. Bramhall SR, Allum WH, Jones AG, et al. Incidence, treatment and survival in 13,560 patients with pancreatic cancer: an epidemiological study in the West Midlands. Br J Surg 1995; 82:111–115.
5. Neoptolemos JP, Russell RCG, Bramhall SR, et al. Low mortality following resection for pancreatic and periampullary tumours in 1026 patients: UK survey of specialist pancreatic units. Br J Surg 1997; 84:1370–1376.
6. Wong T, Howes N, Threadgold J, et al. Molecular diagnosis of pancreatic ductal adenocarcinoma in high-risk patients. Pancreatology 2001; 1:486–509.
7. Kalser MH, Ellenberg SS. Pancreatic cancer: adjuvant combined radiation and chemotherapy following curative resection. Arch Surg 185; 120:899–903.
8. Douglass HO. Further evidence of effective adjuvant combined radiation and chemotherapy following curative resection of pancreatic cancer. Cancer 1987; 59:2006–2010.
9. Bakkevold KE, Arnesjo B, Dahl O, et al. Adjuvant combination chemotherapy (AMF) following radical resection of carcinoma of the pancreas and papilla of Vater: results of a controlled, prospective, randomised multicenter study. Eur J Cancer 1993; 5:698–703.
10. Klinkenbijl JH, Jeekel J, Sahmoud T, et al. Adjuvant radiotherapy and 5-fluorouracil after curative resection of cancer of the pancreas and periampullary region. Phase III trial of the EORTC Gastrointestinal Tract Cancer Cooperative Group. Ann Surg 1999; 230:776–784.
11. Magee CJ, Ghaneh P, Neoptolemos JP. Surgical and medical therapy for pancreatic carcinoma. Best Pract Res Clin Gastroenterol 2002; 16:435–55.
12. Jones L, Mosca F, Russell C, et al. Standard Kausch-Whipple pancreatoduodenectomy. Dig Surg 1999; 16:297–304.
13. Pedrazzoli S, Di Carlo V, Dionigi R, et al. Standard versus extended lymphadenectomy associated with pancreatoduodenectomy in the surgical treatment of adenocarcinoma of the head of the

pancreas: a Multicenter, prospective, randomized study. Lymphadenectomy Study Group. Ann Surg 1998; 228:508–517.
14. Mosca F, Giulianotti PC, Balestracci T, et al. Long-term survival in pancreatic cancer: pylorus-preserving vs Whipple pancreatoduodenectomy. Surgery 1997; 122:553–566.
15. Trede M, Schwall G, Saeger H-D. Survival after pancreatoduodenectomy: 118 consecutive resections without an operative mortality. Ann Surg 1990; 211:447–458.
16. Allema JH, Reinders ME, Vangulik TM, et al. Prognostic factors for survival after pancreaticoduodenectomy for patients with carcinoma of the pancreatic head region. Cancer 1995; 75:2069–2076.
17. Yeo C, Abrams R, Grochow L, et al. Pancreaticoduodenectomy for pancreatic adenocarcinoma: postoperative adjuvant chemoradiation improves survival: a prospective, single institution experience. Ann Surg 1997; 225:621–633.
18. Snow J. On the mode of communication of cholera. 2nd edn. London: John Churchill, 1860 (facsimile of 1936 reprinted edition published in 1965 by Hafner, New York).
19. Streptomycin in Tuberculosis Trials Committee, Medical Research Council. Streptomycin treatment in pulmonary tuberculosis: a Medical Research Council investigation. BMJ 1948; ii:769–82.
20. van der Wijden CL, Overbeke JA. Audit of reports of randomised clinical trials published in one journal over 45 years. BMJ 1995; 311:918.
21. Moher D, Schulz KF, Altman DG. The CONSORT statement: revised recommendations for improving the quality of reports of parallel group randomized trials. Lancet 2001; 357:1191–4.
22. Moher D, Jones A, Lepage L, et al. Use of the CONSORT statement and quality of reports of randomized trials: a comparative before-and-after evaluation. JAMA 2001; 285:1992–1995.
23. Peto R, Baigent C. Trials: the next 50 years. Large scale randomised evidence of moderate benefits. BMJ 1998; 317:1170–1.
24. ISIS-2 (Second International Study of Infarct Survival) Collaborative Group. Randomised trial of intravenous streptokinase, oral aspirin, both, or neither among 17,187 cases of suspected acute myocardial infarction. Lancet 1988; ii:349–360.
25. Jadad AR, Moore RA, Carroll D, et al. Assessing the quality of reports of randomized clinical trials: is blinding necessary? Control Clin Trials 1996; 17:1–12.
26. Neoptolemos JP, Dunn JA, Stocken DD, et al. European Study Group for Pancreatic Cancer. Adjuvant chemoradiotherapy and chemotherapy in resectable pancreatic cancer: a randomised controlled trial. Lancet 2001; 358:1576–85.
27. Neoptolemos JP, Stocken DD, Dunn JA, et al. European Study Group for Pancreatic Cancer. Influence of resection margins on survival for patients with pancreatic cancer treated by adjuvant chemoradiation and/or chemotherapy in the ESPAC-1 randomized controlled trial. Ann Surg 2001; 234:758–68.
28. Link KH, Formentini A, Leder G, et al. Resection and radiochemotherapy of pancreatic cancer – the future? Langenbecks Arch Surg 1998; 383:134–144.
29. Abbruzzese JL. Past and present treatment of pancreatic adenocarcinoma: chemotherapy as a standard treatment modality. Semin Oncol 2002; 29:2–8.
30. Neoptolemos JP, Cunningham D, Friess H, et al. Adjuvant therapy in pancreatic cancer: historical and current perspectives. Ann Oncol 2003; 14:675–92.

6 Gemcitabine: a Systematic Review

Susan E. Ward, Eva Morris and Nick Bansback

Pancreatic cancer is the eighth most common cancer in the UK, accounting for 6562 deaths in the UK in 1998.[1] One-year survival rates are in the order of 12% and less than 3% of patients survive to 5 years.[2] Its symptoms are wide-ranging, but may only appear towards the latter stage of the disease and so the vast majority of patients present with advanced disease.

Health resources are scarce. Choices have to be made concerning their deployment. The technology appraisal process for new and existing health technologies, undertaken by the National institute for Clinical Excellence, addresses this decision-making process by considering two key questions: first, "Does the health technology work?" (the evaluation of effectiveness), and second, "Is it worth doing compared to other things that could be done with the same resources?" (the economic evaluation).

A review of the effectiveness and cost-effectiveness of gemcitabine in the treatment of pancreatic cancer is indeed timely. Uncertainty continues to exists about the role of chemotherapy in pancreatic cancer and the optimal regimen. Survival of patients with pancreatic cancer remains poor and therapeutic options are limited. The use of chemotherapy in the UK varies by geographical location and between different providers. Recent guidance on the management of upper GI cancers recommended the use of palliative chemotherapy, but did not provide specific guidance on the most effective regimen. Over recent years some Centres and Units in the UK had obtained funding for gemcitabine, whilst funding had been refused at a number of hospitals, including a number of specialist centers.[3]

It is estimated that less than 15% of patients in England and Wales currently receive palliative chemotherapy. (Crellin, A., Yorkshire Centre for Clinical Oncology, Cookridge Hospital, Leeds: personal communication, 2000). This proportion is expected to increase over the next few years, following the recent introduction of new guidance on the management of upper gastro-intestinal (GI) cancers,[4] which recommends the consideration of palliative therapy with chemotherapy for patients with advanced disease.

The standard chemotherapy used for patients with pancreatic cancer in the UK over recent years has been 5-fluorouracil (5-FU). Evidence shows a small survival advantage and improvement in quality of life (QoL) in a proportion of patients treated with 5-FU.[5]

Gemcitabine offers an alternative to these patients. It is a novel nucleoside analogue which inhibits DNA synthesis. It is indicated for the treatment of adults with locally advanced or metastatic adenocarcinoma of the pancreas and for patients with 5-FU refractory pancreatic cancer and offers the advantage of simple administration on an outpatient basis. Given the relatively poor efficacy of current treatments and the anticipated rise in the use of chemotherapy for patients with pancreatic cancer it was timely to review both the effectiveness and the cost-effectiveness of this treatment option.

Undertaking the Systematic Review

A systematic review of the evidence on gemcitabine was undertaken. The search strategy aimed to identify all papers relating to gemcitabine and pancreatic cancer. Keyword strategies were developed using key references retrieved through initial scoping searches. Search strategies did not include search terms or filters that would limit results to specific publication types or study designs. Date and language restrictions were not used.

Full searches of the bibliographic databases along with further current research and grey literature sources were undertaken in August 2000. Searches of the following databases were undertaken; Medline, Embase, Science Citation Index (SCI), Cochrane Database of Systematic Reviews (CDSR), Cochrane Controlled Trials Register (CENTRAL/CCTR), the NHS Centre for Reviews and Dissemination databases (DARE, NHS EED, HTA) and the OHE Health Economics Database (HEED). A search of the previous six months of PubMED was undertaken to identify recent studies not yet indexed on Medline. Hand and citation searches were undertaken in November 2000. Search strategies are detailed elsewhere.[6]

The Evidence on Effectiveness

The searches undertaken retrieved a total of 458 studies. These included a total of seven randomized controlled trials (RCTs) and 57 phase II studies. Phase I studies were excluded.

Of the seven RCTs, only one fully published trial of gemcitabine compared with standard chemotherapy treatment (5-FU) was identified.[7] The other two full RCTs related to adjuvant therapy.[8;9] The remaining four studies were only available in abstract form.[10–13] Only one of these, a comparison of gemcitabine with the matrix metalloproteinase inhibitors, BAY 12-9566 conducted by Moore et al.,[10] provided survival data on gemcitabine.

No RCTs of gemcitabine versus best supportive care (BSC) were identified. In addition, no high quality randomised trials of gemcitabine as a second line treatment were identified.

Survival

Gemcitabine as a First Line Therapy

The best evidence available relating to the use of gemcitabine as a first line therapy comes from Burris et al.[7] This study compares the use of gemcitabine to 5-FU in 126 patients with locally advanced or metastatic pancreatic cancer. Patients randomised to gemcitabine had significantly better one-year survival (18% *vs* 2%, p = 0.0025), significantly better median survival (5.65 *vs* 4.41 months, p = 0.0025), improved median progression free survival (2.33 *vs* 0.92 months, p = 0.0002) and a longer time to treatment failure (2.04 *vs* 0.92 months, p = 0.0004.) However, no difference was observed in partial tumour response rates between the two treatment arms.

No description of the method of randomisation was available and the investigation was single blind, resulting in a low Jadad score of 2 for this study. In addition questions exist which cast doubt on the validity of its results. Firstly, it can be criticised due to the small sample size involved. Only 126 individuals are included in the analysis and results based on such a small patient population sample cannot be regarded as definitive. Secondly the control arm of 5-FU alone was administered as a bolus infusion. This has been shown to be a sub-optimal method of administration in other types of gastrointestinal cancers[14] and, as such, may not be a valid control against which to evaluate gemcitabine. The one-year survival rate in the 5-FU arm was unusually low, at 2%. The median survival for the 5-FU arm may also be considered to be low at 4.41 months (mean 4.52 months). In trials by Glimelius et al. and Palmer et al., comparing 5-FU combined with other chemotherapy agents to BSC, the median survival for 5-FU was 6.0 and 7.6 months, respectively.[5;15] It is possible that had 5-FU been given in a more active form, the comparatively significant benefit attributed to gemcitabine could have been reduced.

The only RCT in abstract form which provided survival data for gemcitabine was Moore et al.,[10] a randomised comparison of gemcitabine and BAY12-9566, involving 277 patients. The median survival rate of gemcitabine was 6.4 months, comparable to the figure obtained by Burris of 5.65 months.

Other evidence is limited. Storniolo et al.,16 in a study of open-label single-arm design with patients with locally advanced or metastatic pancreatic cancer, reported median survival to be 4.8 months (95% CI, 4.5–5.1 months) for 2380 patients. All of the remaining studies identified are of a phase II or retrospective cohort design. The majority are published in abstract form and, so, the data available is limited. In addition, they frequently contain only a very small number of patients. Given the heterogeneity of the interventions evaluated and the study population characteristics and outcome measures no attempt has been made to pool outcomes or conduct any form of meta-analysis. However, from these studies one-year survival for gemcitabine is seen to range between 15% and 26% and median survival between 4.7 and 8.8 months.

In summary this is a very poor evidence base by which to assess the efficacy of gemcitabine as a first line therapy. Whilst it would appear that gemcitabine offers similar survival to 5-FU based regimes, the validity of the only RCT which compares gemcitabine to the standard treatment of 5-FU has been questioned and the results of the Burris trial cannot be regarded as definitive. In addition, due to the experimental comparisons used and the limited results reported, it is exceedingly difficult to evaluate or validate the other relevant RCTs. Further detailed, high quality studies are required before the role of gemcitabine in first line therapy can be fully determined.

Gemcitabine as a Second Line Therapy

Rothenberg et al.[17] is the only trial to involve exclusively individuals with relapsed disease. It examines the effect of gemcitabine in patients with metastatic pancreatic cancer that had progressed despite the administration of 5-FU. The study only involved 74 patients and, of these, only 63 were evaluated for clinical benefit response (CBR) and 54 for response. The study demonstrated a median survival of 4 months and one-year survival of 4%.

Although these results look promising for gemcitabine in second line treatment, no additional evidence is available to support this trial and phase II trials alone should not form the basis of the establishment of standard therapy.

Other Applications of Gemcitabine

Additional studies were identified which examined the role of gemcitabine as adjuvant chemotherapy, gemcitabine in combination chemotherapy, and the role of gemcitabine plus radiation and gemcitabine plus hormonal therapy. These studies are detailed elsewhere.[6] The current evidence base is insufficient to assess fully the use of gemcitabine in these applications. Further studies, involving more participants and of higher methodological quality, are required before its full impact on survival in these applications can be assessed.

Quality of Life

As pancreatic cancer is such a devastating disease, with a particularly dismal prognosis, maintenance of quality of life is the major goal of palliation. Severe pain is a common symptom. Pancreatic cancer also causes jaundice, weight loss, poor appetite, vomiting, general GI problems and diabetes.4 The role of chemotherapy in pancreatic cancer and its impact on quality of life is not clear cut. Benefits in terms of survival time and alleviation of symptoms may be outweighed by the cost of toxicity and deterioration in quality of life.[18]

Once again the Burris RCT7 provides the best evidence in relation to the efficacy of gemcitabine in terms of improving this quality of life in advanced pancreatic cancer patients. In the absence of a validated quality of life tool Burris et al.[7] used clinical benefit response (CBR) in an attempt to determine how well tumour-related symptoms are controlled.

The measurement of CBR is based on the assessment of four parameters; pain intensity (a daily assessment on a linear analog scale), analgesic intake (assessed by consumption of morphine or its equivalent), Karnofsky performance status and weight change (a secondary parameter). In order for a patient to be designated a clinical benefit responder they must show a significant and sustained 50% improvement in at least one of the three assessed parameters, with no deterioration in any of the others. If patients remain stable in all parameters, they are considered to be a responder if they have not lost 7% of their body weight, and a non-responder if there has been greater weight loss.

The Burris trial 7 demonstrated that the administration of gemcitabine led to significantly more clinical benefit responders compared to those randomised to 5-FU (23.8% *vs* 4.8%, $p = 0.0022$). Other identified evidence included six phase II studies, 19 20 17 21 22 23 which demonstrated CBR rates much higher than that obtained in the Burris study, ranging between 27% and 48%.

Rothenberg et al.[17] assessed CBR in patients with metastatic pancreatic cancer refractory to 5-FU. They demonstrated a CBR rate of 27%. No other supporting evidence was identified.

It should, however, be noted that the use of CBR to assess quality of life is not a validated tool and a number of criticisms of the technique have been made.[24–26] For example, the primary criteria for this response are based on patient self-reports. As such, the subjective nature of this patient self-reporting could lead to a 'placebo effect'.[27] Furthermore, the CBR endpoint requires follow-up to be long enough for a response to be observed. This is an issue for the Burris study, where the possibility exists that 5-FU patients were removed from the study earlier than the gemcitabine patients and, as such, the results are not entirely reliable.

Based on the available evidence, the value of gemcitabine in improving quality of life, over and above other forms of treatment, remains inconclusive. The Burris trial shows a significant benefit over 5-FU but, due to cautions over the administration of 5-FU and concerns over the outcome measure used, this cannot be considered to be a definitive result. Further evidence, in the form of high quality randomised trials, are required to assess fully the benefit of gemcitabine as first line and second line therapy over other forms of treatment, in terms of quality of life.

Adverse Effects of Intervention

Two studies which reviewed the safety and toxicity of gemcitabine were identified.[28;29] Aapro et al.[28] reviewed data from 979 patients in 22 completed clinical studies using 800–1250 mg/m2 on days 1, 8, 15 every 28 days. Similarly, Tonato et al.[29] assessed the toxicity profile of the drug in 790 patients from phase II trials. Both studies consisted of a cohort or individuals with a range of solid tumours.

Both these reviews conclude that gemcitabine is well tolerated with a mild toxicity profile. Interestingly, in the Burris trial, gemcitabine was shown to have a higher toxicity profile than 5-FU. This once again may point to the possibility that a sub-optimal dose of 5-FU was delivered, since the toxicity of bolus 5-FU would generally be expected to be similar to the toxicity relating to gemcitabine.

The Evidence on Cost Effectiveness of Gemcitabine

Two existing economic studies were identified as part of the systematic review. First, a health economic evaluation of the treatment of patients diagnosed with pancreatic cancer in Sweden estimated the incremental cost per life year gained for gemcitabine using a hypothetical analysis of gemcitabine and best supportive care versus best supportive care.[30] Their analysis synthesised the survival rates and resource use (in-patient and out-patient care) from the Burris trial[7] with Swedish epidemiological data. The incremental cost per life year gained (LYG) for gemcitabine was estimated to be 132 286 Swedish Kroner (around £14 000 using December 2000 exchange rates). Second, Trippoli and Messori (1999)[31] using the survival data from the Burris trial[7] and cost data estimated from individual data on the use of resources and morbidity, presented preliminary data, in abstract form, showing the incremental cost of gemcitabine to be less than $20 000 compared with 5-FU. Subsequent analysis (Messori,A., Meta-analysis Study Group of SIFO, Florence: Personal Communication, 2000) produced a preliminary estimate of cost per QALY using the Q-TWiST (Quality Adjusted Time Without Symptoms or Toxicity) approach. The Italian analysis results in an estimated discounted cost per life year gained of $48 000 (£33 500), and a cost per QALY of $52 000(£36 800). The work was not taken beyond the preliminary estimates due to issues relating to the quality of the cost data.

Both of the analyses identified are dependant on outcome results from the single (Eli Lilly sponsored) RCT. The ability to generalise this trial's results are unproven to date. In addition, the Swedish evaluation demonstrated the upward sensitivity of the cost per LYG ratio to decreases in incremental survival benefit from gemcitabine. Given that the effectiveness review presented earlier in this report casts some doubt on the survival benefits demonstrated by the Burris trial, this raises concerns regarding the robustness of cost per LYG figures that have been demonstrated.

Economic Evaluation of Gemcitabine

As part of the rapid review process an economic evaluation was undertaken combining UK costs with the survival evidence from Burris et al[7] to compare the cost-effectiveness of first line treatment with gemcitabine with treatment with fluorouracil (5-FU). The mean treatment cost difference used in conjunction with the mean survival gain was used to give an indication of the cost effectiveness ratio. Full details of this evaluation are reported elsewhere.[6]

Costs

The cost of 5-FU is dependent on the type of delivery. The weekly bolus 5-FU regimen, used in the Burris trial, is not generally used in the UK. However two regimens, commonly used in the UK, were considered. The De Gramont regime, which consists of 5-FU (400 mg/m^2) by bolus intravenous injection plus high dose folinic acid (200 mg/m^2), for 2 days at 14-day intervals. This is the more expensive regimen, with high inpatient and chemotherapy costs. The protracted venous infusion (PVI) 5-FU regime consists of 5-FU (300 mg/m^2/day) administered continually via an ambulatory pump, allowing the drug to be administered in the home setting. Although there are additional costs associated with the pump and the insertion of a central line it offers the advantage of low volumes of inpatient and outpatient visits, which is beneficial to both patient and providers.

The drug cost of gemcitabine is more expensive than 5-FU, but overall costs are partly offset by the simplicity of drug administration, a 30 minute infusion delivered on an outpatient basis. No inpatient admission is required. Costs relating to pump and central line insertion and removal, as required for PVI 5-FU, are avoided, as are the potential complications arising from the use of central venous catheters. In addition, some Cancer Centres and or Units may not have the infrastructure necessary to support infused PVI 5-FU schedules.

Survival

The mean survival gain of gemcitabine over 5-FU was estimated using Area Under the Curve analysis to determine the area between the gemcitabine and 5-FU curves. The mean survival gain estimated in this way gave 2.27 months (6.79 months *vs* 4.52 months), compared with the median survival benefit of

1.24 months (5.65 months *vs* 4.41 months). The median survival, although a useful measure in assessing clinical efficacy, underestimates the area under the curve due to the shape of the survival curves in the Burris trial.

Given the absence of evidence on the effectiveness of alternative 5-FU regimens in pancreatic cancer the mean survival gain of gemcitabine over 5-FU in the economic model is assumed to be the same for the different regimens There is however strong evidence to show that in other treatments of gastro-intestinal cancer the bolus 5-FU alone would be considered inferior in terms of response rates and efficacy.[14] This may well mean that the survival gains for gemcitabine are overstated in the economic modelling.

The mean survival gain for gemcitabine, 2.27 months, was combined with the incremental cost of the gemcitabine over 5-FU to calculate a cost per life year gained (LYG) for gemcitabine. Based on comparison with PVI 5-FU regime the incremental cost of gemcitabine is estimated to be £16 543 per life year gained. Based on the De Gramont regimen the corresponding figure is £7209. These estimates suggest that the cost effectiveness of gemcitabine remains within the levels achieved by treatments currently used in the NHS.

Sensitivity analysis demonstrated that the cost per LYG figure was sensitive to assumptions on survival. Based on comparison with PVI 5-FU regime the incremental cost of gemcitabine is estimated to rise to £25 000 per life year gained if the survival difference fell to 1.5 months.

Uncertainty relating to the evidence of effectiveness means that the cost effectiveness analysis can not be considered to be robust. The evidence for the quality of life benefits of gemcitabine is particularly poor. There is widespread acknowledgment for the need for a RCT to confirm the survival benefits of gemcitabine, and particularly to enable the collation of acceptable quality of life data.[26;27;30] Without better information, the cost-effectiveness of gemcitabine for first and second line treatment of pancreatic cancer remains in doubt.

Conclusion

The prognosis for pancreatic cancer patients remains poor. For patients with poor performance status the emphasis should remain on symptom control and involvement of a palliative care team. For patients with good performance status, chemotherapy may offer benefit. However no chemotherapy drugs have yet demonstrated response rates higher than 20%. Based on the conclusions of this review no standard therapy for the first line treatment of patients with pancreatic cancer can be recommended. Gemcitabine offers, at best, a small increase in survival over 5-FU. It does however increase patient choice, in relation to the mode of administration, in an area where therapeutic options are limited. Preliminary estimates of costs suggest that these are not prohibitively high for gemcitabine.

For the future, further evidence on the survival, quality of life and cost is required before any definite conclusions can be drawn about cost-effectiveness. In reality the use of gemcitabine as part of a combination chemotherapy regime appears to offer the most likely way forward and high quality randomised evidence is awaited. In addition, further RCT evidence is also required for the use of gemcitabine as adjuvant treatment and as second line treatment.

References

1. Northern and Yorkshire Cancer Registry and Information Service. Cancer treatment policies and their effects on survival: pancreas (Key sites study 4). Leeds: Northern and Yorkshire Cancer Registry and Information Service/University of Leeds; 2000.
2. Eli Lilly and Company Limited. Gemzar (Gemcitabine) for Pancreatic Cancer. Confidential Submission; 2000.
3. Cancer Research Campaign. CancerStats - the vital statistics on cancer mortality:UK: Cancer Research Campaign; 2000.
4. NHS Centre for Reviews and Dissemination. Guidance on commissioning cancer services. Improving outcomes in upper gastrointestinal cancers - the manual. London: Department of Health 2001.
5. Glimelius B, Hoffman K, Sjoden P-O, et al. Chemotherapy improves survival and quality of life in advanced pancreatic and biliary cancer. Ann of Oncol 1996; 7:593–600.
6. Ward S, Morris E, Bansback N, et al. A rapid and systematic review of the clinical and cost effectiveness of gemcitabine for the treatment of pancreatic cancer. Health Technology Assessment 2001; 5:No 24.
7. Burris HA, Moore MJ, Andersen J, et al. Improvements in survival and clinical benefit with gemcitabine as first- line therapy for patients with advanced pancreas cancer: A randomized trial. J Clin Oncol 1997; 15:2403–13.
8. Lygidakis NJ, Berberabe AE, Spentzouris N, et al. A prospective randomized study using adjuvant locoregional chemoimmunotherapy in combination with surgery for pancreatic carcinoma. Hepatogastroenterology 1998; 45:2376–81.
9. Lygidakis NJ, Spentzouris N, Theodoracopoulos M, et al. Pancreatic resection for pancreatic carcinoma combined with neo- and adjuvant locoregional targeting immuno-chemotherapy–a prospective randomized study. Hepatogastroenterology 1998; 45:396–403.
10. Moore MJ, Hamm J, Eisenber P, et al. A comparison between gemcitabine and matrix metalloproteinase inhibitor BAY12-9566 (9566) in patients with advanced pancreatic cancer [abstract]. Proc Am Soc Clin Oncol 2000; 19:240a.
11. Rosemurgy A, Buckels J, Charnley R, et al. A randomised study comparing marimastat to gemcitabine as first line therapy in patients with non-resectable pancreatic cancer [abstract]. Proc Am Soc Clin Oncol 1999; 18:261a.
12. British Biotech. Results of Marimistat Study 193 in advanced pancreatic cancer. [Press Release]. Available at: URL: www.britbio.co.uk.
13. Cantore M, Marangolo M, Cavazini G, et al. Preliminary results of arandomised trial in unresectable pancreatic cancer: FUFA vs GEM vs FLEC given intra-arterially [abstract]. Proc Am Soc Clin Oncol 2000; 19:269a.
14. Meta-analysis Group on Cancer. Toxicity of fluorouracil in patients with advanced colorectal cancer: effect of administration schedule and prognostic factors. J Clin Oncol 1998; 16:3537–41.
15. Palmer KR, Kerr M, Knowles G, et al. Chemotherapy prolongs survival in inoperable pancreatic carcinoma. Br J Cancer 1994; 81:882–5.
16. Storniolo AM, Enas NH, Brown CA, et al. An investigational new drug treatment program for patients with gemcitabine: results for over 3000 patients with pancreatic carcinoma. Cancer 1999; 85:1261–8.
17. Rothenberg ML, Moore MJ, Cripps MC, et al. A phase II trial of gemcitabine in patients with 5-FU-refractory pancreas cancer Ann Oncol 1996; 7:347–53.
18. Fitzsimmons D, Johnson CD, George S, et al. Development of a disease specific quality of life (QoL) questionnaire module to supplement the EORTC core cancer QoL questionnaire, the QLQ-C30 in patients with pancreatic cancer. Euro J Cancer 1999; 35:939–41.
19. Kurtz JE, Trillet-Lenoir V, Bugat R, et al. Compassionate use of gemcitabine in advanced pancreatic cancer: a French multicentric study. Bull Cancer 1999; 86:202–6.
20. Petrovic Z, Jovic J, Perisic N, et al. Monotherapy with gemcitabine in patients with advanced pancreatic carcinoma. Ann Oncol 1998; 9:641.
21. Scheithauer W, Kornek G, Ulrich-Pur H, et al. Phase II trial of high-dose gemcitabine in patients with metastatic pancreatic adenocarcinoma [abstract]. Euro J Cancer 1999; 35:538.
22. Spagnuolo P, Roversi R, Rossi G, et al. Phase II study of gemcitabine as locoregional treatment of advanced pancreatic cancer - [abstract]. Proc Am Soc Clin Oncol 1999; 18:300a.
23. Ulrich-Pur H, Kornek GV, Raderer M, et al. A phase II trial of biweekly high dose gemcitabine for patients with metastatic pancreatic adenocarcinoma. Cancer 2000; 88:2505–11.

24. Schaafsma J, Osoba D. The Karnofsky performance status scale re-examined: a cross-validation with EORTC-C30. Quality of Life Research 1994; 3:413–24.
25. Wilkin D, Hallam L, Doggett M. Measures of Need and outcome for primary health care. Oxford: Oxford Medical Publications; 1994.
26. Kokoska ER, Stapleton DR, Virgo KS, et al. Quality of Life measurements do not support palliative pancreatic cancer treatments. Int J Oncology 1998; 13:1323–9.
27. Gelber RD. Gemcitabine for pancreatic cancer: how hard to look for clinical benefit? An American perspective [editorial; comment]. Ann Oncol 1996; 7:335–7.
28. Aapro MS, Martin C, Hatty S. Gemcitabine – a safety review. Anticancer Drugs 1998; 9:191–201.
29. Tonato M, Moscini AM, Martin C. Safety profile of gemcitabine. Anticancer Drugs 1995; 6 (Suppl 6):27–32.
30. Ragnarson-Tennvall G, Wilking N. Treatment of locally advanced pancreatic carcinoma in Sweden – A health economic comparison of palliative treatment with best supportive care versus palliative treatment with gemcitabine in combination with best supportive care. Pharmaco Economics 1999; 15:377–84.
31. Trippoli S, Messori A. Cost-effectiveness of gemcitabine as first-line therapy for patients with advanced pancreatic cancer [abstract]. Value in Health 1999; 2:22.

7 Farnesyl Protein Transferase Inhibitors in Pancreatic Cancer

Helgi van de Velde, Vanina Popova, Irina Mountian and Peter de Porre

Farnesyl Protein Transferase as a Target for Anti-cancer Drug Design

The development of inhibitors of the farnesyl protein transferase enzyme and their potential role as targeted anti-cancer therapies has historically been driven by the recognition of the importance of farnesylation in the activity of normal and mutated Ras proteins. For the Ras proteins to transduce the extracellular signals provided by growth factors and cytokines, they must be anchored to the inner surface of the plasma membrane. This association is facilitated by a series of post-translational chemical modifications, the first one of which is a farnesylation reaction catalyzed by the farnesyl protein transferase enzyme.[45] It was hypothesized that inhibition of this reaction would prevent the association of Ras proteins with the cell membrane, therefore block the constitutive activity of mutated Ras or the growth factor driven activity of wild type Ras, and as such inhibit the growth of tumours, such as pancreatic cancer, in which Ras is thought to play a major role in oncogenesis and tumour growth.[6] Subsequent pre-clinical research has revealed that other intracellular proteins than Ras are involved in the antiproliferative effects of farnesyl protein transferase inhibition; these insights are corroborated by clinical research indicating that antitumour activity is mainly seen in tumour types which do not harbor K-ras mutations. This chapter intends to review the pre-clinical and clinical data of farnesyl protein transferase inhibition in pancreatic cancer, to highlight the current hypotheses regarding the antiproliferative effects of this novel class of agents and to summarize the evidence of antitumour activity in other cancer types.

Mammalian farnesyl protein transferase is a heterodimer zinc metalloenzyme which catalyzes the addition of a farnesyl group to the cysteine residue of the C-terminal CAAX-box of a variety of intracellular proteins[45,33,13] (Fig. 7.1). Farnesyl protein transferase recognizes the 'CAAX motif', consisting of a cysteine residue (C), two aliphatic amino acids (AA) and an amino acid X (usually serine, methionine or glutamine) at the C-terminus of various intracellular proteins. It covalently attaches a 15-carbon farnesyl pyrophosphate (FPP) to the sulfhydryl group of this cysteine residue. Farnesyl pyrophosphate is a 15-carbon isoprenoid moiety and a lipid intermediate of the cholesterol biosynthesis pathway. The farnesyl protein transferase enzyme is closely related to two other prenyltransferases,

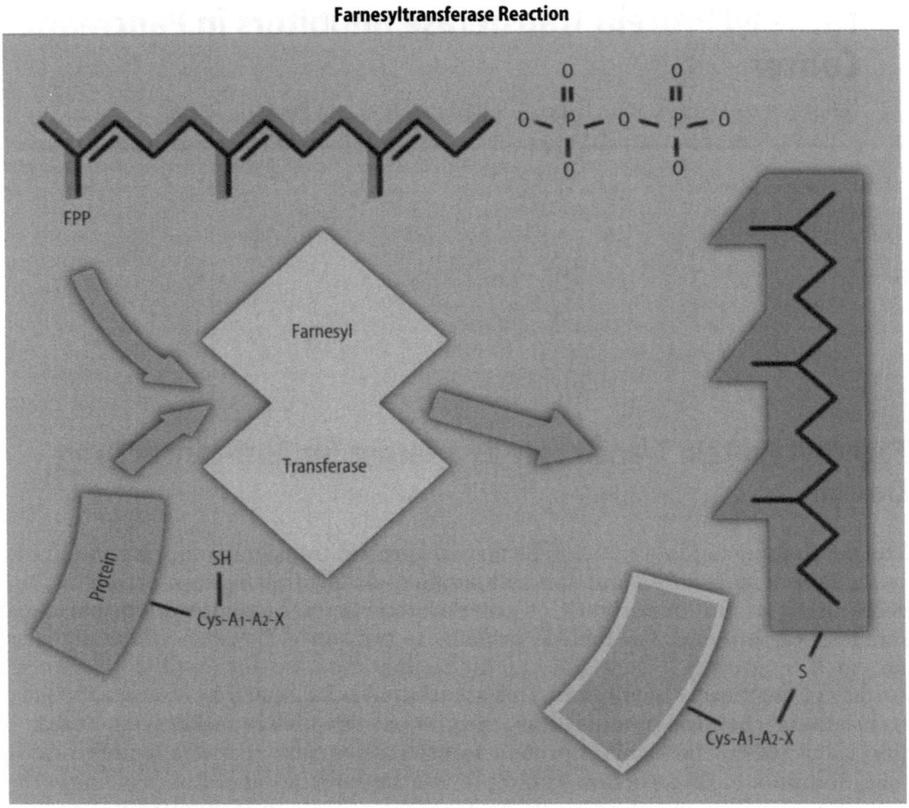

Figure 7.1. The farnesyltransferase reaction. The C-terminal CAAX box of the protein is recognized by the farnesyl protein transferase enzyme. A 15-carbon farnesyl group is then covalently attached by the enzyme to the sulfhydryl group of the cystein residue of the CAAX with release of pyrophosphate (FPP = farnesyl pyrophosphate). This reaction can be blocked in several ways by farnesyl protein transferase inhibitors.

geranylgeranyl protein transferase-I (GGPTase-I) and geranylgeranyl protein transferase-II (GGPTase-II), which catalyze the attachment of a 20-carbon geranylgeranyl isoprenoid moiety to the cysteine of similar c-terminal motifs.[45,33] While GGPTase-II recognizes a CCXX, XXCC or CXC sequence, GGPTase I has a specificity for proteins in which the CAAX motif contains leucine as residue X. This clarifies why some proteins can both be farnesylated and geranylgeranylated.

Cloning of the farnesyl protein transferase gene and the acquisition of detailed information on the enzymatic reaction have led to the identification and/or rational design of farnesyl protein transferase inhibitors. Several approaches have been used: (1) identification of CAAX competitive inhibitors that compete with the CAAX portion of the target substrates for the farnesyl protein transferase enzyme; this group is further subdivided into 'peptidomimetics/CAAX mimetics' (mimicking the CAAX structure) and 'nonpeptidomimetics' (which are structurally or functionally unrelated to the CAAX motif); (2) identification of farnesyldiphosphate (FDP) analogs that compete with the FDP substrate for farnesyl protein transferase; and (3) identification of bisubstrate analogs that combine the features of both FDP analogs and peptidomimetics. The majority of the farnesyl protein transferase inhibitors for which pre-clinical or clinical data in pancreatic cancer have been reported and summarized in this chapter, belong to the first category of nonpeptidomimetic competitive inhibitors; these include R115777 (ZARNESTRA™), SCH66336 and BMS-214662. Other compounds discussed in this review include L-744832 and L-774123, which are peptidomimetic competitive inhibitors, and manumycin, a natural FDP analog.

Mechanism of Action of Farnesyl Protein Transferase Inhibitors

Original Hypothesis: Inhibition of Ras Activity

Farnesyl protein transferase inhibitors were historically developed as a strategy to inhibit Ras-driven tumours, by inhibiting the processing of Ras proteins in tumour cells. Three *ras* genes are present in the human genome (Harvey- or H-*ras*, Kirsten- or K-*ras* and N-*ras*). While the wild-type *ras* gene products have an important function in normal signal transduction, mutations in *ras* genes are associated with tumour development and are found in approximately 20–30% of all human cancers. Pancreatic adenocarcinoma is the tumour type with the highest incidence of *ras* mutations : 85–90 % of pancreatic adenocarcinomas bear a mutation in the K-*ras* gene.[23] Therefore, within this initial hypothesis, pancreatic cancer constituted a rational tumour type in which to test the antitumour potential of farnesyl protein transferase inhibition.

The normal *ras* gene product is a monomeric membrane-localized G protein of 21 kd that functions as a molecular switch linking receptor and nonreceptor tyrosine kinase activation to downstream cytoplasmic or nuclear events. Ras proteins are members of an extended family of GTPases that cycle between an inactive guanosine 5′-diphosphate (GDP)-bound form and an active guanosine 5′-triphosphate (GTP)-bound state. It is in the GTP-bound form that Ras is active in the signal transduction pathway. Ras proteins only remain in this GTP-bound state for a short time, since the Ras protein itself is a GTPase which rapidly cleaves the terminal phosphate group from GTP, thereby returning the Ras protein to its inactive GDP-bound form. The known mutations in the *ras* genes obliterate this GTPase activity and therefore render the Ras proteins constitutively active.[45,1]

Ras proteins are synthesized as a biologically inactive cytosolic propeptide (Pro-Ras) and are attached to the inner surface of the cell membranes only after they have undergone a series of closely linked post-translational modifications at the C-terminal CAAX box (C = cysteine, a = any aliphatic residue and X = any other residue), thereby increasing their hydrophobic properties and facilitating their anchorage to plasma membrane.[18,20] The first and most critical step in this series is the farnesylation reaction during which farnesyl protein transferase adds the 15-carbon farnesyl group derived to the Ras protein C-terminus. Inhibition of this farnesylation reaction prevents the attachment of the Ras proteins to the cell membrane, therefore keeping the Ras proteins as inactive cytosolic proteins.

Consequently, farnesyl protein transferase has become a very attractive target for the development of anticancer agents.

While all three species of Ras are preferentially farnesylated, both K-Ras and N-Ras can also be prenylated by geranylgeranyl protein transferase I (GGPTase), which might serve as a 'shunt pathway'.[53,34] By contrast, H-Ras protein appears to be exclusively prenylated by farnesyl protein transferase.

Identification of Multiple Intracellular Targets of Farnesyl Protein Transferase Inhibition

While tumour growth suppression has indeed been observed in multiple *in vivo* and *in vitro* models of H-*ras*, K-*ras* and N-*ras* transformation as well as in several wild-type *ras* tumour types (see section C), pre clinical research has also produced a growing body of evidence that inhibition of the farnesylation of other intracellular proteins than Ras are also important in the antitumour effect of farnesyl protein transferase inhibitors. The main arguments for the existence of multiple intracellular targets of farnesyl protein transferase inhibition can be summarized in Table 7.1.[40,41]

Several other farnesylated proteins may play a role in the cytotoxic effects of farnesyl protein transferase inhibition. Leading candidates, some of which were already known to participate in cell growth regulation, have been suggested to contribute to this anti-tumour effect. Probably these hypotheses are not mutually exclusive but complementary, and more farnesylated proteins related to cellular growth and differentiation may be identified in the next few years. Interesting candidate proteins currently thought to contribute to these observed anti-tumour properties, include Rho-B, centromere binding proteins E and F (CENP-E/CENP-F), lamin B, protein tyrosine phosphatase (PTP) and TGFbetaRII (Fig. 7.2).

Rho-B, a 21 kD G-protein, has been implicated as the prenylated target of farnesyl protein transferase inhibitors by Prendergast and colleagues.[40] Rho-B is a member of the Rho superfamily of small GTPases involved in regulation of the actin cytoskeleton, vesicle trafficking and numerous other cell processes. Rho-B can either be farnesylated or geranylgeranylated. While farnesylated Rho-B promotes cellular transformation, geranylgeranylated Rho-B has the opposite effect. In the presence of farnesyl protein transferase inhibitors, Rho-B would become exclusively geranylgeranylated and therefore would become growth inhibitory. Although Rho proteins are not mutated in cancer cells, their expression

Table 7.1. Evidence for the existence of multiple intracellular sites of action

- Farnesyl protein transferase inhibitors can inhibit cell transformation by H-ras proteins that are engineered to allow membrane anchorage by N-myristoylation. Despite the intact H-ras protein activity allowed by this alternative membrane anchorage, inhibition of farnesyl protein transferase activity resulted in inhibition of cellular transformation.
- Alternative geranylgeranylation of K-ras and N-ras proteins has been observed in cells treated with farnesyl protein transferase inhibitors. Despite this alternative prenylation pathway, farnesyl protein transferase inhibitors demonstrate antitumour activity in cells with activated K-ras mutations.
- The kinetics of morphological reversion observed in H-ras cells upon treatment with a farnesyl protein transferase inhibitor are too rapid to be explained by depletion of processed H-Ras. Despite the half-life of fully modified H-Ras (24h), reversion of H-ras transformation is achieved within 18–24h of drug treatment, when modified Ras persist at > 50% of their pretreatment level.

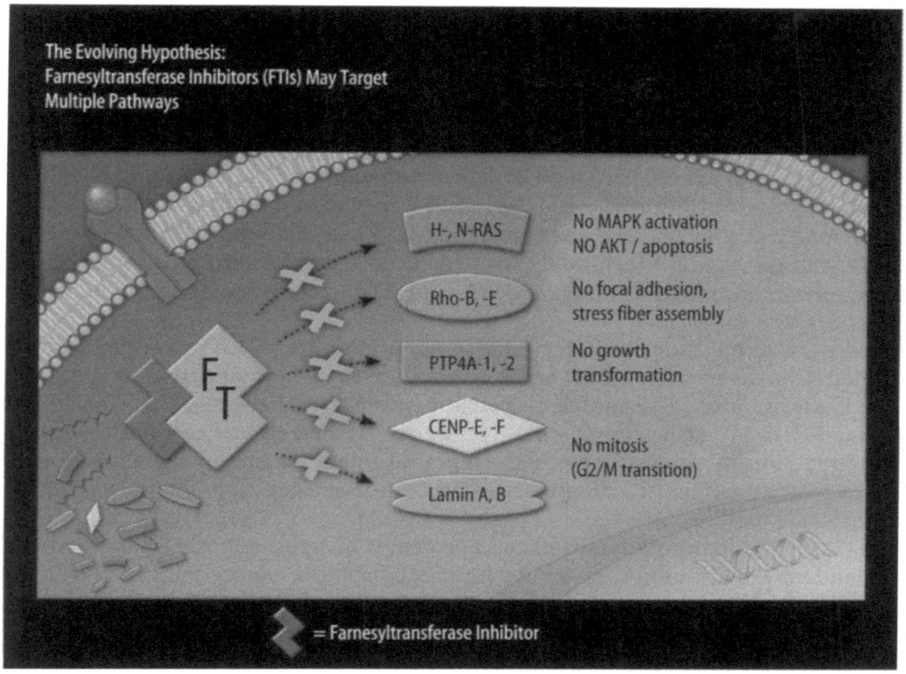

Figure 7.2. The evolving hypothesis: farnesyltransferase inhibitors (ftis) may target multiple pathways. Multiple farnesylated intracellular proteins may contribute to the antiproliferative effects of farnesyl protein transferase inhibition. Besides the Ras family of proteins, these targets include Rho-B and Rho-E, PTP4A-1 and PTP4A-2 (Protein Tyrosine Phosphatase-4A-1 and -4A-2), CENP-E and -F (Centromere- associated proteins-E and F) and lamins. Inhibition of farnesylation of these different targets leads to different downstream effects.

is often elevated, suggesting that Rho dysregulation promotes malignant phenotypes.

CENP-E and CENP-F are centromere associated kinesin motors that play critical roles in mitosis. Inhibition of farnesylation of CENPs would prevent their binding to microtubules and in this way contribute to the G2/M arrest often observed with farnesyl protein transferase inhibitors.[49,3] Why the division of transformed cells should be more susceptible to inhibition of these proteins than that in normal cells is not clear. Other targets, including Rheb[49] and farnesylated proteins associated with the PI3-K/AKT2-mediated cell survival pathway[27] are also being investigated. Altogether, there seems to be a mounting volume of laboratory evidence that multiple relevant proteins beyond Ras determine the cellular responsiveness to farnesyl protein transferase inhibitors.

Activity of Farnesyl Protein Transferase Inhibitors in Pancreatic Cancer in Pre-Clinical Studies

As a result of the initial hypothesis that farnesyl protein transferase inhibition would constitute targeted therapy in tumour types with a high incidence of *ras* mutations, many farnesyl protein transferase inhibitors were tested for antitumour activity in pancreatic cancer cell lines and xenografts.

Manumycin (UCF1-C), a farnesyl diphosphate analog isolated from a strain of Streptomyces and acting as a competitive inhibitor of farnesyl protein transferase, was shown to inhibit the growth of pancreatic cancer cell lines (SUIT-2, MIAPaCa-2, AsPC-1, and BxPC-3) in a dose dependent manner.[29] Interestingly, the IC50 inhibitory concentrations were lower in cell lines with a mutant K-*ras* gene (SUIT-2, MIAPaCa-2, and AsPC-1) than in the BxPC-3 cell line with wild type *ras*. In a nude mouse xenograft model of MIAPaCa-2, intraperitoneal injection of manumycin inhibited tumour growth and DNA synthesis in the inoculated tumours.[26]

Farnesylamine, a derivative of farnesol with inhibitory activity on the farnesyl protein transferase enzyme, revealed cytotoxic activity and induction of apoptosis in a K-ras mutated PK-1 pancreatic cell line (IC50 24 μM) as well as in K-ras transformed NIH/3T3 cells (IC50 5 μM).[50] Subsequent research however indicated that the induction of apoptosis by this compound might be due to the activation of c-jun N-terminal kinase rather than a direct effect of inhibition of farnesyl protein transferase inhibition.[35]

L-744832, a peptidomimetic farnesyl protein transferase inhibitor, showed dose-dependent growth inhibition in five human pancreatic cancer cell lines (AsPC-1, BxPC-3, CAPAN-2, Cfpac-1, Panc-1). The Panc-1 and CAPAN-2 cells were most sensitive to the growth inhibitory effects of L-744, 832 (IC_{50} values of 1.3 and 2.1 μM), AsPC-1 and BxPC-2 were moderately sensitive (IC_{50} 12–15 μM), while in the Cfpac-1 cells the IC_{50} was not reached, even at concentration up to 50 μM. This result indicates that the growth inhibition by L-744832 occurs regardless of *ras* mutation status.[48] In the most sensitive cell lines, a dose dependent increase in cells with a 4n DNA population was observed, consistent with cell cycle arrest either during G2 or during early mitosis (G2/M). In addition, in the sensitive cell lines apoptosis was induced in a p53-independent manner. Interestingly, no change in prenylation of the K-Ras protein could be observed in any of the cell lines, suggesting that farnesylated proteins other than K-Ras may act as the important regulators of the observed G2/M kinetics[48]

R115777, a non-peptidomimetic competitive farnesyl protein transferase inhibitor, was tested in vitro for inhibition of cell proliferation in five K-*ras* mutation-bearing pancreatic cell lines (SU86.86, CAPAN-2, Panc-1, AsPC-1, and CAPAN-1). CAPAN-2 and SU86 were very sensitive to this compound (IC50 9.5-16 nM) while in the other cell lines the IC50 was higher than 500 nM.[16] Oral administration of R115777 to nude mice bearing a subcutaneous pancreatic tumour xenograft (CAPAN-2) inhibited tumour growth at doses of 50 and 100 mg/kg bid (growth inhibition 59% and 76% respectively [Fig. 7.3]). In this CAPAN-2 xenograft, R115777 treatment produced predominantly an antiproliferative effect with inhibition of DNA synthesis, accompanied by an modest induction of apoptosis in the host endothelial cells of the tumour vasculature.[16]

SCH66336, another competitive inhibitor of farnesyl protein transferase, was tested for activity in the pancreatic cancer cell lines MIAPaCa-2, Panc-1 and AsPC-1. MIAPaCa-2 showed moderate sensitivity to SCH66336 (IC50-300nM) with accumulation in G2/M, whereas Panc-1 and AsPC-1 were among the most resistant cell lines tested (IC50 >1000nM).[3] All three cell lines harbor K-*ras* and p53 mutations indicating that this difference in sensitivity cannot be explained by a dif-

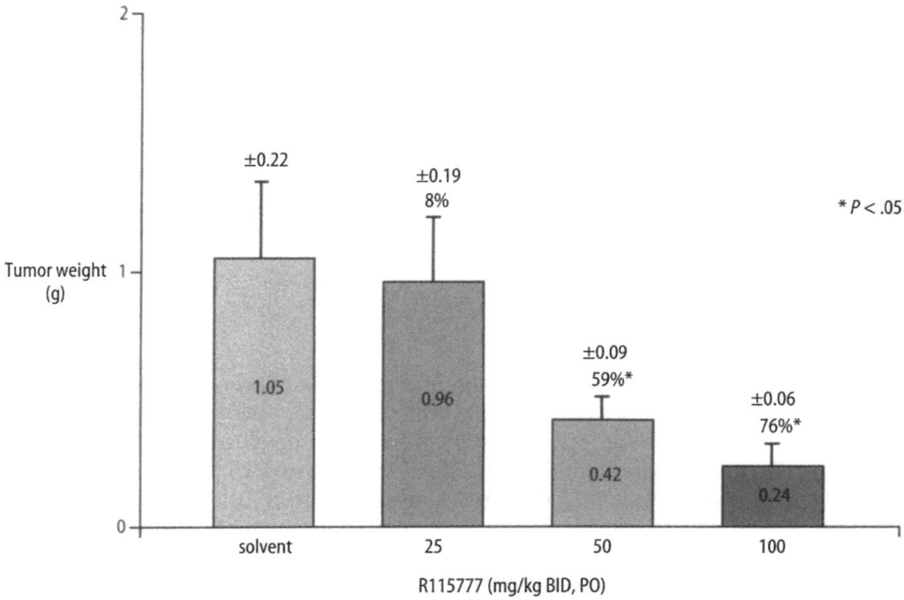

Figure 7.3. Dose-dependent growth inhibition by R115777 in CAPAN-2 pancreatic adenocarcinoma xenografts. Continuous oral administration of ZARNESTRA™ in mice bearing CAPAN-2 pancreatic adenocarcinomas leads to a statistically significant difference in tumor weight as compared to the vehicle control. This growth inhibition is dose-dependent with the highest amount of growth inhibition observed at the 100 mg/kg bid dosing (bid = twice daily).

ference in p53 mutational status or *ras* mutational status. Combination treatment of this farnesyl protein transferase inhibitor and SCH58500 (p53 wild-type adenovirus) was reported to have an additive effect in Panc-1 and a synergistic effect in MIAPaCa-2 *in vitro*.[37] In a different experiment with SCH66336 in a human tumour cloning assay, a positive tumour response was reported in one primary pancreatic cancer specimen at a 0.5 μM concentration.[39]

BMS-214662, another non-peptidomimetic farnesyl protein transferase inhibitor, was reported to inhibit cell growth of MIAPaCa-2 with an IC_{50} of 0.12 μM. In a mouse xenograft model of the same cell line, this compound, given orally for 10 days, was able to induce complete responses in four of seven animals at the highest dose evaluated (600 mg/kg/administration).[44]

For other farnesyl protein transferase inhibitors a limited amount of preclinical information in pancreatic cancer models is available. FTI-276(6) showed significant tumour growth inhibition in the MIAPaCa-2 xenograft model, while ER-51785 showed only modest growth inhibition in the same model.[22,36] BMI-46068 showed significant growth inhibition in MIAPaCa-2 and modest activity in HS-766 (wild-type *ras*) and CFPAC (mutated K-*ras*) pancreatic cancer cell lines.[42]

In summary, when multiple cell lines were tested with the same compound, a variabilility in sensitivity was seen which could not be explained by *ras* mutation status or p53 mutation status. Inhibition of DNA synthesis, arrest in G2/M phase and induction of apoptosis were observed.

Clinical Experience of Farnesyl Protein Transferase Inhibitors in Pancreatic Cancer

R115777 (ZARNESTRA™) was the first farnesyl protein transferase inhibitor to enter clinical trials.[55] Subsequently, L778123, SCH66336 and BMS 214662 have also started clinical evaluation. The following paragraphs summarize published data on the safety profile of these compounds as well as on the clinical experience gathered so far in pancreatic cancer and other tumour types.

Safety Profile

ZARNESTRA™ is an orally available agent which has been explored twice-daily dosing in several schedules (continuous administration, 3 wk on/1 week off, 9 days on/5 days off) in phase I trials.[14,24,55] Reversible myelosuppression (mainly neutropenia) and fatigue were the main dose-limiting toxicities. Other side-effects include mild gastro-intestinal toxicity (nausea, vomiting, diarrhoea), skin rash, and peripheral neurotoxicity upon prolonged continuous daily dosing at doses of 300 mg twice-daily and higher. At the recommended dose of 300 mg twice-daily in the 3-week-on/1-week-off schedule, the drug appeared well tolerated with reversible myelosuppression and mild gastro-intestinal toxicity as its main side-effects.[28] In a placebo-controlled randomized trial, there was no evidence of drug-induced fatigue/asthenia.[15] The combination of ZARNESTRA™ with gemcitabine in its approved dosing schedule (1000 mg/m^2 3 weeks out of 4) also appeared well tolerated at the recommended ZARNESTRA™ dose of 200 mg twice-daily; myelosuppression and fatigue were the dose-limiting toxicities of this combination.[38]

SCH66336 is also an orally available tricyclic farnesyl protein transferase inhibitor explored in twice-daily and once-daily dosing in several schedules (continuous administration, 1 week on/2 week off, 2 week on/2 week off) in phase I trials.[1,17,25] Most important dose-limiting toxicity was gastro-intestinal (mainly diarrhoea); other dose-limiting toxicities included fatigue, neurocortical toxicity and myelosuppression on continuous dosing. Recommended doses for phase II testing are 200 mg twice-daily or 300 mg once daily on the continuous dosing schedule and 200 mg twice daily on the 2 week on/2 week off schedule. At the recommended dose of 200 mg twice-daily further explored in phase II, side effects were also mainly gastro-intestinal (diarrhoea, nausea/vomiting), fatigue and myelosuppression.[12,32] The recommended dose of SCH63666 in combination with gemcitabine was established as 250 mg daily.

BMS-214662 is available as an oral and intravenous agent and has been explored in phase I in several schedules (1h iv q3wk, 24h iv q3wk, 1h iv every week). Main toxicities were gastro-intestinal (nausea, vomiting, diarrhoea), myelosuppression, fatigue and transaminase elevations.[47,52,54] Severe gastro-intestinal and liver toxicities prevent the achievement of adequate systemic exposure following the oral route.[7] Supraventricular tachycardia with QTc prolongation has been reported in one patient.[10]

L778123 is an intravenously available peptidomimetic inhibitor explored in phase I and early phase II studies. Neutropenia/thrombocytopenia and QTc prolongation were the dose-limiting toxicities. Side-effects at the recommended dose were somnolence, fatigue, myelosuppression and nausea/vomiting.[5,46]

Because of the cardiac conduction abnormalities, the clinical development of L778123 has been discontinued.[1,12]

In summary, reversible myelosuppression seems to be a side-effect shared by all farnesyl protein transferase inhibitors currently tested in the clinic.[1,12] For other non-hematologic toxicities, such as high-grade diarrhoea and nausea/vomiting, cardiac, neurocortical and peripheral neurotoxicity, there appear to be marked differences depending on agent and schedule of administration.

Clinical Experience in Advanced Pancreatic Cancer

The largest amount of clinical experience with a farnesyl protein transferase inhibitor in pancreatic cancer so far has been gathered in a randomized phase III study with ZARNESTRA™.[51] The purpose of this trial was to determine whether the addition of ZARNESTRA™ to standard gemcitabine therapy could improve the overall survival in patients with advanced pancreatic cancer. The study was a randomized, double-blind, placebo-controlled trial comparing gemcitabine and ZARNESTRA™ (GEM+Z) versus gemcitabine and placebo in patients with locally advanced or metastatic pancreatic adenocarcinoma previously untreated with systemic therapy. ZARNESTRA™ was given orally at a dose of 200 mg twice daily continuously, gemcitabine at 1000 mg/m2 iv weekly x7 for 8 weeks, then weekly x3 every 4 weeks. Primary endpoint was median overall survival; secondary endpoints included 6-month- and 1-year survival, progression-free survival, safety and quality of life. Six hundred eighty-eight patients were enrolled. Baseline characteristics were well balanced between the two treatment arms and were similar to other large studies. No statistically significant differences in survival parameters were observed. The median overall survival for GEM+Z was 193 days *versus* 182 days for control ($p = 0.75$); 6-month and 1-yr survival rates for GEM+Z were 53% and 27% *versus* 49% and 24% for control; median progression-free survival for GEM+Z was 112 days *versus* 109 days for control. In the subgroup of patients with locally advanced pancreatic cancer, a difference in median overall survival of 71 days in favor of the GEM+Z group was noted (335 days *versus* 264 days). Neutropenia and thrombocytopenia ≥ grade 3 were observed in 40% and 15% in GEM+Z *versus* 30% and 12% in control. With the exception of diarrhoea (38% GEM+Z vs 25% control) and hypokalemia (15% GEM+Z vs 8% control), incidences of non-hematologic adverse events were similar in the two groups. Combination therapy of gemcitabine + ZARNESTRA™ has an acceptable toxicity profile but does not prolong overall survival in advanced pancreatic cancer as compared to single-agent gemcitabine.[51]

Single agent activity of SCH66336 in advanced pancreatic cancer was explored in a randomized phase II trial comparing SCH66366 with gemcitabine in patients with metastatic adenocarcinoma of the pancreas.[32] Patients were randomized to receive treatment with SCH66336 at the daily dose of 200 mg PO bid or gemcitabine 1000 mg/m^2 weekly for 3 weeks followed by one week of rest. The primary endpoint was progression free survival (PFS) at 3 months. Sixty-three patients were randomized. The 3 month PFS rate for the SCH66336 group was 23% *versus* 31% for the gemcitabine group. The median overall survival for the SCH66336 group was 3.3 months *versus* 4.4 months for the gemcitabine group. Two patients with a partial response and six patients with stable disease were reported in the

SCH6366 group versus one partial response and 11 stable diseases in the gemcitabine group.[32]

Although some hints of clinical activity in pancreatic cancer were generated, these studies have not been able to show that farnesyl protein transferase inhibition can improve clinical outcome in advanced pancreatic cancer. One could argue that the same statement can be made about many valuable chemotherapy agents currently in clinical use and that statistically significant improvement in overall survival in advanced pancreatic cancer is a very challenging test given the aggressive nature and notorious chemo-resistance of this disease. In fact, 5-fluorouracil, an agent frequently used in pancreatic cancer, was also not able to statistically improve overall survival in combination with gemcitabine versus gemcitabine alone.[4] Along those lines, one can argue that studies of farnesyl protein transferase inhibitors in less advanced stages of pancreatic cancer, including radiosensitization studies, are warranted before reaching a definite conclusion of the role of farnesyl protein transferase inhibitors in the therapeutic approach in pancreatic cancer.

It is possible that the antitumour activity of farnesyl protein transferase inhibition is independent of *ras* mutation status and that therefore pancreatic cancer with its high incidence of *ras* mutations should not be regarded as a more attractive disease target for farnesyl protein transferase inhibitors than any other tumour type. Indeed, as will be discussed in the next section, promising clinical antitumour activity has been observed in several haematological (refractory AML, CML, myelodysplastic syndromes) and solid tumour types (breast cancer, glioblastoma, squamous cell carcinoma) in which the role of *ras* mutations is limited, if it exists at all.

Clinical Activity in Other Tumour Types

In haematological malignancies, promising clinical data have been gathered in myeloid malignancies (acute myeloid leukemia, chronic myeloid leukemia, and myelodysplastic syndromes). Most of the published evidence of clinical activity in myeloid malignancies to date comes from studies with ZARNESTRA™.[11,12]

In a Phase I trial of ZARNESTRA™ a 32% response rate (including two patients with a complete response) was noted in refractory or relapsed AML.[30] This activity has been confirmed by data of a phase II trial in relapsed AML which reported that seven out of 42 patients achieved a reduction in bone marrow blasts to <5% on ZARNESTRA™ monotherapy.[21] In a Phase II trial in CML, 5 haematological complete responses and two partial responses were noted in 22 patients treated with ZARNESTRA™.[11] In myelodysplastic syndromes, ZARNESTRA™ has been reported to produce hematologic remissions in 6/18 (33%) evaluable patients in phase I and complete remissions in 2/16 (13%) evaluable high-risk patients in phase II.[31] Responses have also been observed in myeloproliferative diseases (MPD) as well as in myelofibrosis (MF) and multiple myeloma (MM).[19,11,2] With SCH66336, responses have been reported in CML and myelodysplastic syndromes.[9,43] Modest clinical activity in relapsed/refractory acute leukemias has also been seen with BMS-214662.[12]

In solid tumours, promising antitumour activity in phase II has been seen with ZARNESTRA™ in advanced breast cancer, with a 11% single agent response rate and a 13% rate of disease stabilization >6 months, irrespective of *ras* mutational status or of HER2 positivity.[28] Partial responses and disease stabilization beyond

6 months have also been observed with single agent ZARNESTRA™ in glioblastoma multiforme.[8]

Conclusion

The development of inhibitors of the farnesyl protein transferase enzyme as targeted anti-cancer therapy has historically been driven by the recognition of the importance of farnesylation in the activity of normal and mutated ras proteins. Over the last years, an increasing body of pre-clinical evidence has been gathered that farnesylated proteins other than ras, such as Rho-B, CENPs, lamins, PTP, Rheb and others, also constitute potential targets for farnesyl protein transferase inhibition and are linked to the antiproliferative effects of farnesyl protein transferase inhibitors.

Consistent with the original *ras* hypothesis, several farnesyl protein transferase inhibitors have been tested for activity in pancreatic cancer both in pre-clinical models and in clinical trials. While in pre-clinical tumour models various farnesyl protein transferase inhibitors were able to inhibit pancreatic cancer growth, generally in a dose-dependent manner, the clinical activity of R115777 (ZARNESTRA™) and SCH66336, the only two compounds tested so far in advanced pancreatic cancer, appeared limited. No clinical data exist to date on activity of farnesyl protein transferase inhibitors in early stage pancreatic cancer.

In line with the pre-clinical data identifying intracellular protein targets other than ras, interesting clinical activity has been observed in tumour types not driven by *ras*, such as AML, CML, myelodysplastic syndromes, glioblastoma multiforme and breast cancer. Further development of these agents in these tumour types is ongoing. The safety profile of these agents, with reversible myelosuppression, fatigue and a variable degree of gastro-intestinal complaints as their main side-effects, appeared to be very acceptable. Therefore, farnesyl protein transferase inhibitors continue to be viewed as a promising novel class of anticancer agents with potential therapeutic benefit in a variety of hematological and solid tumours (Fig. 7.4).

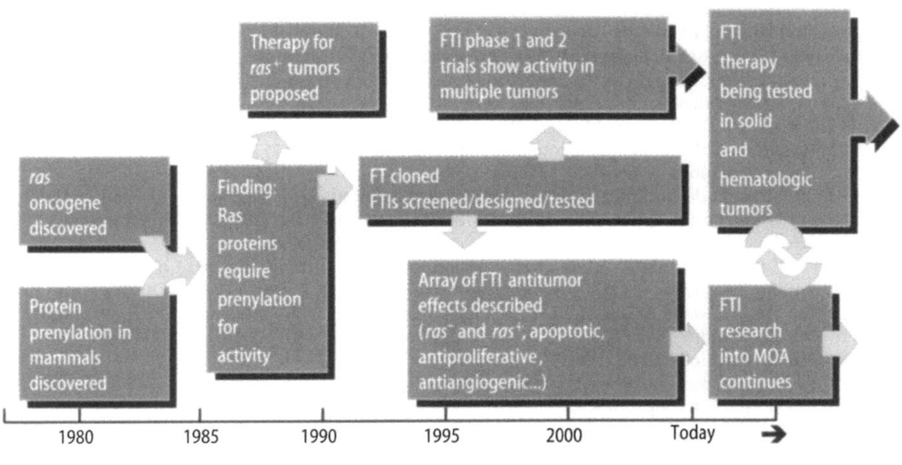

Figure 7.4. The evolving hypothesis – the FTIs may have broad clinical potential.

Acknowledgements

The authors would like to thank Ilse Versmissen and An Van Eyken for excellent editorial assistance.

References

1. Adjei AA, Erlichmann C, Davis JN, et al. A phase I trial of the farnesyl transferase inhibitor SCH66336: Evidence for biological and clinical activity. Cancer Research 2000; 60:1871–1877.
2. Alsina M, Overton R, Belle N, et al. Farnesyl transferase inhibitor FTI-R115777 is well tolerated, induces stabilization of disease and inhibits farnesylation and oncogenic/tumour survival pathways in patients with advanced multiple myeloma. Proceedings of the American Association for Cancer Research 2002 (abstr); 43:1000.
3. Ashar HR, James L, Gray K, et al. The farnesyl transferase inhibitor SCH 66336 induces a G(2) – >M or G(1) pause in sensitive human tumor cell lines. Experimental Cell Research 2001; 262:17–27.
4. Berlin JD, Catalano P, Thomas JP, et al. Phase III study of gemcitabine in combination with fluorouracil versus gemcitabine alone in patients with advanced pancreatic cancer carcinoma: Eastern Cooperative Oncology Group Trial E2297. Journal of Clinical Oncology 2002; 20:3270–3275.
5. Britten C, Rowinsky E, Yao S-L, et al. The farnesyl protein transferase (FTPase) inhibitor L-778, 123 in patients with solid cancers. Proceedings of American Society of Clinical Oncology 1999 (abstr); 18:155a.
6. Butera J, Malachovsky M, Rathore R, et al. Novel approaches in development for the treatment of pancreatic cancer. Frontiers in Bioscience 1998; 3:E226–E229.
7. Caponigro F. Farnesyl transferase inhibitors: a major breakthrough in anticancer therapy? Anti-Cancer Drugs 2002; 13:891–897.
8. Cloughesy TF, Kuhn J, Wen P, et al. Phase II trial of R 115777 (Zarnestra) in patients with recurrent glioma not taking enzyme inducing antiepileptic drugs (EIAED): a North American Brain Tumor Consortium (NABTC) report. Proceedings of American Society of Clinical Oncology 2002 (abstr); 21:80a.
9. Cortes J, Daley G, Talpaz M, et al. Pilot study of SCH66336 (Lonafarnib), a farnesyl transferase inhibitor (FTI), in patients with chronic myeloid leukemia (CML) in chronic or accelerated phase resistant or refractory to Imatinib. Proceedings of American Society Hematology 2002 (abstr); 43:614.
10. Cortes J, Kurzrock R, O'Brien SM, et al. Phase I study of a farnesyl transferase inhibitor (FTI), BMS-214662, in patients with refractory or relapsed acute leukemias. Blood 2001 (abstr); 98:594A.
11. Cortes JE, Albitar M, Thomas D, et al. Efficacy of the farnesyl transferase inhibitor in chronic myeloid leukemia and other hematological malignancies. Blood 101 (5):1692–7.
12. Cortes JE, Kurzrock R, Kantarjian HM. Farnesyltransferase inhibitors: novel compounds in development for the treatment of myeloid malignancies. Semin Hematol 2002; 39:26–30.
13. Cox AD. Farnesyltransferase inhibitors. Drugs 2001; 61:723–732.
14. Crul M, de klerk GJ, Swart M, et al. Phase I Clinical and Pharmacologic Study of chronic oral administration of the farnesyl protein transferase inhibitor R115777 in advanced cancer. Journal of Clinical Oncology 2002; 20:2726–2735.
15. Cunningham D, de Gramont A, Scheithauer W, et al. Randomized double-blind placebo-controlled trial of the farnesyltransferase inhibitor R115777 (Zarnestra™) in advanced refractory colorectal cancer. American Society of Clinical Oncology 2002 (abstr); 21:126a.
16. End DW, Smets G, Todd AV, et al. Characterization of the antitumor effects of the selective farnesyl protein transferase inhibitor R115777 in vivo and in vitro. Cancer Research 2001; 61:131–137.
17. Eskens FALM, Awada A, Cutler DL, et al. Phase I and pharmacokinetic study of the oral farnesyltransferase inhibitor SCH 66336 given twice daily to patients with advanced solid tumors. Journal of Clinical Oncology 2001; 19:1167–1175.
18. Gibbs JB. Lipid modifications of proteins in the Ras superfamily, In: L Birnbaumer and B Dickey (ed): GTPases in biology. New York, Springer-Verlag, 1993; pp. 335–344.
19. Gotlib J, Dugan U, Katamneni K, et al. Phase I/II study of farnesyltransferase inhibitor R115777 (Zarnestra) in patients with myeloproliferative disorders (MPDs): preliminary results. Proceedings of American Society of Clinical Oncology 2002 (abstr); 21:4a.

20. Hancock JF, Paterson H, Marshall CJ. A polybasic domain or palmitoylation is required for the addition of the CAAX motif to localize p21 to the plasma membrane. Cell 1990; 63:139.
21. Harousseau JL, Stone R, Thomas X, et al. Interim results from a phase II study of R115777 (Zarnestra) in patients with relapsed and refractory acute myelogenous leukemia. Proceedings of American Society of Clinical Oncology 2002 (abstr); 21:265a.
22. Henry KJJ, Wasicak J, Tasker AS, et al. Discovery of a series of cyclohexylethylamine-containing protein farnesyltransferase inhibitors exhibiting potent cellular activity. Journal of Medical Chemistry 1999; 42:4844–4852.
23. Hruban RH, Wilentz RE, Goggins M, et al. Pathology of incipient pancreatic cancer. Annals of Oncology 1999; 10:9–11.
24. Hudes GR, Schol J. Phase I trial of oral R115777 in patients with refractory solid tumors, In: SM Sebti and AD Hamilton (ed): Farnesyltransferase inhibitors in cancer therapy. Humana Press, 2000; pp. 251–254.
25. Hurwitz HI, Amado R, Prager D, et al. Phase 1 pharmacokinetic trial of the farnesyl transferase inhibitor SCH66336 plus gemcitabine in advanced cancers. Proceedings of American Society of Clinical Oncology 2000 (abstr); 19:185a.
26. Ito T, Kawata S, Tamura S, et al. Suppression of human pancreatic cancer growth in BALB/c nude mice by manumycin, a farnesyl:protein transferase inhibitor. Japanese Journal of Cancer Research 1996; 87:113–116.
27. Jiang K, Coppola D, Crespo NC, et al. The phosphoinositide 3-OH kinase/AKT2 pathway as a critical target for farnesyltransferase inhibitor-induced apoptosis. Mol Cell Biol 2000; 20:139–148.
28. Johnston SRD, Hickish S, Houston S, et al. Efficacy and tolerability of two dosing regimens of R115777 (Zarnestra), a farnesyl protein transferase inhibitor, in patients with advanced breast cancer. Proceedings of American Society of Clinical Oncology 2002 (abstr); 21:35a.
29. Kainuma O, Asano T, Hasegawa M, et al. Inhibition of growth and invasive activity of human pancreatic cancer cells by a farnesyltransferase inhibitor, manumycin. Pancreas 1997; 15:379–383.
30. Karp JE, Lancet JE, Kaufmann SH, et al. Clinical and biologic activity of the farnesyltransferase inhibitor R115777 in adults with refractory and relapsed acute leukemias: a phase 1 clinical-laboratory correlative trial. Blood 2001; 97:3361–3369.
31. Kurzrock R, Cortes J, Kantarjian HM. Clinical development of farnesyltransferase inhibitors in leukemias and myelodysplastic syndrome. Semin Hematol 2002; 39:20–24.
32. Lersch C, Van Cutsem E, Amado R, et al. Randomized Phase II Study of SCH 66336 and Gemcitabine in the Treatment of Metastatic Adenocarcinoma of the Pancreas. Proceedings of American Society of Clinical Oncology 2001 (abstr); 20:153a.
33. Lobell RB, Kohl NE. Pre-clinical development of farnesyltransferase inhibitors. Cancer and Metastasis Reviews 1998; 17:203–210.
34. Lobell RB, Omer CA, Abrams MT, et al. Evaluation of Farnesyl: Protein Transferase and Geranylgeranyl: Protein transferase inhibitor combination in pre-clinical models. Cancer Research 2001; 61:8758–8768.
35. Mizukami Y, Ura H, Obara T, et al. Requirement of c-Jun N-Terminal kinase for apoptotic cell death induced by farnesyltransferase inhibitor, farnesylamine, in human pancreatic cancer cells. Biochemical and Biophysical Research Communications 2001; 288:198–204.
36. Nakamura K, Yamaguchi A, Namiki M, et al. Antitumor activity of ER-51785, a new peptidomimetic inhibitor of farnesyl transferase: synergistic effect in combination with paclitaxel. Oncology Research 2000; 12:477–484.
37. Nielsen LL, Shi B, Hajian G, et al. Combination therapy with the farnesyl protein transferase inhibitor SCH66336 and SCH58500 (P53 Adenovirus) in pre-clinical cancer models. Cancer Research 1999; 59:5896–5901.
38. Patnaik A, Eckhardt E, Itzbicka E, et al. A phase I and Pharmacokinetic (Pk) Study of the Farnesyltransferase Inhibitor, R115777 in Combination with Gemcitabine (Gem). Proceedings of American Society of Clinical Oncology 2000 (abstr); 19:2a.
39. Petit T, Izbicka E, Lawrence RA, et al. Activity of SCH 66336, a tricyclic farnesyltransferase inhibitor, against human tumor colony-forming units. Annals of Oncology 1999; 10:449–453.
40. Prendergast GC. Farnesyltranferase inhibitors define a role for RhoB in controlling neoplastic pathophysiology. Histology & Histopathology 2001; 16:269–275.
41. Prendergast GC, Rane N. Farnesyltransferase inhibitors: mechanism and applications. Expert Opinion Investig Drugs 2001; 10:2105–2116.
42. Prevost GP, Pradines A, Viossat I, et al. Inhibition of human tumor cell growth in vitro and in vivo by a specific inhibitor of human farnesyltransferase: BIM-46068. Int J Cancer 1999; 83:283–287.

43. Ravoet C, Mineur P, Robin V, et al. Phase I-II study of a farnesyl transferase inhibitor (FTI), SCH66336, in patients with Myelodysplastic syndrome (MDS) or secondary acute myeloid leukemia (sAML). Proceedings of American Society Hematology 2002 (abstr); 43:3136.
44. Rose WC, Lee FY, Fairchild CR, et al. Preclinical antitumor activity of BMS-214662, a highly apoptotic and novel farnesyltransferase inhibitor. Cancer Research 2001; 61:7507–7517.
45. Rowinsky EK, Windle JJ, Von Hoff DD. Ras protein farnesyltransferase: A strategic target for anticancer therapeutic development. Journal of Clinical Oncology 1999; 17:3631–3652.
46. Rubin E, Abbruzzese JL, Morrison BW, et al. Phase I trial of the farnesyl protein transferase (FPTase) inhibitor L-778123 on a 14 or 28-day dosing schedule. Proceedings of American Society of Clinical Oncology 2000 (abstr); 19:178a.
47. Ryan DP, Eder JP, Supko JG, et al. Phase I clinical trial of the farnesyltransferase (FT) inhibitor BMS-214662 in patients with advanced solid tumors. Proceedings of American Society of Clinical Oncology 2000 (abstr); 19:185a.
48. Song SY, Meszoely IM, Coffey RJ, et al. K-Ras-independent effects of the farnesyl transferase inhibitor L-744,832 on cyclin B1/Cdc2 kinase activity, G2/M cell cycle progression and apoptosis in human pancreatic ductal adenocarcinoma cells. Neoplasia 2000; 2:261–272.
49. Tamanoi F, Kato-Stankiewicz J, Jiang C, et al. Farnesylated proteins and cell cycle progression. Journal of Cellular Biochemistry 2001; 37:64–70.
50. Ura H, Obara T, Shudo R, et al. Selective cytotoxicity of farnesylamine to pancreatic carcinoma cells and Ki-ras-transformed fibroblasts. Molecular Carcinogenesis 1998; 21:93–99.
51. Van Cutsem E, Karasek P, Oettle H, et al. Phase III trial comparing gemcitabine + R115777 (Zarnestra) versus gemcitabine + placebo in advanced pancreatic cancer (PC). Proceedings of American Society of Clinical Oncology 2002 (abstr); 21:130a.
52. Voi M, Tabernero J, Cooper MR, et al. A phase I study of the farnesyltransferase (FT) inhibitor BMS-214662 administered as a weekly 1-hour infusion in patients (Pts) with advanced solid tumors: Clinical findings. Proceedings of American Society of Clinical Oncology 2001 (abstr); 20:79a.
53. Whyte DB, Kirschmeier P, Hockenberry TN, et al. K- and N-Ras are geranylgeranylated in cells treated with farnesyl protein transferase inhibitors. J Biol Chem 1997; 30:14459–14464.
54. Zhu AX, Supko JG, Ryan DP, et al. A phase I clinical, pharmacokinetic and pharmacodynamic study of the farnesyltransferase inhibitor BMS-214662 given as a 24 hour continuous intravenous (IV) infusion once weekly x 3 in patients with advanced solid tumors. Proceedings of American Society of Clinical Oncology 2002 (abstr); 21:92a.
55. Zujewski J, Horak ID, Bol CJ, et al. Phase I and pharmacokinetic study of farnesyl protein transferase inhibitor R115777 in advanced cancer. Journal of Clinical Oncology 2000; 18:927–941.

8 Novel Alternatives to Chemotherapy in Advanced Disease: Gastrin Antibodies

Martyn E. Caplin

Pancreatic cancer has an incidence of approximately 10 per 100 000 population per year in Europe and North America and is the fifth most common cause of cancer death.[1] Pancreatic cancer often present with advanced disease and has a poor prognosis.[2] The median survival depends on the stage of the disease at presentation, but may be of the order of 4–6 months for metastatic disease. Current treatments for inoperable pancreatic cancer make little impact on the median survival.[3,4] Gemcitabine is currently recognized as the most effective chemotherapy agent for this condition. The median survival of patients on the first two clinical trials using gemcitabine was between 3.85 months and 5.65 months from the date of the first treatment. However, it has been shown to offer some improvement in symptoms compared with fluorouracil when a symptom score called the 'clinical benefit response' was used.[3,4,5,6]

Strategies for New Pancreatic Cancer Agents

New agents for pancreatic cancer are needed. Several novel strategies are under active investigation. These include attempts to modulate growth factor activity, anti-angiogenic factors, vascular inhibitors, antistromal agents, gene therapy and immunotherapy.[7–13] Anti-hormonal therapy was first suggested over twenty years ago related to anti-androgens and anti-oestrogens and there has been some suggestion of therapeutic efficacy with receptor blockade using tamoxifen and flutamide respectively.[14–16] Recently there has been increasing interest in gastrin as a growth factor and the possible therapeutic effect of anti-gastrin agents.[17]

Gastrin

Gastrin has been shown to promote the growth of both normal gastrointestinal mucosa as well as a variety of malignancies including colorectal, gastric, pancreatic, hepatocellular, renal, lung and brain.[18–24] These same tissues have been shown to demonstrate the CCK-B/gastrin receptor. Most recently it has been shown that gastrin and its CCK-B receptor are activated early in the adenoma-carcinoma sequence for colonic carcinoma.[25,26] This has important implications in terms of not only understanding the process of malignant transformation but also raising the possibility of novel therapeutic approaches including targeting gastrin and its receptor at an early stage.

In vitro and *in vivo* studies have shown that neoplastic cells not only have the ability to respond to circulating forms of gastrin but also respond to the autocrine production of gastrin and its precursors. The post-translational processing of gastrin involves an enzymatic cascade which determines the form of gastrin ultimately produced (Fig. 8.1). In simplistic terms activation of the gastrin gene on chromosome 17q produces mRNA encoding pre-progastrin. Within the endoplasmic reticulum the pre-progastrin is cleaved by endopeptidases to progastrin which passes to the Golgi apparatus and can subsequently be processed to glycine-extended gastrin 34. The glycine-extended gastrin 34 can be amidated by peptidylglycine alpha-amidating monooxygenase to form amidated gastrin 34, or cleaved

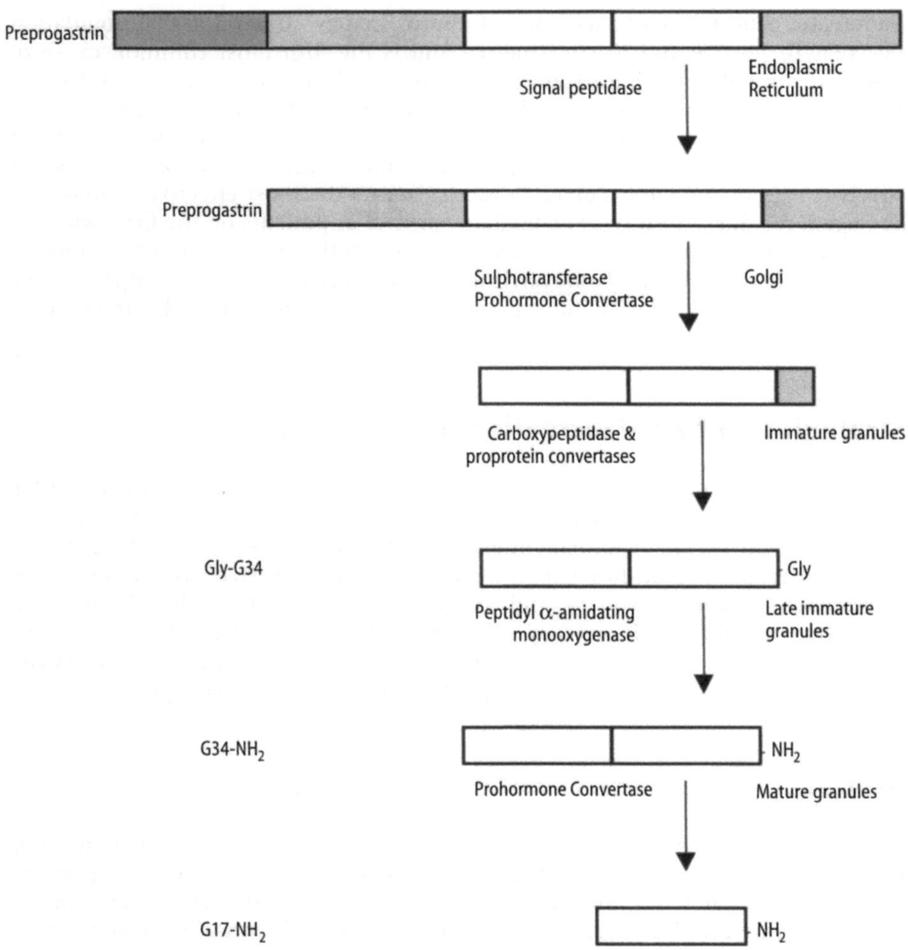

Figure 8.1. Post-translational processing of gastrin

at dibasic residues resulting in the formation of amidated gastrin 17 (G17) and glycine-extended gastrin 17 (gly-G17).[27–30]

There is now good evidence that in addition to the 'mature' amidated gastrin stimulating neoplastic cell growth, the precursor forms including progastrin and glycine-extended gastrin have potent trophic effects. This was first demonstrated by Seva et al comparing the ability of both amidated G17 and glycine-G17 to stimulate DNA activity in the rat pancreatic adenocarcinoma cell line AR42J.[31]

There is now a wealth of evidence for the role of gastrin and its precursors in cancer growth and this is well summarised in recent review articles.[32,33] Many tumours demonstrate oncofetal expression of peptides and this appears to apply to gastrin and the pancreas. Gastrin is transiently expressed in the fetal pancreas and is associated with pancreatic growth and differentiation, however it does not appear to be expressed in the normal adult pancreas.[34,35]

Transgenic mouse models provide supporting evidence for the trophic effects of gastrin at the gene level. This involves the fusion of a Simian virus 40 large tumour antigen (SV40 Tag) gene to a 1.5kb 5′ flanking region of the gastrin gene or the SV40 Tag gene fused to a 10.5kb mid-region of the gastrin gene; both result in the mice developing pancreatic tumours.[36]

In vitro and *in vivo* experiments have shown that gastrin and precursor forms stimulate the growth of pancreatic cancer cell lines and mouse xenograft pancreatic cancer. In addition anti-gastrin agents including anti-gastrin antibodies inhibit both the *in vitro* and *in vivo* proliferative effects of gastrin.[37,38] CCK-B/gastrin receptor antagonists however are only able to inhibit the proliferative effects of amidated gastrin and has no effect on precursor forms confirming that these precursor forms bind to a separate receptor. Recently a unique CCK-C 'cancer' receptor was described functioning as a growth receptor in pancreatic cancer but not being present in normal human pancreas.[39]

It has been previously established that gastrin stimulates the growth of pancreatic cancer by an autocrine mechanism. There is constitutive release of amidated gastrin and its precursor forms, which feed back not only to its own cell but also to neighbouring cells thus having paracrine effect.[31,37]

We have previously shown by immunocytochemistry that the normal pancreas showed no expression of receptor or gastrin isoforms except for occasional cells in the islets. Pancreatic cancer specimens showed definite expression of CCK-B/gastrin receptor in 96%, progastrin 92%, glycine-extended gastrin in 54% and amidated gastrin in 23% of cancer sections.[40] Goetze et al have also recently assessed CCK-B/gastrin receptor and gastrin peptide expression in pancreatic cancer resection specimens, resection margin specimens and normal human pancreatic tissue.[41] They found CCK-BR mRNA present in all carcinomas, resection margins and normal pancreatic tissue. Using radioimmunoassay progastrin was present in all tumours and resection margins and very low amounts in normal pancreatic tissue. Glycine extended gastrin was present in 63% of pancreatic cancers, 74% of resection margins at low concentration and very low levels were detected in normal pancreas. Amidated gastrin was detected in 71% of pancreatic cancers, 75% of resection margins at low concentration and again at very low concentration in some normal pancreatic tissue.

Thus the *in* vitro and in vivo studies showing the proliferative effects of gastrin, as well as demonstration of constitutive formation of gastrin and its precursor forms by pancreatic cancer specimens suggests a role for anti-gastrin agents in the treatment of pancreatic cancer. The anti-gastrin agent G17DT is an immunogen that forms antibodies to human amidated G17 and gly-G17 42. Whereas CCK-B receptor antagonists can only block the effect of amidated gastrin, G17DT induced antibodies can bind both amidated gastrin and glycine extended gastrin. This immunogen has been used in both *in vitro* and *in vivo* studies and shown to inhibit the growth of a number of G.I. cancers.[43–48]

We have performed a phase II study of G17DT in patients with advanced pancreatic cancer. The aims of this study were to determine antibody response of patients with proven pancreatic cancer to G17DT; evaluate safety and tolerability; and look for preliminary evidence of efficacy.[49]

The study was an open, multiple dose, single centre study of G17DT in patients with proven pancreatic cancer. Patients were initially recruited to receive 100micro-grammes of G17DT on weeks 0,2 and 6 weeks. In view of a poor antibody response to 100μg of G17DT a request was subsequently submitted to the ethics committee, after the fourteenth patient was recruited, to increase the dose to 250 μg.

Only 6 of 13 patients (46%) developed anti-gastrin antibodies to the 100μg dose of G17DT and therefore the dose was increased in subsequent patients to 250μg with 14 of 17 patients (82.4%) forming antibodies. Interesting features from the study include: of the antibody producers 5/20 (25%) had an increase in dry weight at week 16; 5/20 (25%) had stable disease as measured by CT imaging at week 16; and 9/20 (45%) had a Karnofsky performance score of ≥80 at week 16. The median survival from first injection of the whole group was 187 days, 217 days for antibody producers and 121 for antibody negative patients (log rank 0.0035). Three patients developed a sterile abscess following G17D immunisation. Most patients just had mild discomfort at the injection site.

A similar study from Nottingham by Gilliam et al compared the effect of G17DT 250 μg at 0, 1 and 3 weeks versus a matched control group of palliative therapy with best supportive care.[50] The antibody response was 89%. The side-effect profile was negligible except for some minor local injection site reactions. The group quote a significant increase in 50% median survival (297 days *vs* 108 days). There was again a description of weight gain in a proportion of patients.

These phase 2 studies are therefore very encouraging in terms of antibody response and tolerability with apparent benefits to patient's biological function and perhaps survival. Phase3 studies are now completing comparing G17DT in combination with Gemcitabine *versus* Gemcitabine alone. Other groups are assessing the effects of CCK-B receptor antagonist given as a continuous intravenous infusion however the results and peer review articles are awaited. Another approach is the development of anti-gastrin antisense oligonucleotides with preliminary studies ongoing.[51]

In conclusion gastrin is a trophic factor for a number of cancers including pancreatic cancer. The understanding of the gastrin post-translational pathway and autocrine/paracrine effects has led to the development of the anti-gastrin agent G17DT. Agents targeting gastrin and its receptor may well be of therapeutic significance and pragmatically will most likely be used in conjunction with chemotherapy.

Acknowledgement

Dr Caplin's research team receives a research grant, BXB8 from Aphton Corporation, Woodland, Ca, USA.

References

1. Fernandez E, La Vecchia C, Porta M, et al. Trends in pancreatic cancer mortality in Europe, 1955–1989. Int J Cancer 1994; 15: 57 (6):786–92.
2. Bramhall SR, Allum WH, Jones AG, et al. Treatment and survival in 13,560 patients with pancreatic cancer, and incidence of the disease, in the West Midlands: an epidemiological study. Br J Surg 1995; 82 (1):111–5.
3. Burris HA 3rd, Moore MJ, Andersen J, et al. Improvements in survival and clinical benefit with gemcitabine as first-line therapy for patients with advanced pancreas cancer: a randomized trial. J Clin Oncol 1997; 15 (6):2403–13.
4. Rothenberg ML, Moore MJ, Cripps MC, et al. A phase II trial of gemcitabine in patients with 5-FU-refractory pancreas cancer. Ann Oncol 1996; 7 (4):347–53.
5. Burris H, Storniolo AM. Assessing clinical benefit in the treatment of pancreas cancer: gemcitabine compared to 5-fluorouracil. Eur J Cancer 1997; 33:S18–22 (Suppl 1).
6. Burris HA 3rd. Objective outcome measures of quality of life. Oncology 1996 (Suppl 11); 10:131–5.
7. McKenzie IF, Aposolopoulos V. Towards immunotherapy of pancreatic cancer. Gut 1999; 44 (6):767–9.
8. Bramhall SR. Novel non-operative treatment and treatment strategies in pancreatic cancer. Expert Opin Investig Drugs 2000; 9 (6):1179–95.
9. Kroep JR, Pinedo HM, van Groeningen CJ, et al. Experimental drugs and drug combinations in pancreatic cancer. Ann Oncol 1999; 10:234–8 (Suppl 4).
10. Rosemurgy A, Harris J, Langleben A, et al. Marimastat in patients with advanced pancreatic cancer: a dose-finding study. Am J Clin Oncol 1999; 22 (3):247–52.
11. Rosemurgy A, Harris J, Langleben A, et al. Marimastat, a novel matrix metalloproteinase inhibitor in patients with advanced carcinoma of the pancreas. Proc Am Soc Clin Oncol 1996; 15:207 (abstr 470).
12. Yang L, Hwang R, Pandit L, et al. Gene therapy of metastatic pancreas cancer with intraperitoneal injections of concentrated retroviral herpes simplex thymidine kinase vector supernatant and ganciclovir. Ann Surg 1996 Sep; 224 (3):405–14.
13. Sunamura M, Oonuma M, Motoi F, et al. Gene therapy for pancreatic cancer targeting the genomic alterations of tumor suppressor genes using replication-selective oncolytic adenovirus. Hum Cell 2002 Sep; 15 (3):138–50.
14. Taylor OM, Benson EA, McMahon MJ. Clinical trial of tamoxifen in patients with irresectable pancreatic adenocarcinoma. The Yorkshire Gastrointestinal Tumour Group. Br J Surg 1993 Mar; 80 (3):384–6.
15. Wong A, Chan A. Survival benefit of tamoxifen therapy in adenocarcinoma of pancreas. A case-control study. Cancer 1993; 71 (7):2200–3.
16. Greenway BA. Effect of flutamide on survival in patients with pancreatic cancer: results of a prospective, randomised, double blind, placebo controlled trial. BMJ 1998 Jun 27; 316 (7149):1935–8.
17. Brett BT, Caplin ME. Towards immunotherapy for pancreatic cancer. Gut 2000; 46 (4):582–3.
18. Johnson LR. Regulation of gastrointestinal growth. In Physiology of the gastrointestinal tract, Vol. LR Johnson, J Christensen, MI Grossman, et al. (eds). New York, Raven Press 1981; pp. 169–196.
19. Townsend CM, Beauchamp RD, Singh P, et al. Growth factors and intestinal neoplasms. Am J Surg 1988; 155:526–536.
20. Watson SA, Durrant LG, Crosbie JD, et al. The in vitro growth response of primary human colorectal and gastric cancer cells to gastrin. Int J Cancer 1989; 43:692–696.
21. Seva C, Scemama JL, Bastie MJ, et al. Lorgumide and loxiglumide inhibit gastrin-stimulated DNA synthesis in a rat tumoral pancreatic cell line (AR42J). Cancer Res 1990; 5829–5833.
22. Yao CZ, Bold RJ, Ishizuka J, et al. Growth of mouse hepatocytes is stimulated by gastrin. J Cell Physiol 1995; 163:532–537.
23. Blackmore M, Doherty E, Manning JE, et al. Autocrine growth stimulation of human Wilms tumour G401 cells by a gastrin-like peptide. Int J Cancer 1994; 57:385–391.
24. Rehfeld JF, Bardram L, Hilsted L. Gastrin in human bronchogenic carcinomas: constant expression but variable processing of progastrin. Cancer Res 1989; 49:2840–2843.
25. Smith AM, Watson SA. Gastrin and gastrin receptor activation: an early event in the adenoma-carcinoma sequence. Gut 2000; 47 (6):820–4.
26. Watson SA, Morris TM, McWilliams DF, et al. Potential role of endocrine gastrin in the colonic adenoma carcinoma sequence. Br J Cancer 2002; 87 (5):567–73.

27. Dickinson CJ, Sawada JM, Guo YJ, et al. Specificity of prohormone convertase endoproteolysis of progastrin in AtT-20 cells. J Clin Invest 1995; 96:1425–1431.
28. Marino LR, Takeuchi T, Dickinson CJ, et al. Expression and post-translational processing of gastrin in heterologous endocrine cells. J Biol Chem 1991; 266:6133–6.
29. Dickinson CJ, Yamada T. Gastrin amidating enzyme in the porcine pituitary and antrum: characterization of molecular forms and substrate specificity. J Biol Chem 1991; 266:334–338.
30. Hilsted L, Rehfeld JF. Carboxyamidation of antral progastrin: relation to other posttranslational modifications. J Biol Chem 1987; 262:16953–16957.
31. Seva C, Dickinson CJ, Yamada T. Growth-promoting effects of glycine-extended progastrin. Science 1994; 265:410–412.
32. Smith AM, Watson SA. Review article: gastrin and colorectal cancer. Aliment Pharmacol Ther 2000; 14 (10):1231–47.
33. Rozengurt E, Walsh JH. Gastrin, CCK, signaling, and cancer. Annu Rev Physiol 2001; 63:49–76.
34. Larsson LI, Rehfeld JF, Sundler F, et al. Pancreatic gastrin in foetal and neonatal rats. Nature 1976; 262:609–610.
35. Brand SJ, Fuller PJ. Differential gastrin gene expression in rat gastrointestinal tract and pancreas during neonatal development. J Biol Chem 1988; 263:5341–5347.
36. Montag AG, Oka T, Baek KH, et al. Tumours in hepatobiliary tract and pancreatic islet tissues of transgenic mice harboring gastrin simian virus 40 large tumour antigen fusion gene. Proc Nat Acad Sci USA 1993; 90:6696–6700.
37. Smith JP, Fantaskey AP, Liu G, et al. Identification of gastrin as a growth peptide in human pancreatic cancer. Am J Physiol 1995; 268:R135–R141.
38. Smith JP, Shih A, Wu Y, et al. Gastrin regulates growth of human pancreatic cancer in a tonic and autocrine fashion. Am J Physiol 1996; 270:R10878–1084.
39. Smith JP, Verderame MF, McLaughlin P, et al. Characterization of the CCK-C (cancer) receptor in human pancreatic cancer. Int J Mol Med 2002; 10 (6):689–94.
40. Caplin M, Savage K, Khan K, et al. Expression and processing of gastrin in pancreatic adenocarcinoma. Br J Surg 2000; 87 (8):1035–40.
41. Goetze JP, Nielsen FC, Burcharth F, et al. Closing the gastrin loop in pancreatic carcinoma: co-expression of gastrin and its receptor in solid human pancreatic adenocarcinoma. Cancer 2000; 88 (11):2487–94.
42. Watson SA, Gilliam AD. G17DT – a new weapon in the therapeutic armoury for gastrointestinal malignancy. Expert Opin Biol Ther 2001; 1 (2):309–17.
43. Watson SA, Michaeli D, Grimes S, et al. Gastrimmune raises antibodies that neutralise amidated and glycine-extended gastrin-17 and inhibit the growth of colon cancer. Cancer Res 1996; 56:880–885.
44. Caplin M, Khan K, Grimes S, et al. Effect of gastrin and anti-gastrin antibodies on proliferation of hepatocyte cell lines. Dig Dis Sci 2001; 46 (7):1356–66.
45. Watson SA, Morris TM, Varro A, et al. A comparison of the therapeutic effectiveness of gastrin neutralisation in two human gastric cancer models: relation to endocrine and autocrine/paracrine gastrin mediated growth. Gut 1999; 45 (6):812–7.
46. Watson SA, Smith AM. Hypergastrinemia promotes adenoma progression in the APC(Min-/+) mouse model of familial adenomatous polyposis. Cancer Res 2001 Jan 15; 61 (2):625–31.
47. Smith AM, Justin T, Michaeli D, et al. Phase I/II study of G17-DT, an anti-gastrin immunogen, in advanced colorectal cancer. Clin Cancer Res 2000; 6 (12):4719–24.
48. Gilliam AD, Henwood M, Smith AM, et al. A phase II study of G17DT in gastric carcinoma. Gut 2001; 48 (Suppl 1):A36.
49. Brett BT, Smith SC, Bouvier CV, et al. Phase II study of anti-gastrin-17 antibodies, raised to G17DT, in advanced pancreatic cancer. J Clin Oncol 2002; 20 (20):4225–31.
50. Gilliam AD, Henwood M, Watson SA, et al. G17DT may improve survival of patients with advanced pancreatic carcinoma. J Clin Oncol 2001; 29:533.
51. Smith JP, Verderame MF, Zagon IS. Antisense oligonucleotides to gastrin inhibit growth of human pancreatic cancer. Cancer Lett 1999; 8: 135 (1):107–12.

9 Novel Alternatives to Chemotherapy in Advanced Disease: Gene Transfer

Paula Ghaneh, Christopher M. Halloran, Eithne Costello and John P. Neoptolemos

Pancreatic cancer remains one of the most difficult cancers to treat effectively. It is one of the largest cancer killers with universally poor survival rates. It claims over 6,500 lives per year in the U.K.,[1] over 40 000 in Europe,[1,2] nearly 19 000 in Japan[3] and almost 30 000 annually in the United States.[4–7] The median survival for all stages of pancreatic cancer is less than 3–5 months from diagnosis, with a five year survival of 0.4–3%.[1,7,8]

Surgical resection offers the potential of a cure, but even after successful surgery the prognosis remains poor, with median survival of around 13–15 months and five year survival rates of 15–20%.[9–13] The majority of patients present with advanced disease that is not amenable to surgical resection, or with widespread metastatic disease. Resection rates of only 10–15% are achieved even in specialised centres.[14] There is a lack of effective therapies for those patients unsuitable for surgery. Conventional chemotherapy and radiotherapy approaches have been used to improve survival in patients with resectable or advanced disease. 5-fluorouracil (5-FU) with folinic acid as a modulator has been the mainstay of chemotherapy. No combination of agents has been shown to be superior to 5-FU alone in randomised trials.[15] The use of 5-FU/folinic acid or chemoradiotherapy has been assessed in the adjuvant setting in the ESPAC-1 trial and encouraging survival results were observed for patients who received 5-FU/folinic acid chemotherapy.[16] Recently the nucleoside analogue gemcitabine has been utilised in patients with advanced pancreatic cancer to produce some improvement in survival over 5-FU.[17] The effect of gemcitabine versus 5-FU or surgery alone in the adjuvant setting will be examined in the ESPAC-3 study which is currently ongoing. These studies will be pivotal in providing a structured approach to adjuvant therapy. It is apparent, however that the survival of these patients is still very poor overall.

There is a clear need for novel therapies to be developed to provide an effective treatment for these patients. A sound understanding of the molecular events which are important in the development of pancreatic cancer may help provide some of the answers.

Molecular Mechanisms in Pancreatic Cancer

In cancer cells there is a stepwise accumulation of genetic lesions which confer a selective growth advantage that can result in tumour formation and metastatic spread. Pancreatic intraepithelial neoplasia (PanIN) represent progressive stages of neoplastic growth which are the precursors to pancreatic adenocarcinomas.[18] Molecular and pathological analysis of evolving pancreatic adenocarcinoma (including PanINs) has demonstrated a characteristic pattern of genetic lesions.[19] The majority affect the oncogene K-ras and tumour suppressor genes p16, p53 and SMAD4. The accumulation of these genetic changes leads to a profound disturbance in cell cycle control and continuous growth. Activating K-ras mutations are the first genetic changes that are detected and are found in over 80% of pancreatic adenocarcinomas.[20] These mutations can affect proliferation, cell survival and invasion through several effector pathways. There is also evidence for an important early contribution of the autocrine epidermal growth factor (EGF) family signalling. Pancreatic adenocarcinomas overexpress EGF ligands and receptors and EGFR and ERBB2 induction has been found in low grade PanINs.[21]

Loss of function of p16 due to mutation, deletion or promoter hypermethylation occurs in 80–85% pancreatic cancers.[22] The p16 locus encodes two tumour suppressor genes p16 and ARF via distinct first exons and alternative reading frames in shared downstream exons.[19] Many pancreatic cancers sustain a loss of both transcripts thereby disrupting both the retinoblastoma (RB) and p53 tumour suppressor pathways. P16 promotes cell cycle arrest in G1 and ARF stabilises p53. P16 mutations are also seen in dysplastic lesions.[19]

P53 is mutated, generally by missense alterations of the DNA binding domain, in more than 50% of pancreatic cancers.[22] These also arise in later stage PanINs with severe dysplasia.[19] Loss of p53 promotes severe genetic instability.

Another frequent alteration in pancreatic adenocarcinoma is the loss of SMAD4 which encodes a transcriptional regulator which is a component in the transforming growth factor β (TGF-β) signalling cascade.[23] TGF-β inhibits the growth of normal cells by blocking the cell cycle or promoting apoptosis; the cellular responses are partly dependent on SMAD4. SMAD4 loss is found in the later PanINs possibly associating it with tumour progression.[24]

Disruption of apoptotic pathways also contributes to the malignant phenotype.[25] The ability of tumour cells to invade and metastasize indicates an important role for factors controlling cell/cell/stromal interactions and tumour angiogenesis. Imbalances are found in the expression of matrix metalloproteinases (MMPs) and tissue inhibitors of MMPs (TIMPs).[26] There is over expression of vascular endothelial factors (VEGFs) and fibroblast growth factors which contribute to tumour cell growth and invasion.[27]

Genomic and proteomic strategies are now being employed to identify key/causative genes in sporadic pancreatic tumourigenesis.[28] Up to 5–10% of pancreatic cancers may have a hereditary component and identification of germline mutations which may be implicated in familial pancreatic cancer[29] will also be vital in identifying important therapeutic targets.

Overall these accumulated genetic abnormalities contribute to the malignant phenotype and represent possible therapeutic targets for gene therapy.

Gene Therapy

Gene therapy may be defined as the transfer and expression of exogenous genetic material into human cells to produce a therapeutic response. At the present time clinical protocols are directed at somatic gene therapy only. There are over 400 clinical trials worldwide assessing gene therapy in patients with cancer. The gold standard of cancer gene therapy is to selectively and efficiently kill tumour cells only. Targeting techniques may incorporate the gene delivery system, tissue or tumour specific promoters and physical delivery of the gene of interest to the tumour by direct injection or regional delivery. There are major obstacles to achieving these goals and this may be reflected in the encouraging but not hugely effective results seen so far in clinical trials. There has been early adoption of gene therapy strategies before targeting and efficiency has been optimised and this may have contributed to some poor early results. There have been well publicised adverse reactions and complications of some gene therapy protocols[30,31] and the lessons have been learnt from these studies.

The main methods of gene delivery are viral, non-viral and physical. The most commonly used viral vectors are those based on retroviruses, adenoviruses and adeno-associated viruses. Non-viral vector systems include the use of naked DNA, cationic lipid–DNA complexes and DNA condensed with cationic polymers. Physical approaches involve needle-free injection and electroporation. To date, the most efficient gene transfer is achieved with viral vectors and hence these are the most commonly used gene delivery systems in cancer gene therapy protocols.

Viral Vectors

Retroviral Vectors

Vectors based on oncoretroviruses have been developed as tools for gene therapy because they have a fairly large cloning capacity, they do not transfer viral genes (and are thus relatively non-immunogenic) and stably integrate the transferred therapeutic gene into the chromosome of the host cell.[32] The main drawback of these vectors is the difficulty in achieving high titres. Retroviruses are usually manufactured in titres up to around 10^8 particles per ml. The safety of retroviral vectors has been improved by the creation of self-inactivating (SIN) vectors.[33] However, retroviral integration into the host genome can lead to insertional mutagenesis and unpredictable expression of the transgene. There is also direct experimental evidence that retroviral vectors can induce leukaemia in mice and humans.[30] These effects are unpredictable and represent a major challenge to overcome.

Gene delivery to tumour cells of pancreatic origin has been achieved with oncoretroviral vectors such as the Moloney murine leukaemia virus (MoMLV).[34, 35] The main limitation of oncoretroviral vectors is their inability to infect non-dividing cells which may represent a relatively small proportion of tumour cells at any one time, this poses a problem for efficient gene transfer but does confer a level of specificity.

To increase tumour or tissue specificity of retroviral vectors it is possible to manufacture vectors from a wide variety of packaging cells lines that exhibit tissue specific promoters and inducible promoters.[36, 37]

Retroviral tropism can be redirected by insertion of short peptide ligands at multiple locations in the envelope. Moloney murine leukemia virus (MLV) envelope derivatives bearing short peptide ligands for gastrin-releasing protein (GRP) have been developed which selectively transduce human cancer cell lines that overexpress the receptor.[38] Another study incorporated EGFR specific ligands into a series of chimeric env proteins of the Moloney murine leukaemia virus in an attempt to increase tumour selectivity of these vectors.[39]

Adenoviral Vectors

Adenoviruses are double stranded DNA viruses that enter cells by receptor-mediated endocytosis, eventually being released to the cytoplasm in a pH dependant manner. Vectors based on these viruses have many attributes that render them attractive for cancer gene therapy. They can be purified to high titres (up to 10^{13} particles per ml) and infect a wide variety of dividing and non-dividing cells to achieve good rates of transduction. Adenoviruses can incorporate up to 37Kb of foreign DNA. Adenovirus DNA does not integrate into the host chromosome but remains episomal in the nucleus – subsequent expression, at least for early generation vectors, is transient. Since by and large the aim of cancer gene therapy protocols is to kill the target cancer cells, long-term expression is not essential. Early-generation adenoviral vectors elicit a significant immune response in vivo,[40] while this immunogenicity is seen as a disadvantage for some gene therapy applications, for cancer treatment it may serve to increase the rate of elimination of cancer cells. The precise response of the host immune system to the virus is unknown as exemplified by the recent death of a patient in a phase 1 clinical trial.[41]

Attempts to increase the specificity of adenoviral vectors for pancreatic cancer have been directed at cellular receptors which are overexpressed in pancreatic cancer. One study used a bispecific fusion protein formed by a recombinant soluble form of truncated Coxsackie and Adenovirus Receptor (sCAR) genetically fused with human EGF (sCAR-EGF) to redirect the vector to the EGFR which is overexpressed in pancreatic cancer. This same study also used a genetically modified Ad vector to allow efficient CAR-independent infection by binding to cellular integrins. This resulted in a dramatic enhancement of gene transfer.[42]

Pancreatic ductal adenocarcinomas overexpress the type I high-affinity fibroblast growth factor receptor (FGFR-1). A conjugate consisting of fibroblast growth factor (FGF)-2 linked to a Fab' fragment against the adenovirus knob region was evaluated in human pancreatic cancer cell lines treated with an adenoviral vector. This combination was associated with high levels of transduction efficiency.[43]

Adeno-Associated Viral Vectors

Adeno-associated viruses (AAV) are non-pathogenic single stranded DNA viruses. AAV integrates its genome almost exclusively into a specific location on human chromosome 19.[44] For efficient replication, they require co-infection with a helper virus, usually adenoviruses or herpesviruses. Vectors based on AAV however integrate much less efficiently and more randomly than the parent virus. Unlike adenoviruses they do not efficiently stimulate the immune response. The vector tropism is sufficiently broad to allow transfer of genes to most tissue types and in certain of these tissues expression of the transgene has been relatively long lived.[45] The drawbacks to AAV include packaging cell lines which are sensitive to the toxic effects of the gene responsible for replication of AAV (the 'REP' gene) and also to helper viruses. Moreover this system is incapable of producing high titres of the vector with a stably incorporated therapeutic gene. AAV-based vectors have a very low capacity, accomodating only ~4.5kb of foreign DNA. A way around this latter problem is to co-deliver two AAV's, each carrying half the desired protein. Once delivered, head-to-toe splicing (concatomerisation) will occur allowing reconstitution of a functional larger transgene.[46,47] AAV vectors have been used for gene transfer to pancreaitic carcinoma cells.[48,49]

Lentivral vectors

Lentiviruses can replicate in non-dividing cells. Vectors based on these viruses may prove an attractive alternative for gene therapy of pancreatic cancer. The development of lentiviral vectors has been facilitated by the enormous body of research on HIV-1 and the accumulated knowledge on their oncoretroviral predecessors.[50] Third generation vectors are multiply attenuated, containing three of the original nine genes of HIV-1, and thus, 40% of its genome only. Like retroviral vectors, the transfer vector containing the therapeutic gene is the only genetic material delivered to target cells. Since no virus derived coding sequences are transferred, immune responses to viral proteins are avoided. A major disadvantage is that these vectors will integrate at random chromosomal sites. Lentiviral vectors already have an established role in the transduction of T-cells[51] and haematopoietic stem cells.[52, 53] Lentiviral vectors have been used to treat solid tumours in pre-clinical studies with good effect.[54] Although there are no clinical trials using lentiviral vectors at present there is continued interest in this method of gene delivery.

Alphaviral Vectors

Replication defective alphavirus vectors are currently being developed for gene therapy approaches. The Semliki Forest virus (rSFV), is a member of the alphavirus genus. Recombinant SFV particles contain a self-replicating RNA molecule that carries the genes coding for the viral replicase. The genes encoding the virus structural proteins are replaced by the therapeutic gene. Most individuals lack pre-existing immunity against SFV and the immune response is limited or non-existent. SFV mediated antigen expression is transient as infected cells die by apoptosis. This represents an exciting new vector.[55]

Hybrid Vectors

Hybrid vectors utilise desirable properties of current viral systems such as prolonged expression, elevation in titre and immunogenic response. There are several examples of this although none as yet has made a significant impact on cancer gene therapy. Hybrid adenovirus and Epstein-Barr virus (EBV) allowed high titre and long-term expression of transgene due to the stable maintenance of episomal EBV.[56] Alternatively, chimeras of adenovirus and retrovirus can be used to convert in-vivo target cells into retroviral producer cells.[57]

Replication Competent Vectors

All the vectors discussed so far are replication incompetent. A means of increasing the number of cells transduced in a tumour is to use replication competent vectors that depend on the transformed phenotype of the tumour cell to replicate. The ONYX-015 is a mutant adenovirus that preferentially replicates in cells lacking functional p53 (a property of many tumour cells), due to a deletion in the adenovirus E1B gene.[58] There is no intrinsic therapeutic domain in these constructs. Tumour cell killing is a virtue of the general lytic action of the replicating adenoviruses within their cells. The use of ONYX-015 has proved safe enough to reach Phase III trials. Unfortunately, its relatively low efficiency means that it is unlikely to be used on its own.[59]

A recent study[60] showed that co-transduction of a pancreatic cancer cell line with an E1B deleted adenovirus (similar to the ONYX-015 virus) and a replication incompetent adenovirus carrying a human IL-2 transgene increased the IL-2 production by 370-fold. Moreover, the combination resulted in complete regression of established pancreatic tumours in SCID mice. This is a promising use of replication competent vectors. Recently onco-lytic effects of Herpesvirus saimiri have been observed in pancreatic cancer cell lines. This virus appears to be selectively cytopathic for pancreatic cancer cell lines when compared with colon cancer cell lines.[61]

Non-Viral Vectors

Naked DNA

Naked DNA in the form of plasmid DNA, is easily manufactured in bacteria and has a limitless therapeutic insert size. The delivery efficiency is far less than that of adenoviral or AVV systems. If feasible, reasonable levels of transduction can be achieved by direct local injection. Tumour cell targeting is not specific and transgene expression is brief. Naked DNA vectors possess un-methylated CpG islands, which stimulate cytokine cascades in animal models. This feature is an obvious advantage for genetic-vaccines in terms of recruitment of antigen presentation.[62]

Attempts to increase the efficiency of transfer have included the use of therapeutic ultrasound which induces cell membrane permeabilization. This approach enhanced the transfection efficiency of naked plasmid DNA in vivo as well as in vitro.[63]

Cationic Lipids

Cationic lipids are synthetic spherical lipid bi-layers that bind DNA by electrostatic interaction enabling endocytosis of the lipid-DNA complex whilst offering protection of the DNA. This vector system suffers from instability and it lacks specificity for cell targeting. Entrance of cationic lipids into the nucleus is more tightly controlled than that of entry to the cytoplasm. This results in mainly cytoplasmic delivery – hence transient transgene expression, although such expression may be all that is required.[64]

Condensed DNA Particles

Cationic polymers such as oligopeptides[65] heterologous polylysine[66] or polyethylene imine (PEI)[67] can be used to condense DNA by electrostatic interaction into small particles. The resulting particles are resistant to degredation and exhibit enhanced endosome uptake.[68] Unfortunately DNA delivered into the cell by this method may become trapped in endosomes and be targeted for lysosomal degradation. Condensed DNA particles have a marginal superiority over that of naked DNA with lower immunogenicity and an ability to retarget tissue.

The size of condensed DNA particles is a key determinant for *in vivo* diffusion, as well as for gene delivery to the cell nucleus. A recent study produced particles measuring approximately 30 nm, which corresponds to the volume of a single molecule of plasmid DNA, resulting in improved *in vivo* diffusion.[69]

Improved tumour targeting through cell surface receptors has been demonstrated. Complexes of a chimeric protein targeted to the EGF receptor (EGFR) and a reporter plasmid produced by condensation with poly-L-lysine resulted in elevated reporter plasmid expression in EGFR expressing cells compared with poly-L-lysine DNA complexes alone.[70]

Artificial Chromosomes

The construction of vectors based on chromosomal elements may represent a more stable method of gene transfer. The vectors may be stably maintained and replicated as an episome in the target cell. A number of prototype small circular vectors and artificial chromosome vectors have been developed but so far none of these constructs has been actually used in gene therapy trials. Artificial chromosomes have the undoubted advantage of being mitotically stable and have an indefinite cloning capacity allowing the insertion of all control elements for correct expression of the transgene. The drawbacks include their large size so that they are difficult to handle and can be recovered only in small quantities. Small circular non-viral vectors have the advantage that they can be handled with ease and obtained in large quantities, but their cloning capacity may be restricted.[71]

Tumour and Tissue Specific Promoters

It is an obvious advantage for the vector system to exhibit tissue or tumour specificity to optimise targeting. This can include viral/vector modifications as outlined previously or focus on transcriptional regulatory elements relevant to pancreatic cancer. There have been various studies which have assessed tumour specific promoters in a number of gene therapy approaches.

Midkine (MK), a heparin binding growth factor, and cyclooxygenase-2 (COX-2), are both up-regulated at the mRNA or protein level in many human malignant tumors including pancreatic cancer. One study assessed the expression of a reporter gene (luciferase) under the control of the COX-2 or MK promoter. A high level of luciferase activity was seen in this construct compared to the control promoter. This may represent a promising method of tumour targeting.[72]

Pancreatic cancer cells overexpress cell surface antigens such as carcinoembryonic antigen (CEA) and MUC1. The promoters for these genes have been utilised in adenoviral and retroviral vectors for in vitro and in vivo studies of pancreatic cancer. Significant increases in transduction efficiency were observed using the vectors under control of the CEA promoter. This strategy may provide a useful tool for treating pancreatic cancer.[73]

Gene Therapy Approaches

Gene therapy approaches for pancreatic cancer include those directed against activated oncogenes or dominant mutated genes, restoration of tumour suppressor gene function, augmentation of anti-tumour immunity, gene directed enzyme prodrug therapy (GDEPT), manipulation of MMPs and TIMPs and growth factors, promotion of apoptosis and endocrine manipulation.

Oncogene Directed Gene Therapy

Kras Oncogene

Over 80% of pancreatic cancer cases exhibit 'constitutive' mutational activation of K-ras which results in the activation of effector pathways that may differ from those involved in the normal K-ras signalling system.[74,75] Several approaches have been used to target the K-ras pathway in pancreatic cancer cells.

Dominant-Negative Strategy

One study[76,77] used an adenovirus expressing a dominant negative H-ras mutant derived from the v-H-ras oncogene containing an asparagine residue at codon 116 (in the GTP binding domain) in place of tyrosine (N116Y). This mutant competes with oncogenic ras for a guanine nucleotide exchange factor. Expressed under the control of the tumour specific carcinoembryronic antigen (CEA) promoter, N116Y suppressed the progression of liver metastasis by a human pancreatic cancer cell line in a nude mouse model.

The activation of downstream pathways of ras, MEK-ERK and MEKK1-JNK and their roles in cell survival and proliferation identify them as possible targets for dominant mutant gene therapy. Dominant negative-MEKK strongly inhibits the survival of colonies of pancreatic cancer cells and this was not seen in non-pancreatic cancer cells.[78]

Antisense and Ribozyme Strategies

Gene therapy strategies may be used to alter transcription, processing and translation of mutated K-ras by the development of anti-sense (*AS*) RNA or ribozymes.[82] *AS* RNAs act by binding to the complimentary mRNA of the targeted gene to block translation. Ribozymes are small catalytic RNA species that exhibit site-specific cleavage activity and are involved in the repair of point mutations. Pancreatic cancer cell lines with mutant K-ras when treated with plasmids that express *AS* RNA show a reduction in p21-ras protein and growth suppression but not in cell lines containing wt K-ras.[83] Plasmids containing *AS* RNA transfected into nude mice with a liposome system also showed an inhibition of pancreatic tumour development.[84] The combination of antisense kras and over expression of the melanoma differentiation associated gene-7 (mda-7) has been shown to be more effective than either agent used alone.[85]

In another study, anti-K-ras ribozyme targeted against a mutated codon 12 caused a reduction in the levels of mutant K-ras mRNA.[86] The disadvantage of both these approaches is that both of these RNA species are susceptible to endonuclease degradation. There is no doubt that this has contributed to the fact that clinical trials, so far, have been very disappointing.

RNA interference (RNAi) is a newly discovered cellular pathway for the silencing of sequence-specific genes at the mRNA level by the introduction of the cognate double-stranded (ds) RNA. A recent study demonstrated that RNAi may be more potent than AS RNA in reducing target gene expression in human cancer cell lines.[87]

Immunotherapy

A clinical study demonstrated specific cytotoxic T lymphocyte (CTL) responses against a mutant ras peptide in patients with pancreatic cancer.[88] Clones of these T cells were able to transiently kill pancreatic cancer cell lines obtained from the same patient and maintained in culture. CD4+ and CD8+ T-cell subsets were able to identify the tumour cells harbouring the initial ras mutation. In Phase I/II studies two out of five patients with K-ras mutations given synthetic ras peptides had transient T cell responses.[89] Pancreatic tumour peptide vaccines that lead to the secretion of granulocyte-macrophage colony stimulating hormone (GM-CSF) might augment recruitment of antigen presenting cell types and enhancement of the CTL rsponse.[83]

Cancer-associated Sm-like Oncogene (CaSm)

CaSm is present in up to 88% of pancreatic tumours and is important in the 'malignant' phenotype.[90] Adenoviral expression vectors containing anti-sense constructs have shown dramatic effects both *in vitro* and *in vivo* in pancreatic cancer models. Cellular proliferation *in vitro* was decreased and *in vivo* there was reduced expression of CaSm in the tumour tissue and a reduction in tumour volume resulting in increased survival time.[91]

The combination of an adenovirus expressing antisense RNA to CaSm (Ad-alpha CaSm) and gemcitabine has been examined in pancreatic cancer both in vitro and in vivo. This combination of Ad-alpha CaSm with gemcitabine was more effective in killing tumour cells than either agent used separately.[92]

Tumour Suppressor Gene Therapy

p16INK4a Tumour Suppresser Gene

Loss of normal cell cycle control is a key feature of tumour cells. The association of cyclins and cyclin-dependent kinases are necessary for cell cycle progression. Cyclin D1 forms an active complex with either cyclin dependant kinase (CDK) 4 or 6 resulting in phosphorylation of the retinoblastoma protein (pRb) and subsequent progression from G_1 to S phase of the cell cycle. The $p16^{INK4a}$ gene belongs to the INK4 group of tumour suppresser genes which are specific inhibitors of the complex cyclinD1-CDK4/6 and serves to arrest the cell cycle up-stream of the restriction point maintaining cells in a quiescent state.[22] $p16^{INK4a}$ function is lost in >80% of human pancreatic adenocarcinomas and is thus an important target for potential genetic correction.

$p16^{INK4}$ requires functional Rb to exert a cytostatic effect. Gene therapy strategies using re-introduction of $p16^{INK4a}$ are therefore more likely to succeed if the recipient cell has functional Rb. Studies have shown that pancreatic cancers rarely contain mutant Rb[93] if $p16^{INK4}$ is mutated. $p16^{INK4a}$ is among the most potent CDK inhibitors (CDK-I) involved in cell cycle arrest. Adenoviral introduction of $p16^{INK4a}$ produces apoptosis in-vitro as well as growth arrest in an in-vivo mouse model.[94] $p16^{INK4a}$ was the only CDK-I that delayed growth following direct tumour injection.

A $p16^{INK4a}$ expressing adenovirus vector (Adp16), gives rise to mRNA in pancreatic cells after only one hour and significant inhibition of growth after seven days.[95] Direct injection of Adp16 into the pancreatic bed or via the portal vein to the liver could be an advantageous adjunct to limit metastases after resection. Transfection of pancreatic cancer cells in-vitro with $p16^{INK4a}$ fusion peptides resulted in cell cycle arrest at G_1 that was associated with hypophosphorylation of Rb.[96] Pancreatic cancer cells in culture underwent G_1 arrest and apoptosis following transduction with Adp16 and caused significant growth arrest in human pancreatic tumours grown in nude mice.[97] Simultaneous adenoviral transduction of $p16^{INK4a}$ and p53, may enhance apoptotic cell death in tumour cells in-vitro, whilst inhibiting tumour growth in nude mice.[98]

The p53 and $p16^{INK4a}$ status of a tumour may also affect its response to chemotherapy and ionising radiation.[99] G_1 cell cycle arrest induced by $p16^{INK4a}$ has been shown to confer resistance against chemotherapeutic drugs that act predominantly in the S phase of the cycle.[100–103]

p53 Tumour Suppresser Gene

p53 is a transcription factor, induced either by DNA damage or inappropriate mitogenic stimuli, which functions as a tumour suppressor gene. Activation of p53 up-regulates p21, a member of the CIP/KIP group of tumour suppressor genes acting specifically upon cyclin E/CDK2 complex and hence promoting cell cycle arrest at G1/S phase. p53 either initiates cell repair or apoptosis via transcriptional or non-transcriptional pathways. A downstream target for p53 is its negative regulator MDM2 (HDM2 in humans) that abrogates p53-transactivation[104] and targets p53 for nuclear export and cytosolic degradation.[105, 106] Recent work has shown the existence of a novel cellular protein

MDM2 Binding Protein (MTBP), which induces G_1 arrest and is in turn regulated by MDM2.[107,108] Functional loss of p53 may result through mutational inactivation of p53 or over-expression of MDM2. Functional loss of p53 occurs in 50–75% of pancreatic cancer cases.[109]

We and others have observed that adenoviral-mediated introduction of p53 into pancreatic cancer cell lines with mt-p53 results in reduction in cell growth and induction of apoptosis *in vitro*, along with tumour growth inhibition in nude mice models.[97,110] A recent study[111] observed that pancreatic cancer cells regardless of genotype showed growth arrest after Adp53 administration although apoptosis could not be induced in cells with wild-type p53. It was also demonstrated that cells containing wild-type p16INK4a transduced with Adp53 underwent greater levels of apoptosis than cells with mutant p16INK4a. These same mt-p16INK4a mutant cells when transfected with Adp16 prior to Adp53 showed equivalent apoptosis levels to wt-p16INK4a cells. This may suggest that co-operation between p53 and p16INK4a is required for full cell cycle control.

Following transduction with Adp53 we were able to elicit both inhibition of cell growth and apoptosis, even in wt p53 pancreatic cancer cell lines.[97] Furthermore enhanced levels of apoptosis were observed in-vivo following dual infection with Adp53 and Adp16. From these data it can be concluded that there is co-operation at least in terms of apoptosis induction when combining introduction of p16INK4a and p53 in pancreatic cancer models. The precise nature of this co-operation remains to be elucidated. It has been suggested that some tumour lines have by-passed the need for mutant p53 by possessing defective down stream apoptotic pathways.[111]

The p53 status of a tumour has a bearing upon the responsiveness to chemotherapy and ionising radiation.[112] Patients with tumours that possess wt-p53 may be more likely to undergo a complete clinical response to chemotherapy (reviewed in ref.111). The evidence favours a link between the loss of functional p53 and thus of apoptosis in response to drug treatment.

There is conflicting data from studies exploring the effects of combining standard chemotherapeutic drugs and introduction of p53. It has been concluded that p53-mediated cell cycle arrest and apoptosis are independent of one another but are dependant upon the type of drug used, the concentration of that drug, the level of accumulated p53, the type of tissue examined and the order of administration.[113,114] Gemcitabine and cisplatin have been combined with Adp53 or Adp16 in pancreatic cancer models. This study showed that cells treated with vector then gemcitabine had reduced susceptibility to the drug, which was consistent with the observation that more cells were shifted towards G1 and away from the S phase where gemcitabine (nucleoside analogue) is active. Conversely, cells treated with gemcitabine then vector had increased susceptibility, suggesting that gemcitabine-induced DNA damage augmented p53 or p16INK4a dependent apoptosis.[115]

E2F-1 Gene

The cellular transcription factor E2F1 promotes apoptosis in various systems independent of the endogenous p53 status.[116] This has led to the suggestion that E2F1 may act as a potent tumour suppressor by engaging apoptotic pathways. E2F-1 has been overexpressed in pancreatic cancer cells both on its own and in combination with chemotherapeutic agents such as etoposide and gemcitabine. Increased rates of apoptosis and sensitivity to the chemotherapeutic agents used were observed.[117,118]

Immunotherapy

Pancreatic tumour cells are poorly immunogenic: vaccination of unmodified tumour cells usually fails to elicit a potent immune response. Systemic immunity is dependent largely on CD4+ T helper cells and CD8+ cytotoxic T lymphocytes (CTL). Immunotherapy attempts to augment the immune response in favour of CTL. Tumour cells genetically engineered to produce various cytokines have been shown to generate an antitumour response. Pancreatic cell lines transduced with interleukins (IL-2, IL-4, IL-6, IL-12, IL-15), tumour necrosis factor alpha (TNF-α or granulocyte-macrophage colony stimulating factor (GMCSF) have each been shown to inhibit growth, or in some cases result in complete tumour regression in subcutaneous nude mice models.[119–121] A recombinant vaccinia virus encoding the human interleukin-1-β (IL-1β) given intravenously or intratumorally in a subcutaneous pancreatic cancer nude mouse model, resulted in significant tumour growth inhibition.[122]

CTL activation requires the presentation of a relevant peptide-MHC class I complex together with co-stimulatory signals from antigen presenting cells (APCs). Pancreatic tumour cells express low levels of these co-stimulatory molecules. Irradiated tumour cells engineered to produce GM-CSF, which recruits APCs, can produce a systemic anti-tumour immune response.[123]

An alternative approach uses dendritic cells (DC) which are APCs, and can be isolated from the peripheral blood of patients. These purified DC can be pulsed with exogenously added peptides to tumour associated antigens such as ras, p53, HER2/neu and CEA, to elicit specific CTL response.

Vaccination of dendritic cells pulsed with peptides for the HER2/neu protein and the CEA antigen, induces HLA class I restricted CTL responses which are capable of lysing human pancreatic cell lines.[124] Irradiated purified DC pulsed with the CEA peptide have been used to generate CEA specific CTLs in the presence of IL-7, in pancreatic and breast carcinoma patients.[124] In another study an immunological response induced by autologous dendritic cells (DCs) pulsed with allogeneic tumor lysate in a pancreatic cancer patient demonstrated a dramatic increase of the PMNC killing capacity against pancreatic cancer cell lines in vitro.[125]

The αGal epitope is known to be a major xeno-antigen. The αGal epitope, when expressed on the cell surface, binds to natural antibodies in human serum. This binding activates the complement cascade, leading to complement dependent cell lysis. Cancer cell specific transcription of the alphaGal epitope, was achieved under the control of a promoter region of the human telomerase reverse transcriptase (hTERT) in one study in pancreatic cancer. These cells were susceptible to antibody mediated killing.[126]

GDEPT

Genetically directed enzyme producing therapy (GDEPT) involves the delivery of a non-mammalian gene into tumour cells which, when expressed, can convert a systemically administered non-toxic prodrug to a toxic metabolite. This produces a high concentration of the toxic metabolite at the site of the tumour and reduces systemic toxicity. It is currently impossible to achieve transfer of the gene to all cells within a solid tumour or to disseminated metastases. A feature of all currently used GDEPT approaches is that administration of the prodrug results not only in the death of the transfected cell but also in the death of surrounding cells in a phenomenon known as the 'bystander effect'. This bystander effect may work via the toxic metabolite freely diffusing or moving through gap junctions to neighbouring non-transfected cells or by activation of the immune response.

The most widely used enzyme-prodrug strategy is the herpes simplex virus thymidine kinase-ganciclovir system (HSV-TK/GCV). The thymidine kinase gene phosphorylates GCV to an intermediate that is then phosphorylated by cellular kinases into a potent DNA synthesis inhibitor. Both retroviral and adenoviral vectors have been used to deliver the TK gene under the control of the CEA promoter into pancreatic CEA producing cell lines and increase their sensitivity to GCV.[127] A recent report has shown that an improved reduction in tumour volume in an *in vivo* model, was obtained using a combination of an adenovirus and retroviral producing cell line both of which contained the HSV-TK construct, than either viral vector alone.[128]

Cytosine deaminase (CD) is found in bacteria and fungi and converts the non-toxic prodrug 5-fluorocytosine (5FC) to 5-FU, an S phase cytotoxic agent. An adenoviral vector containing a cytomegalovirus promoter fused to the CD gene was used to infect the murine pancreatic cell line Panc02, resulting in expression of CD and sensitivity to 5FC *in vitro*.[129] When the construct was injected directly into the tumour mass, followed by systemic administration of 5FC, a 70% reduction in tumour mass was observed compared to controls.

The *E.coli* enzyme nitroreductase (NTR) can convert CB1954 (5-(aziridin-1-yl)-2,4-dinitrobenzamide) a weak monofunctional alkylating agent into a potent difunctional alkylating agent which crosslinks DNA. Retroviral transduction of this gene into colorectal and pancreatic cell lines increased their sensitivity to CB1954 compared to parental cell lines.[130] A marked bystander effect was observed when only 10% of SUIT2 pancreatic cancer cells expressed nitroreductase. In a subcutaneous nude mouse model, mice were transfected with SUIT2 NTR cells and then treated with intraperitoneal injections of CB1954.

Another approach to GDEPT against pancreatic cancer is the use of the prodrug isofamide. This is normally converted in the liver by cytochrome P450 to phosphoramide mustard and acroleim, which alkylates DNA and protein, respectively. Cells which have been genetically modified to express cytochrome P450 were encapsulated in cellulose sulphate and injected directly into subcutaneous tumours derived from human pancreatic cells.[131] Administration of isofamide resulted in partial or complete regression of the tumour.

A phase I/II trial in 14 patients with pancreatic cancer used encapsulated genetically modified allogeneic cells, which expressed cytochrome P450. These were delivered by supraselective angiography to the tumour vasculature. This approach showed some tumour responses.[132]

A recent novel GDEPT strategy has used the methionase gene (MET) in combination with selenomethionine prodrug. Tumour cell killing was significantly increased due to an impressive bystander effect.[133]

MMPS, TIMPS and Angiogenesis Factors

Pancreatic cancer is characterised by local invasion and early metastases. As with other highly invasive cancers this is dependent on the capacity to degrade the basement membrane and extracellular matrix (ECM). Matrix metalloproteinases (MMPs) are a large family of zinc containing proteinases which degrade the ECM. A variety of these MMPs are highly expressed in pancreatic cancer compared to normal pancreatic tissue.[26] The activity of these proteinases are tightly controlled by transcriptional regulation, latent proform activation and the binding of pro and active MMPs to natural tissue inhibitors (TIMP 1–4 s).[26] These inhibitors bind specifically to MMPs in a 1:1 molar ratio, and have a potential application in preventing invasion of tumour cells.

TIMP1 or TIMP2 have been introduced in pancreatic tumor and it has been demonstrated in vitro that the TIMP-expressing pancreatic tumor cells were significantly less invasive than cells transfected with a control vector. In vivo, adenoviral delivery of TIMP1 or TIMP2 to nude mice harbouring intraperitoneal human pancreatic cancers resulted in prolonged survival compared with control mice.[134]

Vascular endothelial growth factor (VEGF) plays an important role in tumor angiogenesis. The soluble form of flt-1 VEGF receptor inhibits VEGF activity in a dominant-negative manner. Adenoviral mediated transfer of this receptor was associated with growth suppression in pancreatic cancer cells.[135]

Growth Factors

Human pancreatic cancers over-express EGFR and its ligands (EGF, transforming growth factor alpha (TGF-, amphiregulin, heparin binding EGF like growth factor and betacellulin).[27] Introduction of an antisense oligonucleotide to amphiregulin in pancreatic cell lines reduced the level of amphiregulin released into the medium and inhibited cell growth in a dose dependent manner, even though levels of EGFR were also elevated.[136] Amplification and over-expression of c-erbB2 occurs in 20–30% of pancreatic cancers. The c-erbB2 protooncogene encodes a 185 KDa putative growth factor receptor that is homologous, but distinct from the EGF receptor. An antisense oligodeoxynucleotide against erbB2 reduced expression and resulted in growth arrest of human mammary carcinoma cell lines.[137]

NK4 acts as a competitive antagonist of hepatocyte growth factor (HGF) and is an inhibitor of angiogenesis. Overexpression of NK4 was associated with decreased tumour progression possibly as a result of its function as an angiogenesis inhibitor.[138]

Apoptosis

Programmed cell death or apoptosis can be mediated by several gene therapy approaches, such as over-expression of p16 and p53, which have been used alone or in combination with chemotherapy or irradiation.[97]

Bax is a strong pro-apoptotic gene that induces programmed cell death when expressed. Adenoviral mediated transfer of the bax gene under control of the human telomerase reverse transcriptase (hTERT) promoter was used in pancreatic cancer cells in a recent study. High levels of bax expression were observed which induced apoptosis.[139]

The N5 gene encodes a death-domain-containing protein (p84N5) that can trigger atypical apoptosis from within the nucleus, suggesting it may be a candidate for use as a gene therapy for cancer. Adenoviral-mediated N5 gene transfer reduced the growth and metastasis of primary human tumors in subcutaneous and orthotopic xenograft mouse models.[140]

Endocrine Gene Therapy

Gastrin is a regulatory peptide responsible for the secretion of gastric acid and cell turnover in the gastrointestinal tract. It has been shown to stimulate growth of cancers arising from it such as colon, stomach and pancreatic. An antisense oligonucleotide designed to bind to gastrin mRNA at the start codon and thereby disrupting mRNA translation has been shown to significantly inhibit growth of pancreatic cancer *in vitro* and *in vivo*.[141]

Somatostatin is a cyclic neuropeptide that negatively regulates a number of processes such as epithelial cell proliferation and exocrine and endocrine secretions. Studies have shown that somatostatin and its stable analogues suppress the growth of various normal and cancer cells. Five subtypes of somatostatin receptors have been cloned from human, mouse, and rat. Among them, the subtypes sst1, sst2, and sst5 are responsible for the antiproliferative effect of somatostatin and its analogues in vitro. Adenoviral mediated overexpression of somatostatin receptor subtype 2 (sst2) gene resulted in decreased pancreatic tumour growth and local antitumor bystander effects in vivo.[142]

Conclusion

Pancreatic cancer is a highly aggressive disease resulting in early invasion and metastasis. There is only a moderate improvement in long term survival in patients who are suitable for resection. Genomic and proteomic strategies will hopefully increase our knowledge of the key molecular events involved in pancreatic tumourigenesis. The molecular study of familial pancreatic cancer patients may hold the key to future therapies.

Most of the gene therapy strategies outlined above work well in vitro and in vivo models. The clinical situation demands efficient and safe delivery methods, selective expression of the gene of interest and toxicology. There is no ideal delivery system at the moment. Direct transfer of the vector by percutaneous, laparoscopic, angiographic or endoscopic administration will be required in Phase I/II clinical trials to obtain direct access to the pancreatic tissue. These delivery systems combined with tumour specific promoters should increase specific gene expression and selective tumour cell killing.

There have been two clinical trials, so far, of gene therapy in pancreatic cancer. The results have been encouraging but further studies are needed. It remains likely that gene therapy will be used in combination with conventional treatments and this will form the basis of future clinical trials.

References

1. Parkin DM, Bray FI, Devesa SS. Cancer burden in the year 2000. The global picture. Eur J Cancer 2001; 37:pp. S4–S66.
2. Fernandez E, et al. Trends in pancreatic cancer mortality in Europe. Int J Cancer 1994; 57: pp. 786–92.
3. Cancer Statistics in Japan 2001, in Foundation for the promotion of cancer research. National Cancer Center, Tokyo, 2001; p. 37.
4. Greenlee RT, et al. Cancer Statistics, 2001. Cancer Journal for Clinicians, 2001; 51 (6):pp. 15–36.
5. Carter D, C. Etiology and epidemiology of pancreatic and periampullary cancer, in Surgery of the pancreas, 2nd Edition, D Carter, C, Editor. 1997, Churchill Livingstone: New York, pp. 427–442.
6. Jemal A, et al. Cancer statistics 2002. Ca-a Cancer Journal for Clinicians 2002; 52:pp. 23–47.
7. Bramhall S, Dunn J, Neoptolemos JP. Epidemiology of pancreatic cancer., in The Pancreas, HG Beger, et al., Editors. 1998, Blackwell Scientific: Boston, pp. 889–906.
8. Bramhall SR, et al. Treatment and survival in 13,560 patients with pancreatic cancer, and incidence of the disease, in the West Midlands: an epidemiological study. Brit J Surg 1995; 82 (1):pp. 111–115.
9. Mosca F, et al. Long-term survival in pancreatic cancer: pylorus-preserving versus Whipple pancreatoduodenectomy. Surgery 1997; 122 (3):pp. 553–566.
10. Allema JH, et al. Prognostic factors for survival after pancreaticoduodenectomy for patients with carcinoma of the pancreatic head region. Cancer 1995; 75 (8):pp. 2069–2076.
11. Allison D, et al. DNA content and other factors associated with ten year survival after resection of pancreatic cancinoma. J Surg Oncol 1998; 67:pp. 151–9.
12. Nitecki S, et al. Long term survival after resection for ductal adenocarcinoma of the pancreas. Is it really improving? Ann Surgery 1995; 221:pp. 59–66.
13. Yeo CJ, et al. Pancreaticoduodenectomy for pancreatic adenocarcinoma: postoperative adjuvant chemoradiation improves survival. A prospective, single-institution experience. Ann Surgery 1997; 225 (5):pp. 621–33; discussion 633–6.
14. Neoptolemos JP, et al. Low mortality following resection for pancreatic and periampullary tumours in 1026 patients. Brit J Surg 1997; 84:pp. 1370–1376.
15. Ghaneh P, Slavin J, Sutton R, et al. Adjuvant therapy in pancreatic cancer. World J Gastroenterol 2001; 7:482–9.
16. Neoptolemos JP, Dunn JA, Stocken DD, et al. European Study Group for Pancreatic Cancer. Adjuvant chemoradiotherapy and chemotherapy in resectable pancreatic cancer: a randomised controlled trial. Lancet 2001; 10; 358:1576–85.
17. Burris HA, et al. Improvements in survival and clinical benefit with gemcitabine as first-line therapy for patients with advanced pancreas cancer: a randomized trial. J Clin Oncol 1997; 15 (6):pp. 2403–2413.
18. Hruban RH, Adsay NV, Albores-Saavedra J, et al. Pancreatic intraepithelial neoplasia: a new nomenclature and classification system for pancreatic duct lesions. Am J Surg Pathol 2001; 25:579–86.
19. Bardeesy N, DePinho RA. Pancreatic cancer biology and genetics. Nat Rev Cancer 2002; 2:897–909.
20. Almoguera C, Shibata D, Forrester K, et al. Most human carcinomas of the exocrine pancreas contain mutant c-K-ras genes. Cell 1988; 53:549–54.
21. Day JD, Digiuseppe JA, Yeo C, et al. Immunohistochemical evaluation of HER-2/neu expression in pancreatic adenocarcinoma and pancreatic intraepithelial neoplasms. Hum Pathol 1996; 27:119–24.
22. Rozenblum E, Schutte M, Goggins M, et al. Tumor-suppressive pathways in pancreatic carcinoma. Cancer Res 1997; 57:1731–4.
23. Hahn SA, Schutte M, Hoque AT, et al. DPC4, a candidate tumor suppressor gene at human chromosome 18q21.1. Science 1996; 271:350–3.
24. Wilentz RE, Iacobuzio-Donahue CA, Argani P, et al. Loss of expression of Dpc4 in pancreatic intraepithelial neoplasia: evidence that DPC4 inactivation occurs late in neoplastic progression. Cancer Res 2000; 60:2002–6.
25. Evans JD, Cornford PA, Dodson A, et al. Detailed tissue expression of bcl-2, bax, bak and bcl-x in the normal human pancreas and in chronic pancreatitis, ampullary and pancreatic ductal adenocarcinomas. Pancreatology 2001; 1:254–62.

26. Bramhall SR, Neoptolemos JP, Stamp GW, et al. Imbalance of expression of matrix metalloproteinases (MMPs) and tissue inhibitors of the matrix metalloproteinases (TIMPs) in human pancreatic carcinoma. J Pathol 1997; 182:347–55.
27. Keleg S, Buchler P, Ludwig R, et al. Invasion and metastasis in pancreatic cancer. Mol Cancer 2003; 2:14.
28. Crnogorac-Jurcevic T, Efthimiou E, Nielsen T, et al. Expression profiling of microdissected pancreatic adenocarcinomas. Oncogene 2002; 21:4587–94.
29. Eberle MA, Pfutzer R, Pogue-Geile KL, et al. A new susceptibility locus for autosomal dominant pancreatic cancer maps to chromosome 4q32–34. Am J Hum Genet 2002; 70:1044–8.
30. Marshall E. Gene therapy. Second child in French trial is found to have leukaemia. Science 2003; 299:320.
31. Lehrman S. Virus treatment questioned after gene therapy death. Nature 1999; 401:517–8.
32. Kurian KM, Watson CJ, Wyllie AH. Retroviral vectors. Molecular Pathology 2000; 53 (4): 173–6.
33. Morgan RA, Anderson WF. Human gene therapy. Annual Review in Biochemistry 1993; 62:191–217.
34. Yu SF, Von Ruden T, Kantoff PW, et al. Self inactivating retroviral vectors designed for transfer of whole genes into mammalian cells. Proceedings of the National Academy of Science USA 1986; 83 (10):3194–98.
35. Humphreys MJ, Greenhalf W, Neoptolemos JP, et al. The potential for gene therapy in pancreatic cancer. International Journal of Pancreatology 1999; 1:5–21.
36. Burns JC, Friedman T, Driever W, et al. Vesicular stomatitis virus G glycoprotein psudotyped retroviral vectors: concentration to very high titre and efficient gene transfer into mammalian and non-mammalian cells. Proceedings of the National Academy of Science USA 1993; 90 (17):8033–37.
37. Friedman T (ed). The development of human gene therapy. Cold spring harbour laboratory press, New York, 1999.
38. Gollan TJ, Green MR. Selective targeting and inducible destruction of human cancer cells by retroviruses with envelope proteins bearing short peptide ligands. J Virol 2002; 76:3564–9.
39. Erlwein O, Wels W, Schnierle BS. Chimeric ecotropic MLV envelope proteins that carry EGF receptor-specific ligands and the Pseudomonas exotoxin A translocation domain to target gene transfer to human cancer cells. Virology 2002; 302:333–41.
40. Yang Y, Su Q, Wilson JM. Role of viral antigens in destructive cellular immune response to adenoviral vector transduced cells in mouse lung. Journal of Virology 1996; 70 (10):7209–12.
41. Somia N, Verma IM. Gene therapy: Trials and Tribulations. Nature Genetics 2000; 92:91–99.
42. Wesseling JG, Bosma PJ, Krasnykh V, et al. Improved gene transfer efficiency to primary and established human pancreatic carcinoma target cells via epidermal growth factor receptor and integrin-targeted adenoviral vectors. Gene Ther 2001; 8:969.
43. Kleeff J, Fukahi K, Lopez ME, et al. Targeting of suicide gene delivery in pancreatic cancer cells via FGF receptors. Cancer Gene Ther 2002; 9:522–32.
44. Kotin RM, Siniscalo M, Samulski RJ, et al. Site specific integration of adeno-associated virus. Proceedings of the National Academy of Science USA 1990; 87 (6):2211–15.
45. Carter PJ, Samulski RJ. Adeno associated viral vectors as gene delivery vehicles. International Journal of Molecular Medicine 2000; 6 (1):17–27.
46. Yan Z, Zhang Y, Duan D, et al. Trans splicing vectors expand the utility of adeno-associated virus for gene therapy. Proceedings of the National Academy of Science USA 2000; 97 (12):6716–21.
47. Nakai H, Storm TA, Kay MA. Increasing the size of rAAV-mediated expression cassettes in vivo by intermolecular joining of two complimentary vectors. Nature Biotechnology 2000; 18 (5):527–32.
48. Peng L, Sidner RA, Bochan MR, et al. Construction of recombinant adeno-associated virus vector containing the rat preproinsulin II gene. Journal of Surgical Research 1997; 69: 193–8.
49. Kasuya H, Mizuno M, Yoshida J, et al. Combined effects of adeno-associated virus vector and a herpes simplex virus mutant as neoplastic therapy. Journal of Surgical Oncology 2000; 74 (3):214–8.
50. Aspinall RJ, Lemoine NR. Gene therapy for pancreatic and billiary malignancy. Annals of Oncology 1999; 10 (Suppl 4):188–92.
51. Costello E, Munoz M, Buetti E, et al. Gene transfer into stimulated and unstimulated T lymphocytes by HIV-1-derived lentiviral vectors. Gene Therapy 2000; 7:596–604.

52. Mityoshi H, Smith KA, Mosier DE, et al. Transduction of human CD34+ cells that mediate long term-term engraftment of NOD/SCID mice by HIV vectors. Science 1999; 283 (540Z):682–686.
53. Case SS, Price MA, Jordan CT, et al. Stable transduction of quienscent CD34+ CD38- human haematopoetic cells b HIV-1-based lentiviral vectors. Proc Natl Acad Sci USA 1999; 96 (6):2988–93.
54. Pfeifer A, Kessler T, Silletti S, et al. Suppression of angiogenesis by lentiviral delivery of PEX, a noncatalytic fragment of matrix metalloproteinase 2. Proceeding of the National Academy of Science USA 2000; 97 (22):12227–32.
55. Colmenero P, Chen M, Castanos-Velez E, et al. Immunotherapy with recombinant SFV-replicons expressing the P815A tumor antigen or IL-12 induces tumor regression. Int J Cancer 2002; 98:554–6.
56. Tan BT, Wu L, Berk AJ. An Adenovirus-Epstein Barr virus hybrid that stably transforms cultured cells with high efficiency. Journal of Virology 1999; 73 (9):7582–89.
57. Feng M, Jackson WH, Goldman KR, et al. Stable in vivo transduction via a novel adenoviral/retroviral chimeric vector. Nature Biotechnology 1997; 15 (9):866–70.
58. Bischoff J, Kim DH, Williams A, et al. An adenovirus mutant that replicates selectively in p53-defecient human tumour cells. Science 1996; 274 (5286):373–6.
59. Mulvihill S, Warren R, Venook A, et al. Safety and feasibility of injection with an E1B-55 kDa gene-deleted, replication-selective adenovirus (ONYX-015) into primary carcinomas of the pancreas: a phase I trial. Gene Ther 2001; 8:308–15.
60. Motoi F, Sunamura M, Ding L, et al. Effective gene therapy for pancreatic cancer by cytokines mediated by restricted replication competent adenovirus. Human Gene Therapy 2000; 11 (2):223–35.
61. Stevenson AJ, Giles MS, Hall KT, et al. Specific oncolytic activity of herpesvirus saimiri in pancreatic cancer cells. Br J Cancer 2000; 83 (3):329–32.
62. Krieg AMJ. Direct immunologic activities of CpG DNA and implications for gene therapy. Journal of Gene Medicine 1999; 1:56–63.
63. Taniyama Y, Tachibana K, Hiraoka K, et al. Development of safe and efficient novel nonviral gene transfer using ultrasound: enhancement of transfection efficiency of naked plasmid DNA in skeletal mus. Gene Ther 2002; 9:372–80.
64. Farwood H, Gao X, Son K, et al. Cationic liposomes for direct gene transfer in therapy of cancer and other diseases. Annals of the New York Academy of Science 1994; 31:23–34.
65. Gottschalk S, Sprawwow JT, Hauer J, et al. A novel DNA-peptide complex for efficient gene transfer and expression in mammalian cells. Gene Therapy 1996; 3:448–57.
66. Wagner E, Zenke M, Cotton M, et al. Transferrin-polycation conjugates as carriers for DNA uptake into cells. Proceeding of the National Academy of Science USA 1990; 87 (9):3410–14.
67. Boussif O, Zanta MA, Behr JP. Optimised galenics improve in-vitro gene transfer by cationic molecules up to 1000-fold. Gene Therapy 1996; 3:1074–8.
68. Schmid RM, Weidenbach H, Yamagushi H, et al. Direct gene transfer into the rat pancreas using DNA-liposomes. Eur J Clin Invest 1998; 28 (3):220–26.
69. Dauty E, Behr JP, Remy JS. Development of plasmid and oligonucleotide nanometric particles Gene Ther 2002; 9:743–8.
70. Fominaya J, Ukerek C, Wels W. A chimeric fusion protein containing transforming growth factor-alpha mediates gene transfer via binding to the EGF receptor. Gene Therapy 1998; 5:521–30.
71. Lipps HJ, Jenke AC, Nehlsen K, et al. Chromosome-based vectors for gene therapy. Gene 2003; 304:23–33.
72. Wesseling JG, Yamamoto M, Adachi Y, et al. Midkine and cyclooxygenase-2 promoters are promising for adenoviral vector gene delivery of pancreatic carcinoma. Cancer Gene Ther 2001; 8:990.
73. Ohashi M, Kanai F, Tanaka T, et al. In vivo adenovirus-mediated prodrug gene therapy for carcinoembryonic antigen-producing pancreatic cancer. Jpn J Cancer Res 1998; 89:457–62.
74. Van Weering DH, de Rooij J, Marte B, et al. Protein kinase B activation and lamellipodium formation are independent phosphoinositide 3-kinase-mediated events differentially regulated by endogenous ras. Molecular Cell Biology 1998; 18 (4):1802–11.

75. Balmain A. Target genes and target cells in carcinogenesis. Br J Cancer 1999; 80:28–33.
76. Katoh H, Kuzumaki N, Shichinohe T, et al. Suppression of pancreatic cancer by the dominant negative ras mutant, N116Y. J Surg Res 1996; 66:125–30.
77. Takeuchi M, Shichinohe T, Senmaru N, et al. The dominant negative H-ras mutant, N116Y, suppresses growth of metastatic human pancreatic cancer cells in the liver of nude mice. Gene Therapy 2000; 7 (6):518–26.
78. Hirano T, Shino Y, Saito T, et al. Dominant negative MEKK1 inhibits survival of pancreatic cancer cells. Oncogene 2002; 21:5923–8.
79. Gjertsen M, Bjorheim J, Saeserdal I, et al. Cytotoxicity CD4+ and CD8+ T lymphocytes generated by mutant p21-ras (12 val) peptide vaccination of a patient recognise 12 val dependant nested epitopes present with in the vaccine peptide and kill autologous tumour cells carrying this mutant. International J Cancer 1997; 72:784–90.
80. Gjertson M, Saeserdal I, Thorsby E, et al. Characterisation of immune response in pancreatic cancer patients after mutant p21-ras peptide vaccination. Br J Cancer 1996; 74:1828–33.
81. Jaffee EM, Schutte M, Gossett J, et al. Development and characterisation of a cytokine-secreting pancreatic adenocarcinoma vaccine from primary tumours for use in clinical trials. Cancer Journal Science American 1998; 4:194–203.
82. Mukhopadhyay T, Roth JA. Antisense regulation of oncogenes in human cancer. Critical Review in Oncogenesis 1996; 7:151–90.
83. Aoki K, Yoshida T, Matsumoto N, et al. Suppression of p21-ras levels leading to growth inhibition of pancreatic cancer cell lines with Ki-ras muations but not those with out Ki-ras mutations. Molecular Carcinogenesis 1997; 20:251–58.
84. Aoki K, Yoshida T, Sugimura T, et al. Liposome-mediated in vivo gene transfer of antisense K-ras construct inhibits pancreatic tumour dissemination in the murine peritoneal cavity. Cancer Research 1995; 55:3810–16.
85. Su Z, Lebedeva IV, Gopalkrishnan RV, et al. A combinatorial approach for selectively inducing programmed cell death in human pancreatic cancer cells. Proc Natl Acad Sci USA 2001; 98:10332–7.
86. Kijima H, Scanlon KJ. Ribozyme as an approach for growth suppression of human pancreatic cancer. Molecular Biotechnology 2000; 14:59–72.
87. Aoki Y, Cioca DP, Oidaira H, et al. RNA interference may be more potent than antisense RNA in human cancer cell lines. Clin Exp Pharmacol Physiol 2003; 30:96–102.
88. Lemoine NR, Jain S, Hughes CM, et al. Ki-ras oncogene activation in pre-invasive pancreatic adenocarcinoma. Gastoenterology 1992; 102:230–6.
89. Mukhopadhyay T, Roth JA. Antisense regulation of oncogenes in human cancer. Critical Review in Oncogenesis 1996; 7:151–90.
90. Schweinfest CW, Grabber MW, Chapman JM, et al. CaSm: an Sm like protein that contributes to the transformed state in cancer cells. Cancer Research 1997; 57 (14):2961–5.
91. Kelley JR, Brown JM, Frasier MM, et al. The cancer-associated Sm-like oncogene: A novel target for the gene therapy of pancreatic cancer. Surgery 2000; 128 (2):353–60.
92. Kelley JR, Fraser MM, Schweinfest CW, et al. CaSm/gemcitabine chemo-gene therapy leads to prolonged survival in a murine model of pancreatic cancer. Surgery 2001; 130:280–8.
93. Barton CM, McKie MB, Hogg A, et al. Abnormalities of the rb1 and dcc tumour suppresser genes-uncommon in human pancreatic adenocarcinoma. Molecular Carcinogenesis 1995; 13 (2):61–9.
94. Schreiber M, Muller WJ, Singh G, et al. Comparison of the effectiveness of adenovirus vectors expressing cyclin kinase inhibitors $p16^{INK4A}$, $p18^{INK4C}$, $p19^{INK4D}$, $p21^{WAF1/CIP1}$ and $p27^{KIP1}$inin-ducing cell cycle arrest, apoptosis and inhibition of tumourigenicity. Oncogene 1999; 18:1663–76.
95. Kobayashi S, Shirasawa H, Sashiyama H, et al. $p16^{INK4a}$ expression adenovirus vector to suppress pancreas cancer cell proliferation. Clin Cancer Res 1999; 5 (12):4182–85.
96. Fujimoto K, Hosotani R, Miyamoto Y, et al. Inhibition of pRb phosphorylation and cell cycle progression by an antennapedia-p16 (INK4A) fusion peptide in pancreatic cancer cells. Cancer Letters 2000; 159 (2):151–8.

97. Ghaneh P, Greenhalf W, Humpreys M, et al. Adenovirus mediated transfer of p53 and $p16^{INK4A}$ results in pancreatic cancer regression in vitro and in vivo. Gene Therapy 2001; 8:199–208.
98. Sandig V, Brand K, Herwig S, et al. Adenovirally transferred $p16^{INK4A}$ and p53 genes cooperate to induce apoptotic tumour cell death. Nat Med 1997; 3 (3):313–19.
99. King TC, Estalilla OC, Safran H. Role of p53 and p16 gene alterations in determining response to concurrent paclitaxel and radiation in solid tumour. Seminars in Radiation Oncology 1999; 9:4–11.
100. Stone S, Dayananth P, Kamb A. Reversible, p16 mediated cell cycle arrest as protection from chemotherapy. Cancer Research 1996; 56:3199–3202.
101. Fueyo J, Gomez-Manzano C, Puduvalli VK, et al. Adenovirus-mediated p16 transfer to glioma cells induces G_1 arrest and protects from praclitaxel and topptecan: implications for therapy. Intl J Oncology 1998; 12:665–69.
102. Fukuoka K, Adachi J, Nishio K, et al. p16INK4A expression is associated with the increased sensitivity of human non-small cell lung cancer cells to DNA topoisomerse inhibitors. Japan J Cancer Res 1997; 88 (10):1009–16.
103. Chow LSN, Wang X, Kwong DLW, et al. Effect of $p16^{INK4A}$ on chemosensitivity in nasopharygeal carcinoma cells. Intl J Oncology 2000; 17:135–140.
104. Oliner JD, Pietenpol JA, Thiagallingam S, et al. Oncoprotein MDM2 conceals the activation domain of tumour suppresser p53. Nature 1993; 362 (29):857–60.
105. Momand J, Zambetti GP, Olson DC, et al. The mdm-2 Oncogene product forms a complex with the p53 protein and inhibits p53-mediated transactivation. Cell 1992; 69:1237–45.
106. Roth J, Dobbelstein M, Freedman DA, et al. Nucleo-cytoplasmic shuttling of the hdm2 oncoprotein regulates the levels of the p53 protein via a pathway used by the human immunodeficiency virus rev protein. Eur Mol Bio J 1998; 17 (2):554–64.
107. Boyd MT, Vlatkovic N, Haines DS. A novel cellular protein (MTBP) binds to MDM2 and induces a G_1 arrest that is suppressed by MDM2. J Bio Chem 2000; 275 (41):31883–31890.
108. Boyd MT, Zimonjic DB, Popescu NC, et al. Assaignment of the MDM2 binding protein gene (MTBP) to human chromosome band 8q24 by in situ hybridisation. Cytogentetics and Cell Genetics 2000; 90:64–5.
109. Barton CM, Staddon SL, Hughes CM, et al. Abnormalities of the p53 tumour suppressor gene in human pancreatic cancer. Bri J Cancer 1991; 64:1076–82.
110. Bouvet M, Bold RJ, Lee J, et al. Adenovirus-mediated wild-type p53 tumour suppresser gene therapy induces apoptosis and suppresses growth of human pancreatic cancer. Ann of Surg Oncology 1998; 5 (8):681–88.
111. Cascallo M, Mercade E, Capella G, et al. Genetic background determines the response to adenovirus-mediated wild-type expression in pancreatic tumour cells. Cancer Gene Therapy 1999; 6 (5):428–36.
112. Chang EH, Pirollo KF, Bouker KB. Tp53 gene therapy: a key to modulating resistance to anticancer therapies. Molecular Medicine Today 2000; 6:358–65.
113. Osaki S-I, Nakanishi Y, Takayama K, et al. Alteration of drug chemo sensitivity caused by the adenovirus-mediated transfer of the wild-type p53 gene in human lung cancer cells. Cancer Gene Therapy 2000; 7 (2):300–7.
114. Merlin Thomas, Brandner G, Hess RD. Cell cycle arrest in ovarian cancer cell lines does not depend on p53 status upon treatment with cytostatic drugs. Intl J Oncology 1998; 13:1007–16.
115. Cascalló M, Calbo J, Lluis Gelpi J, et al. Modulation of drug cytotoxicity by reintroduction of wild-type p53 gene (Ad5CMV-p53) in human pancreatic cancer. Cancer Gene Therapy 2000; 7 (4):545–56.
116. Phillips AC, Vousden KH. E2F-1 induced apoptosis. Apoptosis 2001; 6:173–182.
117. Elliott MJ, Farmer MR, Atienza C Jr, et al. E2F-1 gene therapy induces apoptosis and increases chemosensitivity in human pancreatic carcinoma cells. Tumour Biol 2002 Mar–Apr; 23 (2):76–86.
118. Rodicker F, Stiewe T, Zimmermann S, et al. Therapeutic efficacy of E2F1 in pancreatic cancer correlates with TP73 induction. Cancer Res 2001 Oct 1; 61 (19):7052–5.
119. Clary BM, Coveney EC, Philip R, et al. Inhibition of established pancreatic cancers following specific active immunotherapy with interleukin-2 gene-transduced tumour cells. Cancer Gene Ther 1997; 4:97–104.

120. Kimura M, Tagawa M, Takenaga K, et al. Loss of tumorigenicity of human pancreatic carcinoma cells engineered to produce interleukin-2 or interleukin-4 in nude mice: a potentiality for cancer gene therapy. Cancer Letts 1998; 128:47–53.
121. Yoshida Y, Tasaki K, Kimurai M, et al. Anti-tumour effect of human pancreatic cancer cells transduced with cytokine genes which activate Thl helper T cells. Anticancer Res 1998; 18:333–336.
122. Peplinski GR, Tsung K, Meko JB, et al. In vivo gene therapy of a murine pancreatic tumour with recombinant vaccina virus encoded human interleukin 1 beta. Surgery 1995; 118:185–191.
123. Jaffee EM, Abrams R, Cameron J, et al. A phase I clinical trial of lethally irradiated allogeneic pancreatic tumour cells transfected with GM-CSF gene for treatment of pancreatic adenocarcinoma. Humna Gene Ther 1998; 9 (13):195–71.
124. Alters SE, Gadea JR, Philip R. Immunotherapy of cancer-generation of CEA specific cytotoxic T lymphocytes using CEA pulsed dendritic cells. Adv Exp Med Biol 1997; 417:519–524.
125. Stift A, Friedl J, Dubsky P, et al. In vivo induction of dendritic cell-mediated cytotoxicity against allogeneic pancreatic carcinoma cell. Int J Oncol 2003 Mar; 22 (3):651–6.
126. Sawada T, Yamada O, Yoshimura N, et al. Xenoantigen, an alphaGal epitope-expression construct driven by the hTERT-promoter, specifically kills human pancreatic cancer cell line. Cancer Cell Int 2002; 2:14.
127. DiMaio JM, Clary BM, Dan FV, et al. Directed enzyme pro-drug gene therapy for pancreatic cancer in vivo. Surgery 1994; 116:205–213.
128. Carrio M, Romagosa A, Mercade E, et al. Enhanced pancreatic tumour regression by a combination of adenovirus and retrovirus-mediated delivery of the herpes simplex virus thymidine kinase gene. Gene Ther 1999; 6:547–553.
129. Evoy D, Hirschowitz EA, Naama HA, et al. In vivo adenoviral-mediated gene transfer in the treatment of pancreatic cancer. J Sur Res 1997; 69:226–231.
130. Green NK, Youngs DJ, Neoptolemos JP, et al. Sensitization of colorectal and pancreatic cancer cell lines to the prodrug 5-(aziridin-1-yl)-2, 4-dinitrobenzamide (CB1954) by retroviral transduction and expression of the E. coli nitroreductase gene. Cancer Gene Ther 1997; 4:229–238.
131. Lohr M, Muller P, Karle P, et al. Targeted chemotherapy by intratumoral injection of encapsulated cells engineered to produce CYP2B1, an isofamide activating cytochrome P450. Gene Ther 1998; 5:1070–1078.
132. Lohr M, Hoffmeyer A, Kroger J, et al. Microencapsulated cell-mediated treatment of inoperable pancreatic carcinoma. Lancet 2001; 357:1591–2.
133. Miki K, Xu M, Gupta A, et al. Methioninase cancer gene therapy with selenomethionine as suicide prodrug substrate. Cancer Res 2001 Sep 15; 61 (18):6805–10.
134. Rigg AS, Lemoine NR. Adenoviral delivery of TIMP1 or TIMP2 can modify the invasive behavior of pancreatic cancer and can have a significant antitumor effect in vivo. Cancer Gene Ther 2001 Nov; 8 (11):869–78.
135. Hoshida T, Sunamura M, Duda DG, et al. Gene therapy for pancreatic cancer using an adenovirus vector encoding soluble flt-1 vascular endothelial growth factor receptor. Pancreas 2002 Aug; 25 (2):111–21.
136. Funatomi H, Itakura J, Ishiwata I, et al. Amphiregullin antisense oligonucleotide inhibits the growth of T3M4 human pancreatic cancer cells and sensitizes the cells to EGF receptor-targeted therapy. Int J Cancer 1997; 72:512–517.
137. Brysch WE, Magal JC, Louis M, et al. Inhibition of p185c-erbB-2 proto-oncogene expression by antisense oligodeoxynucleotide down-regulates p185-associated tyrosine-kinase activity and strongly inhibits mammary tumour-cell proliferation. Cancer Gene Ther 1994; 1:99–105.
138. Saimura M, Nagai E, Mizumoto K, et al. Tumor suppression through angiogenesis inhibition by SUIT-2 pancreatic cancer cells genetically engineered to secrete NK4. Clin Cancer Res 2002; 8:3243–9.
139. Pirocanac EC, Nassirpour R, Yang M, et al. Bax-induction gene therapy of pancreatic cancer. J Surg Res 2002; 106:346–???.
140. Yin S, Bailiang W, Xie K, et al. Adenovirus-mediated N5 gene transfer inhibits tumor growth and metastasis of human carcinoma in nude mice. Cancer Gene Ther 2002; 9:665–72.

141. Palmer Smith J, Verderame MF, Zagon IS. Antisense oligonucleotides to gastrin inhibit growth of human pancreatic cells. Cancer Letts 1999; 135:107–112.
142. Vernejoul F, Faure P, Benali N, et al. Antitumor effect of in vivo somatostatin receptor subtype 2 gene transfer in primary and metastatic pancreatic cancer models. Cancer Res 2002; 62:6124–31.

10 Suicide Gene Therapy for Pancreatic Cancer

Amor Hajri

Pancreatic cancer is the fifth most common cause of cancer death in Europe and USA. Despite increasing interest and research focusing on pancreatic cancer, the prognosis is still poor and less than 10% of patients survive five years even when conventional treatment can be accomplished.[1,2] Operability is relatively low and the majority of patients present with advanced and metastatic disease in which radiotherapy and chemotherapy are ineffective.[3,4] The efficacy of the conventional approaches is often hampered by an insufficient therapeutic index, lack of specificity, and the emergence of drug-resistant cell subpopulations. One approach aimed at enhancing the selectivity of cancer chemotherapy for solid tumors relies on the application of gene therapy technologies. Gene therapy, one of the most progressive and exciting areas of biomedical research, has undergone rapid development over the past decade. Significant research progress has been made in the development and refinement of viral and non-viral vectors for gene transfer in vitro and in vivo.[5–8]

Strategies in Cancer Gene Therapy

The essential strategies in cancer gene therapy are: expression of suicide genes, expression of cytokines and chymokines to stimulate antitumoral cellular immune response, genes enhancing the tumor-cell immunogenicity, blocking of oncogenes, introduction of tumor suppressor genes, and blocking tumor angiogenesis.[5,9]

Chemotherapy using cytotoxic drugs is one of the mainstays of current cancer therapy. Although it is effective in various cancer cases, patients often suffer serious adverse events due to non-specific damage of healthy cells. Doses must therefore be limited for safety reasons. The objective is to develop a safer chemotherapeutic approach using gene delivery to target the cytotoxic drug into tumor cells. New strategies are necessary to treat pancreatic cancer and gene therapy offers hope in this regard. Many studies have shown promising results of gene therapy in the treatment of pancreatic cancer in rodent models. A remarkable research effort has recently focused on the possibility of rendering cancer cells more sensitive to chemotherapeutics by introducing 'suicide genes'.

Suicide Gene Therapy

Suicide genes encode for enzymes that metabolize non toxic prodrugs into highly toxic substances thereby killing the transduced cells. Gene therapy of malignant tumors using suicide genes is performed in two steps. First, the tumor cells are transduced with the vector expressing the suicide gene and, in the second step, the non toxic prodrug is administrated systemically (Fig. 10.1). The suicide gene/prodrug system also known as gene-directed enzyme prodrug therapy (GDEPT) or virus-directed enzyme prodrug therapy (VDEPT),[10–13] may be used in isolation or combined with other strategies. VDEPT using selectively replicating viruses as vectors represents a promising means to target suicide genes specifically to tumor cells, an approach that is only beginning to be explored. Ideally, the gene encoding the enzyme should be expressed exclusively in the tumor cells and should reach the concentration sufficient to activate the prodrug for clinical benefit.

HSV-TK Gene

A variety of suicide genes encoding different types of enzymes have been investigated for their potential use in cancer gene therapy (Table 10.1). To date, the most commonly used suicide gene for the treatment of various cancers is herpes simplex virus thymidine kinase (HSV-TK) with the prodrug gancyclovir

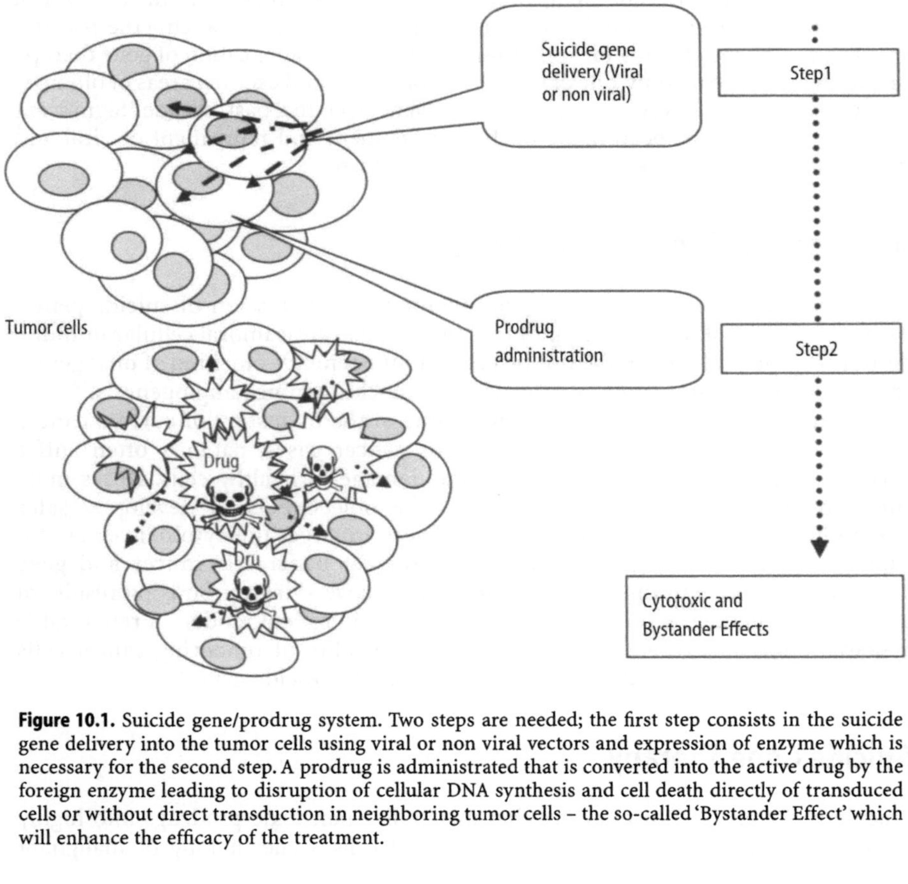

Figure 10.1. Suicide gene/prodrug system. Two steps are needed; the first step consists in the suicide gene delivery into the tumor cells using viral or non viral vectors and expression of enzyme which is necessary for the second step. A prodrug is administrated that is converted into the active drug by the foreign enzyme leading to disruption of cellular DNA synthesis and cell death directly of transduced cells or without direct transduction in neighboring tumor cells – the so-called 'Bystander Effect' which will enhance the efficacy of the treatment.

Table 10.1. Suicide gene encoding for enzymes which have been investigated for use in cancer gene therapy

Suicide gene	Prodrug
HSV-TK	GCV, ACV, BvdU
CD (E.coli,yeast)	5-FC
XGPRT (E. coli gpt)	6-TX
NT (Nitorreductase)	CB1954
PNP (E.coli DeoD)	6-MePdR
Cytochrome P450 2B1	CFA
dCK	ara-C

(GCV) (14, 15). The drug GCV is nontoxic as long as it is not metabolized. It is a poor substrate for human TK but is metabolized to monophosphate GCV (MP-GCV) by HSV-TK. Subsequently, cellular enzymes convert MP-GCV to triphosphate-GCV, which is incorporated into DNA and RNA. This confers cytotoxicity and cell death by termination of DNA and RNA synthesis. Therefore, tumor cells expressing HSV-TK may be selectively killed by GCV treatment.

Makinen et al.[16] have reported that HSV-TK gene transfer followed by GCV treatment is efficient in killing pancreatic cancer cells in vitro, in a transduced subcutaneous tumor model, as well as in in vivo transduced pancreatic tumors using an immunocompetent animal model. These results highlight the potential of gene therapy to treat experimental pancreatic cancer. Rosenfeld et al.[17] demonstrated that pancreatic carcinoma cells are highly susceptible to transduction with recombinant adenoviral vector expressing HSV-TK gene and elicit a potent bystander effect on neighboring tumor cells. In this experiment, pancreatic tumor cells injected intraperitoneally into nude mice resulted in significant tumor formation. The treatment of animals with Ad-CMV/HSV-TK and GCV induced a dramatic decrease in overall tumor burden for up to 8 weeks post-GCV treatment.

CD Gene

Another widely used suicide gene is the bacterial, fungal and yeast genes encoding cytosine deaminase (CD), which deaminate cytosine to uracil and 5-fluorocytosine (5-FC) to 5-fluorouracil (5-FU). Due to a lack of CD in mammalian cells, the CD gene has become an attractive candidate for chemogene cancer therapy.[18] Transfer of the CD gene to tumor cells allows conversion of relatively non-toxic 5-FC to 5-FU. The latter inhibits both RNA and DNA synthesis and leads to cell death. Several reports have demonstrated that the anti-cancer effect of CD/5-FC system gene therapy provides a strong bystander effect that does not require direct cell-to-cell contact.[19] It was shown that CD/5-FC gene therapy system can enhance the effect of radiation in vitro and in vivo.[20–23]

In our laboratory, we have demonstrated that both HSV-TK/GCV and eCD/5-FC systems have an effective antitumor activity on different pancreatic adenocarcinoma models. These suicide gene/prodrug systems inhibit the pancreatic tumor cell growth in a dose and time-dependent manner as indicated by the [^{3}H]thymidine incorporation and MTT toxicity tests (Fig. 10.2).

The antiproliferative effect could be directly via the inhibition of protein, RNA and DNA synthesis and/or indirectly via apoptosis induction as shown by the Hoechst reaction and the DNA ladder analysis (Fig. 10.3 and 10.4).

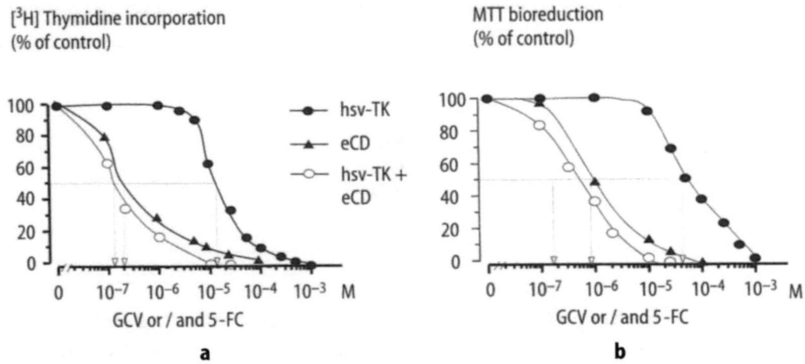

Figure 10.2. **a** Effects of increasing concentrations of specific prodrugs of suicide gene on rat pancreatic tumor cell DNA synthesis and **b** viability transduced with suicide genes encoding *herpes virus simplex* thymidine kinase (●), *Escherichia coli* cytosine deaminase (▲) or a combination of the two enzymes (○). HA-RPC cell proliferation was assayed via [^{3}H]thymidine incorporation into DNA and cell viability by measuring the reduction of biomass using MTT. Data, expressed as a percentage of the mean value of untreated control cells, are the means from three independent experiments.

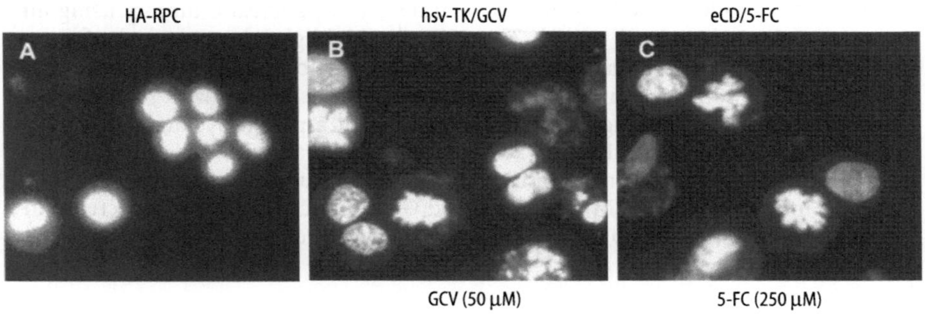

Figure 10.3. Identification of apoptotic bodies on fluorescence micrographs of parental HA-RPC tumor cells (A) or after suicide gene transduction with HSV-TK (B) or eCD (C). Cells were managed for apoptosis detection with either Hoechst 33342 processing. The parental cell line showed after staining well-shaped nuclei. After addition of their specific substrates the presence of a suicide gene expression gave numerous condensed nuclei corresponding to apoptotic bodies.

In different experimental studies on pancreatic tumor cell lines, we have shown that eCD/5-FC is more efficient than HSV-TK/GCV system (Fig. 10.2 and 10.3).

The therapeutic index of HSV-TK/GCV system is higher, but its bystander effect is lower than that of eCD/5-FC system (Fig. 10.5). *In vivo*, we used a rat hepatic metastasis model to investigate the effect of eCD gene transfer into rat pancreatic adenocarcinoma expressing eCD. The hepatic metastasis model was developed after injection of pancreatic adenocarcinoma HA-RPC cell line stably transfected with eCD. All the animals treated with 5-FC (250 mg/kg) were metastases free. The actuarial survival study indicated that all the animals injected with the pancreatic tumor cells HA-RPC expressing eCD in combination with 5-FC treatment were alive after 150 days. These results indicate that eCD/5-FC system could be very efficient in inhibiting the pancreatic tumor growth and the development of metastases. In this experiment we observed that one third of the animals receiving the eCD/HA-RPC cells without 5-FC treatment survived (Fig. 10.6). Indirectly, these results suggest that the eCD gene expression induces an anti-tumor immune response.

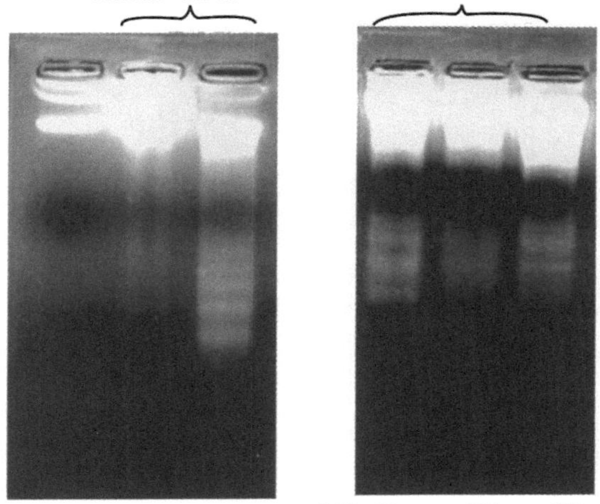

Figure 10.4. Agarose gel electrophoresis of DNA showing the substrate dose-dependence of DNA fragmentation of HSV-TK and eCD-transduced HA-HPC tumor cells. The characteristic pattern of internucleosomal DNA cleavage (*e.g.* DNA ladder), indicative of nuclease activation, was from 100 μM of Ganciclovir and from 40 μM of 5-fluorocytosine.

UPRT Gene

More recently, it was demonstrated that uracil phosphoribosyltransferase (UPRT) gene, encoding enzyme to convert 5-FU to 5-fluoroluridine 5'-monophosphaste, renders the tumor cells more sensitive to 5-FU treatment.[24] In the same way, it is conceivable that the UPRT gene coexpression with eCD gene and 5-FC treatment could be more efficient than the eCD gene expression alone. This approach significantly inhibits the tumor cell growth, and prolonged animal survival in different tumor models.[25,26]

Following these observations, we have decided to apply a double suicide gene therapy strategy to incoporate these interacting therapies using one recombinant vector expressing both the fusion gene eCD:UPRT and HSV-TK.

DeoD Gene

The Escherichia Coli DeoD gene encodes the purine nucleoside phosphorylase (ePNP), another suicide gene which metabolizes certain adenosine analogs like 6-methyl-Purine deoxy-riboside (MePdR) or fludarabine, the mammalian analog is inactive in this regard. E. coli PNP, unlike mammalian PNP, accepts not only oxopurine analogs, but also 6-aminopurine (adenine) analogs as substrates, and hence can be used to selectively cleave certain nontoxic purine nucleosides to very toxic purines and purine analogs.[27] We have constructed a vector expressing ePNP (pCI-ePNP-Neo) and studied its effect in different

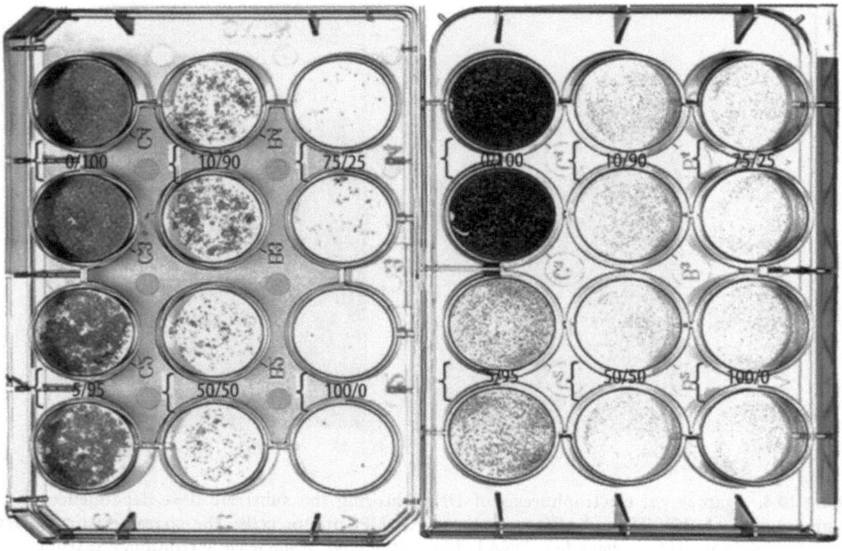

Figure 10.5. Suicide gene bystander-effects were investigated by clonogenicity tests. Ten days after seeding an increasing proportion (from right to left of the 12-well plate) of transduced pancreatic tumor cells mixed with parental cells, viable cells were revealed by Giemsa staining. Significant bystander effect started with at least 5% of transduced cells with both suicide genes. There are more survival cell colonies with 10% transduced tumor cells with hsv-TK/ GCV than eCD/ 5-FC system.

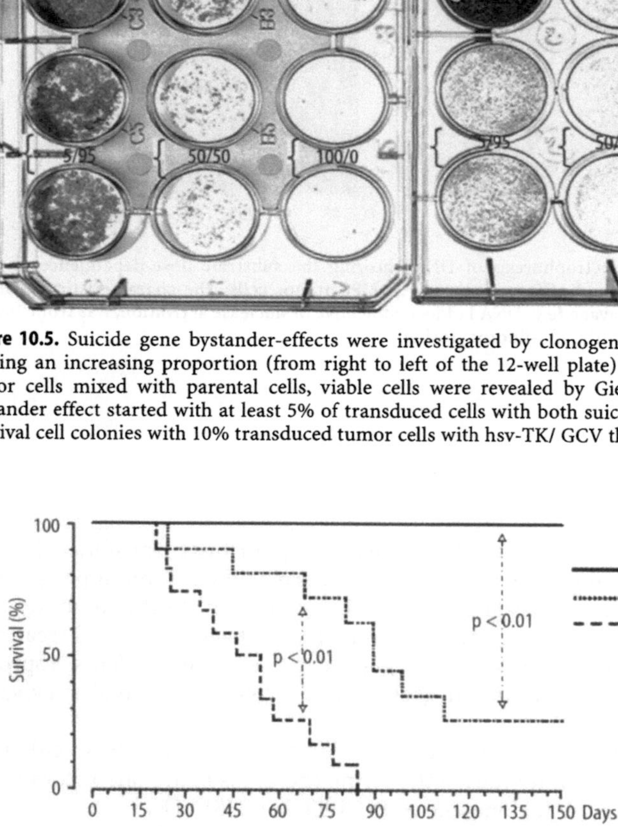

Figure 10.6. Kaplan-Meyer survival curves of rats with hepatic metastasis of an exocrine pancreatic tumor. Survival of rats bearing eCD-transduced HA-RPC metastasis, with or without 5-FC supply, was significantly greater (log rank test) than rats bearing parental pancreatic tumor cells HA-RPC.

pancreatic tumor cell lines. In cell culture, the cytotoxic and proliferative tests revealed a marked and high sensitivity of ePNP-transduced pancreatic tumor cells to MePdR treatment (*manuscript in press; pancreas*). E. coli PNP differs fundamentally from the HSV-TK/GCV system, since direct cell-to-cell contact or gap junctions are not required for ePNP/MePdR system to kill cells. The ePNP enzyme cleaves MePdR to liberate 6-methyl purine (MeP), a potent membrane permeant and freely diffusible toxin. A strong bystander effect is a hall-mark of this approach in different tumor models.

Bystander Effect

Because this therapeutic gene cannot be easily introduced into the whole cell population of a tumor, the successful eradication of tumors depends on a phenomenon called the 'bystander effect', by which the introduced gene can affect cells in which it is not itself present. From a therapeutic point of view, it may be crucial to enhance this phenomenon through various means to achieve tumor eradication.[28,29]

In cancer gene therapy, several reports have demonstrated that even using efficient viral vectors, it is extremely unlikely that every cell in a solid tumor mass could be infected in vivo. The expression of the suicide gene leads to the accumulation of the prodrug-activating enzyme in the transduced cancer cells. Subsequent administration of the prodrug leads to its 'activation' in the cells which contain the enzyme, leading at the site of production to a high local concentration of the cytotoxic species. Importantly, there is local diffusion of the active drug from cells in which it is produced to neighboring cells. In this way, potentially all the cells (or the majority) could be killed in a tumor mass, without requiring that 100% of the tumor cells should be targeted by the suicide gene vector.[23,30–32]

The suicide gene expression will enable transfected cells to metabolize the non-toxic prodrugs into toxic metabolites. These active products can freely diffuse across the cell membrane or can be transferred to neighboring tumor cells via gap junctions causing apoptosis without direct transduction (bystander effect). Neighboring untransduced pancreatic tumor cells will be affected by the suicide gene/ prodrug system-induced bystander effect.

Suicide Gene Expression and Pancreatic Tumor Cell Targeting

The major objective is to develop a safer approach to chemotherapy using gene delivery to target the cytotoxic drug to the tumor cells. Unfortunately, a current limitation of nearly all cancer gene therapy approaches is that the *in vivo* efficiency reached by the therapeutic genes is too low to make them efficacious against most human cancers. Moreover, the suicide gene system requires accurate targeting since gene expression in normal cells followed by exposure to GCV, 5-FC or other prodrug treatment will result in cell death. This problem has been addressed by placing the suicide gene under control of a tissue-specific (or preferably a tumor-specific) promoter so that the gene will be expressed only in a select population of targeted cells. Several experimental studies were made using recombinant vectors in which suicide gene expression is controlled by the DF3/Muc1, CEA or ErbB2 promoters. This appears to provide the appropriate specificity of suicide gene expression for tumor marker-positive pancreatic cancers, although the level of expression probably needs improvement to be really useful. The ideal candidate for transcriptional targeting would be a tumor specific promoter and/or enhancer and its activation will be strong enough to achieve therapeutic levels of the desired transcript.

The possibility of regulating the transgene expression would be a highly desirable feature. There is another considerable interest in molecular-based therapy directed at the K-ras, p16, DPC-4 and p53 proteins. The K-ras proto-oncogene has been identified mutated in 75–90% of pancreatic tumors. The tumor suppressor gene p53 has received much interest due to its high incidence of mutation in cancers.[33] Mutations in p53 occur in about 70% of pancreatic adenocarcinoma.[34] Restoration of the tumor suppressor activity and development of agents interfering with K-ras expression or its biologic activity may provide a significant step forward in the treatment of pancreatic cancer,[35,36] resulting in a far greater therapeutic index than can be achieved by systemic administration of conventional chemotherapy.

Future Directions

Gene therapy is an exciting and promising approach. However, a realistic view is necessary to use the maximum of information from the cell and molecular biology of pancreatic cancer to develop new therapeutic strategies. A key constraint in gene therapy is the vector design for gene delivery and therapeutic gene expression targeting. Only optimization of each of these will result in therapeutic benefit. Improved targeting is based on the development of viral and non-viral methods of delivery and transcriptional promoters of the therapeutic gene that is specific to the tumor. The experimental gene therapy strategies currently employed in the fight against pancreatic cancer include antisense and ribozyme strategies (K-ras), suicide gene/prodrug system, oncolytic viral therapy and promoter gene strategies. It is evident that considerable interest and effort in cancer gene therapy in the next few years would be focused on the targeting and the delivery of therapeutic genes specifically to tumor cells in the patient. To achieve this goal, the suicide gene therapy vector will need (among others requests) to concentrate in the tumor, be selectively activated in the tumor, have a high bystander effect, selectively kill tumor cells, have no adverse effect when expressed in normal cells, and be deactivated once the therapeutic goal is achieved. The first experimental results indicate that the use of double suicide gene prodrug system or the combination of suicide gene with cytokine (IL2) gene expression can lead to a synergistic effect and can be a powerful approach for treatment of cancer.[37–40] Hopefully, one of these novel strategies may extend the current therapeutic repertoire for pancreatic cancers and provide a treatment option for otherwise untreatable patients.

We believe that the combination of different therapeutic gene expressions should be more efficient for the treatment of many cancers including pancreatic cancer. It is conceivable to associate suicide gene expression with other susceptible therapeutic genes such as cytokines, p53 and anti-angiogenesis genes. Cancer gene therapy approaches are often designed as monogene expression; however, the multigenic therapeutic strategy should be more effective. The suicide gene/prodrug system can be used either alone or as an adjuvant to other treatment modalities. Certain genes can sensitize tumor cells to radiation or drugs and hence can be used to enhance the therapeutic effect. Gene therapy continues to represent a challenge to basic science and clinical investigators and there are various approaches being examined in clinical trials to evaluate the success of these gene therapy regimens in humans.

References

1. Ries LAG, Eisner M, Kosary CL, et al. (Eds) SEER Cancer Statistics Review, 1973–1998. Bethesda, Md: National Cancer Institute; 2001.
2. Anderson KE, Potter JD, Mack TM. Pancreatic cancer. In: Schottenfeld D, Fraumani JF, eds. Cancer Epidemiology and Prevention. 2nd ed. New York, NY: Oxford University Press; 1996; 725–771.
3. Graziano F, Catalano G, Cascinu S. Chemotherapy for advanced pancreatic cancer: the history is changing. Tumori 1998; 84:308–11.
4. Bramhall SR, Neoptolemos JP. Adjuvant chemotherapy in pancreatic cancer. Int J Pancreatol 1997; 21:59–63.
5. Mulherkar R. Gene therapy for cancer. Current science 2001; 81:555–560.
6. Pearson AS, Bouvet M, Evans DB, et al. Gene therapy and pancreatic cancer. Frontiers in Bioscience 1998; 1:230–237.
7. Dachs GU, Dougherty GJ, Stratford IJ, et al. Progress in gene therapy for cancer. Oncology Res 1997; 9:313–325.
8. Tuting T, Storkus WJ, Lotze MT. Gene -based strategies for the immunotherapy of cancer. J Mol Med 1997; 75:478–491.
9. Holloran CM, Ghaneh P, Neoptolomos JP, et al. Gene therapy for pancreatic cancer- current and prospective strategies. Surgical Oncology 2000; 9:181–191.
10. Speinger CJ, and Niculescu-Duvaz I. Prodrug-activating systems in suicide gene therapy. The J clinical investigation 1999; 105:1161–1167.
11. Marais R, Spooner RA, Light Y, et al. Gene-directed enzyme prodrug therapy with a mustard prodrug/carboxypeptidase G2 combination. Cancer Res 1996; 56:4735–4742.
12. Bridgewater JA, et al. Expression of the bacterial nitroreductase enzyme in mammalian cells renders them selectively sensitive to killing by the prodrug CB1954. Eur J Cancer 1995; 31A:2362–2370.
13. Huber BE, Richards CA, Austin EA. VDEPT: an enzyme/prodrug gene therapy approach for the treatment of metastatic colorectal cancer. Advanced Drug Delivery 1995; 17:279–292.
14. Whartenby KA, Darnowski JW, Freeman SM, et al. Recombinant interferon alpha2a synergistically enhances ganciclovir-mediated tumor cell killing in the herpes simplex virus thymidine kinase system. Cancer Gene Ther 1999; 6:402–8.
15. Hasegawa H, Shimada M, Yonemitsu Y, et al. Preclinical and therapeutic utility of HVJ liposomes as a gene transfer vector for hepatocellular carcinoma using herpes simplex virus thymidine kinase. Cancer Gene Ther 2001; 8:252–258.
16. Makinen K, Loimas S, Wahlfors J, et al. Evaluation of herpes simplex thymidine kinase mediated gene therapy in experimental pancreatic cancer. J Gene Med 2000; 2:361–367.
17. Rosenfeld ME, Vickers SM, Raben D, et al. Pancreatic carcinoma cell killing via adenoviral mediated delivery of the herpes simplex virus thymidine kinase gene. Ann Surg 1997; 225:609–18.
18. Freeman SM. Suicide gene therapy. Adv Exp Med Bio 2000; 465:411–22.
19. Ichikawa T, Tamiya T, Adachi Y, et al. In vivo efficacy and toxicity of 5-fluorocytosine/cytosine deaminase gene therapy for malignant gliomas mediated by adenovirus. Cancer gene therapy 2000; 7:74–82.
20. Pederson LC, Buchsbaum DJ, Vickers SM, et al. Molecular chemotherapy combined with radiation therapy enhances killing of cholangiocarcinoma cells in vitro and in vivo. Cancer Res 1997; 57:4325–4332.
21. Rogulski KR, Wing MS, Paielli DL, et al. Double suicide gene therapy augments the antitumor activity of a replication-competent lytic adenovirus through enhanced cytotoxicity and radiosensitization. Hum Gene Ther 2000; 11:67–76.
22. Freytag SO, Rogulski KR, Paielli DL, et al. A novel three-pronged approach to kill cancer cells selectively: concomitant viral, double suicide gene, and radiotherapy. Human Gen Ther 1998; 9:1323–1333.
23. Huber BE, Austin EA, Richards CA, et al. Metabolism of 5-fluorocytosine to 5-fluorouracil in human colorectal tumor cells transduced with the cytosine deaminase gene: significant antitumor effects when only a small percentage of tumor cells express cytosine deaminase. Proc Natl Acad Sci USA 1994; 91:8302–83026.
24. Kanai F, Kawakami T, Hamada H, et al. Adenovirus-mediated transduction of Escherichia coli uracil phosphoribosyltransferase gene sensitizes cancer cells to low concentrations of 5-fluorouracil. Cancer Res 1998; 1; 58:1946–1951.
25. Koyama F, Sawada H, Hirao T, et al. Combined suicide gene therapy for human colon cancer cells using adenovirus-mediated transfer of Escherichia coli cytosine deaminase gene and Escherichia coli uracil phosphoribosyltransferase gene with 5-fluorocytosine. Cancer Gene Ther 2000; 7:1015–22.

26. Koyama F, Sawada H, Fuji H, et al. Adenoviral-mediated transfer of Escherichia coli uracil phosphoribosyltransferase (UPRT) gene to modulate the sensitivity of the human colon cancer cells to 5-fluorouracil. Eur J Cancer 2000; 36:2403–2410.
27. Parker WB, King SA, Allan PW, et al. In vivo gene therapy of cancer with E. coli purine nucleoside phosphorylase. Hum Gene Ther 1997; 8:1637–1644.
28. Pope IM, Poston GJ, Kinsella AR. The role of the bystander effect in suicide gene therapy. Eur J Cancer 1997; 33:1005–1016.
29. Imaizumi K, et al. Bystander tumoricidal effect and gap junctional communication in lung cancer cells. Am J Respir Cell Mol Biol 1998; 18:205–212.
30. Friedlos F, Court S, Ford M, et al. Gene-directed enzyme prodrug therapy: quantitative bystander cytotoxicity and DNA damage induced by CB1954 in cells expressing bacterial nitroreductase. Gene Ther 1998; 5:105–112.
31. Boucher PD, Ruch RJ, Shewach DS. Differential ganciclovir- mediated cytotoxicity and bystander killing in human colon carcinoma cell lines expressing herpes simplex virus thymidine kinase. Hum Gene Ther 1998; 9:801–814.
32. Touraine RL, Vahanian N, Ramsey WJ, et al. Enhancement of the herpes simplex virus thymidine kinase/ganciclovir bystander effect and its antitumor efficacy in vivo by pharmacologic manipulation of gap junctions. Hum Gene Ther 1998; 9:2385–91.
33. Sakorafas GH, Tsiotou AG, Tsiotos GG. Molecular biology of pancreatic cancer; oncogenes, tumor suppressor genes, growth factors, and their receptors from a clinical perspective. Cancer Treat Rev 2000; 26:29–52.
34. Berrozpe G, Shaeffer J, Peinado MA, et al. comparative analysis of mutations in the p53 and k-ras genes in pancreatic cancer. Int J Cancer 1994; 58:185–191.
35. Bouvet M, Bold RJ, Lee Evans DB, et al. Adenovirus-mediated wild type p53 tumor suppressor gene therapy induces apoptosis and suppresses growth of human pancreatic cancer. Ann Surg Oncol 1998; 5:681–688.
36. Sakorafas GH, Tsiotos GG. Molecular biology of pancreatic cancer: potential clinical implications. BioDrugs 2001; 15:439–52.
37. Ju DW, Cao X, Tao Q, et al. Augmentation of antitumor effect of adenovirus-mediated CD suicide gene therapy by cotransfer of interleukin 2 gene in melanoma-bearing mice. Chin Med J 1999; 112:162–5.
38. Majumdar AS, Zolotorev A, Samuel S, et al. Efficacy of herpes simplex virus thymidine kinase in combination with cytokine gene therapy in an experimental metastatic breast cancer model. Cancer Gene Ther 2000; 7:1086–99.
39. Chen SH, Kosai K, Xu B, et al. Combination suicide and cytokine gene therapy for hepatic metastases of colon carcinoma: sustained antitumor immunity prolongs animal survival. Cancer Res 1996; 56:3758–62.
40. Palu G, Cavaggioni A, Calvi P, et al. Gene therapy of glioblastoma multiforme via combined expression of suicide and cytokine genes: a pilot study in humans. Gene Ther 1999; 6:330–7.

Pancreatic Cystic Tumours

11 Pancreatic Cystic Lesions and Neoplasms

Markus Kosmahl and Günter Klöppel

The prognosis of the common ductal adenocarcinoma of the pancreas[32] is so poor that proper recognition of those few pancreatic tumours that have a favourable prognosis is of particular importance. The category of cystic lesions and neoplasms of the pancreas includes cystic forms of differing morphology, pathology and biology. All of these tumours are uncommon compared with ductal adenocarcinoma. However, they are of importance because they belong to the curable pancreatic tumours. Until the end of the 1970s the spectrum of cystic diseases of the pancreas was relatively narrow and consisted mainly of serous and mucinous neoplasms.[16,17,26] In the 1980s, the development and widespread use of new imaging techniques led to the discovery and delineation of new categories of cystic and pseudocystic tumours, such as intraductal papillary-mucinous neoplasms (also known as mucinous tumours, mucinous ductal ectasia or intraductal papillary and mucin-hypersecreting tumours)[6] and solid and pseudopapillary neoplasms (also known as solid and cystic tumours).[33] In the past ten years, improvements in imaging techniques and their systematic application in patients suffering from unexplained abdominal symptoms led to a further increase in the number of resected cystic lesions. This in turn advanced our knowledge about these lesions. New entities (such as macrocystic serous cystadenoma,[37] serous oligocystic and ill-demarcated tumour,[19] solid variant of serous cystadenoma,[48] intraductal papillary oncocytic neoplasm,[2] mucinous nonneoplastic cyst[35] and acinar cell cystadenoma[10,15,72] were described and the pathogenesis, morphology and biology of the already known entities were studied in more detail.

From studies of large series of pancreatic lesions and neoplasms with a cystic appearance it is obvious that some entities are much more frequent than others.[5] In our series of 418 cases (Kosmahl and Klöppel, unpublished observations), pseudocysts (16%), intraductal papillary-mucinous neoplasms (IPMNs) (18.3%), mucinous cystic neoplasms (MCNs) (7.6%), serous cystic neoplasms (SCNs) (11%), solid pseudopapillary neoplasms (SPNs) with cystic changes (21.2%) and ductal adenocarcinomas (DACs) with cystic changes (8%) were most frequent. The remaining uncommon cystic tumours included such lesions as lymphoepithelial cysts, cystic endocrine tumours and cystic nonepithelial neoplasms.

In this chapter the currently available information on the clinicopathological features of the common pancreatic cystic lesions# and neoplasms will be reviewed, while the uncommon cystic lesions are only briefly dealt with.

Pseudocysts

A pseudocyst presents as a grossly visible and well demarcated cystic lesion, which contains necrotic-haemorrhagic material and/or turbid fluid rich in pancreatic enzymes. The cystic contents are enclosed by a wall of inflammatory and fibrous tissue devoid of an epithelial cell lining. Pseudocysts usually occur attached to the pancreas and are a sequel of extensive confluent autodigestive tissue necrosis caused by acute pancreatitis.[31]

Pseudocysts are thought to be the most common type of cystic lesions of the pancreas, with an estimated relative frequency of 75%.[24] In our series, pseudocysts account for only 17% of the cases, most likely because this is a series from a referral centre, which accumulates more tumours than pseudocyst cases. The correct prevalence figures may therefore be higher than 17% but probably also lower than 75%, since the 75% figure was generated at a time when only large cystic lesions in the pancreas were detected with certainty.

Pseudocysts develop as a consequence of an episode of severe acute pancreatitis, often in the setting of alcoholic pancreatitis.[31] Most of the patients are men with an age range of 35 to 60 years (Table 11.1). If children and adolescents are affected by pseudocysts, they are caused by hereditary or traumatic pancreatitis.

The most common differential diagnosis of pseudocyst is versus IPMN, MCN and SPN, because the gross appearance of the latter neoplasms may be similar to that of pseudocysts. Histologically and cytologically, however, pseudocysts differ from the cystic neoplasms in that they lack any epithelial lining but display haemorrhagic debris and inflammatory cells. Moreover, pseudocysts contain pancreatic enzymes, such as amylase and lipase, and lack elevated levels of CEA and CA 19-9.[5]

Intraductal Papillary-Mucinous Neoplasms

Among the uncommon exocrine tumours of the pancreas, IPMNs have received increasing attention in recent years because of their clinical picture, favourable prognosis, unclear nature and their obscure relationship to DAC.[6,39] While the diagnosis of IPMNs has improved considerably during the past years, because the

Table 11.1. Clinicopathological features of pseudocysts in the pancreas

- Men : women = 3:1
- Age range, 35–60 years
- Localisation, extrapancreatic > intrapancreatic
- Morphology, no epithelial lining, haemorrhagic debris
- Pathogenesis, caused by severe episodes of acute pancreatitis

The term cystic lesions is used throughout the text to designate any nonneoplastic tumorous change, while the term cystic tumour denotes any cystic lump, regardless of whether it is neoplastic or not.

disease is being recognised better,[6,12,27,30,38,51] the nature of these neoplasms, their pathogenesis and their relationship to DAC have remained obscure. Recent studies, however, seem to throw some light on these issues.

IPMNs are characterised by intraductal proliferation of mucin-producing cells, which are arranged in papillary patterns. In many IPMNs hypersecretion of mucin leads to a cystic dilatation of the involved ducts. In a few IPMNs, focal or diffuse intraductal papillary growth causes duct dilatation. The cytological atypia in IPMNs ranges from minimal to severe; consequently they can be divided into adenomas, borderline tumours and intraductal carcinomas. In addition, intestinal, pancreatobiliary and oncocytic differentiation may be distinguished.[6] Although these neoplasms are usually slow growing tumours, approximately 30% may eventually become invasive and metastasise.[22,30,56] IPMNs are most frequently localised in the main duct of the head region of the pancreas. Those IPMNs that arise from secondary ducts seem to have an even better prognosis than the IPMNs of the main duct.[61]

IPMNs were thought to be very rare, accounting for 1% or less of pancreatic exocrine tumours.[29] However, in recent years better recognition of this neoplasm has led to an increase in its incidence figures. In our series of exocrine pancreatic tumours, the incidence of IPMNs is approximately 3%, and among the cystic neoplasms IPMNs account for 17%. IPMNs occur slightly more frequently in men than in women and the age ranges from 40 to 80 with a mean of 65 years (Table 11.2). Symptoms of acute and/or chronic pancreatitis are most common, but IPMNs may also be detected incidentally. Recently, it was reported that a number of IPMN patients showed an increased rate of extrapancreatic malignancies.[58]

The cause and pathogenesis of IPMN are obscure, but it is interesting to note that in IPMNs that are associated with invasive carcinoma, the invasive component shows either a tubular or a mucinous invasive component. The tubular invasion pattern resembles DAC, while the mucinous pattern shows the features of colloid (mucinous noncystic) carcinoma.

Recent studies in which the mucin production in IPMNs was typed[41,68] have shown that IPMNs with a mucinous invasive component that has the appearance of a colloid (mucinous noncystic) carcinoma produce MUC2, but not MUC1, whereas IPMNs that show an invasive tubular DAC-like component lack MUC2 expression but may stain for MUC1.[7,41,45] In addition to these distinct types of IPMNs, a third type co-expressing MUC 1 and MUC2 was distinguished. This type included the recently described oncocytic subtype of IPMN.[2] From these studies it appears that IPMNs form a heterogeneous group of neoplasms, which can be divided into at least three types on the basis of their mucin immunophenotype, one common MUC2+ type and two less frequent, either MUC2-/MUC1+ or MUC1+/MUC2+ types. While the common MUC2+ IPMNs form one group together with MUC2+ colloid (mucinous noncystic) carcinoma and may be considered to be the precursor of this carcinoma,[8,54] MUC2-/MUC1+ IPMNs

Table 11.2. Clinicopathological features of intraductal papillary-mucinous neoplasms of the pancreas

- Men : women, 1.5 : 1
- Age range: 40–80 years (mean 65)
- Localisation, 80% in the head region
- Morphology, intraductal papillary growth and mucin production
- Prognosis, favourable in at least 70% of patients

appear to have a close relationship to DACs.[41] The third IPMN type, the oncocytic type, may represent a group of its own. The molecular mechanisms involved in the altered regulation of MUC genes in IPMNs are not yet known, but they may be related to a different cell lineage-associated tumorigenesis in these neoplasms. It also appears that the various types of IPMNs also differ in prognosis, since MUC2+ IPMNs obviously fare better than the other IPMNs.[9,45] Recently, IPMNs were observed in two patients with Peutz-Jeghers syndrome.[53]

Mucinous Cystic Neoplasms

MCNs of the pancreas afflict women almost exclusively, involve predominantly the body-tail of the pancreas, do not communicate with the ductal system, and may be unilocular or multilocular.[70] Since the seminal paper by Compagno and Oertel in 1978,[17] there has been a debate about the prognosis and origin of these neoplasms.[62] Two recent studies seem to have settled the first issue.[66,71] On the second issue a hypothesis has been advanced.[71]

More than 90% of MCNs occur in the body and tail of the pancreas, where they form large round cystic tumours showing a unilocular or multilocular cut surface and diameters between 6 and 23 cm.[70] Multilocularity, localisation in the head region and presence of papillary projections and stromal nodules, all correlate with an associated invasive component.[66,71] The cystic spaces are lined by mucin-producing epithelial cells that are supported by an ovarian-like stroma which may be focally hyalinised. MCNs composed of cells exhibiting only minimal atypia are adenomas, those with moderate or even severe atypia are borderline tumours and carcinomas, respectively.[11,34,57] Invasive MCNs show the pattern of either a DAC or an undifferentiated carcinoma with osteoclast-like giant cells. The stroma may also contain sarcomatous nodules.[65]

MCNs comprise approximately 1% in our series of pancreatic exocrine tumours and among the cystic neoplasms they account for approximately 7%. The higher frequencies that have been reported in some previous studies are probably due to the fact that IPMNs and MCNs were not clearly distinguished from each other or were still interpreted as a single entity. The clear differentiation of MCNs from IPMNs also revealed that MCNs are extremely rare in men.[67, 71] The age at diagnosis ranges from 45 to 50 years, though patients with invasive carcinoma are often older than 50 years (Table 11.3). More than 60% of the patients experience abdominal discomfort or pain or present with a palpable tumour. In the remaining patients the tumour is an incidental finding. The cyst fluid is usually rich in CEA and CA 19-9 and contains columnar cells.[50]

The prognosis of MCNs has found to be excellent if the tumours are completely resected, and this can be achieved today in more than 90% of cases 64. Two recent studies based on extensive tumour sampling have shown that recurrence and tumour-related death were features of deeply invasive MCNs only.[66,71]

Table 11.3. Clinicopathological features of mucinous cystic neoplasms

- Women : men = 9 : 1
- Age range, 20–80 years (mean 49)
- Localisation, > 90% in the body-tail region
- Morphology, mucinous cyst without duct communication
- Prognosis, excellent after complete resection

MCNs of the pancreas resemble the same tumour category in the ovary. Like ovarian MCNs, the epithelial cells of pancreatic MCNs show gastroenteropancreatic differentiation[55] and the stromal cells may express oestrogen and progesterone receptors as well as inhibin, which has been recommended as a marker for certain ovarian neoplasms including MCN.[25, 71] Because of this similarity between the pancreatic and ovarian MCNs the 'genital ridge hypothesis' has been advanced, which infers that cellular stromal elements from the genital ridge may associate with the dorsal pancreatic anlage, or rarely the ventral anlage, and might thus later give rise to an MCN.[71]

The differential diagnosis of MCNs is especially versus IPMNs. IPMNs, in contrast to MCNs, communicate with the duct system, are mainly localised in the pancreatic head and occur more often in men than in women. Immunocytochemically, non-invasive MCNs are negative for MUC1 or MUC2 (except for single MUC2 positive goblet cells). Only in cases with an invasive component was MUC1 expression observed.[4]

Serous Cystic Neoplasms

SMAs, SOIAs and VHL-CNs are composed of the same cell type. This cell is characterised by glycogen-rich cytoplasm and a ductal immunoprofile.[13, 16, 19] However, despite these cytological similarities, the three types of SCNs differ in their localisation in the pancreas, their gross appearance, gender distribution and genetic alterations[13], suggesting that they represent different entities (Table 11.4). The role of the solid variant of serous cystic adenoma[48] and of serous cystadenocarcinoma[23] in the spectrum of SCNs is not yet clear, mainly owing to the small number of cases that have been reported so far.[18]

In our series, SMAs equal MCNs in frequency (5.5% *versus* 6.9% of cases). If SOIAs and VHL-CNs are added, the group of SCNs accounts for approximately 10% of all pancreatic cystic lesions and neoplasms. The most common SCN is SMA, which make up 60% of all SCNs. They present as single, well circumscribed, slightly bosselated round tumours, with diameters ranging from 2.5–16 cm. Their cut surface shows numerous small (honeycomb-like) cysts arranged around a (para)central stellate scar, which may contain calcifications. About two thirds of the

Table 11.4. Clinicopathological features of serous cystic tumours of the pancreas

Serous microcystic adenoma (SMA)
- Women : men = 9 : 1
- Age, range 35–90 years (mean 65)
- Localisation, more than 80% in body-tail region, stellate scar
- Prognosis, good

Serous oligocystic adenoma (SOIA)
- Women and men alike
- Age, range 30–70 years (mean 65)
- Localisation, head region
- Prognosis, good

Von Hippel-Lindau associated cystic neoplasms (VHL-CN)
- Women and men alike
- Age range: 30–70 years (mean 42)
- Localisation, diffuse involvement
- Prognosis, good

SMAs occur in the body-tail region and almost all in women.[13] They are usually found incidentally. SOIAs, which account for 30% of SCNs, are composed of few relatively large cysts (for which reason they have also been described as macrocystic serous adenoma),[37] lack the stellate scar and round shape and occur predominantly in the head of the pancreas, where they may obstruct the common bile duct and cause jaundice.[19] They show no sex predilection. In VHL patients the SCNs arise at multiple sites, and in advanced stages of the disease they may merge and involve the entire pancreas.[42,57] Because the VHL-associated cystic lesions affect the pancreas diffusely, they differ markedly from the gross features of both SMAs and SOIAs. Biologically, it is also important to note that VHL patients, like SOIA patients, but in contrast to SMA patients, are not predominantly female. This suggests that SMAs differ in their pathogenesis from VHL-CNs and SOIAs. Recently reported molecular data support this assumption. While VHL-CNs were found to be characterised by both LOH at chromosome 3p (which contains the VHL gene) and a VHL gene germ line mutation, only 40% of SMAs had LOH at chromosome 3p and of these tumours only two (22%) exhibited a somatic VHL gene mutation.[43] Interestingly, more than 50% of SMAs showed LOH at 10q. It appears therefore that VHL-gene alterations are of minor importance in SMAs, while gene changes at 10q may play a major role. Whether the VHL gene is involved in the pathogenesis of SOIAs remains to be elucidated. The same also holds for the extremely rare serous cystadenocarcinomas.[57]

The differential diagnosis of SMAs is primarily versus multiloculated MCNs, although their honeycomb appearance and stellate scar distinguish them quite clearly. SOIAs are more difficult to differentiate from other cystic lesions because of their variegated gross appearance. Recently we found that inhibin is expressed in the epithelial cells of all types of SCNs, but not in the epithelial lining of MCNs (Kosmahl and Klöppel, unpublished observation). In MCNs inhibin only occurs in stromal cells,[52, 71] making inhibin a good marker for use in differentiating SCNs from MCNs.

Solid Pseudopapillary Neoplasms

SPNs are round tumours whose diameters may range from 2–17 cm). They are found in any region of the pancreas or loosely attached to it. The cut surface typically shows friable tan-coloured tumour tissue, the centre of which is undergoing haemorrhagic cystic degeneration, thereby forming irregular bloody cavities. Usually SPNs appear to be demarcated by a pseudocapsule in which calcifications may occur. Histologically, there are three main features. First, solid areas merge with pseudopapillary, haemorrhagic and pseudocystic structures. Second, the tumour tissue shows a delicate microvasculature that forms pseudorosettes or may be accompanied by hyalinised or myxoid stroma. The third feature concerns the tumour cell itself. It is unique because it does not resemble any of the known cell types in the pancreas. It shows eosinophilic or foamy cytoplasm (often containing PAS-positive globules) and a hybrid immunophenotype combining mesenchymal (vimentin, alpha-1-antitrypsin), endocrine (neuron specific enolase, synaptophysin, progesterone receptor) and epithelial (cytokeratin) differentiation.[36]

Once thought to be very rare, SPNs have distinctly increased in frequency as they came to be better recognised, and in our series they account for approximately

Table 11.5. Clinicopathological features of solid pseudopapillary neoplasms

Women : men = 9 : 1
• Age range: 8–60 years (mean 26)
• Localisation, no preference
• Morphology, haemorrhagic pseudocyst in tumour
• Prognosis, rarely malignant (5%–10%)

6% of all exocrine pancreatic tumours. If only the cystic tumours are considered, SPNs (with cystic changes) are the most common type (24%). They occur predominantly in young women (15–35 years of age), but may occasionally also be encountered in men[28,33] (Table 11.5). Many SPNs are detected incidentally. However, the patients may also present with sudden pain (because of bleeding into the tumour) or symptoms related to compression of adjacent organs.

In 85% to 90% of the patients the prognosis of SPN is excellent. In the remaining patients metastases (e.g. peritoneum, liver) are present at the time of diagnosis or occur later after removal of the primary. Even if metastases have developed, many of them are amenable to resection, usually resulting in long-term survival of the affected patients. There are still no prognostic factors that could help in the distinction between SPNs with or without malignant potential. It is therefore necessary to treat all SPNs by complete surgical resection.

The pathogenesis of SPNs is obscure. Because of its complex and hybrid immunoprofile the cellular phenotype is not consistent with any of the known pancreatic cell types. In view of their striking female preponderance and the known close approximation of the genital ridges to the pancreatic anlage during embryogenesis, it has been hypothesised that SPNs, like MCNs, might derive from genital ridges/ovarian anlage-related cells, which were attached to the pancreatic tissue during early embryogenesis.[36] Recently it was found that most SPNs show nuclear expression of β-catenin, associated with β-catenin mutations.[1,60]

The differential diagnosis of cystic SPNs includes pseudocysts and cystic forms of endocrine tumours of the pancreas. Apart from the typical histological features of SPNs, the expression of such markers as vimentin and neuron specific enolase in the absence of chromogranin A and the very faint expression of cytokeratin and synaptophysin distinguish this most enigmatic neoplasm of the pancreas from all other tumours.

Ductal Adenocarcinomas and Variants with Cystic Features

DACs and variants thereof showing cystic features are relatively frequent. In our series of cystic tumours they account for 8%. Three pathological mechanisms may explain the development of cystic changes in these primarily solid neoplasms.[4] Well-differentiated DACs may show ectatic duct-like structures that acquire a microcystic, grossly visible appearance. The cysts, however, are usually no larger than 0.5 cm. The second mechanism by which DACs and their variants can become cystic is central tumour necrosis. This may occur in large tumours and especially in poorly differentiated or undifferentiated sarcomatoid carcinomas.[57] Finally, DACs may obstruct not only the main pancreatic duct but also single secondary ducts, thereby producing small non-neoplastic retention cysts. While in the first and third case, the cystic changes are so subtle that they are usually not revealed by imaging techniques, a central tumour necrosis may produce a radiographically visible cystic cavity.

Uncommon Cystic Neoplasms and Lesions

Among the uncommon cystic tumours of the pancreas are a variety of neoplastic and non-neoplastic changes. The neoplasms include such tumours as cystic acinar cell carcinomas, cystic endocrine tumours, cystic metastases (i.e. from renal cell carcinoma), dermoid cysts and a number of cystic nonepithelial tumours.[46] The rare benign cystic changes consist of lymphoepithelial cysts,[3] para-ampullary duodenal wall cysts,[21] ciliated foregut cysts,[47] enteric duplication cysts,[49] dermoid cysts,[44] multicystic hamartoma,[20] congenital cysts,[14] endometrial cysts,[59,63] parasitic cysts[69] and the recently briefly mentioned mucinous nonneoplastic cyst[35] and acinar cell cystadenoma.[10,15,72] While the prognosis of the cystic epithelial neoplasms depends on the malignant potential of the respective type of tumour, the prognosis of the nonneoplastic cystic lesions is good.

References

1. Abraham SC, Klimstra DS, Wilentz RE, et al. Solid-pseudopapillary tumors of the pancreas are genetically distinct from pancreatic ductal adenocarcinomas and almost always harbor β-catenin mutations. Am J Pathol 2002; 160:1361–1369.
2. Adsay NV, Adair CF, Heffess CS, et al. Intraductal oncocytic papillary neoplasms of the pancreas. Am J Surg Pathol 1996; 20:980–994.
3. Adsay NV, Hasteh F, Cheng JD, et al. Lymphoepithelial cysts of the pancreas: a report of 12 cases and a review of the literature. Mod Pathol 2002; 15:492–501.
4. Adsay NV, Klimstra DS. Cystic lesions of the pancreas. Saunders, Philadelphia, 2000.
5. Adsay NV, Klimstra DS, Compton CC. Cystic lesions of the pancreas. Introduction. Semin Diagn Pathol 2000; 17:1–6.
6. Adsay NV, Longnecker DS, Klimstra DS. Pancreatic tumors with cystic dilatation of the ducts: intraductal papillary mucinous neoplasms and intraductal oncocytic papillary neoplasms. Semin Diagn Pathol 2000; 17:16–30.
7. Adsay NV, Merati K, Andea A, et al. The dichotomy in the preinvasive neoplasia to invasive carcinoma sequence in the pancreas: differential expression of MUC1 and MUC2 supports the existence of two separate pathways of carcinogenesis. Mod Pathol 2002; 15:1087–1095.
8. Adsay NV, Pierson C, Sarkar F, et al. Colloid (mucinous noncystic) carcinoma of the pancreas. Am J Surg Pathol 2001; 25:26–42.
9. Adsay V, Conlon K, Brennan M, et al. Intraductal papillary-mucinous neoplasms of the pancreas (IPMN): an analysis of in situ and invasive carcinomas associated with 23 cases. Mod Pathol 1997; 10:143A.
10. Albores-Saavedra J. Acinar cystadenoma of the pancreas: a previously undescribed tumor. Ann Diagn Pathol 2002; 6:113–115.
11. Albores-Saavedra J, Gould EW, Angeles-Angeles A, et al. Cystic tumors of the pancreas. In: PP Rosen, RE Fechner (eds) Pathology annual, volume 25, part 2. Appleton & Lange, East Norwalk, 1990; pp. 19–50.
12. Azar C, Van de Stadt J, Rickaert F, et al. Intraductal papillary mucinous tumours of the pancreas. Clinical and therapeutic issues in 32 patients. Gut 1996; 39:457–464.
13. Capella C, Solcia E, Klöppel G, et al. Serous cystic neoplasms of the pancreas. In: SR Hamilton, LA Aaltonen (eds) Pathology and Genetics of Tumours of the Digestive System. WHO Classification of Tumours. IARC Press, Lyon, 2000; pp. 231–233.
14. Casadei R, Campione O, Greco VM, et al. Congenital true pancreatic cysts in young adults: case report and literature review. Pancreas 1996; 12:419–421.
15. Chatelain D, Paye F, Mourra N, et al. Unilocular acinar cell cystadenoma of the pancreas an unusual acinar cell tumor. Am J Clin Pathol 2002; 118:211–214.

16. Compagno J, Oertel JE. Microcystic adenomas of the pancreas (glycogen-rich cystadenomas): a clinicopathologic study of 34 cases. Am J Clin Pathol 1978; 69:289–298.
17. Compagno J, Oertel JE. Mucinous cystic neoplasms of the pancreas with overt and latent malignancy (cystadenocarcinoma and cystadenoma). A clinicopathologic study of 41 cases. Am J Clin Pathol 1978; 69:573–580.
18. Compton CC. Serous cystic tumors of the pancreas. Semin Diagn Pathol 2000; 17:43–55.
19. Egawa N, Maillet B, Schröder S, et al. Serous oligocystic and ill-demarcated adenoma of the pancreas: a variant of serous cystic adenoma. Virchows Arch 1994; 424:13–17.
20. Flaherty MJ, Benjamin DR. Multicystic pancreatic hamartoma: a distinctive lesion with immunohistochemical and ultrastructural study. Hum Pathol 1992; 23:1309–1312.
21. Fléjou JF, Potet F, Molas G, et al. Cystic dystrophy of the gastric and duodenal wall developing in heterotopic pancreas: an unrecognized entity. Gut 1993; 34:343–347.
22. Fukushima N, Mukai K, Sakamoto M, et al. Invasive carcinoma derived from intraductal papillary-mucinous carcinoma of the pancreas: clinicopathologic and immunohistochemical study of 8 cases. Virchows Arch 2001; 439:6–13.
23. George DH, Murphy F, Michalski R, et al. Serous cystadenocarcinoma of the pancreas: a new entity? Am J Surg Pathol 1989; 13:61–66.
24. Hastings PR, Nance FC, Becker WF. Changing patterns in the management of pancreatic pseudocysts. Ann Surg 1975; 181:546–551.
25. Healy DL, Burger HG, Mamers P, et al. Elevated serum inhibin concentrations in postmenopausal women with ovarian tumors. N Engl J Med 1993; 329:1539–1542.
26. Hodgkinson DJ, ReMine WH, Weiland LH. A clinicopathologic study of 21 cases of pancreatic cystadenocarcinoma. Ann Surg 1978; 188:679–684.
27. Kimura W, Makuuchi M, Kuroda A. Characteristics and treatment of mucin-producing tumor of the pancreas. Hepatogastroenterology 1998; 45:2001–2008.
28. Klimstra DS, Wenig BM, Heffess CS. Solid-pseudopapillary tumor of the pancreas: A typically cystic carcinoma of low malignant potential. Semin Diagn Pathol 2000; 17:66–80.
29. Klöppel G. Pancreatic, non-endocrine tumours. In: G Klöppel, PU Heitz (eds) Pancreatic pathology. Churchill Livingstone, Edinburgh, 1984; pp. 79–113.
30. Klöppel G. Clinicopathologic view of intraductal papillary-mucinous tumor of the pancreas. Hepato-Gastroenterology 1998; 45:1981–1985.
31. Klöppel G. Pseudocysts and other non-neoplastic cysts of the pancreas. Semin Diagn Pathol 2000; 17:7–15.
32. Klöppel G, Hruban RH, Longnecker DS, et al. Ductal adenocarcinoma of the pancreas. In: SR Hamilton, LA Aaltonen (eds) Pathology and Genetics of Tumours of the Digestive System. WHO Classification of Tumours. IARC Press, Lyon, 2000; pp. 221–230.
33. Klöppel G, Lüttges J, Klimstra D, et al. Solid-pseudopapillary neoplasm. In: SR Hamilton, LA Aaltonen (eds) Pathology and Genetics of Tumours of the Digestive System. WHO Classification of Tumours. IARC Press, Lyon, 2000; pp. 246–248.
34. Klöppel G, Solcia E, Longnecker DS, et al. Histological typing of tumours of the exocrine pancreas. Second edition. WHO International histological classification of tumours. Springer, Berlin, 1996.
35. Kosmahl M, Egawa N, Schröder S, et al. Mucinous nonneoplastic cyst of the pancreas: a novel nonneoplastic cystic change? Mod Pathol 2002; 15:154–158.
36. Kosmahl M, Seada LS, Jänig U, et al. Solid-pseudopapillary tumor of the pancreas: its origin revisited. Virchows Arch 2000; 436:473–480.
37. Lewandrowski K, Warshaw A, Compton C. Macrocystic serous cystadenoma of the pancreas: a morphologic variant differing from microcystic adenoma. Hum Pathol 1992; 23:871–875.
38. Loftus EV, Jr., Olivares-Pakzad BA, Batts KP, et al. Intraductal papillary-mucinous tumors of the pancreas: Clinicopathologic features, outcome, and nomenclature. Gastroenterology 1996; 110:1909–1918.
39. Longnecker DS, Adler G, Hruban RH, et al. Intraductal papillary-mucinous neoplasms of the pancreas. In: SR Hamilton, LA Aaltonen (eds) Pathology and Genetics of Tumours of the Digestive System. WHO Classification of Tumours. IARC Press, Lyon, 2000; pp. 237–240.
40. Lüttges J, Feyerabend B, Buchelt T, et al. The mucin profile of noninvasive and invasive mucinous cystic neoplasms of the pancreas. Am J Surg Pathol 2002; 26:466–471.
41. Lüttges J, Zamboni G, Longnecker D, et al. The immunohistochemical mucin expression pattern distinguishes different types of intraductal papillary mucinous neoplasms of the pancreas and determines their relationship to mucinous noncystic carcinoma and ductal adenocarcinoma. Am J Surg Pathol 2001; 25:942–948.
42. Mohr VH, Vortmeyer AO, Zhuang Z, et al. Histopathology and molecular genetics of multiple cysts and microcystic (serous) adenomas of the pancreas in von Hippel-Lindau patients. Am J Pathol 2000; 157:1615–1621.

43. Moore PS, Zamboni G, Brighenti A, et al. Molecular characterization of pancreatic serous microcytic adenomas. Evidence for a tumor suppressor gene on chromosome 10q. Am J Surg Pathol 2001; 158:317–321.
44. Morohoshi T, Hamamoto T, Kunimara T, et al. Epidermoid cyst derived from an accessory spleen in the pancreas. A case report with literature survey. Acta Pathol Jpn 1991; 41:916–921.
45. Nakamura A, Horinouchi M, Goto M, et al. New classification of pancreatic intraductal papillary-mucinous tumour by mucin expression: its relationship with potential for malignancy. J Pathol 2002; 197:201–210.
46. Paal E, Thompson LD, Heffess CS. A clinicopathologic and immunohistochemical study of ten pancreatic lymphangiomas and a review of the literature. Cancer 1998; 82:2150–2158.
47. Pappas S, Diaz L, Talamonti M. A cystic pancreatic mass discovered in a patient with ileocecal carcinoid (Pathologic quiz case). Arch Pathol Lab Med 2002; 126:229–230.
48. Perez-Ordonez B, Naseem A, Lieberman PH, et al. Solid serous adenoma of the pancreas. The solid variant of serous cystadenoma? Am J Surg Pathol 1996; 20:1401–1405.
49. Pilcher CS, Bradley ELI, Majmudar B. Enterogenous cyst of the pancreas. Am J Gastroenterol 1982; 77:576–577.
50. Rattner DW, Fernandez-del Castillo C, Warshaw AL. Cystic pancreatic neoplasms. Ann Oncol 1999; 10 (Suppl ?):S104–S106.
51. Rickaert F, Cremer M, Devière J, et al. Intraductal mucin-hypersecreting neoplasms of the pancreas. A clinicopathologic study of eight patients. Gastroenterology 1991; 101:512–519.
52. Ridder GJ, Maschek H, Flemming P, et al. Ovarian-like stroma in an invasive mucinous cystadenocarcinoma of the pancreas positive for inhibin. A hint concerning its possible histogenesis. Virchows Arch 1998; 432:451–454.
53. Sato N, Rosty C, Jansen M, et al. STK11/LKB1 Peutz-Jeghers gene inactivation in intraductal papillary-mucinous neoplasms of the pancreas. Am J Pathol 2001; 159:2017–2022.
54. Seidel G, Zahurak M, Iacobuzio-Donahue CA, et al. Almost all infiltrating colloid carcinomas of the pancreas and periampullary region arise from in situ papillary neoplasms. A study of 39 cases. Am J Surg Pathol 2002; 26:56–63.
55. Sessa F, Bonato M, Frigerio B, et al. Ductal cancers of the pancreas frequently express markers of gastrointestinal epithelial cells. Gastroenterology 1990; 98:1655–1665.
56. Sessa F, Solcia E, Capella C, et al. Intraductal papillary-mucinous tumours represent a distinct group of pancreatic neoplasms: an investigation of tumour cell differentiation and K-ras, p53, and c-erbB-2 abnormalities in 26 patients. Virchows Arch 1994; 425:357–367.
57. Solcia E, Capella C, Klöppel G. Tumors of the pancreas. AFIP Atlas of Tumor Pathology, Third series, fascicle 20. Armed Forces Institute of Pathology, Washington, D.C., 1997.
58. Sugiyama M, Atomi Y. Extrapancreatic neoplasms occur with unusual frequency in patients with intraductal papillary mucinous tumors of the pancreas. Am J Gastroenterol 1999; 94:470–473.
59. Sumiyoshi Y, Yamashita Y, Maekawa T, et al. A case of hemorrhagic cyst of the pancreas resembling the cystic endometriosis. Int Surg 2000; 85:67–70.
60. Tanaka Y, Kato K, Notohara K, et al. Frequent β-catenin mutation and cytoplasmic/nuclear accumulation in pancreatic solid-pseudopapillary neoplasm. Cancer Res 2001; 61:8401–8404.
61. Terris B, Ponsot T, Paye F, et al. Intraductal papillary mucinous tumors of the pancreas confined to secondary ducts show less aggressive pathologic features as compared with those involving the main pancreatic duct. Am J Surg Pathol 2000; 24:1372–1377.
62. Thompson LD, Becker RC, Przygodzki RM, et al. Mucinous cystic neoplasm (mucinous cystadenocarcinoma of low-grade malignant potential) of the pancreas: a clinicopathologic study of 130 cases. Am J Surg Pathol 1999; 23:1–16.
63. Verbeke C, Harle M, Sturm J. Cystic endometriosis of the upper abdominal organs. Report on three cases and review of the literature. Pathol Res Pract 1996; 192:300–304.
64. Warshaw AL, Compton CC, Lewandrowski K, et al. Cystic tumors of the pancreas. New clinical, radiologic, and pathologic observations in 67 patients. Ann Surg 1990; 212:432–443.
65. Wilentz RE, Albores-Saavedra J, Hruban RH. Mucinous cystic neoplasms of the pancreas. Semin Diagn Pathol 2000; 17:31–42.
66. Wilentz RE, Albores-Saavedra J, Zahurak M, et al. Pathologic examination accurately predicts prognosis in mucinous cystic neoplasms of the pancreas. Am J Surg Pathol 1999; 23:1320–1327.
67. Wouters K, Ectors N, Van Steenbergen W, et al. A pancreatic mucinous cystadenoma in a man with mesenchymal stroma, expressing oestrogen and progesterone receptors. Virchows Arch 1998; 432:187–189.
68. Yonezawa S, Taira M, Osako M, et al. MUC-1 mucin expression in invasive areas of intraductal papillary mucinous tumors of the pancreas. Pathol Int 1998; 48:319–322.

69. Yorganci K, Iret D, Sayek I. A case of primary hydatid disease of the pancreas simulating cystic neoplasm. Pancreas 2000; 21:104–105.
70. Zamboni G, Klöppel G, Hruban RH, et al. Mucinous cystic neoplasms of the pancreas. In: SR Hamilton, LA Aaltonen (eds) Pathology and Genetics of Tumours of the Digestive System. WHO Classification of Tumours. IARC Press, Lyon, 2000; pp. 234–236.
71. Zamboni G, Scarpa A, Bogina G, et al. Mucinous cystic tumors of the pancreas. Clinicopathological features, prognosis and relationship to other mucinous cystic tumors. Am J Surg Pathol 1999; 23:410–422.
72. Zamboni G, Terris B, Scarpa A, et al. Acinar cell cystadenoma of the pancreas. A new entity? Am J Surg Pathol 2002; 26:698–704.

12 Pancreatic Involvement in Von Hippel–Lindau Disease

Pascal Hammel, Benoît Terris, Valérie Vilgrain, Philippe Ruszniewski and Stéphane Richard

Genetic Basis

Von Hippel–Lindau (VHL) disease is characterized by a dominant autosomal predisposition to develop hemangioblastomas of the retina and central nervous system (CNS), renal cell carcinoma, pheochromocytoma and endolymphatic sac tumors with marked phenotypic variability.[1,2] The VHL gene, located on chromosome 3p25–26, is composed of three exons, encoding for a 213 amino acid protein which is widely expressed in both fetal and adult human tissues. A hallmark of VHL tumours is their high degree of vascularization, which arises from overexpression of the vascular endothelial growth factor (VEGF), a crucial factor in angiogenesis.[2] The VHL gene is a multifunctional tumour suppressor gene which is principally involved in negative regulation of hypoxia-inducible mRNAs such as the mRNA encoding for VEGF. The activity of VHL protein has been linked to the targeting of specific proteins for ubiquitin-dependent proteolysis.[1,2] Lack of degradation of this factor due to absence of the VHL protein results in uncontrolled production of factors promoting formation of blood vessels such as VEGF.[2] Reintroduction of wild-type VHL protein in renal cell carcinoma cell lines lacking wild-type VHL protein suppresses their high level of VEGF mRNA accumulation. In addition, reintroduction of wild-type VHL protein prevents the development of tumours in nude mouse xenografts, confirming the tumour suppressive function the VHL gene. Germ-line mutations in the VHL gene are extremely heterogeneous and are distributed widely throughout the coding sequence.[1–3] They are now identifiable in virtually all families with VHL.[3] Some constitutional mosaicisms were recently reported in parents of patients with apparent *de novo* mutations.[4] Genotype–phenotype correlations are emerging confirming the clinical pheochromocytoma-based distinction.[5] In VHL type I (without pheochromocytoma) up to 96% of gene alterations are deletions, insertions, nonsense, or splice site mutations resulting in a truncated protein. In type IIA (with pheochromocytoma and low risk of renal cell cancer), up to 92% are missense mutations. In type IIB, mutations affect the critical contact region between VHL protein and elongin C.[1,2] Finally, a type IIC was recently individualized, which is characterized by the familial occurrence of isolated pheochromocytomas only.[1] Pancreatic involvement is present in type I and IIB, but rare or absent in type IIA and IIC. Hence, genetic factors may also influence the estimation of pancreatic involvement in VHL patients. For example, Neumann et al.[6] reported a 17% prevalence of pancreatic involvement in a series of 66 patients. After genotyping the 22 families from their series, a common founder effect mutation at codon 98 of the VHL gene (Tyr98His) was identified.[7] The latter is known to be associated with a VHL phenotype in which pheochromocytomas are frequent but renal and pancreatic lesions less so.[3] In contrast, patients in our series were from 94 different families originating from several regions in France and exhibited various types of mutations in the VHL gene (Ref 8 and unpublished data).

Pancreatic Lesions

Pancreatic lesions described in VHL patients consist of cysts or serous cystadenomas,[6,9–14] neuroendocrine tumours (NET),[6,9,12,15–19] adenocarcinomas,[9] hemangioblastomas[20] or renal-cell cancer metastasis.[21,22] In contrast with VHL lesions of other organs, pancreatic lesions were formerly thought to have no clinical relevance as they tended to be infrequently symptomatic.[9] However, cystic lesions may compress neighbouring organs[14] and NET can metastasize.[6,9,12,15–17] The frequency of pancreatic involvement in living patients studied by imaging was estimated as approximately 50% when pooling the largest series[6,10,11] whereas the single earlier autopsy series of 29 VHL patients cited a 72% prevalence.[23] In the largest prospective study recently published by our group, the prevalence of pancreatic involvement in 158 patients was significantly higher (77%), similar to the latter autopsy report.[12] Two main reasons probably explain this high rate: 1) systematic examination of the pancreas using helical computed tomography (CT) scan with appropriate contrast injection or magnetic resonance imaging and review by an experienced radiologist optimized the detection of small pancreatic lesions[10–12]; 2) examination of all aymptomatic patients at risk (i.e. with VHL gene mutation) likely improved the detection of pancreatic involvement.

Most pancreatic lesions in VHL disease are asymptomatic and discovered during systematic screening of VHL family members.[6,10–12] However, the size of lesions may evolve with time as we observed in half of our patients during 30 months follow-up.[12] Radiological evidence of compression of the main pancreatic duct or neighboring organs was seen in about 20% of patients. Acute pancreatitis secondary to stenosis of the main pancreatic duct by cysts or tumours has been described.[24,25] VHL disease can be diagnosed in approximately 5% of patients after the chance discovery of pancreatic lesions during abdominal imaging performed for unrelated reasons.[12] Thus, the possibility of VHL disease should be evoked by gastroenterologists, surgeons and/or radiologists on discovering an unusual pancreatic lesion in yong patients (<40 years) without a family history of multiple endocrine neoplasia. These patients should be screened for VHL disease germline mutations. In addition, pancreatic involvement is the only phenotypic expression in 8% of cases and represents a key factor in establishing the diagnosis of VHL disease in relatives of affected patients in whom mutation has not been identified.[1]

Pancreatic Cysts

Cystic lesions are prominent in patients with pancreatic involvement of VHL. Hyperproduction of VEGF may favour pancreatic and/or renal cyst formation.[2]

Interestingly, a high female ratio in patients with serous cystadenoma is also found in VHL patients (80%). The size of cysts in VHL patients varies. Cystadenomas are often large in size (>5 cm) and even panglandular (Fig. 12.1). In our experience of five patients who underwent surgery to treat NET and in whom multiple cysts were also diagnosed on CT scan, histological examination of the resected specimen revealed cystic lesions to be mainly multifocal serous cystadenomas.[26] Finally, the distinction between true cysts and serous cystadenomas is of no practical significance academic as it does not change the therapeutic approach. Radiological discrimination between multiple cysts and serous cystadenomas is probably not accurate from histological and genetic points of view. Mohr et al[27] have shown that various subtypes of cystic lesions seem to represent architectural and histological variants of the same molecular genetic process. Isolated cysts are not rare in VHL disease, they accounted for 15% of cystic lesions in our experience. Congenital solitary cysts represent a very small proportion of sporadic cystic pancreatic lesions.[28,29] In patients with VHL disease, it is not excluded that these cysts represent serous cystadenomas in a rare macrocystic form.[26]

Pancreatic calcifications are frequent in VHL patients with multiple cysts. There are often few (<5), thin-walled and peripheral and thus clearly differ from those seen in chronic pancreatitis.[30] In contrast, serous cystadenomas in VHL have

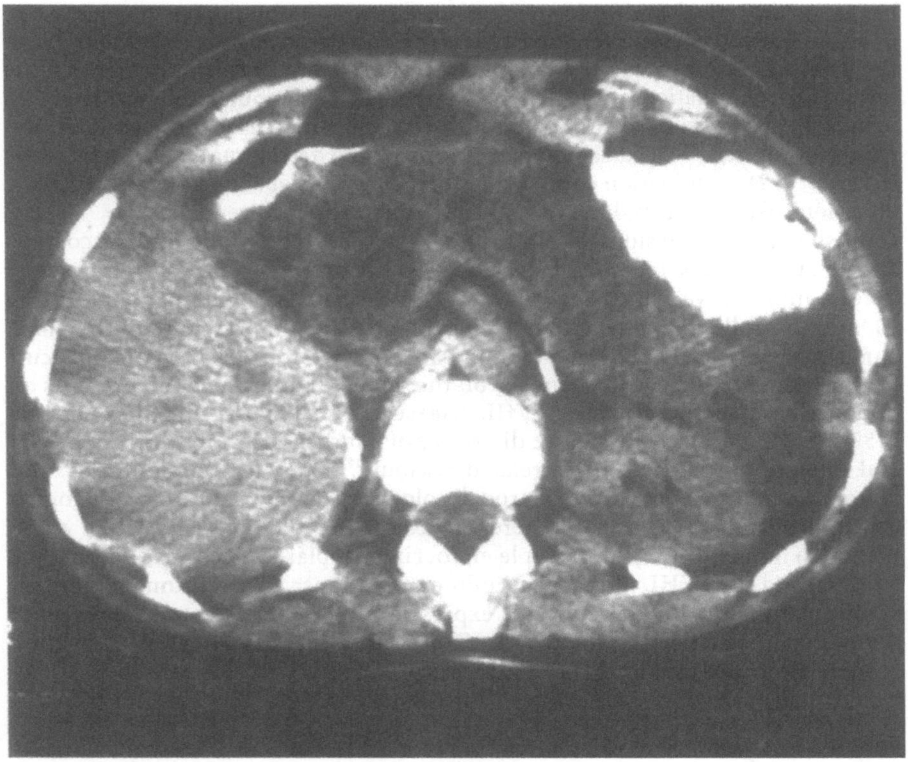

Figure 12.1. CT scan with contrast injection. The pancreas contains countless hypodense lesions of various sizes corresponding to cysts.

prominent calcifications.[12] Low contents of pancreatic enzymes and tumor markers found in cystic fluid as analysed in a small number of patients is similar to that found in sporadic serous cystadenomas.[31]

Pancreatic Symptoms

Even though pancreatic involvement with cysts or serous cystadenomas occurs frequently, the prevalence of pain, acute pancreatic or jaundice due to pancreatic or biliary duct compression is low.[12] Likewise, diabetes is rare even when the pancreatic parenchyma is completely replaced with cysts or cystadenomas.[12,32]

Risk of Malignancy

A correlation between renal cyst and cancer was proposed due to the presence of allelic loss in both lesions.[33] In contrast, this possibility is less likely in pancreatic lesions knowing that cystic lesions originate from exocrine tissue whereas solid tumours are neuroendocrine. Pancreatic resections in asymptomatic VHL patients with cystic lesions should not be proposed as there is a risk of causing pancreatic endocrine and exocrine insufficiency due to the necessity to remove a large amount of pancreatic parenchyma when attempting to remove the totality of lesions.[12] In patients with symptoms, careful analysis is required to assess the mechanisms resulting in symptoms from cystic lesions. Although therapeutic experience is still limited, endoscopic or surgical drainages are probably preferable to resections whenever possible.

Neuroendocrine Tumours

NET are the most important pancreatic lesions in VHL disease. They account for 10–17% of pancreatic involvement.[10,12,17] NET are multiple (2 to 5 tumours) in 50% of cases.[12,17] Countless microadenomas and nesidioblastosis can be encountered at histological examination.[12] Thus, the combination of multiple NET and pheochromocytoma is not only confined to the multiple endocrine neoplasia type 2. A positive association between NET and pheochromocytoma but a negative association between NET and renal involvement have been suggested. An isolated NET can represent the first manifestation of VHL disease.[18] NET are often asymptomatic but can occasionally cause acute pancreatitis or pain caused by compression of the main pancreatic duct.[12] Hormone hypersecretion, especially somatostatin, may occur but it is clinically silent.[12,15,18–19]

Lubensky et al.[16] have described the pathological characteristics of 30 NET in 14 patients with VHL disease. Clarification of neuroendocrine cells, thought to be due to the accumulation of fat and myelin as shown using electronic microscopy, is present in 60% of cases in VHL patients, a feature not found in sporadic NET.[16,26] Focal positivity on immunochemistry with various markers (somatostatin, pancreatic polypeptide, insulin and/or glucagon) was present in 35% of cases.[16]

Differential Diagnosis

The differential diagnosis between NET and other vascular tumors of the pancreas in VHL is limited.[10,12] When presentation is typical (i.e. well limited and highly vascular solid tumour), the diagnosis is easily made on imaging. Sometimes, NET can be difficult to distinguish from solid forms of vascularized serous cystadenomas on CT examination (Fig. 12.2).[10,12,17] In this situation, endoscopic ultrasonography may be helpful showing small (e.g. 1 mm) cysts within the tumour.[12] Endoscopic ultrasonography also appears to be the most accurate in demonstrating the multiplicity of NET by detecting multiple lesions below 10 mm in size. Somatostatin receptor scintigraphy may also help in establishing a diagnosis.[12] Cases of pancreatic hemangioblastomas have been reported in the literature but immunohistochemistry data are lacking to exclude a NET.[20] Despite the frequent occurrence of renal cancer in patients with VHL, which accounts for a high mortality rate, only two cases of pancreatic metastasis from such cancer have been reported.[21,22] These solid and well vascularized tumours may mimick NET (Fig. 12.2). CT or ultrasonography guided fine-needle aspiration can be proposed in doubtful cases.[12] Immunohistochemical analysis may help in the differential diagnosis showing the lack of positive staining with neuroendocrine markers (chromogranin A and synaptophysin).

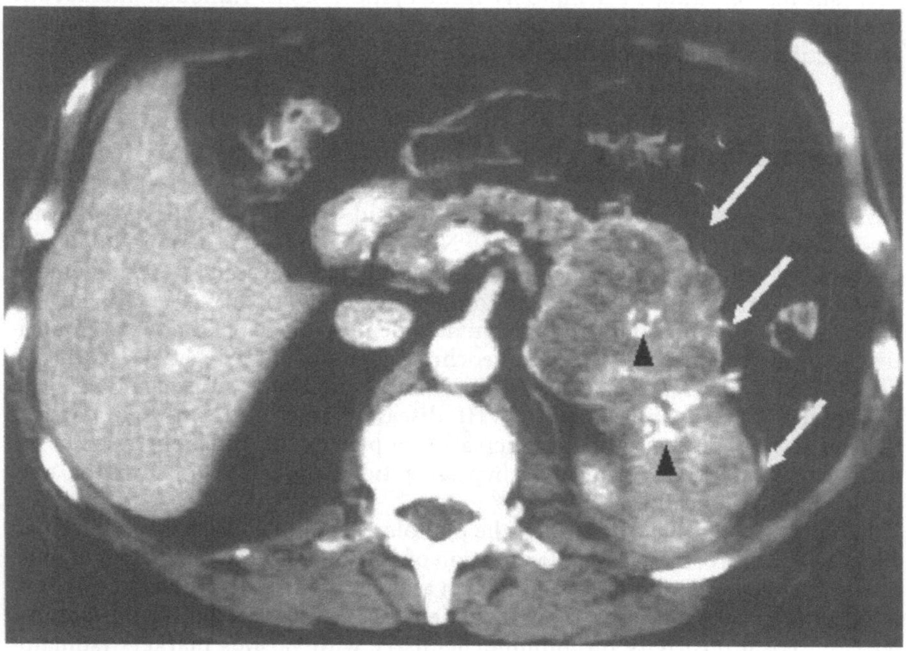

Figure 12.2. CT scan with contrast injection. Large serous cystadenoma (arrows) with calcification (arrow heads) located in the body and tail of the pancreas.

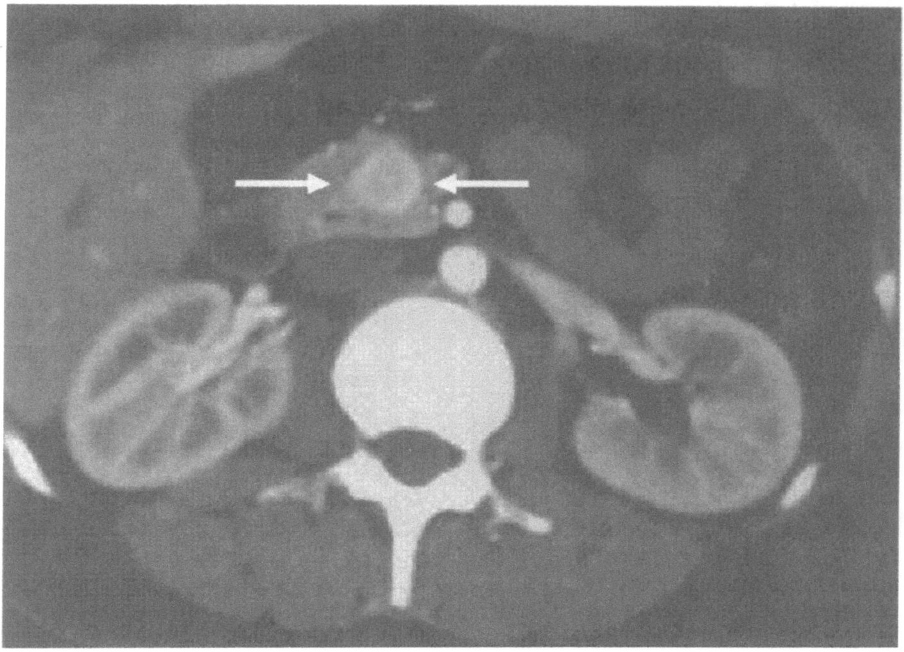

Figure 12.3. CT scan with contrast injection. Typical appearance of endocrine tumour in the pancreatic head. Due to the size (3 cm) and metastatic potential, a surgical resection is appropriate.

Metastatic Potential

Metastasis of NET has been shown to occur in 25% of cases in VHL patients.[6,9,12,17] In the series of Libutti et al.,[17] the size of the primary tumour was significantly higher in patients with liver metastases than in those without (median : 5 cm and 2 cm, respectively). These authors recommended a preventive resection in VHL patients with NET greater than 3 cm. Our experience is similar in that all patients with NET larger than 3 cm, histological features of tumour aggressivity, i.e. invasion of the duodenum, lymph nodes or liver metastases, were found.[12]

Management

The management of smaller NET is not well defined and poses difficulties as these lesions are often multiple and disseminated throughout the pancreas (Figures 12.3 and 12.4). Conservative management in patients with multiple and small NET is probably more appropriate than subtotal or total pancreatectomy. Closer imaging follow-up may be reasonable in an effort to detect rapid increase in tumour size and propose resection of the larger tumours. Limited resections such as enuclation is theoretically preferable to preserve exocrine and endocrine functions.[17] Finally, the therapeutic decision requires multidisciplinary discussion as VHL patients are generally simultaneously affected by various life-threatening tumors of the CNS, adrenal glands or kidneys which may have a greater priority for treatment.

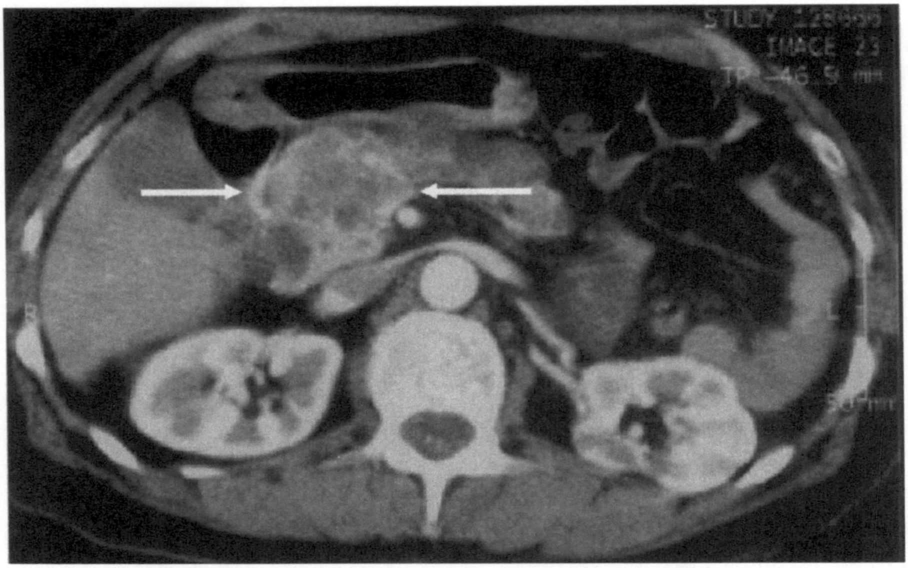

Figure 12.4. CT scan with contrast injection. Serous cystadenoma in the head of pancreas (arrows). Notice the strong enhancement after contrast injection mimicking a well vascularized tumour. Such pseudo-solid forms of serous cystadenoma may be difficult to distinguish with an endocrine tumour thus somatostatin receptor scintigraphy and/or biopsy are required.

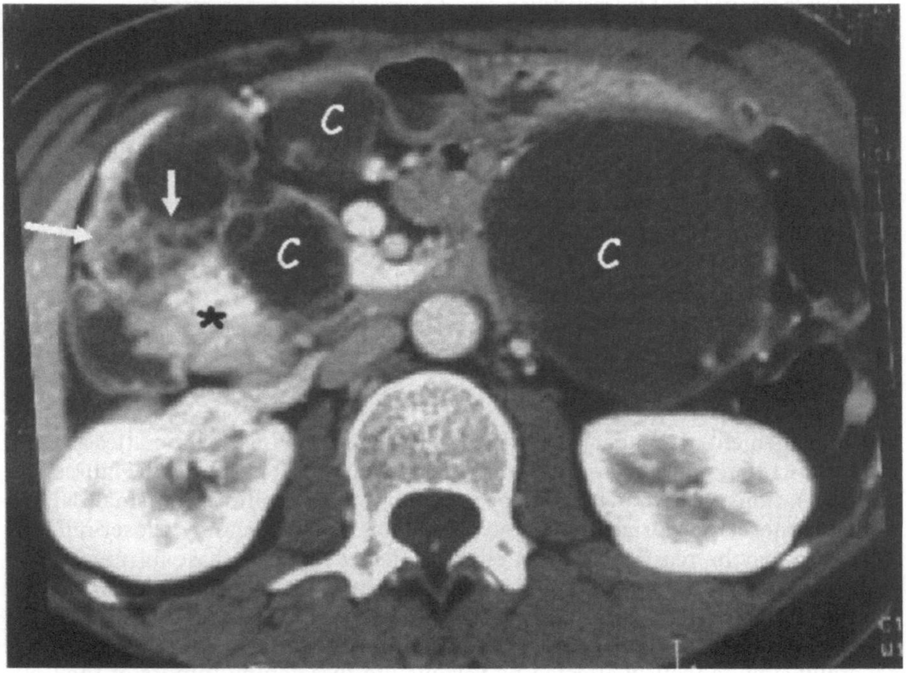

Figure 12.5. CT scan with contrast injection. Combination of all typical pancreatic lesions in a patient with VHL disease: endocrine tumour (black asterisk), serous cystadenoma (arrows) and cysts (C).

Pancreatic Adenocarcinoma

Earlier reports associated pancreatic adenocarcinoma with VHL.[9] Recently, our group and others, did not find an association of VHL disease and pancreatic adenocarcinoma.[12,16] Loss of heterozygosity of the VHL gene has been found in NET, renal cancer and pheochromocytoma. In contrast, Lubensky et al.[12] have recently reported a patient affected by both pancreatic adenocarcinoma and NET, that genetic heterozygosity was preserved in the former lesion whereas deletion of the non-mutated allele was found in the latter.

Conclusion

In conclusion, pancreatic involvement occurs in most patients with VHL disease and consists of true cysts, serous cystadenomas and NET, often in combination. To assess genotype-phenotype correlations in patients with VHL and pancreatic involvement requires further studies. To identify such rare lesions in a patient without a family history requires genetic study and exhaustive investigations to search for other VHL organ involvement. Medical or surgical treatment is required in about 10% of patients with VHL to treat symptomatic pancreatic lesions or to remove NET of large size which are at risk of metastatic progression. The frequent multiplicity of NET and presence of other organ involvement often make therapeutic decisions difficult. A multidisciplinary approach is required to optimize the treatment.

References

1. Zbar B, Kaelin W, Maher E, et al. Third international meeting on von Hippel-Lindau disease. Cancer Res 1999; 59:2251–3.
2. Richard S, David P, Marsot-Dupuch K, et al. Central nervous system hemangioblastomas, endolymphatic sac tumors, and von Hippel-Lindau disease. Neurosurg Rev 2000; 23:1–22.
3. Stolle C, Glenn G, Zbar B, et al. Improved detection of germline mutations in the von Hippel-Lindau disease tumor suppressor gene. Hum Mutat 1998; 12:417–23.
4. Sgambati MT, Stolle C, Choyke PL, et al. Mosaicism in von Hippel-Lindau disease: lessons from kindreds with germline mutations identified in offspring with mosaic parents. Am J Human Genet 2000; 66:84–91.
5. Neumann HPH, Wiestler OD. Clustering of features and genetics of von Hippel-Lindau syndrome. Lancet 1991; 338:258.
6. Neumann HPH, Dinkel E, Brambs H, et al. Pancreatic lesions in the von Hippel-Lindau syndrome. Gastroenterology 1991; 101:465–71.
7. Brauch H, Kishida T, Glavac D, et al. Von Hippel-Lindau disease with pheochromocytoma in the Black Forest region in Germany: evidence for a founder effect. Hum Genet 1995; 95:551–6.
8. Olschwang S, Richard S, Boisson C, et al. Germline mutation profile of the VHL gene in von Hippel-Lindau disease and in sporadic hemangioblastoma. Hum Mutat 1998; 12:424–30.
9. Lamiell JM, Salazar FG, Hsia YE. Von Hippel-Lindau affecting 43 members of a single kindred. Medicine 1989; 68:1–29.
10. Choyke PL, Glenn GM, Walther MM, et al. Von Hippel-Lindau disease: genetic, clinical and imaging features. Radiology 1995; 146:629–42.
11. Hough DM, Stephens DH, Johnson CD, et al. Pancreatic lesions in von Hippel-Lindau disease: prevalence, clinical significance and CT findings. AJR Am J Roentgenol 1994; 162:1091–94.
12. Hammel P, Vilgrain V, Terris B, et al. Pancreatic involvement in von Hippel-Lindau disease. Gastroenterology 2000; 119:1087–95.

13. Girelli R, Bassi C, Falconi M, et al. Pancreatic cystic manifestations in von Hippel-Lindau disease. Int J Pancreatol 1997; 22:101–9.
14. Beerman MH, Fromkes JJ, Carey LC, et al. Pancreatic cystadenoma in von Hippel-Lindau disease: an unusual cause of pancreatic and common bile duct obstruction. J Clin Gastroenterol 1982; 4:537–40.
15. Cornish D, Pont A, Minor D, et al. Metastatic islet-tumor in von Hippel-Lindau disease. Am J Med 1984; 77:147–50.
16. Lubensky IA, Pack S, Ault D, et al. Multiple neuroendocrine tumors of the pancreas in von Hippel-Lindau disease patients. Am J Pathol 1998; 153:223–31.
17. Libutti SK, Choyke PL, Bartlett DL, et al. Pancreatic neuroendocrine tumors associated with von Hippel-Lindau disease: diagnostic and management recommendations. Surgery 1998; 124:1153–9.
18. Mount SL, Weaver DL, Taatjes DJ, et al. Von Hippel-Lindau disease presenting as pancreatic neuroendocrine tumour. Virchows Arch 1995; 426:523–8.
19. Maki M, Kaneko Y, Ohta Y, et al. Somatostatinoma of the pancreas associated with von Hippel-Lindau disease. Internal Medicine 1995; 34:661–5.
20. Fill WL, Lamiell JM, Polk NO. The radiographic manifestations of von Hippel-Lindau disease. Radiology 1979; 133:289–95.
21. Chambers TP, Fishman EK, Hruban RH. Pancreatic metastases from renal cell carcinoma in von Hippel-Lindau disease. Clin Imaging 1997; 21:40–2.
22. Sugiyama M, Katsura M, Yamamoto K, et al. Pancreatic metastasis from renal cell carcinoma causing massive gastrointestinal bleeding in von Hippel-Lindau disease. Hepatogastroenterology 1999; 46:1199–201.
23. Horton WA, Wong V, Eldridge R. Von Hippel-Lindau disease: clinical and pathological manifestations in nine families with 50 affected members. Arch Intern Med 1976; 136:769–77.
24. Klein I, Arrivé L, Tiret E, et al. Maladie de von Hippel-Lindau révélée par une pancréatite aiguë secondaire à une multikystose pancréatique. Gastroenterol Clin Biol 1998; 22:102–3.
25. Tenner S, Roston A, Lichtenstein D, et al. Von Hippel-Lindau disease complicated by acute pancreatitis and Evan's syndrome. Int J Pancreatol 1995; 18:271–5.
26. Terris B, Hammel P. Atteinte pancréatique de la maladie de von Hippel-Lindau. Ann Pathol 2000; 20:124–9.
27. Mohr VH, Vortmeyer AO, Zhuang Z, et al. Histopathology and molecular genetics of multiple cysts and microcystic (serous) adenomas of the pancreas in von Hippel-Lindau patients. Am J Pathol 2000; 157:1615–21.
28. Kimura W, Nagai H, Kuroda A, et al. Analysis of small cystic lesions of the pancreas. Int J Pancreatol 1995; 18:197–206.
29. Sperti C, Pasquali C, Costantino V, et al. Solitary true cyst of the pancreas in adults. Report of three cases and review of the literature. Int J Pancreatol 1995; 18:161–7.
30. Luetmer PH, Stephens DH, Ward EM. Chronic pancreatitis: reassessment with current CT. Radiology 1989; 171:353–7.
31. Hammel P, Lévy P, Voitot H, et al. Preoperative cyst fluid analysis is useful for the differential diagnosis of cystic lesions of the pancreas. Gastroenterology 1995; 108:1230–5.
32. Thompson RK, Peters JI, Sirinek KR, et al. Von Hippel-Lindau syndrome presenting as pancreatic endocrine insufficiency: a case report. Surgery 1988; 105:598–604.
33. Lubensky IA, Gnarra J, Bertheau P, et al. Allelic deletions of theVHL gene detected in multiple microscopic clear cell renal lesions in von Hippel-Lindau disease patients. Am J Pathol 1996; 149:2089–94.

13 Intraductal Papillary Mucinous Tumours of the Pancreas

Christian Partensky, J.Y. Scoazec, B. Napoléon, F.P. Bernard, F. Berger and J. Dumortier

Intraductal papillary mucinous tumours of the pancreas (IPMT) have been recognized as a distinct entity among cystic neoplasms of the pancreas and as a new subdivision among mucinous neoplasms of the pancreas. These tumours have been reported with an increasing frequency[1] since the original description by Ohashi et al. in 1981 in the Japanese literature[2] and by Itaï et al. in English 1986.[3] The pathologic features are replacement of the normal lining of the epithelium by a neoplastic mucus-secreting epithelium along the main pancreatic duct (MPD) or the side branch ducts (SBD), or both main and branch ducts, resulting in cystic dilatation of the MPD or of its major branches.[4] Variable histological lesions range from adenoma, borderline dysplasia to carcinoma without and with invasion, even in the same tumour. Accurate diagnosis necessitates both diagnosis of the IPMT itself and determination of the extent of the neoplasm in the pancreatic ducts which is a critical point to determine the extent of the pancreatic resection. We report, here, a retrospective series of patients who underwent pancreatic resection for IPMT with a critical analysis of the adequacy of the pancreatectomy according to the pathological examination of the operative specimen and to the outcome of patients.

Patients and Methods

Patients

This study included 40 consecutive patients who were operated on by one surgeon (CP) for IPMT from august 1985 to august 2001. They were 26 men and 14 women patients with a mean age at operation of 62.5 ± 1.8 years (median: 64 years with a range: 25–77).

During the same period of time, three other patients with IPMT were treated conservatively. One patient with a concomitant non-resectable lung carcinoma was of the MPD type, and the two other patients, aged 66 and 81 years, had diffuse microcystic lesions of the SBD type.

Preoperative Assessment

Ultrasonography (US) and computed tomography (CT) were performed routinely. Endoscopic retrograde cholangiopancreatography (ERCP) was attempted in 26 patients and was conducted successfully in 24 patients. A total of 28 patients underwent endoscopic ultrasonography (EUS). Endoscopic biopsies through the papilla were taken in ten patients. More sophisticated endoscopic explorations were performed selectively and according to the availability of the procedure in our institution. Transpapillary pancreatoscopy with an ultra-thin endoscope, available since 1996, was used in three patients. Exploration of the MPD by intraductal ultrasonography using a miniprobe has been possible since 1999 and was used for the purpose of diagnosing tumor extension in four patients. Magnetic resonance cholangiopancreatography (MRCP) has been possible since 1997 and was performed routinely after that date. A total of 21 out of 22 patients were examined by MRCP, as one patient was unable to sustain apnoea.

Intraoperative Investigations

Intraoperative ultrasonography (IUS) and frozen sections of the pancreatic margin(s) were performed routinely. Intraoperative pancreatoscopy was performed in 12 patients, using an the ultrathin endoscope (diameter: 2.8 mm): after removal of the operative specimen, the scope was inserted from the cut surface and the MPD of the pancreatic remnant was explored.

Surgical Procedures

Operative procedures included pylorus preserving pancreaticoduodenectomy (PPPD) (except in one patient with a previous distal gastrectomy in whom pancreaticoduodenectomy was performed). Pancreatogastric anastomosis has been used routinely since 1981. When distal pancreatectomy (DP) was performed it was always with preservation of the spleen and of the splenic vessels. Middle pancreatectomy (MP) included resection of the middle part of the pancreas with anastomosis of the pancreatic tail to a Roux-en-Y jejunal loop in the first patient and to the stomach in the following ones. Total pancreatectomy (TP) included preservation of the pylorus, splenic vessels and spleen. All patients underwent a standard lymphadenectomy.

Follow-up

Survival information was available in all 40 patients and was obtained by outpatient follow-up or personal phone interview with the referring physician or with the patient. Abdominal ultrasonography was performed at yearly intervals. CT and/or MRCP were performed selectively according to both clinical and US findings.

Pathologic Examination

Pathologic examination included morphological and histological assessments. Morphologically, the tumour was classified M type if the MPD was involved by the tumour with or without side branch duct invasion and S type if the tumour was localised in SBD without any invasion of the MPD. All specimens were examined histologically and the tumours were classified according to the World Health Organization as having adenomas, borderline tumors, carcinoma without invasion (or intraepithelial neoplasia) and carcinoma with invasion.[5,6,7]

Results

During the 16 years of this study, 40 patients underwent surgical resection for IPMT. Half of them underwent the operation during the last five years.

Clinical Findings

The most common presenting symptom was diarrhoea, followed by abdominal pain and weight loss (Table 13.1). Two patient had an incidental diagnosis by abdominal ultrasonography and one patient was referred by her dermatologist after she developed a Weber–Christian syndrome. A pancreatic endoprosthesis had been inserted in one alcoholic and addicted patient with the presumed diagnosis of chronic pancreatitis and a biliary endoprosthesis in another patient with jaundice.

Preoperative Assessment

Issue of mucus through the papilla was present in 17 patients, among 25 (68%) who had the papilla examined endoscopically (23 by ERCP and two by duodenoscopy). Transpapillary biopsies showed necrotic tissue in one case, mucinous proliferation without carcinoma in five cases, and mucinous carcinoma in four cases. The diagnosis of IPMT was established retrospectively in the first patient of the series who underwent surgery in 1985, after the publication from Itaï et al. one year later. It was established or at least strongly suggested in the 39 other patients at the end of the preoperative investigations. One patient who was alcoholic and addicted to opioids had a previous erroneous diagnosis of chronic pancreatitis which was corrected by endoscopic transpapillary biopsies.

Operative Treatment

The operative procedures are listed in Table 13.2. The decision to perform TP was taken preoperatively in two patients, according to preoperative work-up, and intra-

Table 13.1. Clinical presentation

Prevalent symptom	N patients
Diarrhoea	11 (27.5%)
Pain	8 (20%)
Weight loss	8 (20%)
Subacute pancreatitis	4 (10%)
Jaundice	3 (7.5%)
Incidental diagnosis by US	2 (5%)
Palpable mass	1 (2.5%)
Inflammatory syndrome	1 (2.5%)
Weber Christian syndrome	1 (2.5%)
Unstable Diabetes	1 (2.5%)

Table 13.2. Operative procedures

Operative procedure	N patients
Pancreaticoduodenectomy*	28 (70%)
Distal pancreatectomy	6 (15%)
Middle pancreatectomy	3 (7.5%)
Total pancreatectomy	3 (7.5%)
Total	40

* one with right colectomy and wedge resection of the portal vein

operatively in one patient according to the presence of adenoma at the frozen section of the pancreatic margin. Frozen sections appeared to be positive for adenoma in two other patients after PD, which led to extension of the pancreatic resection towards the left with a subsequent negative margin. Intraoperative pancreatoscopy failed to reveal any lesion in the MPD of the pancreatic remnant.

Pathology Findings

Morphological assessment revealed the tumour to be of the MPD type in 32 patients (80%) and of the SBD type in eight patients (20%). At histological assessment, the tumour was an adenoma in four patients (10%), a borderline tumour in five patients (12.5%), a carcinoma without invasion in nine patients (22.5%) and a carcinoma with invasion in 22 patients (55%). The relationship between the site of the tumour and the pathological diagnosis is shown in Table 13.3. Three of 22 patients with invasive carcinoma had lymph node involvement. One patient had a regional invasion of the mesocolon and of the resected cuff of portal vein without lymph node invasion. Associated tumours were present in two patients: a serous cystadenoma located in the body of the pancreas was resected by PPPD extended to the left, an adenocarcinoma of the ampulla was resected concomitantly by PPPD. Carcinoma with invasion was significantly more frequent in the MPD type (65.6%) than in the SBD type (12.5%) ($p = 0.01$).

Postoperative Course

One patient with an associated nephrotic syndrome died postoperatively on day 11 from massive digestive bleeding due to fistula of the pancreatic caudal remnant with subsequent rupture of the splenic artery, i.e. an operative mortality: of 2.5%. In this case, frozen section of the pancreatic margin was negative; attempt at intraoperative pancreatoscopy was unsuccessful due to the thin diameter of the MPD; pathologic examination of the operative specimen demonstrated carcinoma with invasion which was located in a SBD; although

Table 13.3. Pathologic findings of the operative specimen

Pathology	N patients	MPD	SBD
Adenoma	4 (10.0%)	2	2
Borderline	5 (12.5%)	1	4
Carcinoma without invasion	9 (22.5%)	8	1
Carcinoma with invasion	22 (55.0%)	21	1
Total	40	32	8

the patient was immediately taken back to the operating room for total pancreatectomy and gastrectomy, he died one day later from septic shock. Pathologic examination of the caudal remnant revealed an adenoma in a SBD which was distant from the pancreatic margin and had been overlooked by preoperative investigations (including EES and MRCP).

Long-term Survival

Nine patients died after discharge during the period of follow-up: six patients died from a cause which was unrelated to the disease and three patients with invasive carcinoma died from metastases.

Three patients underwent a reoperation for completion of the pancreatectomy due to persistence (not recurrence) of the disease in the pancreatic remnant: two after PPPD and one after distal pancreatectomy. The three patients had been explored preoperatively by MRCP and EUS.

In the first case which was of MPD duct type, carcinoma with invasion, a tiny cystic lesion was present in the pancreatic tail at distance from the main tumour on MRCP. Frozen section of the pancreatic margin was positive for adenoma and an additional 15 mm segment of the pancreatic tail was removed with a subsequent negative examination. Endoscopic exploration of the MPD of the pancreatic remnant was negative. Three years later, a 3 cm tumour was present in the splenic hilum. Completion pancreatectomy was undertaken and the pathologic examination of the operative specimen showed non invasive carcinoma. The patient is doing well three years later (Table 13.4).

In the second case, which was a multifocal tumour of SBD type, the head of the pancreas had been intentionally left in place after distal subtotal pancreatectomy. Frozen section of the pancreatic margin was negative. Borderline lesions were present in the operative specimen. Totalization by PPPD was decided because of the increase in size of the cystic lesions in the cephalic remnant at MRCP two years later. Pathologic examination of the operative specimen showed identical borderline lesions. The patient is doing well two years later.

The third patient underwent a PPPD for an invasive carcinoma of the MPD type. Preoperative exploration of the pancreatic tail by EES and MRCP was negative. So was the frozen section of the pancreatic margin and the intraoperative exploration of the distal remnant by pancreatoscopy. Asymptomatic recurrence of the tumour was detected by MRCP and was confirmed by EUS two years later. Totalization by splenopancreatectomy was performed. Pathologic examination concluded to invasive carcinoma. The patient is doing well six months later.

The actuarial 5-year survival for the whole series of 40 patients was 73.5%.

Table 13.4. Types of operation according to morphological findings

Operation	MPD type	SBD type
Pancreaticoduodenectomy	5	23
Distal pancreatectomy	1	5
Middle pancreatectomy	2	1
Total pancreatectomy	0	3

Discussion

IPMT has been described as an indolent neoplasm with a small propensity to invade adjacent structures and to metastasise to lymph nodes, liver and other organs.[8] Recent publications have anticipated that the better prognosis of these tumours compared with ductal adenocarcinoma is due to diagnosis before the stage of invasive carcinoma.[9] Many prognostic factors have been identified according to the local and regional extension of the tumor, and to its morphological type, the SBD-type being less aggressive than the MPD-type. Recently, two distinct patterns of intraductal papillae have been identified: intestinal type papillae which are similar morphologically to colic villous adenomas and pancreatobiliary type papillae which have more complex, branching papillae with cuboidal cells showing abundant cytoplasm. The prognostic significance of these two histological types remains questionable.[10]

Preoperative work-up and analysis of intraoperative findings are of critical importance in order to define the surgical strategy and to perform a successful operation.[11] MRCP is a non-invasive imaging technique which seems to be very promising in the evaluation of biliary and pancreatic ductal systems and in the diagnosis of suspected pancreaticobiliary neoplasms.[12] Moreover, it provides information about the ductal system even when a complete obstruction is present, which ERCP is unable to provide.[13] Precise analysis is essential since small lesions distant from the main tumour can be overlooked as was the case in one patient in this series.

One of the main questions regarding surgical strategy is to define the extent of the pancreatic resection.[14] To resect too much would expose the patient to unexpected diabetes. To resect insufficiently would lead to tumor recurrence. Intraoperative examinations which may help include ultrasonography, frozen sections of the pancreatic margins and pancreatoscopy of the pancreatic remnant.[15,16] Adequate resection needs careful attention to preoperative investigations and to intraoperative findings.[17] Frozen section of the resection margin has been advocated as the way to solve the problem[18] (Table 13.5). However, although it is essential, this procedure cannot be totally reliable, since the disease can spread inside the pancreas with intervals of normal epithelium as it was the case in two of our patients who required subsequent completion pancreatectomy.

In the literature, the proportion of total pancreatectomy ranges from 0–35%.[19] Our three cases of one-step total pancreatectomy were justified after pathologic examination of the operative specimen showing that the disease was disseminated through the gland. The three cases of reoperation to perform completion

Table 13.5. Types of operation according to histopathology

Operation	Adenoma	Borderline	Carcinoma without invasion	Carcinoma with invasion
PPPD	2	3	5	18
DP	1	1	2	2
MP	1	1	0	1
TP	0	0	2	1

PPPD: Pylorus pancreaticoduodenectomy
DP: Distal pancreatectomy
MP: Median pancreatectomy
TP: Total pancreatectomy

pancreatecomy were justified in a similar way. However, in two of the three cases, the preoperative MRCP was retrospectively indicative of multifocal disease and a one-step procedure would have been the procedure of choice. The patient who had an emergency reoperation, subsequently died from a residual microscopic SBD disease in the pancreatic remnant which was not detected either preoperatively or intraoperatively. It cannot be excluded that this residual disease participated in the occurrence of the postoperative acute stump pancreatitis with subsequent fistula and bleeding. Exploration by miniprobe was not attempted in this particular patient considering the absence of dilatation of the MPD at the body and tail of the pancreas.

Taking account of the one-step and two-step procedures, six patients underwent a total pancreatectomy which was justified after histopathological examination of the operative specimen. Total pancreatectomy has been advocated as the treatment of choice for IPMT.[20] However, due to the deleterious consequences of instable diabetes mellitus, there is no doubt that it must be restricted to patients with very specific findings and that any over-treatment should be avoided. In this regard, it is essential to take into account the morphological aspect of the IPMT and to differentiate the SBD type which has less of a chance of developing malignancy than MPD.[21] However, the SBD type does not preclude invasive carcinoma since it was the case in one patient of our series (the patient who died postoperatively).

Long-term follow-up is mandatory after resection and MRCP seems to be very promising for the exploration of the pancreatic stump after partial pancreatectomy. More information is required to determine the rhythm of the surveillance according to the morphological type and to the histopathological characteristics of the tumour.

References

1. Sohn TA, Yeo CJ, Cameron JL, et al. Intraductal papillary mucinous neoplasms of the pancreas: an increasingly recognized clinicopathologic entity. Ann Surg 2001; 234:313–322.
2. Ohhashi K, Murakami Y, Takekoshi T. Four cases of « mucin-producing » cancer of the pancreas on specific findings of the papilla Vater. Prog Dig Endosc 1982; 20:348–51.
3. Itaï Y, Ohhashi K, Nagai H, et al. "Ductectatic" mucinous cystadenoma and cystadenocarcinoma of the pancreas. Radiology 1986; 161:697–700.
4. Rickaert F, Cremer M, Deviere J, et al. Intraductal mucin-hypersecreting neoplasms of the pancreas. Gastroenterology 1991; 101:512–519.
5. Kloppel G, Solcia E, Longnecker DS, et al. Histological typing of tumors of the exocrine pancreas. In: World Health Organization international classification of tumors, 2 ed. Berlin: Springer 1996; 11–20.
6. Hruban RH, Adsay NV, Albores-Saavedra J, et al. Pancreatic intraepithelial neoplasia: a new nomenclature and classification system for pancreatic duct lesions. Am J Surg Pathol 2001; 25:579–86.
7. Longnecker DS, Adler G, Hruban RH, et al. Intraductal papillary-mucinous neoplasms of the pancreas, pp. 237–240, in Hamilton SR, Aaltonen LA (eds) Pathology and Genetics. Tumors of the Digestive System, IARC Press, Lyon, 2000.
8. Kimura W, Makuuchi M, Kuroda A. Characteristics and treatment of mucin-producing tumor of the pancreas. Hepato-Gastroenterology 1998; 45:2001–2008.
9. Falconi M, Salvia R, Bassi C, et al. Clinicopathological features and treatment of intraductal papillary mucinous tumour of the pancreas; Br J Surg 2001; 88:376–381.
10. Adsay NV, Conlon KC, Zee SY, et al. Intraductal papillary-mucinous neoplasms of the pancreas. An Analysis of in situ and invasive carcinomas in 28 patients. Cancer 2002; 94:62–77.
11. Sugiyama M, Atomi Y. Intraductal papillary mucinous tumors of the pancreas. Imaging studies and treatment strategies. Ann Surg 1998; 228:685–91.

12. Grogan JR, Saeian K, Taymor AJ, et al. Making sense of Mucin-Producing Pancreatic Tumors. AJR 2001; 176:921–928.
13. Kripalani J, Somnay K, Katz S, et al. Mucinous ductal ectasia of the pancreas: the diagnostic value of MRCP. HPB 1999; 1:223–225.
14. Partensky C, Laugier R. Tumeurs intracanalaires papillaires mucineuses pancréatiques: quelle chirurgie pour quelle tumeur. Gastroenterol Clin Biol 2000; 24:17–20.
15. Kaneko T, Nakao A, Inoue S, et al. Intraoperative ultrasonography by high-resolution annular array transducer for intraductal papillary mucinous tumors of the pancreas. Surgery 2001; 129:55–65.
16. Kaneko T, Nakao A, Nomoto S, et al. Intraoperative pancreatoscopy with the ultrathin pancreatoscope for mucin-producing tumors of the pancreas; Arch Surg 1998; 133:263–267.
17. Kanazumi N, Nakao A, Kaneko T, et al. Surgical treatment of intraductal papillary-mucinous tumors of the pancreas. Hepato-Gastroenterology 2001; 48:967–971.
18. Paye F, Sauvanet A, Terris B, et al. Intraductal papillary mucinous tumors of the pancreas: Pancreatic resections guided by preoperative morphological assessment and intraoperative frozen section examination. Surgery 2000; 127:536–544.
19. Cuillerier E, Cellier C, Palazzo L, et al. Outcome after surgical resection of intraductal papillary and mucinous tumors of the pancreas. Am J Gastroenterol 2000; 95:441–445.
20. Bendix Holme J, Jacobsen NO, Rokkjaer M, et al. Total pancreatectomy in six patients with intraductal papillary mucinous tumour of the pancreas: the treatment of choice. HPB 2001; 3:257–262.
21. Terris B, Ponsot P, Paye F, et al. Intraductal Papillary mucinous tumors of the pancreas confined to secondary ducts show less aggressive features as compared with those involving the main pancreatic duct. Am J Surg Pathol 2000; 24:1372–1377.

Part 2

Chronic Pancreatitis

14 Endoscopic Ultrasound in the Diagnosis of Chronic Pancreatitis and Pancreatic Cancer

Bernhard Glasbrenner, Stefan Kahl and Peter Malfertheiner

Since its introduction in the 1980s endoscopic ultrasound (EUS) has added significantly to the diagnosis of gastrointestinal diseases.[1] One key function has become the staging of esophageal and gastric tumors.[2–7] In pancreatic diseases EUS offers much better access than transabdominal ultrasound for visualization of the whole pancreas and its surroundings, and pancreatic ductal and parenchymal changes may be detected with high resolution. In experienced hands EUS has the highest detection rate of pancreatic neuroendocrine tumors compared to computed tomography (CT), angiography and somatostatin receptor scintigraphy. In particular insulinomas, which are usually small lesions, are detected with high accuracy by EUS.[8–10] In comparison with endoscopic retrograde cholangiopancreatography (ERCP), the technique of EUS is less invasive and carries no risk of pancreatitis or infection. In recent years EUS has progressed from a purely imaging modality to one that can provide tissue diagnosis by EUS-guided fine needle aspiration (FNA). EUS has also evolved into a treatment modality, for example drainage of pancreatic pseudocysts.[11–17]

This review focuses on EUS in the diagnosis and staging of chronic pancreatitis (CP) and pancreatic cancer (PCa) including cystic lesions.

Chronic Pancreatitis

The diagnosis of chronic pancreatitis is based on clinical history, morphologic abnormalities, and functional impairment of the pancreas. In the lack of histopathology, invasive and non-invasive imaging procedures are the most important diagnostic tools for the primary diagnosis of chronic pancreatitis. Transabdominal ultrasonography is the non-invasive and well-tolerated modality of first choice in a patient with a history and symptoms suggestive of CP. Transabdominal ultrasound is first choice beause of aspects such as costs, availability, lack of complications and exclusion of differential diagnoses. The diagnostic accuracy, of course, depends on the visualization of the organ and the investigator's experience.[18]

Cambridge classification system

The most important criteria of chronic pancreatitis for ultrasonography, computed tomography (CT) and ERCP are listed in the Cambridge classification system.[19,20]

An important drawback of ultrasonography is its limited sensitivity for the diagnosis of an uncomplicated early stage of chronic pancreatitis. The diagnostic criteria are the same for CT, which is more expensive but less dependent on the investigator's skill and experience. CT has probably the best diagnostic accuracy for pancreatic calcifications, a specific sign of advanced chronic pancreatitis. In our hands the main use of CT is for complicated chronic pancreatitis with specific questions concerning the presence of inflammatory masses, pseudocysts or calculi in the main pancreatic duct.

In the absence of histology, endoscopic retrograde pancreatography (ERP) is the gold standard for the diagnosis and staging of CP. If the pancreatic duct and its side branches are displayed in high detail, certain abnormalities of pancreatograms can be considered highly specific findings for chronic pancreatitis. The current international definitions and criteria of pancreatographic diagnosis of CP are the 'heart' of the Cambridge classification system.[21] The accuracy of ERP is superior to that of transabdominal ultrasound and CT, but the technique is invasive and needs more and specialized training. Acute pancreatitis following ERP is reported in up to several per cent of cases investigated.[22, 23] Interpretation of pancreatograms may be difficult in the early follow-up period after acute pancreatitis (reversible or persistent or progressive damage?) and in the elderly (chronic pancreatitis or presbypancreas?).[24]

It still seems unlikely that magnetic resonance pancreatography (MRP) will be able to substitute for ERP in the diagnosis of mild CP, since a sufficient visualization of the side branches will probably not be achieved.[25–27]

EUS in chronic pancreatitis

With regard to our present understanding on the pathophysiology of CP, EUS is a very interesting diagnostic tool because it visualizes both parenchymal and ductal changes with high resolution. Based on the necrosis-fibrosis sequence as a crucial event in the development of chronic pancreatitis,[28–30] it seems logical that the detection of parenchymal necrosis or fibrotic septa by EUS might be achieved earlier in the course of the disease than detection of dilated side branches or irregularities of the main pancreatic duct by ERP.

There are several studies showing that EUS is highly sensitive and specific in detecting chronic pancreatitis.[31–47] Wiersema et al.[31] have described and investigated positive predictive values of parenchymal and ductal signs of chronic pancreatitis detectable by EUS (Table 14.1). The EUS criteria for CP have a diagnostic accuracy depending on the number of criteria which are present in a

Table 14.1. EUS features of chronic pancreatitis[31]

Parenchymal changes	focal areas of reduced echogenicity hyperechoic foci (> 3 mm diameter) gland size, cysts accentuation of lobular pattern (hypoechoic areas surrounded by hyperechoic septae)
Ductal changes	increased duct wall echogenicity irregular caliber of main pancreatic duct dilatation of main pancreatic duct dilatation of side branches calculi

specific case. In a prospective study in 126 patients, the positive predictive value of EUS for CP was >85% if >2 criteria were present for all CP patients and if >6 criteria were present for moderate to severe CP (based on ERP criteria). On the other hand, the negative predictive value for moderate to severe CP was >85% if <3 criteria were present.[37]

The most interesting question remains whether EUS is superior to ERP which was taken as the gold standard in most investigations. As it is a major problem to perform histological studies to confirm findings of imaging procedures, we attempted to use a long term follow-up to confirm the diagnosis of CP suspected on EUS.[47] Among 38 patients (29.2%) with a normal ERP 32 patients (84.2%) presented with morphological features on EUS consistent with early chronic pancreatitis in EUS (Table 14.2). During follow-up (median 18 months, range 6–25 months) chronic pancreatitis was confirmed by repeated ERP in 22 of these 32 patients (68,8%). Based on these follow-up data, the sensitivities of endoscopic ultrasonography and endoscopic retrograde pancreatography at the time of the first examination were calculated as 100% and 81% respectively ($p < 0.001$).[47]

Our present conclusion is that EUS seems to be as good as ERCP in diagnosing chronic pancreatitis in advanced stages. In early stages of the disease, when the ductal system is still normal, EUS appears to be more sensitive in diagnosing alcoholic chronic pancreatitis. The open question that remains in the absence of histopathology: How specific are parenchymal lesions seen on EUS in patients with alcohol abuse with and without a clinical history suggestive for CP?

A possible solution for the future is to combine EUS and fine-needle puncture of the pancreas. It has recently been shown that EUS combined with fine-needle aspiration cytology tends to increase specificity and, in particular, the negative predictive value of EUS alone.[48] However, the diagnosis of CP by cytology is not really settled, and the aim must be to obtain high quality histological samples with a low complication rate in patients with suspected early CP on EUS.

Pancreatic Cancer

Pancreatic cancer is associated with a high mortality rate and a short median survival. The large majority of patients diagnosed with pancreatic cancer display clinical symptoms at an advanced stage of the disease.[49, 50] The value of different imaging methods in the assessment of pancreatic cancer is therefore not only related to their ability to detect the tumor, but also in providing information regarding the involvement of surrounding organs, lymph nodes and blood vessels. It is obvious that a high-resolution ultrasound transducer placed in direct proximity to the pancreas is an interesting diagnostic tool for these purposes.

Table 14.2. Parenchymal and ductal EUS changes of CP in patients with normal ERP in a prospective follow-up study on the diagnosis of early chronic pancreatitis[47]

	n	%
Parenchymal changes	32	100
accentuation of lobular pattern (hypoechoic areas surrounded by hyperechoic septae)	32	100
focal areas of reduced echogenicity	18	56
hyperechoic foci (> 3 mm diameter)	8	25
Ductal changes	5	15
increased duct wall echogenicity	5	15

There are three key issues EUS has to address in the diagnosis and staging of pancreatic tumors:

- to visualize the tumor and lymph nodes,
- to differentiate between benign and malignant tumors,
- to contribute to preoperative tumor staging and predict local irresectability.

Visualization of Pancreatic Tumors and Lymph Nodes

EUS is the most sensitive imaging procedure for identifying small pancreatic tumors. The method can reliably detect tumors of less than 2 cm in diameter, when the chance for curative resection is more likely.[51–53] Sensitivity and specificity of EUS to detect pancreatic tumors in comparison to other imaging methods in a large prospective study are shown in Table 14.3.[53]

Eighty to 90% of patients with pancreatic cancer present with symptoms such as pain, jaundice or weight loss at the time of diagnosis. In this clinical circumstance almost any of the available imaging modalities can confirm the diagnosis and it is questionable if the use of multiple imaging techniques adds significantly to patient management. This should be taken into consideration when deciding the optimal work up for patients with pancreatic cancer.

In a study published by Rosch et al. in patients with a strong suspicion of pancreatic disase only a marginal increase in diagnostic sensitivity was achieved by employing sophisticated imaging methods.[54] However, in this study the specificity was substantially superior if either EUS, ERCP or CT was added to US. From this paper we can conclude that imaging procedures should be used in a stepwise fashion for optimal patient management. In this scenario with clinical evaluation and US, EUS would appear to be the optimal additional diagnostic tool to employ with superior specificity to ERCP and other imaging modalities.

Differentiation between Benign and Malignant Pancreatic Tumors

Pancreatic tumors can be mimicked by focal inflammation and differentiation is a particular challenge. In a group of 27 patients with advanced chronic pancreatitis Barthet et al. identified 5 patients with suspected pancreatic carcinoma. In these patients diagnosis was followed up by surgery: three patients had pancreatic carcinoma and two had inflammatory tumors due to chronic pancreatitis.[55] The sensitivity of EUS was 100% but the positive predictive value for pancreatic carcinoma was only 60%. This corresponds to data from Rosch.[53] We performed a prospective comparison of EUS and ERCP in the assessment of masses in the pancreatic head, and the results for both methods and their combination to predict malignant tumors are shown in Table 14.4.[56] Our major finding was that both methods had

Table 14.3. Parameters of different imaging methods for visualization and characterization of pancreatic tumors in a large prospective study on 132 patients[53]

	EUS	US	CT	ERCP	Angiography
sensitivity all tumors	94%	69%	74%	91%	88%
sensitivity tumors < 3 mm	100%	40%	53%	72%	
specificity	100%	40%	53%	72%	

Table 14.4. Results of EUS, ERCP, and of the combination of both to predict malignancy in a large prospective series of patients with benign (n=45) and malignant (n=50) masses in the pancreatic head[56]

	EUS	ERCP	EUS + ERCP
Sensitivity	78%	81%	92%
Specificity	93%	88%	86%
Positive predictive value	93%	89%	88%
Negative predictive value	78%	80%	90%
Diagnostic accuracy	85%	84%	89%

similar diagnostic accuracies to separate malignant from benign masses in the pancreatic head, and the combination of both procedures was not superior to the use of one modality alone.

The positive predictive value of EUS in pancreatic cancer can be enhanced by adding EUS-guided fine needle aspiration (FNA). The accuracy of EUS-guided FNA for the detection of malignant tumors ranges between 85% and 95%.[57–60] In a large prospective study of 102 patients with suspected pancreatic tumor, EUS-guided FNA was negative in 45 patients. Only 4 of these 45 patients had pancreatic cancer at the time of surgery. Sensitivity of EUS-guided FNA to detect pancreatic cancer was therefore 94%.[59] Cases of tumor seeding have not been reported.[61] An update on the present state of knowledge on FNA in pancreatic masses including expert tips for success has been recently published.[62]

Preoperative Tumor Staging and Prediction of Resectability

Preoperative tumor staging (T- and N-stage) is the key domain of EUS and has been confirmed in a large number of studies. A key study reporting on T- and N-stages by EUS in comparison with CT found EUS to be more accurate than CT in all possible tumor-stages and is reported in Table 14.5.[63] In a meta analysis involving 357 patients from 14 studies, EUS had an overall accuracy in preoperative staging of 83 %.[64] However, to draw the appropriate conclusions for our present clinical practice, EUS results must be compared to modern versions of helical CT or magnetic resonance imaging (MRI) with slice thicknesses of 5 mm. We compared these imaging modalities in a large prospective series of patients.[65] In our hands the accuracy rates for the diagnosis of local nonresectability were 92% for EUS, 92% for MRI and 90% for CT. However, EUS does not contribute to the visualization of small distant liver and peritoneal metastases. At present, we suggest a modern helical CT as the most valuable single method for preoperative tumor staging and prediction of resectability. If either no tumor is despicted on CT or local resectability seems questionable, EUS should be performed.

When this diagnostic approach is applied to patients with suspected pancreatic cancer, vascular invasion should be diagnosed by EUS with criteria providing high specificity. This concept is thought to avoid false-positive results that might exclude resectable patients from the only potentially curative therapeutic procedure. In a recent publication Rosch et al.[66]proposed the following criteria for vascular invasion:

- visualization of tumor in the lumen,
- complete obstruction,

Table 14.5. Comparison of accuracy of EUS vs CT in different T- and N-stages of pancreatic cancer[63]

	T1	T2	T3	N1	N2
CT	65%	67%	38%	52%	100%
EUS	92%	85%	93%	72%	72%

- collateral vessels,
- irregular tumor-vessel relationship.

These authors found a sensitivity of only 43% but a specificity of 91% of EUS to detect venous vascular invasion. EUS seems particularly accurate for the detection of splenoportal venous invasion but less accurate for demonstrating arterial or superior mesenteric vein involvement.[66,67] Our personal strategy is to diagnose vascular invasion only in cases with clear visualization of intravascular tumor growth, resulting in a specificity of 100% and a sensitivity of 50% for venous infiltration.[65] We reported that an irregular tumor-vessel relationship is also often seen in patients with inflammatory masses in the pancreatic head. Furthermore the visualization of vascular structures may be difficult with EUS in patients with large tumors or altered anatomy. With the advance of EUS equipment complemented by doppler ultrasononography sensitivity and specificity for the detection of vascular involvement in pancreatic cancer might be further improved.

Benign and Malignant Lymph Nodes

The pancreas is surrounded by multiple small lymph nodes that are usually not seen on EUS. Determination of lymph node involvement in pancreatic cancer is sometimes important for therapeutic decisions but remains a difficult task. The following characteristics of positive lymph nodes have been described:[68,69]

- increased size of lymph nodes (different cutoffs)
- inhomogeneity
- hypoechogeneity
- round, demarcated appearance.

In large series (Table 14.5) and in the literature EUS N-staging is less accurate than T-staging, with an overall accuracy of 74 % (ranging from 49 % to 94 %) in an analysis of literature results.[64]

It is obvious that results of EUS in lymph node staging largely depend on the control population. In our study on EUS in the preoperative assessment of masses in the pancreatic head, benign lymph nodes in inflammatory masses in chronic pancreatitis occurred up to an EUS size of 12 mm.[56] We tried to overcome this problem by applying different cutoffs of lymph node size to patients with (9 mm) and without (5 mm) CP, resulting in a high specificity (91%) but a low sensitivity (55%) and an accuracy of 81% in the diagnosis of malignant lymph nodes. As already mentioned, our criteria were planned to avoid overstaging, thus promoting understaging. The preoperative differentiation between benign and malignant lymph nodes in populations like ours cannot accurately be done without cytology or histology. Once again, EUS-guided FNA seems to be helpful.[70]

An important issue for the future will be whether EUS will have an impact on the management and outcome of patients with pancreatic cancer. It seems likely that EUS will contribute to avoid the need for diagnostic laparoscopy and laparotomy.[71–73] The 3-months improvement in median survival that was found in a comparison of different time intervalls with and without application of EUS is probably multifactorial but should stimulate further research on this topic.[73]

Cystic Pancreatic Lesions

The necessary clinical distinction in pancreatic cystic lesions is between pseudocysts and cystic neoplasms. Pancreatic pseudocysts develop in 2 % to 10 % of patients with mild and up to 50% of patients with severe acute pancreatitis.[74–76] The pathophysiological mechanisms involved are intrapancreatic necrosis or peripancreatic fluid collections which become demarcated with time. Less than half of known pseudocysts following acute pancreatitis regress spontaneously. Those that persist may become symptomatic depending on their localization and size. Both parenchymal and extrapancreatic pseudocysts occur together in up to 40 % of patients suffering with chronic pancreatitis.[77,78] It is a clinical challenge to differentiate between symptomatic and asymptomatic cystic lesions in a disease which is characterized *per se* by pain.

Neoplastic cysts occur in approximately 10% of all cystic lesions. Koito described six classifications of the internal structures of pancreatic cysts, which can be visualized by EUS (Table 14.6). All neoplastic cysts in this study belonged to the first four types, and all non-neoplastic cysts belonged to the last two types. The accuracy of EUS for the distinction between malignant and benign cystic tumors was 96% and 92%, respectively.[79] These excellent results were only partially confirmed by other groups.[80,81] In a recent study of EUS-guided FNA in cystic pancreatic lesions, cytopathology did not improve diagnostic accuracy 81. Our personal opinion is still that the clinical data of the patient (previous history of acute or chronic pancreatitis?) together with the age and clinical course should also strongly be considered for decision-making in the diagnosis and treatment of cystic pancreatic lesions.[82]

Conclusions

EUS contributes substantially to the diagnosis and staging of patients with chronic pancreatitis and pancreatic cancer. EUS is as good as ERCP in diagnosing chronic pancreatitis in advanced stages. In early stages of the disease when the ductal system remains normal, EUS appears to be a superior diagnostic modality because it can detect features of chronic pancreatitis in the parenchyma not visible by other

Table 14.6. Classification of cystic pancreatic tumors[79]

1	Thick wall type
2	tumor protruding type
3	thick septal type
4	microcystic type
5	thin septal type
6	simple type

techniques. The specificity of these EUS findings for the present definition of chronic pancreatitis based on histopathological grounds remains to be elucidated.

Detection of small lesions and neuroendocrine pancreatic tumors as well as preoperative staging of pancreatic cancer has improved with EUS. For detection of small pancreatic tumors less than 2 cm in diameter EUS is the most sensitive method. In the preoperative assessment of pancreatic cancer, EUS in experienced hands should be performed if no tumor is depicted on CT or if local resectability is questionable on CT. EUS is equivalent to ERCP to separate malignant from benign masses in the pancreatic head. EUS-guided fine needle aspiration is a promising tool to enhance the value of EUS in the diagnosis of pancreatic diseases. Whether the use of EUS will have an impact on the outcome of pancreatic cancer can not be answered at present. EUS is probably valuable but not yet sufficiently evaluated in the differential diagnosis of cystic pancreatic lesions.

Acknowledgement

We thank Dr. D. McNamara for critical review of the manuscript.

References

1. Byrne MF, Jowell PS. Gastrointestinal imaging: endoscopic ultrasound. Gastroenterology 2002; 122:1631–1648.
2. Botet JF, Lightdale CJ, Zauber AG, et al. Preoperative staging of esophageal cancer: comparison of endoscopic US and dynamic CT. Radiology 1991; 181:419–425.
3. Grimm H, Binmoeller KF, Hamper K, et al. Endosonography for preoperative locoregional staging of esophageal and gastric cancer. Endoscopy 1993; 25:224–230.
4. Ziegler K, Sanft C, Zeitz M, et al. Evaluation of endosonography in TN staging of oesophageal cancer. Gut 1991; 32:16–20.
5. Ziegler K, Sanft C, Zimmer T, et al. Comparison of computed tomography, endosonography, and intraoperative assessment in TN staging of gastric carcinoma. Gut 1993; 34:604–610.
6. Botet JF, Lightdale CJ, Zauber AG, et al. Preoperative staging of gastric cancer: comparison of endoscopic US and dynamic CT. Radiology 1991; 181:426–432.
7. Caletti G, Ferrari A, Brocchi E, et al. Accuracy of endoscopic ultrasonography in the diagnosis and staging of gastric cancer and lymphoma. Surgery 1993; 113:14–27.
8. Rosch T, Lightdale CJ, Botet JF, et al. Localization of pancreatic endocrine tumors by endoscopic ultrasonography. N Engl J Med 1992; 326:1721–1726.
9. Glover JR, Shorvon PJ, Lees WR. Endoscopic ultrasound for localisation of islet cell tumours. Gut 1992; 33:108–110.
10. Tenner SM, Banks PA, Wiersema MJ, et al. Evaluation of pancreatic disease by endoscopic ultrasonography. Am J Gastroenterol 1997; 92:18–2.
11. Cremer M, Deviere J, Engelholm L. Endoscopic management of cysts and pseudocysts in chronic pancreatitis: long-term follow-up after 7 years of experience. Gastrointest Endosc 1989; 35:1–9.
12. Sahel J. Endoscopic drainage of pancreatic cysts. Endoscopy 1991; 23:181–184.
13. Binmoeller KF, Seifert H, Walter A, et al. Transpapillary and transmural drainage of pancreatic pseudocysts. Gastrointest Endosc 1995; 42:219–224.
14. Dohmoto M, Rupp KD, Hunerbein M, et al. Endoscopic drainage of pancreatic pseudocysts. Dtsch Med Wochenschr 1995; 120:1647–1651.
15. Pfaffenbach B, Langer M, Stabenow-Lohbauer U, et al. Endosonography controlled transgastric drainage of pancreatic pseudocysts. Dtsch Med Wochenschr 1998; 123:1439–1442.
16. Beckingham IJ, Krige JE, Bornman PC, et al. Long term outcome of endoscopic drainage of pancreatic pseudocysts. Am J Gastroenterol 1999; 94:71–74.
17. Seifert H, Dietrich C, Schmitt T, et al. Endoscopic ultrasound-guided one-step transmural drainage of cystic abdominal lesions with a large-channel echo endoscope. Endoscopy 2000; 32:255–259.

18. Glasbrenner B, Kahl S, Malfertheiner P. Modern diagnostics of chronic pancreatitis. Eur J Gastroenterol Hepatol 2002; 14:935–941.
19. Sarner M, Cotton PB. Classification of pancreatitis. Gut 1984; 25:756–759.
20. Singer MV, Gyr KE, Sarles H. Revised classification of pancreatitis. Gastroenterology 1985; 89:683–69.
21. Axon AT, Classen M, Cotton PB, et al. Pancreatography in chronic pancreatitis: international definitions. Gut 1984; 25:1107–1112.
22. Gottlieb K, Sherman S. ERCP and biliary endoscopic sphincterotomy-induced pancreatitis. Gastrointest Endosc Clin North Am 1998; 8:87–114.
23. Freeman ML, DiSario JA, Nelson DB, et al. Risk factors for post-ERCP pancreatitis: a prospective, multicenter study. Gastrointest Endosc 2001; 54:425–434.
24. Forsmark CE, Toskes PP. What does an abnormal pancreatogram mean? Gastrointest Endosc Clin North Am 1995; 5:105–123.
25. Matos C, Deviere J, Nicaise N, et al. Magnetic resonance cholangiopancreatography (MRCP): a perspective on potential clinical applications. Acta Gastroenterol Belg 1997; 60:268–273.
26. Merkle EM, Nüssle K, Glasbrenner B, et al. MRCP – current status. Z Gastroenterol 1998; 36:215–224.
27. Soto JA, Yucel EK, Barish MA, et al. MR cholangio-pancreatography after unsuccessful or incomplete ERCP. Radiology 1996; 199:91–98.
28. Kloppel G, Maillet B. The morphological basis for the evolution of acute pancreatitis into chronic pancreatitis. Virchows Arch A Pathol Anat Histopathol 1992; 420:1–4.
29. Kloppel G, Maillet B. Chronic pancreatitis: evolution of the disease. Hepatogastroenterology 1991; 38:408–412.
30. Ammann RW, Heitz PU, Klöppel G. Course of alcoholic chronic pancreatitis: a prospective clinicomorphological long-term study. Gastroenterology 1996; 111:224–231.
31. Wiersema MJ, Hawes RH, Lehman GA, et al. Prospective evaluation of endoscopic ultrasonography and endoscopic retrograde cholangiopancreatography in patients with chronic abdominal pain of suspected pancreatic origin. Endoscopy 1993; 25:555–564.
32. Wiersema MJ. Diagnosing chronic pancreatitis: shades of gray. Gastrointest Endosc 1998; 48:102–106.
33. Wiersema MJ, Wiersema LM. Endosonography of the pancreas: normal variation versus changes of early chronic pancreatitis. Gastrointest Endosc Clin N Am 1995; 5:487–496.
34. Buscail L, Escourrou J, Moreau J, et al. Endoscopic ultrasonography in chronic pancreatitis: a comparative prospective study with conventional ultrasonography, computed tomography, and ERCP. Pancreas 1995; 10:251–257.
35. Sahai AV, Hoffman BJ, Hawes RH. More EUS questions: what is the impact of EUS impact studies? Am J Gastroenterol 1997; 92:717–718.
36. Sahai AV, Mishra G, Penman ID, et al. EUS to detect evidence of pancreatic disease in patients with persistent or nonspecific dyspepsia. Gastrointest Endosc 2000; 52:153–159.
37. Sahai AV, Zimmerman M, Aabakken L, et al. Prospective assessment of the ability of endoscopic ultrasound to diagnose, exclude, or establish the severity of chronic pancreatitis found by endoscopic retrograde cholangiopancreatography. Gastrointest Endosc 1998; 48:18–25.
38. Catalano MF. Normal structures on endoscopic ultrasonography: visualization measurement data and interobserver variation. Gastrointest Endosc Clin N Am 1995; 5:475–486.
39. Catalano MF, Geenen JE. Diagnosis of chronic pancreatitis by endoscopic ultrasonography. Endoscopy 1998; 30 (Suppl 1):A111–A115.
40. Catalano MF, Lahoti S, Alcocer E, et al. Dynamic imaging of the pancreas using real-time endoscopic ultrasonography with secretin stimulation. Gastrointest Endosc 1998; 48:580–587.
41. Catalano MF, Lahoti S, Geenen JE, et al. Prospective evaluation of endoscopic ultrasonography, endoscopic retrograde pancreatography, and secretin test in the diagnosis of chronic pancreatitis. Gastrointest Endosc 1998; 48:48–11.
42. Lees WR. Endoscopic ultrasonography of chronic pancreatitis and pancreatic pseudocysts. Scand J Gastroenterol Suppl 1986; 123:123–129.
43. Lees WR, Vallon AG, Denyer ME, et al. Prospective study of ultrasonography in chronic pancreatic disease. Br Med J 1979; 1:162–164.
44. Nattermann C, Goldschmidt AJ, Dancygier H. Endosonography in the assessment of pancreatic tumors. A comparison of the endosonographic findings of carcinomas and segmental inflammatory changes. Dtsch Med Wochenschr 1995; 120:1571–1576.
45. Nattermann C, Goldschmidt AJ, Dancygier H. Endosonography in chronic pancreatitis – a comparison between endoscopic retrograde pancreatography and endoscopic ultrasonography. Endoscopy 1993; 25:565–570.

46. Hastier P, Buckley MJ, Francois E, et al. A prospective study of pancreatic disease in patients with alcoholic cirrhosis: comparative diagnostic value of ERCP and EUS and long-term significance of isolated parenchymal abnormalities. Gastrointest Endosc 1999; 49:705–709.
47. Kahl S, Glasbrenner B, Leodolter A, et al. EUS in the diagnosis of early chronic pancreatitis: A prospective follow-up study. Gastrointest Endosc 2002; 55:507–511.
48. Hollerbach S, Klamann A, Topalidis T, et al. Endoscopic ultrasonography (EUS) and fine-needle aspiration (FNA) cytology for diagnosis of chronic pancreatitis. Endoscopy 2001; 33:824–831.
49. Beger HG, Link KH, Poch B, et al. Pancreatic cancer: recent progress in diagnosis and treatment. In: Neoptolemos JP, Lemonie NR (eds.). Pancreatic cancer: molecular and clinical advances. Blackwell Science, Oxford, 1996; pp. 227–235.
50. Ahmad NA, Lewis JD, Ginsberg GG, et al. Longterm survival after pancreatic resection for pancreatic carcinoma. Am J Gastroenterol 2001; 96:2609–2615.
51. Palazzo L, Roseau G, Gayet B, et al. Endoscopic ultrasonography in the diagnosis and staging of pancreatic adenocarcinoma. Results of a prospective study with comparison to ultrasonography and CT scan. Endoscopy 1993; 25:143–150.
52. Muller MF, Meyenberger C, Bertschinger P, et al. Pancreatic tumors: evaluation with endoscopic US, CT, and MR imaging. Radiology 1994; 190:745–751.
53. Rosch T, Lorenz R, Braig C, et al. Endoscopic ultrasound in pancreatic tumor diagnosis. Gastrointest Endosc 1991; 37:347–352.
54. Rosch T, Schusdziarra V, Born P, et al. Modern imaging methods versus clinical assessment in the evaluation of hospital in-patients with suspected pancreatic disease. Am J Gastroenterol 2000; 95:2261–2270.
55. Barthet M, Portal I, Boujaoude J, et al. Endoscopic ultrasonographic diagnosis of pancreatic cancer complicating chronic pancreatitis. Endoscopy 1996; 28:487–491.
56. Glasbrenner B, Schwarz M, Pauls S, et al. Prospective comparison of Endoscopic ultrasound and endoscopic retrograde cholangio-pancreatography in the preoperative assessment of masses in the pancreatic head. Dig Surg 2000; 17:468–474.
57. Gress FG, Hawes RH, Savides TJ, et al. Endoscopic ultrasound-guided fine-needle aspiration biopsy using linear array and radial scanning endosonography. Gastrointest Endosc 1997; 45:243–250.
58. Wiersema MJ, Vilmann P, Giovannini M, et al. Endosonography-guided fine-needle aspiration biopsy: diagnostic accuracy and complication assessment. Gastroenterology 1997; 112:1087–1095.
59. Gress F, Gottlieb K, Sherman S, et al. Endoscopic ultrasonography-guided fine-needle aspiration biopsy of suspected pancreatic cancer. Ann Intern Med 2001; 134:459–464.
60. Chang KJ, Wiersema MJ. Endoscopic ultrasound-guided fine-needle aspiration biopsy and interventional endoscopic ultrasonography. Emerging technologies. Gastrointest Endosc Clin N Am 1997; 7:221–235.
61. Bhutani MS. Interventional endoscopic ultrasonography: state of the art at the new millenium. Endoscopy 2000; 32:62–71.
62. Binmoeller KF, Rathod VD. Difficult pancreatic mass FNA: tips for success. Gastrointestinal Endoscopy 2002; 56 (Suppl):S86–S91.
63. Gress F, Hawes RH, Savides TJ, et al. Role of EUS in the preoperative staging of pancreatic cancer: a large single-center experience. Gastrointest Endosc 1999; 50:786–791.
64. Rosch T. Staging of pancreatic cancer. Analysis of literature results. Gastrointest Endosc Clin N Am 1995; 5:735–739.
65. Schwarz M, Pauls S, Sokiranski R, et al. Is a preoperative multidiagnostic approach to predict surgical resectability of periampullary tumors still effective? Am J Surg 2001; 182:243–249.
66. Rosch T, Dittler HJ, Strobel K, et al. Endoscopic ultrasound criteria for vascular invasion in the staging of cancer of the head of the pancreas: a blind reevaluation of videotapes. Gastrointest Endosc 2000; 52:469–477.
67. Snady H, Bruckner H, Siegel J, et al. Endoscopic ultrasonographic criteria of vascular invasion by potentially resectable pancreatic tumors. Gastrointest Endosc 1994; 40:326–333.
68. Grimm H, Hamper K, Binmoeller KF, et al. Enlarged lymph nodes: malignant or not? Endoscopy 1992; 24 (Suppl 1):320–323.
69. Catalano MF, Sivak MV, Jr., Rice T, et al. Endosonographic features predictive of lymph node metastasis. Gastrointest Endosc 1994; 40:442–446.
70. Bhutani MS, Hawes RH, Hoffman BJ. A comparison of the accuracy of of echo features during endoscopic ultrasound (EUS) and EUS-guided fine-needle aspiration for diagnosis of malignant lymph node invasion. Gastrointest Endosc 1997; 45:474–479.
71. Rumstadt B, Schwab M, Schuster K, et al. The role of laparoscopy in the preoperative staging of pancreatic carcinoma. Gastrointest Surg 1997; 1:245–250.

72. John TG, Wright A, Allan PL, et al. Laparoscopy with laparoscopic ultrasonography in the TNM staging of pancreatic carcinoma. World J Surg 1999; 23:870–881.
73. Erickson RA, Garza AA. Impact of endoscopic ultrasound on the management and outcome of pancreatic carcinoma. Am J Gastroenterol 2000; 95:2248–2254.
74. Bradley EL, Clements JL, Gonzalez AC. The natural history of pancreatic pseudocysts: a unified concept of management. Am J Surg 1979; 137:135–141.
75. Yeo CJ, Bastidas JA, Lynch-Nyhan A, et al. The natural history of pancreatic pseudocysts documented by computed tomography. Surg Gynecol Obstet 1990; 170:411–417.
76. Wilson C. Management of the later complications of severe acute pancreatitis – pseudocyst, abscess and fistula. Eur J Gastroenterol Hepatol 1997; 9:117–121.
77. Lankisch PG, Lohr-Happe A. Pseudocysts in chronic pancreatitis: natural course. In: Beger HG, Buchler MW, Malfertheiner P, eds. Standards in Pancreatic Surgery. Berlin, Heidelberg: Springer Verlag, 1990; 511–519.
78. Bradley EL. Pseudocysts in chronic pancreatitis: development and clinical implications. In: Beger HG, Buchler MW, Ditschuneit H, et al., eds. Chronic Pancreatitis. Berlin, Heidelberg: Springer Verlag, 1990; 260–268.
79. Koito K, Namieno T, Nagakawa T, et al. Solitary cystic tumor of the pancreas: EUS-pathologic correlation. Gastrointest Endosc 1997; 45:268–276.
80. Ahmad NA, Kochman ML, Lewis JD, et al. Can EUS alone differentiate between malignant and benign cystic lesions of the pancreas? Am J Gastroenterol 2001; 96:3295–3300.
81. Sedlack R, Affi A, Vazquez-Sequeiros E, et al. Utility of EUS in the evaluation of cystic pancreatic lesions. Gastrointest Endosc 2002; 56:543–547.
82. Glasbrenner B, Kahl S, Schulz HU, et al. Review on diagnosis and treatment of pancreatic pseudocysts. Leber Magen Darm 2000; 30:114–123.

15 Natural Course of Chronic Pancreatitis

Paul Georg Lankisch

In the minority of patients (i.e. 5.8–20%), chronic pancreatitis takes a primarily painless course.[1–7] Exocrine and endocrine insufficiency are the dominating symptoms. For the majority of patients, however, pain is the decisive symptom, causing much discomfort in their daily lives.

Some studies have correlated the course of pain in chronic pancreatitis in comparison with the duration of the disease, progressing exocrine and endocrine pancreatic insufficiency and morphological changes, such as pancreatic calcifications and duct abnormalities. Furthermore, the course of pain has been studied following alcohol abstinence and after surgery in some groups.

Pain Decrease with the Duration of Chronic Pancreatitis?

Whether burning-out of the gland, i.e. progressive parenchymal destruction, leads to pain decrease has been repeatedly debated.[8,9] The group of Ammann has claimed that pain decreases with increasing duration of the disease.[3,10,11] In one long-term study, 85% of 145 patients with chronic pancreatitis felt no more pain after 4.5 years (median) duration of the disease.[3]

The reports from Zürich are at variance with the studies from Japan and Germany. Miyake et al.[6] found that only 48.2% of the patients with chronic pancreatitis became free of pain within 5 years, and 66–73% after more than 5 years. That meant that every third or fourth patient still suffered from relapsing pain attacks even after a longer observation time. Our group[7] reported that the incidence of relapsing pain attacks decreased during the observation period, but more than half of the patients (53%) still suffered from relapsing pain attacks even after more than 10 years of observation (Table 15.1).[7]

At present, the course of pain in alcoholic and idiopathic chronic pancreatitis remains unclarified. Layer et al.[12] investigated a group of patients with idiopathic chronic pancreatitis who had never consumed alcoholic beverages during their life time. They found that patients with early-onset pancreatitis (onset at <35 years of age) have initially and thereafter a long course of severe pain, whereas patients with a late-onset pancreatitis (onset at >35 years) have a mild and often painless course. Both forms differ from alcoholic pancreatitis in the equal gender distribution and a much slower rate of calcification. In contrast, our group[13] found that the course of pain is the same in alcohol- and

Table 15.1 Pain in relation to the duration of discase in 311 patients with initially painful chronic pancreatitis

Follow-up years	n	Patients still having pain attacks (n = 202)		Patients who became free from pain (n = 109)	
		n	%	n	%
<5	79	67	33	12	11
5–10	80	54	27	26	24
>10	152	81	40	71	65

With increasing observation time, the number of patients still having attacks of pain or becoming free from pain changed significantly ($p<0.0001$). Even after a follow-up for more than 10 years, the majority of patients (81/152; 53%) still suffered from pain. From Lankisch et al.,[7] with permission.

nonalcohol-induced chronic pancreatitis. Even when we divided the non-alcoholic group into teetotallers and patients with little alcohol consumption, and compared separately their course of pain with alcoholics, there were no differences concerning pain relief among the three groups.[14] Further studies are required.

Pain Decrease with Progressing Exocrine and Endocrine Pancreatic Insufficiency?

The Swiss group repeatedly observed a pain decrease as exocrine and endocrine pancreatic function declined.[8–11] Similarly, Girdwood et al.[15] reported from South Africa that pain decreased as exocrine pancreatic function deteriorated.

Groups from Denmark and Germany reported, on the contrary, the opposite. Thorsgaard Pedersen et al.[16] from Copenhagen found no correlation between pain and exocrine pancreatic function. Our group from Göttingen[7] used the secretin-pancreozymin test and fecal fat analysis to evaluate exocrine pancreatic insufficiency, whereas the Swiss group had used only indirect pancreatic function tests, i.e. chymotrypsin measurements, to evaluate exocrine pancreatic insufficiency.[3] We used a clear-cut grading of the severity of exocrine pancreatic insufficiency: slight impairment was defined as reduced enzyme output; moderate, as a decreased bicarbonate concentration along with reduced enzyme output but normal fecal fat excretion; and severe impairment was equated with an abnormal secretin-pancreozymin test plus steatorrhea. At the end of the observation period, 141 (45%) of 311 patients with painful chronic pancreatitis had severe exocrine pancreatic insufficiency. The majority of them (81/144; 57%) still suffered from pain attacks.

Additionally, we studied the course of pain in correlation to endocrine pancreatic insufficiency. Endocrine pancreatic insufficiency was classified as absent, moderate (diabetes mellitus treated only by diet plus/minus oral medication), and severe (requiring insulin) (Table 15.2).[7,17] At the end of observation time, 117 (38%) patients were classified as having severe endocrine pancreatic insufficiency. The majority of them (69/117; 59%) still suffered from pain attacks.

Thus, according to our results, the progression of exocrine and endocrine pancreatic insufficiency has limited, if any, influence on the course of pain in chronic pancreatitis.

Table 15.2. Influence of exocrine and endocrine pancreatic insufficiency on pain in 311 patients with initially painful chronic pancreatitis

	Pancreatic insufficiency		At end of observation period			
			persisting pain (n = 202)		pain relief (n = 109)	
	n	%	n	%	n	%
Exocrine						
Mild	78	25	53	26	25	23
Moderate	92	30	68	34	24	22
Severe	141	45	81	40	60	55
Endocrine						
Mild	72	23	53	26	19	17
Moderate	122	39	80	40	42	39
Severe	117	38	69	34	48	44

At the end of the observation period, exocrine, but not endocrine pancreatic insufficiency differed significantly between patients with persisting pain and those having obtained pain relief ($p = 0.03$ and 0.121). The majority of patients with severe exocrine (81/141; 57%) and endocrine (69/117; 59%) pancreatic insufficiency still suffered from pain attacks. From Lankisch et al.,[7] with permission.

Pain Decrease and Development of Morphological Changes of the Pancreas (Pancreatic Calcifications and/or Duct Abnormalities)

The Swiss group[3,10] showed an increased incidence of pancreatic calcifications, which in turn was associated with pain decrease. However, later on, the same group[18] reported a regression of pancreatic calcifications in a long-term study of patients with chronic pancreatitis. Thus, the prognostic role of pancreatic calcifications concerning the course of pain is unclear.

Furthermore, the Swiss results are at variance with two other studies. Malfertheiner et al.[19] found that 89% of patients had pain despite pancreatic calcifications observed on computed tomography, and 39% very intense pain. In our study, freedom of pain was significantly higher in the calcification group as compared to the noncalcification group. However, the majority of patients with pancreatic calcifications (56%) still had relapsing pain attacks.[7]

The correlation between pain and pancreatic duct changes or pressure in the duct system is also not clear. Ebbehøj et al.[20,21] measured percutaneously or intraoperatively pancreatic tissue fluid pressure and found a significant correlation with pain in patients with chronic pancreatitis but not with the ERCP results, i.e. the regional pressure tended to be highest in the region of the pancreas with the largest and not with the smallest duct diameter. Jensen et al.[22] found no correlation between pancreatic duct changes and pain. Warshaw et al.[23] found in two of 10 of their patients, one year after a lateral pancreaticojejunostomy, no pain relief in spite of a patent anastomosis detected by ERCP.

Two investigations confirmed the nonparallelism between pancreatic duct changes and pain relief. Malfertheiner et al.[19] found severe pain in only 62% of patients who had advanced pancreatic duct changes demonstrated by ERCP. We[7] found no significant correlation between pancreatic duct abnormalities detected by ERCP and pain in 88 patients with chronic pancreatitis. Severe pancreatic duct abnormalities – as defined by the Cambridge classification[24] – were present in 42 patients, but only 16 (31%) of these became free of pain. Despite a normal pancreatic duct in 14 patients, 10 (71%) of them suffered from persisting pain (Table 15.3).[7]

Table 15.3. Pancreatic duct abnormalities upon ERCP, and pain in 88 patients with chronic pancreatitis

	Pancreatic duct abnormalities (n = 88)		At end of observation period			
			persisting pain (n = 60)		pain relief (n = 28)	
	n	%	n	%	n	%
Absent	14	16	10	17	4	14
Mild	3	3	2	3	1	4
Moderate	29	33	22	37	7	25
Severe	42	48	26	43	16	57

Pain was independent of duct abnormalities ($p = 0.45$, not significant). From Lankisch et al.,[7] with permission.

Thus, morphological changes such as pancreatic calcifications or pancreatic duct abnormalities are not necessarily helpful in making a prognosis of chronic pancreatitis or predicting the course of pain.

Recently it has been shown that smoking has an effect on the natural course of the disease since it increases the risk of pancreatic calcification in late-onset but not early-onset idiopathic chronic pancreatitis.[25]

Pain Decrease with Alcohol Abstinence?

Since alcoholism is the leading etiological factor in chronic pancreatitis, it has also been discussed whether alcohol abstinence influences pain or the progression of the disease. Sarles and Sahel[26] reported for 50% of patients with chronic pancreatitis, and Trapnell[27] for 75%, pain relief when alcohol abuse was discontinued.

Two other investigations confirmed that abstinence can be helpful: Miyake et al.[6] demonstrated pain relief in 60% of their patients who discontinued or reduced alcohol intake, whereas in the group of patients who continued drinking, spontaneous pain relief was only 26%. In another study,[7] 66 (31%) of 214 patients with alcoholic chronic pancreatitis were motivated to stop drinking. Pain relief was obtained in only 52% of these patients, whereas the spontaneous relief in alcoholics was 37%. Thus, alcohol abstinence will probably lead in every second patient with chronic pancreatitis to some improvement of pain, but why exactly abstinence helps in some cases, but not in others, remains to be investigated.

Pain Decrease after Endoscopic Procedures?

Endoscopic treatment of chronic pancreatitis has been increasingly performed during the past 10 years applying techniques originally designed for the biliary system to the pancreatic duct system (Tables 15.4 and 15.5).[28] A frequently discussed theory about the cause of pain in chronic pancreatitis is an increased intraductal and intraparenchymal pressure. To avoid surgical drainage operations, stents have been inserted into the pancreatic duct to relieve the pressure, or extracorporeal shock-wave lithotripsy (ESWL) has been used to fragment pancreatic duct stones possibly responsible for the high pressure in the obstructed duct. The results of studies on these endoscopic procedures are shown in Tables 15.4 and 15.5.[29–37] Obviously, an improvement of symptoms, in this case, of pain is possible in a substantial number of patients. The success rate correlates favorably with a

Table 15.4. Results of pancreatic duct endoprosthesis insertion: from Jakobs et al.,[28] with permission

Reference	n	Mean follow-up months	Improvement of symptoms		Stent patience months	Complications
			n/total	%		
Binmoeller et al.[29]	93	36	69/73	74	6	4 × p, 1 × abscess
Smits et al.[30]	49	34	40/49	82	5	2 × b, 2 × p, 9 × mi
Cremer et al.[31]	75	37	71/74	94	12	3 × ch, 1 × he, 2 × mi, 8 × in
Riemann et al.[32]	23	32	17/23	78	4[1]	1 × ch, 1 × p, 1 × in

p = Pancreatitis; b = bleeding; ch = cholangitis; in = pancreatic duct infection;
mi = prosthesis migration; he = hemobilia.
[1] Partly standardized protocol.

Table 15.5. ESWL: technical and clinical success rates in the treatment of pancreatic duct stones: from Jakobs et al.,[28] with permission

Reference	n	Fragmentation/stone clearance n (%)	Mean follow-up months	Improvement of symptoms n (%)	Mortality
Delhaye et al.[33]	123	122 (99)/72 (58)	14	85 (69)	0
Sauerbruch et al.[34]	24	17 (71)/10 (42)	24	12 (70)	0
Adamek et al.[35]	65	41 (63)/21 (33)	n.g.	24 (58)	0
Schneider et al.[36]	50	43 (86)/30 (60)	20	36 (83)	0
van de Hul et al.[37]	17	13 (76)/7 (41)	30	11 (85)	0

n.g. = not given.

number of theories on which different surgical procedures are based. However, it should be stressed that the follow-up period is still too short to come to another conclusion, and none of these studies has been performed with controls.

Of special interest is the long-term follow-up of patients with chronic pancreatitis and pancreatic stones treated with ESWL. Adamek et al.[38] reported that treatment success was better in the presence of a single rather than of multiple stones. However, pancreatic drainage by endoscopy and ESWL had almost no effect on pain in chronic pancreatitis.

Pain Decrease after Surgery?

During the course of the disease, every 2nd to 4th patient needs surgical treatment because of pain and/or organ complications, such as pancreatic pseudocysts.[3,7] The choice of the surgical procedure is definitely dependent on the special circumstances of each patient. It is, however, unclear to what extent surgical treatment influences the course of pain since the different studies cannot be compared for the following reasons:

The definition of freedom of pain is often vague, pain symptoms are usually not measured, for example on an analogue scale.[17]

Not all patients received the same surgical treatment for the same indication. Several authors recommend not performing an indicated resection operation in alcoholics because of the postoperatively difficult treatment of diabetes mellitus in those patients.[39,40]

Although continued alcohol abuse distinctly worsens the effect of surgical treatment,[41–43] it is still difficult to determine whether a postoperative deterioration results from chronic pancreatitis, or from continued alcohol abuse, or from the surgical treatment.

Evaluation of pain differs very much in the duration of the observation period. Postoperative results independent of the surgical procedure showed that freedom of pain will be obtained in up to 90% of the patients over several years of follow-up (Table 15.6).[7,44–77] However, Taylor et al.[78] (Table 15.7) distinctly showed that in the course of a longer follow-up pain increases. Thus, beneficial effects seen after a shorter observation period may be misleading.

Table 15.6. Freedom of pain after different surgical procedures for chronic pancreatitis

Reference	Surgical procedure	Mean observation time years	n	Pain relief %
Way et al.[44]	drainage/resection	5 (approx.)	37	64
Lankisch et al.[45]	drainage/resection	$2\frac{1}{2}$	40	60
Mangold et al.[46]	partial duodenopancreatectomy	1 8/12	44	73
	total duodenopancreatectomy	2 10/12	18	91
	partial left-sided resection	3 5/12	37	60
	subtotal left-sided resection	2 10/12	17	83
Proctor et al.[47]	pancreaticojejunostomy	11/12	22	50
Rosenberger et al.[48]	resection	6	67	69
	nonresective procedures	6	40	50
Lankisch et al.[49]	pancreaticojejunostomy	3 1/12	17	76
	resection	3 1/12	22	64
Prinz and Greenlee[50]	pancreaticojejunostomy	≤7 11/12	91	35
Sato et al.[51]	pancreaticojcnunostomy	6 6/12	38	68
	left-sided resection	6 6/12	14	79
	Whipple's operation	6 6/12	9	67
Gall et al.[52]	Whipple's operation, duct occlusion	>1	67	93
Morrow et al.[53]	ductal drainage	4–13	46	46
	40–80% left-sided resection	4–13	21	33
	80–95% left-sided resection	4–13	8	100
	drainage	6	46	80
	subtotal pancreatectomy	7	21	24
Sato et al.[54]	left-sided resection	>6/12	21	91
	Whipple's operation	>6/12	11	55
	pancreaticojejunostomy	>6/12	43	91
Bradley III[55]	lateral pancreaticojejunostomy	5 9/12	46	28
	caudal pancreaticojcjunostomy	5 9/12	18	17
Cooper et al.[56]	total pancreatectomy	1 6/12	83	72
Frick et al.[57,58]	left-sided resection	6 6/12	74	50
	partial duodenopancreatectomy	6 6/12	62	45
	total duodenopancreatectomy	6 6/12	22	55
	drainage	4 7/12	156	48
Lambert et al.[59]	duodenum-preserving total pancreatectomy	9 5/12	14	64
Rossi et al.[60]	Whipple's operation	6/12	61	72
		2	44	61
		5	33	61
		10	18	61
		15	6	83
Mannell et al.[61]	drainage/resection	8 6/12	100	77
Stone et al.[62]	Whipple's operation	6 2/12	15	53
	total duodenopancreatectomy	9 1/12	15	27

continued overleaf

Reference	Surgical procedure	Mean observation time years	n	Pain relief %
Beger et al.[63]	duodenum-preserving resection of the head of the pancreas	3 8/12	128	77
Peiper and Köhler[64]	resection	10	51	79
	drainage	10	24	65
Beger and Büchler[65]	duodenum-preserving pancreatic head resection	3 6/12	141	77
Lankisch et al.[7]	drainage/resection	6	70	57
Adams et al.[66]	lateral pancreaticojejunostomy	6 4/12	62	42
Frey et al.[67]	local resection of the head of the pancreas combined with longitudinal pancreaticojejunostomy	6/12	50	75
Büchler et al.[68]	duodenum-preserving resection of the head of the pancreas	6/12	15	40
	pylorus-preserving Whipple's operation	6/12	16	75
Fleming and Williamson[69]	total pancrealectomy	3 6/12	40	79
Izbicki et al.[70]	duodenum-preserving pancreactic head resection:			
	Beger's procedure	1 6/12	20	95
	Frey's procedure	1 6/12	22	94
Martin et al.[71]	pylorus-preserving pancreaticoduodenectomy	5 3/12	45	92
Stapleton and Williamson[72]	proximal pancreaticoduodenectomy pylorus-preserving (n = 45) Whipple's operation (n = 7)	4 6/12	52	80
Rumstadt et al.[73]	Whipple's operation	8 3/12	134	66
Traverso and Kozarek[74]	Whipple's operation	3 6/12	47	76
	total pancreatectomy	3 6/12	10	76
Berney et al.[75]	different procedures of pancreatic resection	6 4/12	61	90
Sakorafas et al.[76]	Whipple's operation	6 6/12	66	89
White et al.[77]	total or completion pancreatectomy	6/12	24	8

Further staging of the postoperative beneficial effect on pain was not considered. Closure of literature research: December 2000.

Table 15.7. Percentage of patients who became free of pain 6 months, 2 and 5 years after different surgical procedures because of chronic pancreatitis: from Taylor et al.,[78] with permission

Follow-up	Whipple's operation, %	Pancreatico-jejunostomy, %	Left-sided resection, %
Alcohol-induced pancreatitis			
6 months	82	87	60
2 years	74	53	39
5 years	71	54	26
Idiopathic pancreatitis			
6 months	50	80	77
2 years	50	60	46
5 years	33	60	20

In a study including 207 patients with alcoholic chronic pancreatitis (91 without and 116 with surgical treatment for pain relief), Ammann et al.[79] discussed the pain pattern of chronic pancreatitis and its surgical implication. Chronic pain in their study was typically associated with local complications (mainly pseudocysts), relieved definitely by single drainage procedure in approximately two-thirds of patients. Additional surgery was required for late pain recurrence in 39 patients, primarily symptomatic cholestasis. All patients achieved complete pain relief in advanced chronic pancreatitis. The authors conclude that in their experience relief of chronic pain regularly follows selective surgery tailored to the presumptive pain cause or occurs spontaneously in uncomplicated advanced chronic pancreatitis.

Exocrine Pancreatic Insufficiency

Exocrine pancreatic insufficiency does not play a major prognostic role. Occasionally, massive steatorrhea leading to cachexia and susceptibility to infection has prognostic significance.

Whether exocrine pancreatic insufficiency deteriorates during the course of the disease is disputed. Ammann et al.[3] found that severe exocrine pancreatic insufficiency (defined as fecal chymotrypsin below 40 μg/g) developed within 5.65 years (median) in 122 (86.6%) of 145 patients, whereas Thorsgaard Pedersen et al.[16] observed no significant changes in exocrine pancreatic insufficiency in their patients within an observation period of 4 years. We found in 66 (46.2%) patients no change in the degree of severity of exocrine pancreatic insufficiency, but a deterioration in 61 (42.6%) patients. Functional improvement was even seen in 16 (11.2%) of our patients, several of whom no longer required pancreatic enzyme substitution.

Several other studies furnish evidence of functional improvement in cases of exocrine pancreatic insufficiency in chronic pancreatitis.[6,80–82] Improvement was observed in patients who stopped drinking and/or where exocrine pancreatic insufficiency was moderate, not severe, prior to conservative and/or surgical treatment.[7]

Endocrine Pancreatic Insufficiency

Whereas almost all patients with chronic pancreatitis have an exocrine pancreatic insufficiency to some degree at the time of diagnosis, this is not the case for endocrine pancreatic insufficiency. We found moderate-to-severe endocrine pancreatic insufficiency in 335 patients with chronic pancreatitis, including 24 patients with painless chronic pancreatitis. In only 28 (8%) patients after almost 10 years observation time, the incidence of diabetes had increased 10-fold: 260 (78%) suffered from diabetes and 133 (40%) needed insulin treatment. However, even after this long observation time 75 (22%) patients, i.e. every 5th, still had no diabetes (Table 15.8).[7]

In a large prospective cohort study, Malka et al.[83] compared patients who underwent elective pancreatic surgery with those who never underwent surgical treatment. The prevalence of diabetes mellitus did not increase in the surgical group overall, but was higher 5 years after distal pancreatectomy than after pancreaticoduodenectomy, pancreatic drainage, or cystic, biliary or digestive drainage. There were no differences between the other operations. Pancreatic drainage did not

Table 15.8. Endocrine pancreatic insufficiency in 335 patients with chronic pancreatitis including 24 patients with painless chronic pancreatitis: from Lankisch et al.[7] with permission

Endocrine pancreatic insufficiency	At onset of disease		At end of observation	
	n	%	n	%
Absent	307	92	75	22
Moderate	13	4	127	38
Severe	15	5	133	40
Total	28	8	260	78

prevent the onset of diabetes mellitus. The risk seemed to be largely caused by progression of the disease because it increased by more than 3-fold after the onset of pancreatic calcifications.

Endocrine complications may play a major prognostic role, especially after surgical treatment of chronic pancreatitis, because of possible hypoglycemia.[84] Hypoglycemia frequently occurs after subtotal left-sided pancreatic resection[40] and may contribute to an unfavorable prognosis.

The frequency of some complications of diabetes mellitus secondary to chronic pancreatitis has been studied. Earlier investigations have shown that diabetic retinopathy is a rare complication of pancreatogenic diabetes with an occurrence rate of 7.4–18%.[85–87] Gullo et al.[88] have shown that the risk of retinopathy and the characteristics of this complication in patients with chronic pancreatitis and secondary diabetes are the same as in patients with type I diabetes. About half of the patients studied in both groups had retinopathy; it was background, minimal, or mild-to-moderate without impairment of visual function. The only significant difference was the longer duration of diabetes in patients with retinopathy when compared with those without this complication. A longer observation time may explain the higher frequency of diabetic retinopathy in this study[88] as compared to the earlier investigations.[85–87] Similarly, Tiengo et al.[89] and Couet et al.[90] had found retinopathy in 31 and 41%, respectively, of patients with chronic pancreatitis. Furthermore, in 1995, Levitt et al.[91] have shown that microvascular complications (retinopathy, nephropathy) in pancreatic diabetes and insulin-dependent diabetes mellitus are equally common and severe.

Nondiabetic retinal lesions and retinal function abnormalities (increased threshold of dark adaptation, difficulty with night vision) are also common in patients with chronic pancreatitis, even in the absence of steatorrhea as compared to healthy controls.[92] Electrocardiographic evidence of ischemic heart disease was found twice as frequently in genetic diabetes as in pancreatic diabetes (37 vs. 18%).[93] Diabetic neuropathy was reported in about 30% of patients with chronic pancreatitis (no control group).[94]

Finally, lower extremity arterial disease occurred in 25.3% of patients with chronic pancreatitis and had the same prevalence and distribution as in idiopathic pancreatitis.[95] Whether these complications have major prognostic significance has not yet been investigated.

Complications

The list of complications in chronic pancreatitis includes pancreatic pseudocysts and abscesses, stenosis of the common bile duct, the duodenum and the colon, development of pleural ascites, and gastrointestinal bleeding. All of these complications surely have severe implications for the prognosis of the disease. However, since these have not been dealt with in larger studies, their exact influence on the outcome of the disease is uncertain and, therefore, not discussed here.

Pancreatic and Extrapancreatic Carcinomas

In clinical studies, varying figures concerning the incidence of pancreatic carcinoma in patients with chronic pancreatitis have been reported reaching from 1.4 to 2.7%.[3,7,16,96,97] A multicenter historical cohort study of 2,015 subjects with chronic pancreatitis involved clinical centers in six countries.[98] The cumulative risk of pancreatic carcinoma in patients who were followed up for at least 2 years increased distinctly, and 10 and 20 years after the diagnosis of pancreatitis it was 1.8 and 4%, respectively (Fig. 15.1).[98] Thus, the risk of pancreatic carcinoma was significantly elevated in patients with chronic pancreatitis, and chronic pancreatitis has to be included in the precancers.[98]

Unfortunately, it is very difficult to diagnose a pancreatic carcinoma in chronic pancreatitis. Carcinoma of the pancreas should be definitely suspected in a patient with chronic pancreatitis if there is increasing abdominal discomfort, progressive weight loss, jaundice, and radiological evidence including nodularity of the duodenal sweep.

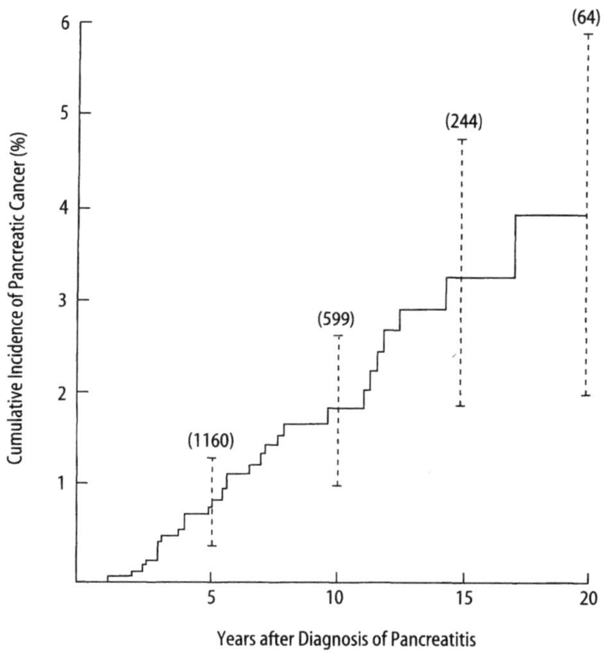

Fig. 15.1. Cumulative incidence of pancreatic cancer in 1,552 subjects with chronic pancreatitis with a minimum of 2 years' follow-up. The vertical lines represent 95% confidence intervals. In parentheses are the numbers of subjects at risk. One additional case of cancer developed after 25 years of follow-up. From Lowenfels et al.[98]

Extrapancreatic carcinomas in chronic pancreatitis are no rare events. They have been reported with varying incidence, reaching from 3.9 to 12.5%.[6,7,16,97,99] In some of these and other studies,[6,7,97,100] a considerable number of extrapancreatic carcinomas involving the upper respiratory tract (oral cavity, larynx, bronchial tree) has been observed. Since alcohol abuse is the dominating etiology of chronic pancreatitis, and probably many alcoholics smoke, extrapancreatic carcinomas involving the upper respiratory tract may reflect the consequences of another abuse habit.

Socio-Economic Situation

Some attention has been paid to the socio-economic situation of the patient with chronic pancreatitis: Gastard et al.[101] found that 1 of 2 male patients continued to work normally, in spite of pain or diabetes; one out of three was regarded as unfit for regular work, being totally incapacitated or absent from work for more than 3 months a year. The figures improved after the 15th year due to the death of patients with severe forms of the disease; at this stage, 68% of the patients were working regularly, and 6% were totally incapacitated.

Thorsgaard Pedersen et al.[16] found a decline during an observation period of 5 years (median). Only 15 (40%) of their 38 surviving patients still worked, whereas the remaining were either on prolonged sick-leave or retired.

Miyake et al.[6] reported that while 63 (71%) of their 89 patients continued to work, almost all other patients, who were either retired or who suffered socio-economically, continued their alcohol abuse.

In our study,[7] the incidence of unemployed patients increased from 3 to 15% and that of the retired, from 3 to 25% during an observation time of about 11 years. Almost half of the retirements were due to pancreatitis.

Mortality

Data on the mortality rate in chronic pancreatitis are difficult to interpret since etiology and mean observation times vary from study to study. Three studies with a comparatively similar observation time (median 6.3–9.8 years) revealed a general death rate of 28.8–35%, but the death rate when related to chronic pancreatitis was only 12.8–19.8%.[3,6,7] Continued alcohol abuse after conservative treatment and/or surgery has been associated with significantly lower survival rates (Fig. 15.2).[3,6,7,39,40,69]

Prognostic Factors

The prognosis of chronic pancreatitis is independent of conservative or surgical treatment. A multicenter investigation in 7 hospitals of 6 countries including 2,015 patients with chronic pancreatitis showed that the mortality rate was 3.6-fold higher than in patients without pancreatitis. The 10-year survival rate was 70%, the 20-year survival rate 45% as compared to 93 and 65%, respectively, in patients without pancreatitis.

The following risk factors were found:

Medium or high age at the time of diagnosis. The mortality rate in patients medium- or high-aged was 2.3- and 6.3-fold, respectively, higher than in patients with chronic pancreatitis, in whom the disease was diagnosed before the age 40.

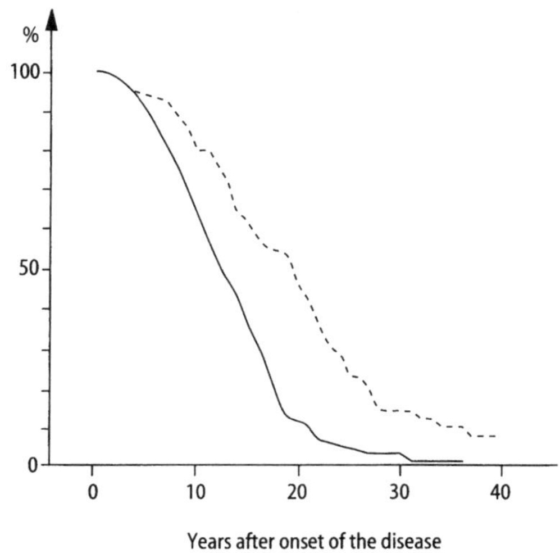

Fig. 15.2. Cumulative survival curve for 230 patients with alcoholic (—) and 105 patients with nonalcoholic (- - -) chronic pancreatitis ($p = 0.0001$). The mean age at onset of the disease (i.e. first pancrearitis-related symptoms) was 37 ± 9 (mean ± SD) years in patients with alcoholic and 39 ± 17 in parients with nonalcoholic chronic pancreatitis. From Lankisch et al.[7]

Consistent alcohol abuse: hazard ratio 1.6.
Smoking: hazard ratio 1.4.
Liver cirrhosis: hazard ratio 2.5.
Neither gender nor surgical history had any influence on the prognosis of the disease.[102]

Outlook

It will not have escaped the attention of the reader of this review that up to now there have only been a few well-performed and valid studies, and even some of them have produced diverging results, in part. More controlled studies with a larger number of patients than any one single center can undertake are necessary. That means we have to consolidate our resources and work out common criteria for the diagnosis of chronic pancreatitis and follow-up of its course. Hence, this review is not only an up-to-date survey of studies on the natural course of chronic pancreatitis, but also an appeal to the reader to take on this task.

Acknowledgement

This chapter was first published in Pancreatology 2001; 1: 3–14.

References

1. Creutzfeldt W, Fehr H, Schmidt H. Verlaufsbeobachtungen und diagnostische Verfahren bei der chronisch-rezidivierenden und chronischen Pankreatitis. Schweiz Mod Wochenschr 1970; 100:1180–1189.

2. Ammann RW, Hammer B. Fumagalli J. Chronic pancreatitis in Zurich, 1963–1972. Clinical findings and follow-up studies of 102 cases. Digestion 1973; 9:404–415.
3. Ammann RW, Akovbiantz A, Largiadèr F, et al. Course and outcome of chronic pancreatitis: Longitudinal study of a mixed medical-surgical series of 245 patients. Gastroenterology 1984; 86:820–828.
4. Gullo L, Costa PL, Labó G. Chronic pancreatitis in Italy. Aetiological, clinical and histological observations based on 253 cases. Rendic Gastroenterol 1977; 9:97–104.
5. Gocbell H. Beginn und Entwicklung der chronischen Pankrcatitis. Internist 1986; 27:172–174.
6. Miyake H, Harada H, Kunichika K, et al. Clinical course and prognosis of chronic pancreatitis. Pancreas 1987; 2:378–385.
7. Lankisch PG, Löhr-Happe A, Otto J, et al. Natural course in chronic pancreatitis: Pain exocrine and endocrine pancreatic insufficiency and prognosis of the disease. Digestion 1993; 54:148–155.
8. Ammann R. Die chronische Pankreatitis. Zur Frage der Operationsindikation und Beitrag zum Spontanverlauf der chronisch-rezidivierenden Pankreatitis. Dtsch Med Wochenschr 1970; 95:1–7.
9. Ammann R. Die Behandlung der chronischen Pankrcaritis. Dtsch Med Wochenschr 1970; 95:1234–1235.
10. Ammann RW, Largiadèr, Akovbiantz A. Pain relief by surgery in chronic pancreatitis? Relationship between pain relief, pancreatic dysfunction, and alcohol withdrawal. Scand J Gastroenterol 1979; 14:209–215.
11. Ammann R. Klinik. Spontanverlauf and Therapie der chronischen Pankreatitis. Unter spezieller Berücksichtigung der Nomenklaturprobleme. Schweiz Med Wochenschr 1989; 119:696–706.
12. Layer P, Yamamolo II, Kalthoff L, et al. The different courses of early- and late-onset idiopathic and alcoholic chronic pancreatitis. Gastroenterology 1994; 107:1481–1487.
13. Lankisch PG, Seidensticker F, Löhr-Happe A, et al. The course of pain is the same in alcohol- and nonalcohol-induced chronic pancreatitis. Pancreas 1995; 10:338–341.
14. Lankisch PG, Seidensticker F, Löhr-Happe A, et al. The course of pain is the same in alcoholics, alcohol consumers, and teetotalers (abstract). Pancreas 1996; 13:446.
15. Girdwood AH, Marks IN, Bornman PC, et al. Does progressive pancreatic insufficiency limit pain in calcific pancreatitis with duct stricture or continued alcohol insult? J Clin Gastroenterol 1981; 3:241–245.
16. Thorsgaard Pedersen N, Andersen BN, Pedersen G, et al. Chronic pancreatitis in Copenhagen: A retrospective study of 64 consecurive patients. Scand J Gastroenterol 1982; 17:925–931.
17. Lankisch PG, Andrén-Sandberg Á. Standards for the diagnosis of chronic pancreatitis and for the evaluation of treatment. Int J Pancreatol 1993; 14:205–212.
18. Ammann RW, Muench R, Otto R, et al. Evolution and regression of pancreatic calcification in chronic pancreatitis: A prospective long-term study of 107 patients. Gastroenterology 1988; 95:1018–1028.
19. Malfertheiner P, Büchler M, Stanescu A, et al. Pancreatic morphology and function in relationship to pain in chronic pancreatitis. Int J Pancreatol 1987; 2:59–66.
20. Ebbehøj N, Borly I, Bülow J, et al. Evaluation of pancreatic tissue fluid pressure and pain in chronic pancreatitis: A longitudinal study. Scand J Gastroenterol 1990; 25:462–466.
21. Ebbehøj N, Borly L, Madsen P, et al. Comparison of regional pancreatic tissue fluid pressure and endoscopic retrograde pancreatographic morphology in chronic pancreatitis. Scand J Gastroenterol 1990; 25:756–760.
22. Jensen AR, Matzen P, Malchow-Møller A, et al. The Copenhagen Pancreatitis Study Group: Pattern of pain, duct morphology, and pancreatic function in chronic panereatitis: A comparative study. Scand J Gastroenterol 1984; 19:334–338.
23. Warshaw AL, Popp JW Jr., Schapiro RH. Long-term patency, pancreatic function, and pain relief after lateral pancreaticojejunostomy for chronic pancreatitis. Gastroenterology 1980; 79:289–293.
24. Axon ATR, Classen M, Cotton PB, et al. Pancreatography in chronic pancreatitis: International definitions. Gut 1984; 25:1107–1112.
25. Imoto M, DiMagno EP. Cigarette smoking increases the risk of pancreatic calcification in late-onset but not early-onset idiopathic chronic pancreatitis. Pancreas 2000; 21:115–119.
26. Sarles H, Sahcl J. Dic chronische Pankreatitis; in Forell M (ed): Handbuch der Inneren Medizin, vol 3/6: Pankreas, ed 5, Berlin, Springer, 1976; pp. 737–844.
27. Trapnell JE. Chronic relapsing pancreatitis: A review of 64 cases. Br J Surg 1979; 66:471–475.
28. Jakobs R, Apel D, Riemann JF. Endoscopic treatment of pain and complications of chronic pancreatitis; in Lankisch PG, DiMagno EP (eds). Pancreatic Disease, State of the Art and Future Aspects of Research. Berlin, Springer, 1999; pp. 146–154.
29. Binmoeller KF, Jue P, Seifert H, et al. Endoscopic pancreatic stent drainage in chronic pancreatitis and a dominant stricture: Long-term results. Endoscopy 1995; 27:638–644.

30. Smits ME, Badiga M, Rauws EAJ, et al. Huibregtse K: Long-term results of pancreatic stents in chronic pancreatitis. Gastrointest Endose 1995; 42:461–467.
31. Cremer M, Devière J, Delhaye M, et al. Stenting in severe chronic pancreatitis: Results of medium-term followup in seventy-six patients. Bildgebung 1992; 19 (Suppl 1):10–24.
32. Riemann JF, Bregenzer N, Msier M, et al. Interventionelle Techniken am Pankreasgangsystem. Chir Gastroenterol 1996; 12:38–42.
33. Delhaye M, Vandermeeren A, Baize M, et al. Extracorporeal shock-wave lithotripsy of pancreatic calculi. Gastroenterology 1992; 102:610–620.
34. Sauerbruch T, Holl J, Sackmann M, et al. Extracorporeal lithotripsy of pancreatic stones in patients with chronic pancreatitis and pain: A prospective follow up study. Gut 1992; 33:969–972.
35. Adamek HE, Jakobs R, Krömer MU, et al. Ultraschallgesteuerte extrakorporale Stosswellenlithotripsie (ESWL) von Pankreasgangsteinen (abstr). Dtsch Med Wochenschr 1996; 121 (Sonderheft 1):73.
36. Schneider T, May A, Benninger J, et al. Piezolelectric shock wave lithotripsy of pancreatic duct stones. Am J Gastroenterol 1994; 89:2042–2048.
37. Van der Hul R, Plaisier P, Jeckel J, et al. Extracorporeal shock-wave lithotripsy of pancreatic duct stones: Immediate and long-term results. Endoscopy 1994; 26:573–578.
38. Adamek HE, Jakobs R, Buttmann A, et al. Schneider ARJ, Riemann JF: Long term follow up of patients with chronic pancreatitis and pancreatic stones treated with extracorporeal shock wave lithotripsy. Gut 1999; 45:402–405.
39. While TT, Keith RG. Long term follow-up study of fifty patients with pancreaticojejunostomy. Surg Gynecol Obstet 1973; 136:353–358.
40. Frey CF, Child CG III, Fry W. Pancreatectomy for chronic pancreatitis. Ann Surg 1976; 184:403–414.
41. Leger L, Lenriol JP, Lemaigre G. Five to twenty year follow-up after surgery for chronic pancreatitis in 148 patients. Ann Surg 1974; 180:185–191.
42. Holmberg JT, Isaksson G, Ihso I. Long term results of pancreaticojejunostomy in chronic pancreatitis. Surg Gynecol Obstet 1985; 160:339–346.
43. Capitaine Y, Roche B, Wiesner L, et al. Pancréatitc chronique: Histoire naturelle et evolution en relation avec l'alcoolisme. Schweiz Med Wochenschr 1988; 118:817–820.
44. Way LW, Gadsez T, Goldman L. Surgical treatment of chronic pancreatitis. Am J Surg 1974; 127:202–209.
45. Lankisch PG, Fuchs K, Schmidt H, et al. Ergebnisse der operativen Behandlung der chronischen Pankrearitis mit besonderer Berücksichtigung der exokrinen und endokrinen Funktion. Dtsch Med Wochenschr 1975; 100:1048–1060.
46. Mangold G, Neher M, Oswald B, et al. Ergebnisse der Resektionshehandlung der chronischen Pankreatitis. Dtsch Med Wochenschr 1977; 102:229–234.
47. Proctor HJ, Mendos OC, Thomas CG Jr., et al. Surgery for chronic pancreatitis. Drainage versus resection. Ann Surg 1979; 189:664–671.
48. Rosenberger J, Stock W, Altmann P, et al. Spätergebnisse nach organerhaltenden und resezierenden Eingriffen wegen chronischer Pankreatitis. Leber Magen Darm 1980; 10:22–27.
49. Lankisch PG, Fuchs K, Peiper H-J, et al. Pancreatic function after drainage or resection for chronic pancreatitis: in Mitchell CJ, Kelleher J (eds). Pancreatic Disease in Clinical Practice. London, Pitman Books, 1981; 362–369.
50. Prinz RA, Greenlee HB. Pancreatic duct drainage in 100 patients with chronic pancreatitis. Ann Surg 1981; 194:313–320.
51. Sato T, Noto N, Matsuno S, et al. Follow-up results of surgical treatment for chronic pancreatitis: Present status in Japan. Am J Surg 1981; 142:317–323.
52. Gall FP, Gebhardt C, Zirngibl H. Chronic pancreatitis: Results in 116 consecutive, partial duodenopancreatectomies combined with pancreatic duct occlusion. Hepatogastroenterology 1982; 29:115–119.
53. Morrow CE, Cohen JI, Sutherland DER, et al. Chronic pancreatitis: Long-term surgical results of pancreatic duct drainage, pancreatic resection, and near-total pancreatectomy and islet autotransplantation. Surgery 1984; 96:608–616.
54. Sato T, Miyashita E, Matsuno S, et al. The role of surgical treatment for chronic pancreatitis. Ann Surg 1986; 203:266–271.
55. Bradley EL III. Long-term results of pancreatojejunostomy in patients with chronic pancreatitis. Am J Surg 1987; 153:207–213.
56. Cooper MJ, Williamson RCN, Benjamin IS, et al. Total pancreatectomy for chronic pancreatitis. Br J Surg 1987; 74:912–915.

57. Frick S, Jung K, Rückert K. Chirurgie der chronischen Pankreatitis, I. Spätergobnissc nach Rescktionsbehandlung. Disch Med Wochenschr 1987; 112:629–635.
58. Frick S, Ebert M, Rückert K. Chirurgie der chronischen Pankreatitis. II. Spätergebnissc nach nicht resezierenden Operationen. Dtsch Med Wochenschr 1987; 112:832–837.
59. Lambert MA, Lineban IP, Russell RCG. Duodenum-preserving total pancreatectomy for end stage chronic pancreatitis. Br J Surg 1987; 74:35–39.
60. Rossi RL, Rothschild J, Braasch JW, et al. Pancreatoduodenectomy in the management of chronic pancreatitis. Arch Surg 1987; 122:416–420.
61. Mannell A, Adson MA, McIlrath DC, et al. Surgical management of chronic pancreatitis: Long-term results in 141 patients. Br J Surg 1988; 75:467–472.
62. Stone WM, Sarr MG, Nagorney DM, et al. Chronic pancreatitis. Results of Whipple's resection and total pancreatectomy. Arch Surg 1988; 123:815–819.
63. Beger HG, Büchler M, Bittner RR, et al. Duodenum-preserving resection of the head of the pancreas in severe chronic pancreatitis. Early and late results. Ann Surg 1989; 209:273–278.
64. Peiper H-J, Kakohler H. Chirurgische Therapic der chronischen Pankreatitis. Schweiz Med Wochenschr 1989; 119:712–716.
65. Beger HG, Büchler M. Duodenum-preserving resection of the head of the pancreas in chronic pancreatitis with inflammatory mass in the head. World J Surg 1990; 14:83–87.
66. Adams DB, Ford MC, Anderson MC. Outcome after lateral pancreaticojejunostomy for chronic pancreatitis. Ann Surg 1994; 219:481–489.
67. Frey CF, Amikura K. Local resection of the head of the pancreas combined with longitudinal pancreaticojejunostomy in the management of patients with chronic pancreatitis. Ann Surg 1994; 220:492–507.
68. Büchler MW, Friess H, Müller MW, et al. Randomized trial of duodenum-preserving pancreatic head resection versus pylorus-preserving Whipple in chronic pancreatitis. AM J Surg 1995; 169:65–70.
69. Fleming WR, Williamson RCN. Role of total pancreatectomy in the treatment of patients with end-stage chronic pancreatitis. Br J Surg 1995; 82:1409–1412.
70. Izbicki JR, Bloechle C, Knoefel WT, et al. Duodenum-preserving resection of the head of the pancreas in chronic pancreatitis. A prospective, randomized trial. Ann Surg 1995; 221:350–358.
71. Martin RF, Rossi RL, Leslie KA. Long-term results of pylorus-preserving pancrearodundenectomy for chronic pancracatitis. Arch Surg 1996; 131:247–252.
72. Stapleton GN, Williamson RCN. Proximal pancreatoduodenectomy for chronic pancreatitis. Br J Surg 1996; 83:1433–1440.
73. Rumstadt B, Forssmam K, Singer MV, et al. The Whipple partial duodenopancreatectomy for the treatment of chronic pancreatitis, Hepatogastroenterology 1997; 44:1554–1559.
74. Traverso LW, Kozarek RA. Pancreatoduodenectomy for chronic pancreatitis. Anatomic selection criteria and subsequent long-term outcome analysis. Ann Surg 1997; 226:429–438.
75. Berney T, Rüdisühli T, Oberholzer J, et al. Long-term metabolic results after pancreatic resection for severe chronic panereatitis. Arch Surg 2000; 135:1106–1111.
76. Sakorafas GH, Farnell MB, Nagorney DM, et al. Pancreatoduodenectomy for chronic pancreatitis: Long-term results in 105 patients. Arch Surg 2000; 135:517–524.
77. White SA, Sutton CD, Weymss-Holden S, et al. The feasibility of spleen-preserving pancreatectomy for end-stage chronic pancreatitis. Am J Surg 2000; 179:294–297.
78. Taylor RH, Bagley FH, Brausch JW, et al. Ductal drainage or resection for chronic pancreatitis. Am J Surg 1981; 141:28–33.
79. Ammann RW, Muellhaupt B. Zurich Pancreatitis Study Group: The natural history of pain in alcoholic chronic pancreatitis. Gastroenterology 1999; 116:1132–1140.
80. Kondo T, Hayakawa T, Noda A, et al. Follow-up study of chronic pancreatitis. Gastroenterol Jpn 1981; 16:46–53.
81. Begley CG, Roberts-Thomson IC. Spontaneous improvement in pancreatic function in chronic pancreatitis. Dig Dis Sci 1985; 30:1117–1120.
82. Garcia-Pugés AM, Navarro S, Ros E, et al. Reversibility of exocrine pancreatic failure in chronic pancreatitis. Gastroenterology 1986; 91:17–24.
83. Malka D, Hammel P, Sauvanct A, et al. Risk factors for diabetes mellitus in chronic pancreatitis. Gastroenterology 2000; 119:1324–1332.
84. Linde J, Nilsson LHS, Bárány FR. Diabetes and hypoglycemia in chronic pancreatitis. Scand J Gastroenterol 1977; 12:369–373.
85. Sevel D, Bristow JH, Bank S, et al. Diabetic retinopathy in chronic pancreatitis. Arch Ophthalmol 1971; 86:245–250.

86. Creutzfeldt W, Perings E. Is the infrequency of vascular complications in human secondary diabetes related to nutritional factors? Acta Diabetol Lat 1972; 9 (Suppl 1):432–445.
87. Verdonk CA, Palumbo PJ, Gharib H, et al. Diabetic microangiopathy in patients with pancrearic diabetes mellitus. Diaberologia 1975; 11:395–400.
88. Gullo L, Parenti M, Monti L, et al. Diabetic retinopathy in chronic pancreatitis. Gastroenterology 1990; 98:1577–1581.
89. Tiengo A, Segato T, Briuni G, et al. The presence of retinopathy in patients with secondary diabetes following pancreatectomy or chronic pancreatitis. Diabetes Care 1983; 6:570–574.
90. Couct C, Genton P, Pointel JP, et al. The prevalence of retinopathy is similar in diabetes mellitus secondary to chronic pancreatitis with or without pancreatectomy and in idiopathic diabetes mellitus. Diabetes Care 1985; 8:323–328.
91. Levill NS, Adams G, Salmon J, et al. The prevalence and severity of microvascular complications in pancreatic diabetes and IDDM. Diabetes Care 1995; 18:971–974.
92. Toskes PP, Dawson W, Curington C, et al. Non-diabetic retinal abnormalities in chronic pancreatitis. N Engl J Med 1979; 300:942–946.
93. Joffe BI, Novis B, Scftel HC, et al. Ischaemic heart disease and pancreatic diabetes. Lancet 1971; ii:269.
94. Bank S, Marks IN, Vinik AI. Clinical and hormonal aspects of pancreatic diabetes. Am J Gastroenterol 1975; 64:13–22.
95. Ziegler O, Candiloros H, Guerei B, et al. Lower-extremity arterial disease in diabetes mellitus due to chronic pancreatitis. Diabet Metab 1994; 20:540–545.
96. Möhr P, Ammann R, Largiadèr F, et al. Pankreaskarzinom bei chronischer Pankrealitis. Schwciz Med Wochenschr 1975; 105:590–592.
97. Ammann RW, Knoblauch M, Möhr P, et al. High incidence of extrapancreatic carcinoma in chronic pancreatitis. Scand J Gastroenterol 1980; 15:395–399.
98. Lowenfels AB, Maisonneuve P, Cavallini G, et al. International Pancreatitis Study Group: Pancreatitis and the risk of pancreatic cancer. N Engl J Med 1993; 328:1433–1437.
99. Rocca G, Gaia E, Iuliano R, et al. Increased incidence of cancer in chronic pancreatitis. J Clin Gastroenterol 1987; 9:175–179.
100. Marks IN, Girdwood AH, Bank S, et al. The prognosis of alcohol-induced calcific pancreatitis. S Afr Med J 1980; 57:640–643.
101. Gastard J, Joubaud F, Farbos T, et al. Etiology and course of primary chronic pancreatitis in Western France Digestion 1973; 9:416–428.
102. Lowenfels AB, Maisonncuve P, Cavallini G, et al. International Pancreatitis Study Group: Prognosis of chronic pancreatitis: An international multicenter study. Am J Gastroenterol 1994; 89:1467–1471.

16 Autoimmune Pancreatitis

Günter Klöppel, Matthias Löhr and Daniel Longnecker

In the mid-1990s it became apparent that there is a form of chronic pancreatitis whose clinicopathological features are distinct from alcoholic chronic pancreatitis.[6] This pancreatitis seems to be autoimmune related.

In 1950, Ball, Baggenstoss and collaborators[2] described patients with pancreatitic changes in conjunction with ulcerative colitis. In 1961, Sarles et al.[19] reported patients who suffered from chronic inflammatory sclerosis of the pancreas associated with hypergammaglobulinemia. Later reports drew attention to the association between autoimmune diseases such as Sjögren's syndrome and primary sclerosing cholangitis with chronic sclerosing pancreatitis.[4, 14, 21, 23–25, 28] In 1991, Kawaguchi et al.[13] gave the first detailed description of this special type of pancreatitis and called it lymphoplasmacytic sclerosing pancreatitis. The first report that clearly distinguished between alcoholic chronic pancreatitis and lymphoplasmacytic pancreatitis appeared in 1997 and concerned a series of 12 cases.[6] The term autoimmune pancreatitis (AIP) was coined in the 1990s.[31] Here we will adhere to the name autoimmune pancreatitis, since this term has recently received wide recognition, although so far the evidence for an autoimmune pathogenesis is only circumstantial. This short review will first deal with the pathology of AIP and then discuss its clinical and functional features.

Pancreatic Pathology

The gross appearance of autoimmune pancreatitis mimics pancreatic ductal carcinoma because the inflammatory process, like the carcinoma, commonly focuses on the head of the pancreas, leads to enlargement and a gray to yellowish–white induration of the affected tissue with loss of its normal lobular structure (Fig. 16.1). These changes are associated with obstruction of the pancreatic ducts and usually also of the distal common bile duct. In a minority of cases, the inflammatory process concentrates in the body, or tail, of the pancreas or involves the pancreas diffusely. In contrast to other types of chronic pancreatitis, such as alcoholic chronic pancreatitis, hereditary pancreatitis and tropical pancreatitis, there are no pseudocysts or calculi (i.e. intraductal calcifications).

The histological changes are characterized by an intense infiltration of mononuclear cells, and to some extent granulocytes, around medium-sized and large interlobular ducts that narrows the ducts, occasionally leads to disruption and destruction of duct epithelium and finally causes periductal fibrosis[6, 13] (Fig. 16.2). In areas

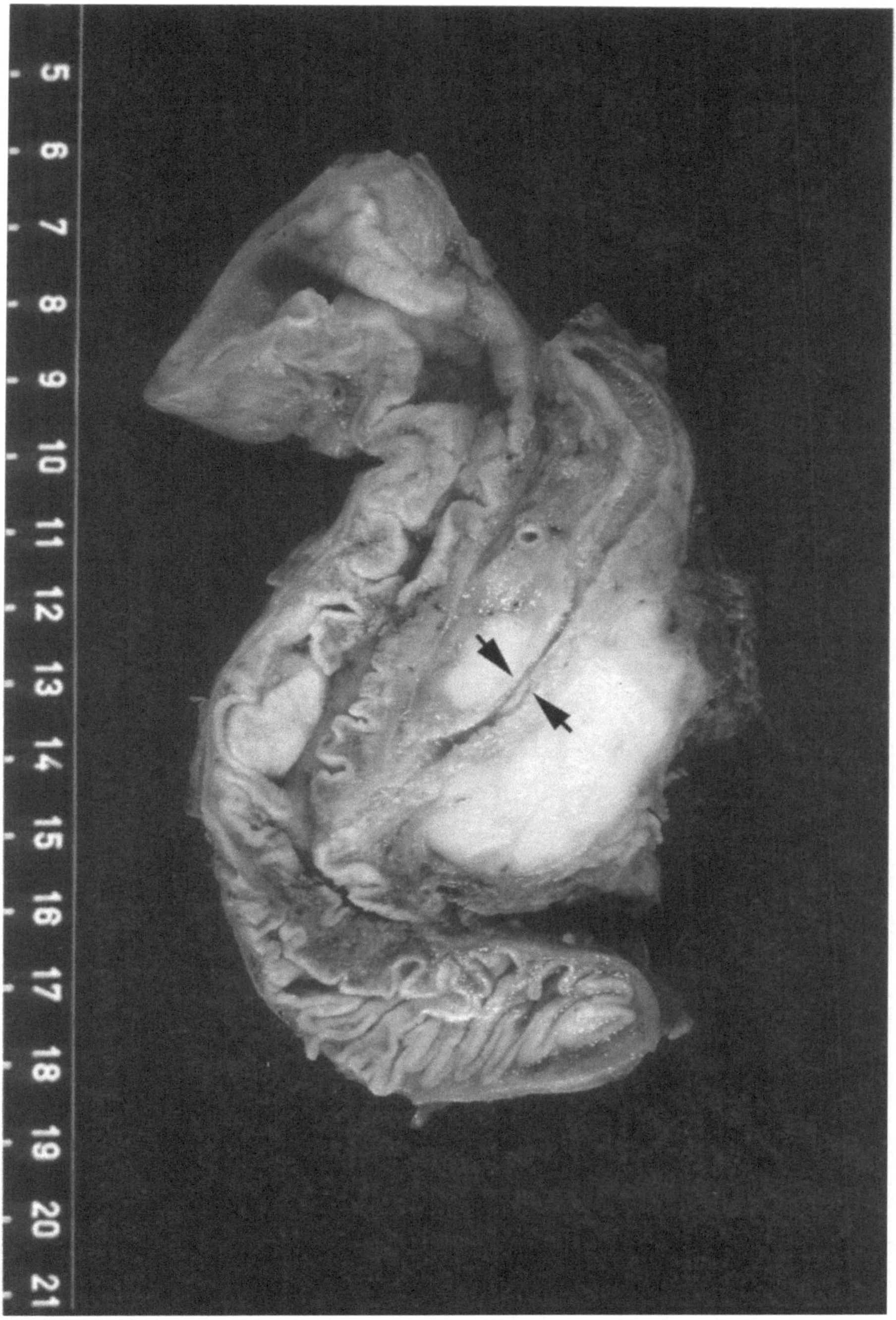

Figure 16.1. Gross appearance of autoimmune pancreatitis. The duodeno-hemipancreatectomy specimen shows an enlarged pancreatic head with homogeneously structured tissue. The intrapancreatic segment of the distal bile duct is narrowed (arrows).

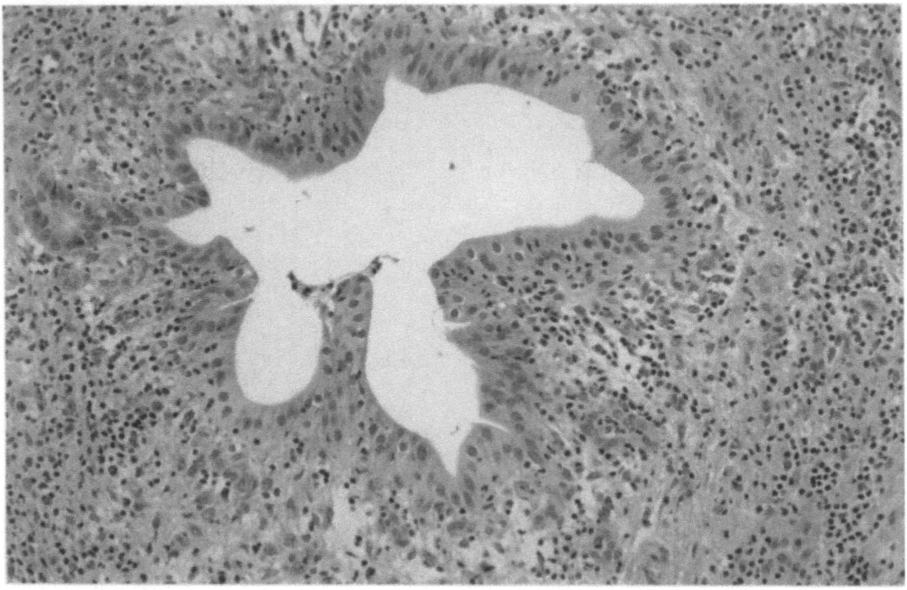

a

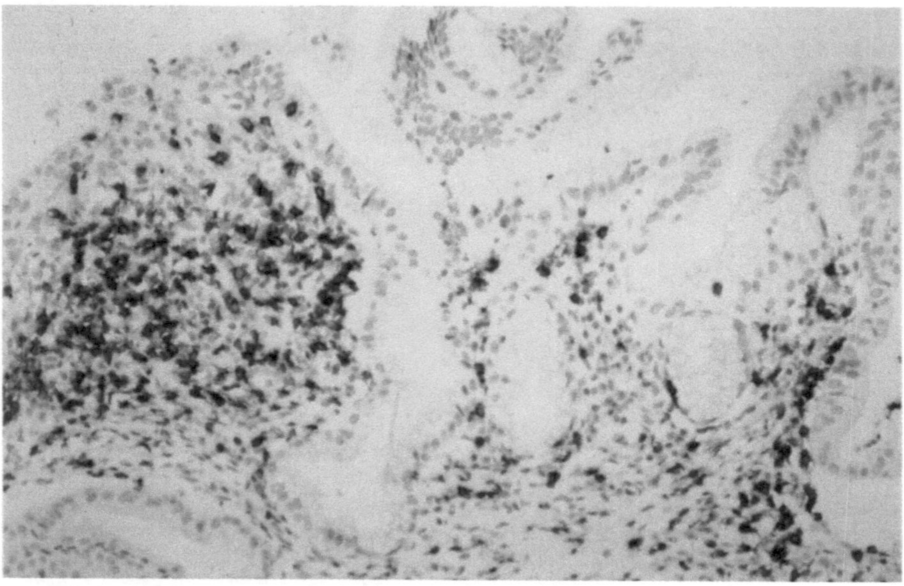

b

Figure 16.2. **a** Medium-sized pancreatic duct surrounded by a dense subepithelial inflammatory infiltrate composed of lymphocytes, plasma cells and occasionally granulocytes. Single inflammatory cells invade the duct epithelium. H&E, ×120. **b** Wall of a pancreatic duct showing numerous CD8-immunostained T lymphocytes, some of them invading the duct epithelium. ×240. **c** Pancreatic duct surrounded by mononuclear inflammatory cells and peripancreatic fibrosis. Goldner, ×60.

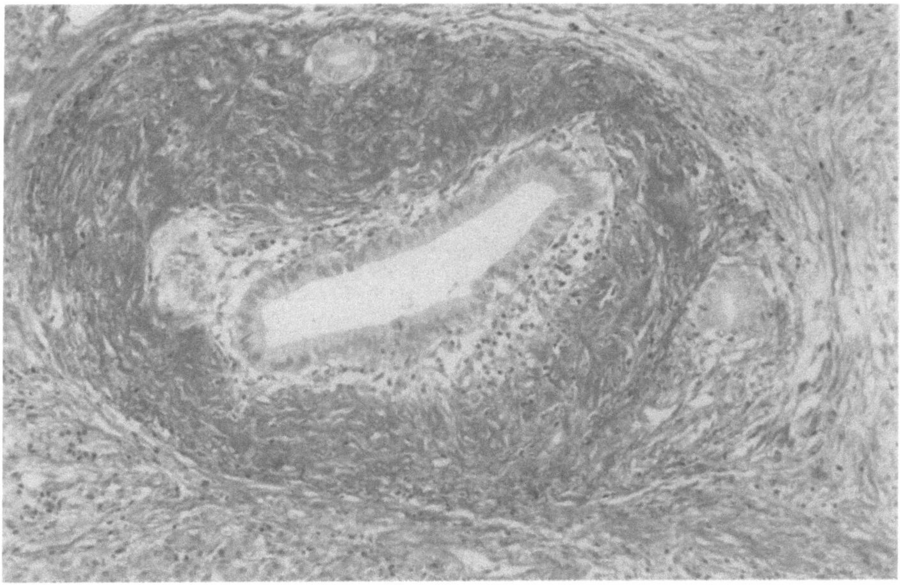

c

Figure 16.2. (*Continued*)

with severe duct involvement the inflammatory process also affects the acinar parenchyma, which may be infiltrated by inflammatory cells and partly replaced by fibrosis (Fig. 16.3). The extent of ductal and periductal inflammation may differ from duct to duct and in some cases advanced inflammation and fibrosis alternate abruptly with areas in which only periductal inflammation is found (Fig. 16.4). If the inflammatory process affects the head of the gland, it usually also involves the distal common bile duct.

The inflammatory infiltrate consists of lymphocytes and plasma cells as well as some macrophages and occasionally also eosinophils. Neutrophils may be present when there is destruction of acinar or ductal cells (Fig. 16.5). Immunocytochemical typing of the lymphocytes reveals that most of them are CD8 and CD4 positive T lymphocytes with fewer B lymphocytes (Fig. 16.2 b). Apart from the involvement of the ducts and acini, an obliterative vasculitis that usually affects the veins may be observed (Fig. 16.6).

The constant features are ductal inflammation and sclerosing pancreatitis with a mononuclear cell infiltrate consisting primarily of lymphocytes and plasma cells. Other features are variable from case to case.

Pathogenesis

Lymphoplasmacytic infiltrates around the ducts and granulo-epithelial lesions in the duct epithelium are the histological hallmarks of AIP in the pancreas.[6,13] They point to potential antigens within the duct epithelium that have become targets of an immune process. As already mentioned, typing of the inflammatory duct-associated

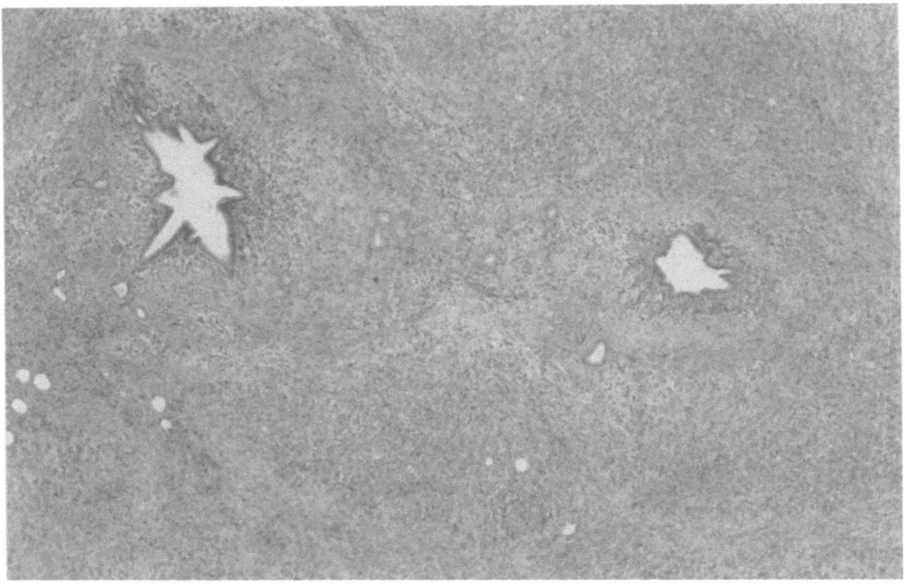

Figure 16.3. Advanced autoimmune pancreatitis involving large interlobular ducts as well as the surrounding tissue, which is largely replaced by inflammatory cells and fibrosis. H&E, ×60.

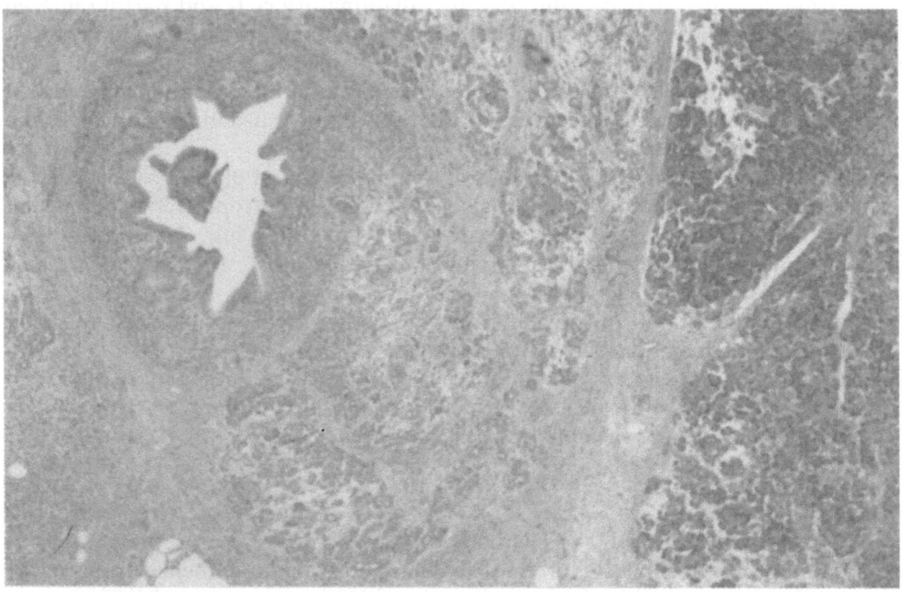

Figure 16.4. Focally accentuated autoimmune pancreatitis involving a large interlobular duct. Note the adjacent normal acinar tissue.

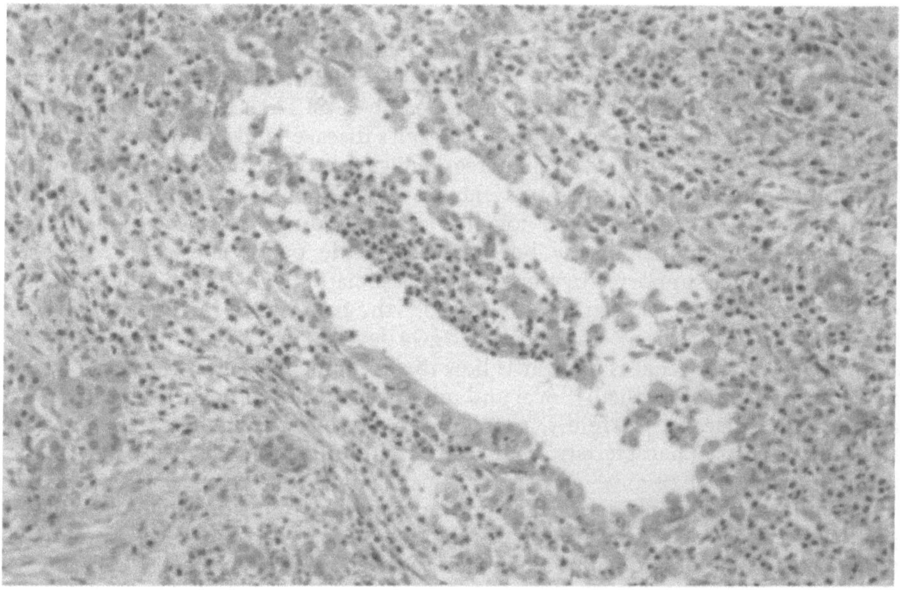

Figure 16.5. Medium-sized pancreatic duct showing invasion and destruction of the duct epithelium by neutrophil granulocytes, which also infiltrate the surrounding tissue. H&E, ×120.

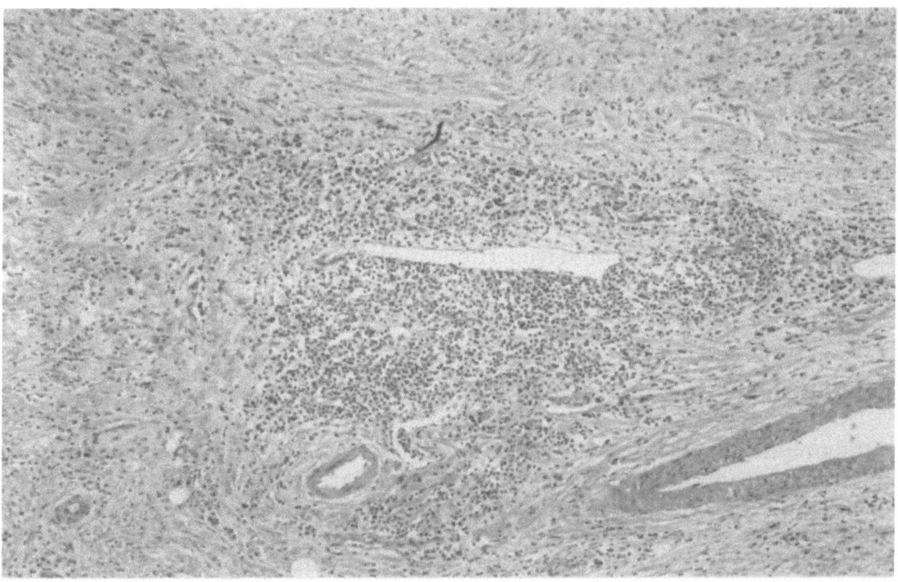

Figure 16.6. Advanced autoimmune pancreatitis showing perivenulitis.

cells revealed that most of them are T-lymphocytes consisting of CD4+ and CD8+ cells.[6,26] Increased numbers of these T-cells bearing HLA-DR were also found in the peripheral blood.[18] Subtyping of the CD4+ cells according to their cytokine production profiles revealed a predominance of CD4+Th1 cells over Th2 cells in some cases,[18] similar to the findings in Sjögren's disease[1] and PSC.[5] HLA-DR antigens have also been detected on pancreatic duct cells.[6,26] Finally, similar to other autoimmune diseases, AIP patients show a particular HLA haplotype, namely DRB1*0405-DQB1*0401.[12] Taken together these findings strongly suggest that autoimmune mechanisms may be involved in the pathogenesis of AIP. This concept is further supported by the common association of AIP with other autoimmune diseases, notably Sjögren's syndrome,[31] the frequent occurrence of various autoimmune antibodies,[18] the elevated IgG4 levels[9] and the responsiveness to steroid therapy.[8,16] What is unclear is how this immune process is triggered in the pancreas and why it is usually focal and not diffuse, as might be expected from an autoimmune disease. Currently, proteomic analysis is being used to find out whether there are characteristic changes in the protein content of the pancreatic juice.[29]

Recently an animal model was introduced with which it is possible to study the pathogenesis of AIP. Using neonatally thymectomized BALB/c mice immunized with CAII or LF and nude mice which had received immunized spleen cells, it was shown that CD4+ Th1 cells are mainly involved in the early development of murine AIP.[27]

Clinical Features

Autoimmune pancreatitis occurs in both sexes, but men are more often affected (male : female ratio 2 : 1). The age ranges from 20–70 years; the peak incidence, however, lies between 50 and 70 years. There are no specific symptoms in patients with autoimmune pancreatitis, and some patients may be pain-free. Usually, the patient may experience abdominal discomfort, but acute attacks as are typical for pancreatitis of other origin are rare. Since obstructive jaundice is common in autoimmune pancreatitis, such patients are often thought to suffer from pancreatic carcinoma, a suspicion that is supported by the imaging results (see below). In a few patients the symptoms of other associated autoimmune disorders such as autoimmune sialadenitis or retroperitoneal fibrosis may be more obvious than those of the pancreatitis.[9]

Relationship with Other Diseases

Autoimmune pancreatitis has been reported in association with a number of other autoimmune and related diseases, such as Sjögren's syndrome (autoimmune sialadenitis), sclerosing extrahepatic cholangitis interpreted as a variant of primary sclerosing cholangitis (PSC), chronic idiopathic inflammatory bowel disease (Crohn's disease and ulcerative colitis), systemic lupus erythematosus, scleroderma, inflammatory pseudotumor, retroperitoneal fibrosis, Hashimoto's thyroiditis and various combinations of these conditions.[6,11,17,20]

The most commonly associated autoimmune disease is Sjögren's syndrome. This association has been called systemic exocrinopathy.[9] Most of the patients affected by both diseases seem to be women,[20] whereas in the autoimmune pancreatitis without Sjögren's syndrome men predominate.[31]

Inflammatory and sclerosing changes of the distal bile duct (which sometimes also involve the gall bladder) are very frequent and are almost an integral part of autoimmune pancreatitis. Because of their similarity with extrahepatic PSC, a relationship with this autoimmune liver disease has been discussed. However, the PSC-like changes in the extrahepatic bile duct system have so far never been found to be accompanied by intrahepatic PSC. Moreover, unlike typical PSC, they appear to respond to steroid therapy. Therefore it is likely that autoimmune pancreatitis, even if it involves the extrahepatic bile ducts, is a different disease and distinct from PSC.

There are a number of reports of inflammatory (myofibroblastic) pseudotumors occurring in the head of the pancreas that involve the pancreatic duct as well as the distal common bile duct.[30] Judging from the descriptions and illustrations of these cases, these changes appear to be compatible with those seen in autoimmune pancreatitis. As the clinical features of the reported inflammatory pseudotumors are also very similar, the possibility has to be considered that the reported inflammatory pseudotumors of the pancreas might represent an advanced stage of autoimmune pancreatitis in which the fibrotic changes predominate. The fact that inflammatory pseudotumors showing sclerosing cholangitis have been observed in the liver hilus[15] suggests that there is possibly an idiopathic pancreatobiliary inflammatory disease complex whose facets include autoimmune pancreatitis, extrahepatic sclerosing cholangitis and inflammatory pseudotumor of the pancreas and/or the common bile duct.

It has long been known that there is a relationship between pancreatitis and inflammatory bowel disease (IBD), particularly Crohn's disease (CD). Pancreatic changes associated with IBD are rare events compared with other extraintestinal lesions, but the overall incidence may range from 1.5%–5%. The two symptomatic conditions are acute (relapsing) pancreatitis and exocrine pancreatic insufficiency. Overt acute pancreatitis is rare in IBD patients, being estimated at 1.5% to 4.5% of all IBD cases.[10] Exocrine pancreatic insufficiency may be found in up to 40% of IBD cases. To date it is unclear whether this represents a distinct second autoimmunopathy, an extraintestinal manifestation of CD, or a direct extension of the disease involving the papilla of Vater and the pancreatic ducts. Since the detection of pancreatic autoantibodies, which are found in about 13% of patients with CD, it has been debated whether a distinctive secretory defect of the pancreas exists in IBD.[22] Exocrine pancreatic insufficiency can be present without any further signs of pancreatic disease. Occasionally there is an asymptomatic elevation of serum amylase and lipase.[3]

As primary biliary cirrhosis (PBC) is commonly associated with Sjögren´s syndrome, there may be also a relationship between PBC and AIP. Although pancreatic hyposecretion was found in patients with PBC,[7] so far AIP has never been observed in association with PBC.

Diabetes mellitus occurring in conjunction with AIP has generally been considered to be of Type 2. In recent years, however, more detailed studies have shown that patients with AIP and diabetes mellitus may have antibodies against islet cells, glutamic acid decarboxylase and tyrosine phosphatase-like protein. This suggests that AIP may also be associated with Type 1 diabetes.

Imaging Findings

Ultrasound reveals a reduction in the echo signal, as seen in pancreatic cancer. Moreover, the borders of such lesions, which are typically localized in the head of the pancreas, may be irregular. These findings are paralleled by those of computed tomography (CT) demonstrating a pancreatic mass, usually with enlarged peripancreatic lymph nodes. Here, in contrast to ultrasound, the enlargement of the pancreas may appear more general, leading to the term 'sausage-like' pancreas. The most pathognomonic finding is the contrast enhancement around the low-density pancreatic lesions mimicking a capsule. An identical phenomenon has been described in magnetic resonance (MR) imaging MRI with a hypointense margin (T2) and delayed enhancement during dynamic MR (FLASH sequence). Pancreatic calcifications or pseudocysts are typically absent in autoimmune pancreatitis. PET scans employing F18-2-deoxyglucose have also been applied in AIP patients and have shown in increased uptake of the tracer, similar to pancreatic cancer. Endoscipic rectograde cholangiopancreatography ERCP shows irregular narrowing of the main pancreatic ducts and narrowing of the bile duct passing through the pancreatic head.[11] In summary, the imaging findings in both CT and MR can be described as 'mass forming pancreatitis'. The differential diagnosis vs. pancreatic carcinoma may be difficult, if not impossible.

Conclusions

AIP is a novel inflammatory entity of the pancreas with distinctive clinical, pathological, laboratory and imaging features. AIP bears a resemblance to primary sclerosing cholangitis, with which it shares morphological similarities. However, the two diseases PSC and AIP differ in their responsiveness to steroid therapy. As in other autoimmune diseases, an inflammatory infiltrate rich in T-lymphocytes can be identified and various autoantibodies are detected. An association with certain HLA haplotypes, at least in East Asian populations, has also been described. Finally, a recently established animal model may allow us to study the etiology and pathology of AIP in more detail. The recognition of AIP makes the disease spectrum of the pancreas comparable to that of the bile ducts and liver.

References

1. Ajjan RA, McIntosh RS, Waterman EA, et al. Analysis of the T-cell receptor Valpha repertoire and cytokine gene expression in Sjögren's syndrome. Br J Rheumatol 1998; 37:179–185.
2. Ball WP, Baggenstoss AH, Bargen JA. Pancreatic lesions associated with chronic ulcerative colitis. Arch Pathol 1950; 50:347–358.
3. Bokemeyer B. Asymptomatic elevation of serum lipase and amylase in conjunction with Crohn's disease and ulcerative colitis. Z Gastroenterol 2002; 40:5–10.
4. Borum M, Steinberg W, Steer M, et al. Chronic pancreatitis: A complication of systemic lupus erythematosus. Gastroenterology 1993; 104:613–615.
5. Dienes HP, Lohse AW, Gerken G, et al. Bile duct epithelia as target cells in primary biliary cirrhosis and primary sclerosing cholangitis. Virchows Arch 1997; 431:119–124.
6. Ectors N, Maillet B, Aerts R, et al. Non-alcoholic duct destructive chronic pancreatitis. Gut 1997; 41:263–268.

7. Epstein O, Chapman RWG, Lake-Bakaar G, et al. The pancreas in primary biliary cirrhosis and primary sclerosing cholangitis. Gastroenterology 1982; 83:1177–1182.
8. Erkelens GW, Vleggaar FP, Lesterhuis W, et al. Sclerosing pancreato-cholangitis responsive to steroid therapy. Lancet 1999; 354:43–44.
9. Hamano H, Kawa S, Horiuchi A, et al. High serum IgG4 concentrations in patients with sclerosing pancreatitis. N Engl J Med 2001; 344:732–738.
10. Heikius B, Niemela S, Lehtola J, et al. Elevated pancreatic enzymes in inflammatory bowel disease are associated with extensive disease. Am J Gastroenterol 1999; 94:1062–1069.
11. Horiuchi A, Kawa S, Hamano H, et al. ERCP features in 27 patients with autoimmune pancreatitis. Gastrointest Endosc 2000; 55:494–499.
12. Kawa S, Ota M, Yoshizawa K, et al. HLA DRB10405-DQB10401 haplotype is associated with autoimmune pancreatitis in the Japanese population. Gastroenterology 2002; 122:1264–1269.
13. Kawaguchi K, Koike M, Tsuruta K, et al. Lymphoplasmacytic sclerosing pancreatitis with cholangitis: variant of primary sclerosing cholangitis extensively involving pancreas. Hum Pathol 1991; 22:387–395.
14. Laszik GZ, Pap A, Farkas G. A case of primary sclerosing cholangitis mimicking chronic pancreatitis. Int J Pancreatol 1988; 3:503–508.
15. Nonomura A, Minato H, Shimizu K, et al. Hepatic hilar inflammatory pseudotumor mimicking cholangiocarcinoma with cholangitis and phlebitis – a variant of primary sclerosing cholangitis? Pathol Res Pract 1997; 193:519–525.
16. Okazaki K. Autoimmune-related pancreatitis. Curr Treat Options Gastroenterol 2001; 4:369–375.
17. Okazaki K, Chiba T. Autoimmune related pancreatitis. Gut 2002; 51:1–4.
18. Okazaki K, Uchida K, Ohana M, et al. Autoimmune-related pancreatitis is associated with autoantibodies and a Thl/Th2-type cellular immune response. Gastroenterology 2000; 118:573–581.
19. Sarles H, Sarles JC, Muratore R, et al. Chronic inflammatory sclerosis of the pancreas – an autoimmune pancreatic disease? Am J Dig Dis 1961; 6:688–698.
20. Sartori N, Löhr M, Basan B, et al. Pancreatitis in systemic scleroderma. Z Gastroenterol 1997; 35:677–680.
21. Scully RE, Mark EJ, McNeely BU. Weekly clinicopathological exercises – case 6, 1982. N Engl J Med 1982; 306:349–358.
22. Seibold F, Mörk H, Tanza S, et al. Pancreatic autoantibodies in Crohn's disease: a family study. Gut 1997; 40:481–484.
23. Sjögren I, Wengle B, Korsgren M. Primary sclerosing cholangitis associated with fibrosis of the submandibular glands and the pancreas. Acta Med Scand 1979; 205:139–141.
24. Smith MP, Loe RH. Sclerosing cholangitis – review of recent case reports and associated diseases and four new cases. Am J Surg 1965; 110:239–246.
25. Sood S, Fossard DP, Shorrock K. Chronic sclerosing pancreatitis in Sjögren's syndrome: A case report. Pancreas 1995; 10:419–421.
26. Uchida K, Okazaki K, Konishi Y, et al. Clinical analysis of autoimmune-related pancreatitis. Am J Gastroenterol 2000; 95:2788–2794.
27. Uchida K, Okazaki K, Nishi T, et al. Experimental immune-mediated pancreatitis in neonatally thymectomized mice immunized with carbonic anhydrase II and lactoferrin. Lab Invest 2002; 82:411–424.
28. Waldram R, Kopelman H, Tsantoulas D, et al. Chronic pancreatitis, sclerosing cholangitis, and sicca complex in two siblings. Lancet 1975; 550–552.
29. Wandschneider S, Fehring V, Jacobs-Emeis S, et al. Autoimmune pancreatic disease: Preparation of pancreatic juice for proteome analysis. Electrophoresis 2001; 22:4383–4390.
30. Wreesmann V, van Eijck CHJ, Naus DCWH, et al. Inflammatory pseudotumour (inflammatory myofibroblastic tumour) of the pancreas: a report of six cases associated with obliterative phlebitis. Histopathology 2001; 38:105–110.
31. Yoshida K, Toki F, Takeuchi T, et al. Chronic pancreatitis caused by an autoimmune abnormality. Proposal of the concept of autoimmune pancreatitis. Dig Dis Sci 1995; 40:1561–1568.

Pancreatic Stellate Cells

17 What's New in Pancreatic Stellate Cell Biology?

Minoti Apte and Jeremy Wilson

Fibrosis is a key pathological feature of chronic pancreatitis.[1] It is also a major component of the prominent desmoplastic (stromal) reaction observed around a majority of pancreatic cancers.[2] It is now generally accepted that, far from being an inevitable end point of chronic injury, fibrosis is an active, dynamic process that is reversible in its early stages. Therefore, an understanding of the initial events in fibrogenesis may allow identification of novel therapeutic targets to prevent or retard its progression.

The pathogenesis of pancreatic fibrosis has received increasing attention in recent years, largely due to the identification and characterisation of stellate cells in the pancreas. Evidence is now accumulating to support a key role for these cells in pancreatic fibrogenesis.[3–10] The ability to isolate and culture pancreatic stellate cells (PSCs)[3, 6] has provided a valuable *in vitro* tool, adding further impetus to studies of their biology. Data from both *in vivo* and *in vitro* studies indicate that pancreatic stellate cells are similar in morphology and function to their hepatic counterparts (i.e. hepatic stellate cells [HSCs] which are well established as the principal effector cells in hepatic fibrosis).[3,6,9] It is postulated that one of the major mechanisms for the production of pancreatic fibrosis is the transformation of PSCs from their quiescent state (in health) to an activated phenotype (during organ injury) that can synthesise and secrete increased amounts of extracellular matrix proteins (particularly fibrillar collagens).

This Chapter outlines our most recent studies with respect to the following aspects of pancreatic stellate cell biology: embryologic origin; migration; matrix degradation; endogenous cytokine production; signalling pathways mediating cell activation; and their role in pancreatic cancer.

Embryologic Origin

The embryologic origin of PSCs (as well as hepatic stellate cells) has been the subject of some debate. Hepatic stellate cells were initially considered to be of mesenchymal origin due to their ability to express vimentin, desmin and, when activated, alpha smooth muscle actin (αSMA).[11] However, this concept has required some revision, given the finding that HSCs also express neural crest cell markers such as glial fibrillary acidic protein (GFAP), nestin, neural cell adhesion molecule (NCAM) and neurotrophins.[12–16] While GFAP expression has been demonstrated in rat PSCs,[3, 17] the expression by these cells of the other neural

Table 17.1. Primers used in RT-CPR of neuotropin mRNA from rat PSC

NGF:	Forward primer 5' CTGC TGA ACC AAT AGC TGC CCG 3' Reverse primer 5' CGC CTT GAC AAA GGT GTG AGT CG 3'
BDNF:	Forward primer 5' TGG ATG AGG ACC AGA AGG TTC GGCC 3' Reverse primer 5' CGA TTG GGT AGT TCG GCA TTG CG 3'
Neurotrophin 3:	Forward primer 5' GAT TAT GTG GGC AAC CCG GTG G 3' Reverse primer 5' GTG TCT ATT CGT ATC CAG CGC CAGC 3'
Neurotrophin 4/5:	Forward primer 5' GTA CTT CTT CGA GAC GCG CTGC 3' Reverse primer 5' GCC CGC ACA TAG GAC TGT TTA GC 3'
Trk A:	Forward primer 5' TCC TTT CTG CCC TCC TCC TAG TGC 3' Reverse primer 5' GTA CTC GAA GAC CAT GAG CAA TGG G 3'
Trk C:	Forward primer 5' AAC GCC AGC ATC AAC ATC ACG G 3' Reverse primer 5' CCT TCT CGG ACA GTC AGG TTC ACG 3'
p75:	Forward primer 5' TGC AGT GTG CAG ATG TGC CTA TGG C 3' Reverse primer 5' AGG AAT GAG GTT GTC GGT GGT GCC G 3'

markers (noted above) is undetermined. We aimed to study the expression of neurotrophins and their receptors in PSCs using RT-PCR.

Neurotrophins are a family of soluble factors essential for the development and maintenance of the mammalian nervous system.[18] The best studied among these factors is the NGF family of neurotrophins which includes nerve growth factor (NGF), brain derived neurotrophic factor (BDNF), neurotrophins 3, 4/5, 6 and 7.[19] These factors mediate the growth of central and peripheral nerves and act via two types of cell surface receptors – the high affinity tyrosine kinase receptors Trk A, B and C and the low affinity receptor p75, a member of the TNF receptor superfamily.[20] In order to determine whether pancreatic stellate cells exhibit expression of NGF, BDNF, neurotrophins 3, 4/5 and their high and low affinity receptors, the following studies were performed.

Rat pancreatic stellate cells were isolated and cultured. Total cellular RNA was extracted from passaged PSCs and reverse transcribed to obtain cDNA using the first strand cDNA synthesis kit (MBI Fermentas, Vilnius, Lithuania). Specific forward and reverse primers for NGF, BDNF, neurotrophin 3, neurotrophin 4/5, TrkA, TrkC and p75[16] were obtained from Geneworks (Adelaide, Australia) as shown in Table 17.1.

Regions of interest were amplified as follows: Cycling was preceded by denaturation at 94°C for 2 minutes followed by 8 minutes at 72°C. Amplification was performed for 30 seconds at 94°C, 30 seconds at annealing temperature, 1 minute at 72°C for 35 cycles. Annealing temperatures used were NGF 59°C; BDNF 54°C, NT3 54°C, NT4/5 60°C, TrkA 58°C; TrkC 54°C, p75 63°C. PCR products obtained were separated on a 2% agarose gel and visualised by ethidium bromide staining.

Bands of expected sizes were observed for NGF (426bp), BDNF (428bp) and NT4/5 (135bp) (Fig. 17.1a). NT3 expression was absent in PSCs. With regard to neurotrophin receptors, positive expression was observed for TrkA and p75 (Fig 17.1b), but not for TrkC. The above results were highly reproducible, observed in RNA extracted from four separate stellate cell preparations.

The finding that PSCs have the capacity to synthesise neurotrophic factors (in addition to their well established ability to express GFAP) provides support for the hypothesis that these cells may have a neural crest origin. The expression of NGF, in particular, may be of additional relevance in chronic pancreatitis. Friess et al[21] have reported a close association between upregulation of NGF expression in the

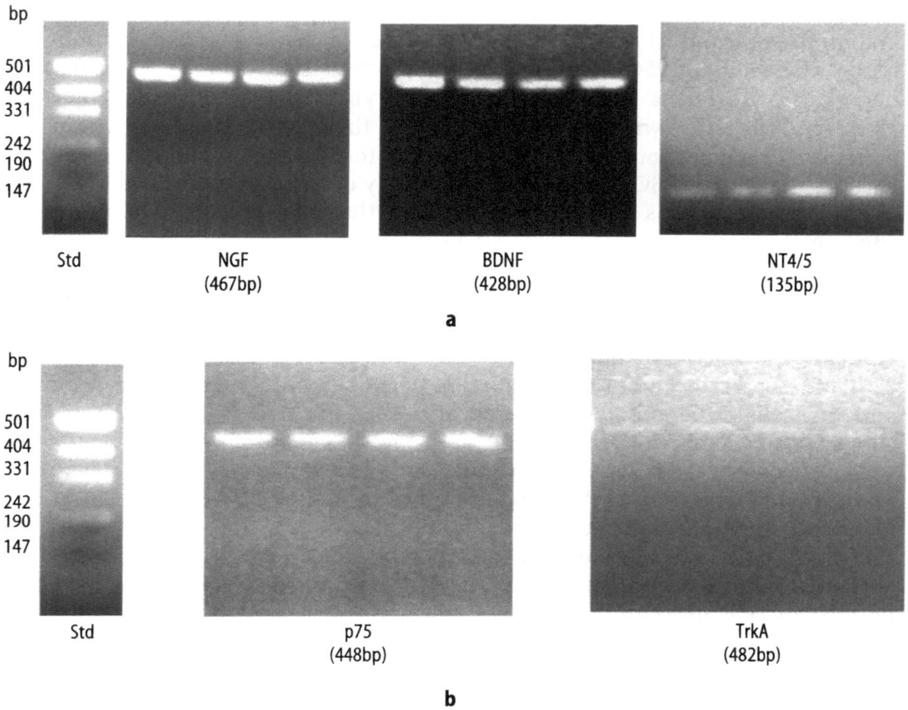

Figure 17.1. Expression of neurotrophins and their receptors in pancreatic stellate cells. RT-PCR of RNA extracted from four separate PSC preparations demonstrated the expression of **a** the neurotrophins nerve growth factor (NGF), brain derived neurotrophic factor (BDNF), and neurotrophin 4/5; and **b** the neurotrophin receptors p75 and tyrosine kinase A (TrkA).

pancreas and the presence of neural hypertrophy in the pancreas of patients with chronic pancreatitis. The latter change is thought to play a role in the pain of chronic pancreatitis.[21] Our finding that PSCs have the ability to synthesise NGF, suggests that in addition to their role in the fibrosis of chronic pancreatitis, PSCs may also have a part in mediating another characteristic feature of chronic pancreatitis, namely, neural hypertrophy.

The expression of the receptors TrkA (which specifically recognises NGF) and p75 is of interest because it suggests that PSCs may be responsive to NGF (via a paracrine and/or an autocrine loop). Studies regarding the effects of NGF and other neurotrophic factors on PSCs have not yet been reported. However, cultured HSCs have been shown to express the low affinity receptor p75 and to undergo apoptosis on exposure to NGF for 24 h.[22]

Migration

In vivo studies using tissue from patients with chronic pancreatitis tissue as well as from experimental models of pancreatic fibrosis have demonstrated the presence of increased numbers of pancreatic stellate cells in fibrotic areas within the gland.[7,9,17] This increase in PSC number could be due to two factors: i) local proliferation of PSCs and ii) migration of PSCs to the affected areas from surrounding tissue. The ability of PSCs to proliferate when activated by factors such as platelet derived growth factor and proinflammatory cytokines is well documented.[4,10] However, little is known about the capacity of these cells to migrate within the pancreas. The aim of our studies was therefore to examine the migration characteristics of cultured PSCs using the methodology described below.

PSC migration was assayed by culturing the cells in cell culture inserts (Becton-Dickinson, Bedford, MA, USA) placed in 24-well culture plates. The inserts have a translucent, uncoated, porous membrane (pore size 8 μm). Freshly isolated or passaged rat PSCs suspended in Iscove's medium were placed in the inserts (30 000 cells/insert), and the inserts in turn were placed in culture wells containing the same medium. Cells were cultured for periods of 12, 24, 48 and 72 h at 37°C. At the end of the incubation period, culture medium was removed and the cells adherent to the membrane were fixed in 100% methanol and subjected to Giemsa staining.[23]

The effect of platelet derived growth factor (PDGF, a known chemotactic factor) on the rate of migration of PSCs was examined by adding PDGF at concentrations of 10 and 20 ng/ml to the culture medium in the lower chamber of the well. The rate of migration was assessed at 12 and 24 h of exposure to PDGF.

Giemsa-stained cells on the membranes were examined by light microscopy. The number of cells on the upper surface and undersurface of the membrane were counted in the same microscopic field (magnification Œ400) by changing the focus of the objective. Five randomly selected microscopic fields were examined for each membrane. The rate of migration of PSCs was expressed as a migration index (%) – number of cells on undersurface of membrane divided by total number of cells on both surfaces of the membrane ×100.

The assessment of cell migration by the above method may be confounded by two factors: a) differences in the rates of proliferation of PSCs on the two surfaces of the membrane and b) the effect of gravity. To address these factors, cell proliferation on both surfaces of the membrane was assessed by an *in situ* proliferation assay, while the effect of gravity was assessed by inverting the insert in the culture well.

Cell proliferation on both sides of the membrane was measured by labelling nuclei with 5-bromo-2'-deoxyuridine (BrdU) using a modification of the method described by Ikeda et al.[24] This method involves incubation of cells in culture medium containing $5x10^{-5}$M BrdU for 16 h. Cells were then washed in cold phosphate buffered saline (PBS) and fixed in ethanol : acetic acid (95:5 vol/vol) for 30 min at 37°C. The DNA from fixed cells was denatured using formamide dissolved in 0.8 M NaCl, 20 mM Tris-HCl (pH 8.0) for 45 min at 70°C. Cells were then washed and incubated with a monoclonal antibody for BrdU (1:100, DAKO corporation, Carpintaria, CA) for one hour at room temperature followed by incubation with a biotinylated secondary antibody (1:100, DAKO corporation, Carpintaria, CA) for one hour at room temperature. After washing in PBS, cells were incubated with an avidin–biotin–peroxidase complex (ABC Kit, Vector Laboratories, Burlingame, CA, USA). Immunocomplexes were visualised by DAB staining (Sigma Chemical Company, St Louis, MO, USA). The number of BrdU positive cells on both surfaces of the membrane in the same microscopic field was counted as described earlier. Data are expressed as the proportion of BrdU positive cells on each side of the membrane.

To examine the possibility that any observed movement of cells from the upper to the undersurface of the membrane may be gravity dependent, the migration assay was repeated with inversion of the inserts in the culture medium. Cells were seeded into the inserts as before (30–000 cells / insert) and allowed to adhere to the membrane for 3 h at 37°C. The insert was then inverted in the culture wells and incubated for a further 9 or 21 h. At the end of the incubation, the membranes were stained with Giemsa solution and cells on both surfaces of the membranes counted as described above.

Migration of passaged pancreatic stellate cells was evident at 12 h; the rate of migration increased over the incubation period of 48 h (Fig 17.2a). Freshly isolated cells also exhibited migration, but this was delayed compared to passaged cells and observed first at 48 h (Fig 17.2a). The delayed migration of freshly isolated PSCs was of interest, given that the time point of 48 h coincides with the first appearance of the expression of α-smooth muscle actin (αSMA, a contractile cytoskeletal protein) in freshly isolated cells cultured on plastic [3]. In contrast to freshly isolated cells, passaged cells examined in these studies were pre-activated (i.e. αSMA positive) from the time of seeding into the inserts. These findings suggest that αSMA expression may play a role in cell motility.

Cell proliferation assays using BrdU demonstrated that the rates of cell proliferation on the top and undersurface of the membranes were similar (42.3 ± 0.8 and 43.8 ± 1.2% respectively; $n = 3$ separate cell preparations), indicating that the observed increase in migration over time could not be attributed to differences in proliferation of cells on the two sides of the membranes. With regard to the effect of gravity on cell movement, experiments with inverted inserts demonstrated that the cells continued to migrate to the 'undersurface' of the membrane at rates similar to those observed with upright inserts (Fig 17.2b).

The presence of PDGF (10 and 20 ng/ml) in the incubation medium in the lower chamber significantly increased the migration rate at 12 and 24 h of incubation, compared to cells not exposed to the growth factor (Fig 17.2c), while rates of cell proliferation on both sides of the membrane were similar. PDGF at a concentration of 20 ng/ml did not increase migration rates above those observed with PDGF at the concentration of 10 ng/ml. This may reflect saturation of cell surface PDGF receptors or maximal stimulation of PSCs at the lower concentration of the growth factor.

The novel finding that PSCs are capable of migration may be important insofar as it suggests an additional explanation for the observed increase in PSC numbers in areas of injury. Thus, the increase in PSC numbers may be due not only to local proliferation but also to migration of PSCs to affected areas from surrounding tissue in response to factors released during tissue injury such as cytokines and oxidant stress. Further studies are needed to characterise directional migration of PSCs and to identify other putative stimuli of PSC migration. In addition, studies to determine the signalling pathways regulating PSC migration would be important to enable identification of potential molecular targets for therapy.

Matrix Degradation

It is now well known that pancreatic stellate cells can synthesise and secrete the extracellular matrix proteins that comprise both normal extracellular matrix and

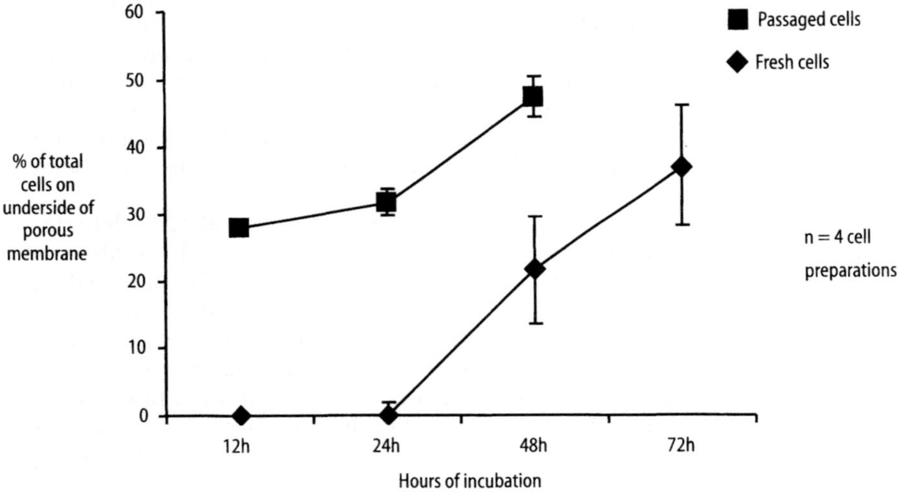
Passaged cells
Fresh cells
% of total cells on underside of porous membrane
60
50
40
30
20
10
0
n = 4 cell preparations
12h
24h
48h
72h
Hours of incubation

a

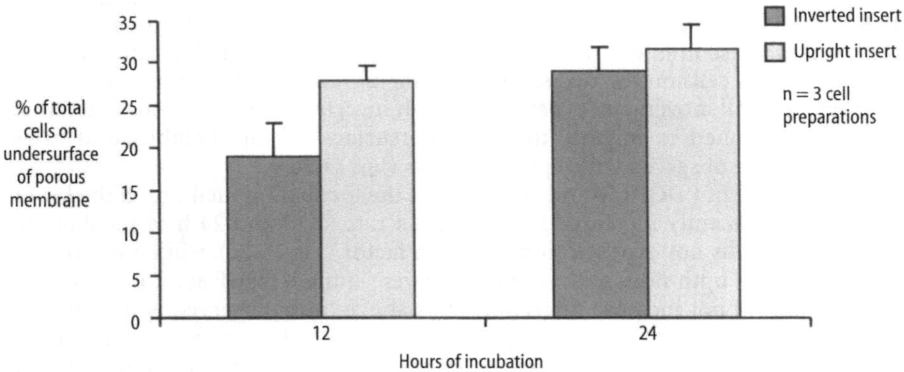
Inverted insert
Upright insert
n = 3 cell preparations
% of total cells on undersurface of porous membrane
35
30
25
20
15
10
5
0
12
24
Hours of incubation

b

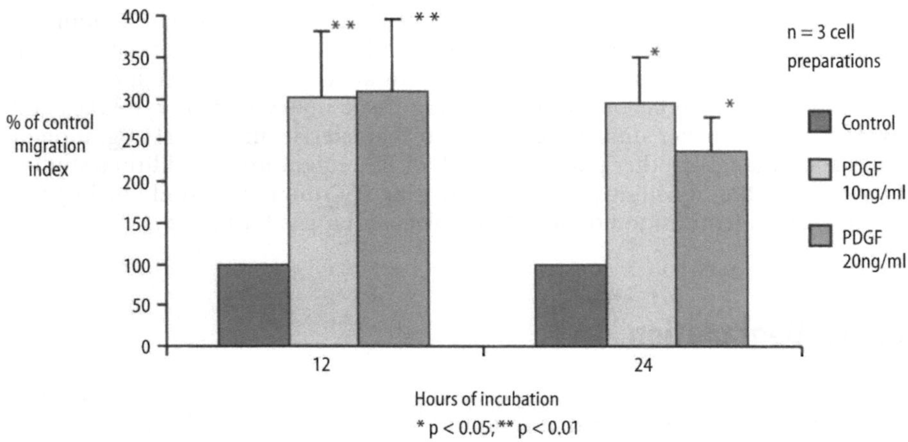
400
350
300
250
200
150
100
50
0
% of control migration index
* *
* *
*
*
n = 3 cell preparations
Control
PDGF 10ng/ml
PDGF 20ng/ml
12
24
Hours of incubation
* p < 0.05; ** p < 0.01

c

pathological fibrous tissue. These include basement membrane collagen, fibrillar collagen, laminin and fibronectin.[3–6] Since the maintenance of normal extracellular matrix in health depends on a fine balance between ECM protein synthesis and degradation, it is important to determine whether PSCs, in addition to their role in ECM synthesis, also play a role in ECM degradation.

The key enzymes responsible for matrix degradation are matrix metalloproteinases (MMPs). These are a family of about 20 zinc-dependent enzymes that are secreted in a latent (inactive) form.[25, 26] Activation occurs via the actions of proteases such as plasmin and trypsin.[27] The activity of MMPs can be inhibited by tissue inhibitors of metalloproteinases (TIMPs). Four subtypes of TIMPs (TIMP1-TIMP4) have been identified to date.[28–31] TIMP1 inhibits the activity of several MMPs (MMP1, 3, 8, 9, 10, 11, 13, 18), while TIMP2 is particularly important in the inhibition of MMP2. MMP2 and MMP9 both degrade basement membrane collagen (Type IV) and are associated with ECM remodelling in wound healing, development, inflammation, fibrosis, angiogenesis and tumour invasion.[32] Degradation of normal basement membrane collagen (collagen Type IV) is thought to facilitate the deposition of pathological fibril-forming collagen.[33]

We wished to determine whether PSCs had the capacity to synthesise MMPs and their inhibitors, and if so to assess the effect of known PSC activating factors such as cytokines, ethanol (a major association of chronic pancreatitis) or its metabolite acetaldehyde on the expression of MMP2 in cell secretions.

Pancreatic stellate cells were cultured in serum-free Iscove Dulbecco's medium for 24 h and the conditioned medium (cell secretions) was collected for assessment of MMP and TIMP expression. Total MMP expression was assessed by zymography. MMP2 was identified by western blotting, while RT-PCR using specific primers was employed to examine the expression of MMP9, TIMP1 and TIMP2.

Zymography

This method, described by Herron et al,[34] allows the detection of both latent and active forms of MMPs. The technique involves the separation of proteins by electrophoresis through a polyacrylamide gel containing a substrate (such as gelatin) that can be readily cleaved by MMPs. The presence of MMPs in the sample can be detected as white bands of lysis against the Coomassie Blue stained gel. For this study, zymogram gels were prepared by addition of type I gelatin to the standard Laemmli acrylamide polymerisation mixture at a final concentration of 1 mg/ml (0.1%). PSCs were incubated for 24 h in serum free medium, which was then

◀ **Figure 17.2.** Migration of pancreatic stellate cells. **a** Freshly isolated (◆) and culture passaged (■) PSCs were cultured for varying periods in inserts consisting of a porous membrane at its base. Passaged cells demonstrated migration from the top to the undersurface of the membrane at 12 h and the rate of migration increased over time. Freshly isolated cells also exhibited increasing rates of migration across the porous membrane over time, however the initial migration was delayed as compared to passaged cells. **b** The influence of gravity on the experimental set-up for studies on PSC migration was assessed by inverting the inserts after cell seeding. The rates of migration (at 12 h and 24 h of incubation) of cells in the inverted inserts were similar to those of cells in upright inserts, indicating that the results of the migration studies were not confounded by gravity. **c** Platelet derived growth factor (PDGF) at concentrations of 10 and 20 ng/ml in the culture medium, significantly increased the rates of PSC migration compared to control PSCs incubated with culture medium alone.

collected, centrifuged for 10 min at 1500 rpm to remove cells and debris and mixed with non-reducing sample buffer (0.4 M Tris pH 6.8, 5% SDS, 20% glycerol, 0.03% bromophenol blue). Samples were electrophoresed at 60 V through a 4% stacking gel and then at 100 V through a 10% resolving gel. Following electrophoresis, gels were washed in 2.5% Triton X-100 with gentle shaking for 30 min and then incubated for 30 min at room temperature in developing buffer (40mM Tris-HCl pH 7.8, 0.2 mM NaCl, 6.67 mM $CaCl_2$, 0.1% Triton X-100). The developing buffer was replaced with fresh developing buffer and the gels incubated overnight at 37°C. The gels were then stained with freshly made 0.5% Coomassie Blue R-250 in 10% acetic acid and 40% methanol for 2–3 h and destained using fresh Coomassie destaining solution (45% ethanol, 10% acetic acid). Gels were washed three times with the destaining solution replaced at 15 min, 30 min, and 1 h and then placed in storage solution (5% methanol, 0.75% acetic acid).

Western Blotting for MMP2

The immunoreactivity of MMP2 was detected by western blotting using a purified mouse monoclonal antibody (Calbiochem-Novabiochem, Cambridge, MA). Cultured PSCs (passages 1–3) were used for all experiments. Quadruplicate wells of cells were exposed to TNFα (5, 10 and 25 U/mL), TGFβ1 (0.5 and 1 ng/ml), IL6 (0.001, 0.1 and 10 ng/mL), ethanol (10 and 50 mM) or acetaldehyde (150 and 200 μM) in serum free culture medium for 24 h at 37°C. Cells incubated with serum free culture medium alone served as controls. Rat recombinant TNFα, TGFβ1 and IL6 were purchased from Peprotech, Rocky Hill, NJ.

The protein concentrations of stellate cell secretions were measured by the method of Lowry et al[35] using bovine serum albumin as the standard. Proteins (100 μg) from each sample were separated by gel electrophoresis using a 10% SDS polyacrylamide gel. Known molecular weight protein standards (Biorad, Richmond, CA, USA) were run alongside the samples. Separated proteins were transferred onto a nitrocellulose membrane using a commercial semi-dry blotting apparatus (Biorad, Richmond, CA, USA). The membranes were blocked in 5% skim milk in Tris buffered saline (TBS; pH 7.6) with 0.05% Tween-20 (TTBS) for 1 h to prevent non-specific binding of antibody. The membranes were then incubated for 1 h at room temperature with monoclonal anti-MMP2 (1 μg/ml) in 5% skim milk in TTBS. After 3 washes of 5 min each with TTBS, the membranes were incubated with the horseradish peroxidase (HRP) – conjugated secondary antibody (1:500; DAKO Corporation, Carpintaria, CA) for 60 min at room temperature. The membrane was then rinsed with TTBS (3 × 5 minutes) and finally with TBS. MMP2 bands were detected by the enhanced chemiluminescence (ECL) technique using the Amersham ECL kit (Amersham Pharmacia Biotech, Sydney, Australia). MMP2 expression was quantified by densitometry of scanned autoradiographs (Scion Image, Maryland, USA). Densitometer readings were expressed as integrated optical densities (arbitrary densitometer units calculated from the density as well as the size of each band) per μg protein loaded onto the gel.

MMP9 and TIMP1/TIMP2 expression: Expression of messenger RNA (mRNA) for MMP9 and for the inhibitors TIMP1 and TIMP2 in PSCs was examined using RT-PCR. Total cellular RNA was extracted from PSCs by a modification of the method described by Chomczynski and Sacchi[36] using the Tri-reagent kit (Sigma Chemical

Table 17.2. Primer sequences for MMP, TIMP and RT-PCR

Rat MMP9:	forward primer: 5' AAG GAT GGT CTA CTG GCA C 3', reverse primer: 5' AGA GAT TCT CAC TGG GGC 3' [38].
Rat TIMP1:	forward primer: 5' ACA GCT TTC TGC AAC TCG 3', reverse primer: 5' CTA TAG GTC TTT ACG AAG GCC 3' [37].
Rat TIMP2:	forward primer: 5' ATT TAT CTA CAC GGC CCC 3', reverse primer: 5' CAA GAA CCA TCA CTT CTC TTG 3' [39].
Rat GAPDH:	forward primer: 5' AAT CCC ATC ACC ATC TTC CA 3', reverse primer: 5' CAA GAA CCA TCA CTT CTC TTG 3'.

Company, St Louis, MO, USA) as described previously[5]. Total cellular RNA was reverse transcribed using a first strand cDNA synthesis kit (MBI Fermentas, Vilnius, Lithuania) according to the manufacturers instructions. The resulting cDNA was amplified using the MasterTaq Kit (Eppendorf Scientific, Westbury, NY, USA) using previously reported primers for MMP9, TIMP1 and TIMP2[37–39] and GAPDH (internal control). Primer sequences as shown in Table 17.2.

The reaction mix contained 4 μl of cDNA, 50 pmol of each primer (forward and reverse), 2 mM $MgCl_2$, 0.2 mM dNTPs, and 2.5 U Taq DNA polymerase. PCR was performed on a Perkin-Elmer thermal cycler with a 2 min predenaturation at 94°C, and 35 cycles of amplification consisting of 94°C for 1 min (denaturation), 55°C (TIMP1 and TIMP2) and 56°C (MMP9) for 1 min (annealing), and 72°C for 1 min (extension).

Zymography revealed the presence of several gelatinolytic bands on the gel representing areas of MMP activity (Fig 17.3a). Most of the activity appeared to be concentrated in an area of the gel corresponding to a molecular weight range of 60–82 kDa (72 kDa is the molecular size of MMP2, while 57 kDa corresponds to MMP13). A distinct band corresponding to a molecular weight of 92 kDa (the known size for MMP9) was also observed. The presence of MMP2 in PSC secretions was confirmed by western blotting (Fig 17.3b). Using a monoclonal antibody against both latent and active forms of MMP2 revealed a single discrete band corresponding to the control (recombinant rat MMP2) band at a molecular size of 72 kDa (the known molecular weight of latent MMP2). RT-PCR studies allowed identification of mRNA for MMP9 in accordance with the band observed on zymography for MMP protein (Fig 17.3c). RT-PCR also revealed that PSCs express mRNA for the MMP inhibitors TIMP1 and TIMP2 (Fig 17.3d). Our finding that PSCs express matrix metalloproteinases as well as their inhibitors concurs with reports in hepatic stellate cells.[40–42]

PSC activating factors such as the cytokines TNF_{α} and IL6 (known to be upregulated in acute pancreatitis[43]) as well as $TGF_{\beta}1$ (an important profibrogenic cytokine upregulated during chronic pancreatitis[44, 45]) were examined for their effects on MMP2 secretion by PSCs. Both TGFß1 and IL6 significantly increased MMP2 expression in PSCS (Figs 17.3e and f), while TNFα had no effect on MMP2 secretion (data not shown). Ethanol (10 and 50 mM) and its metabolite acetaldehyde (150 and 200 μM) also increased MMP2 secretion by PSCs (Fig 17.3g).

The above studies have shown that PSCs are capable of producing a variety of MMPs as well as the inhibitors TIMPs 1 and 2. These findings point to a role for PSCs in ECM degradation, in addition to their well established role in ECM synthesis. It would be reasonable therefore to speculate that, i) in health, PSCs serve to maintain normal tissue architecture; ii) when activated during pancreatic injury,

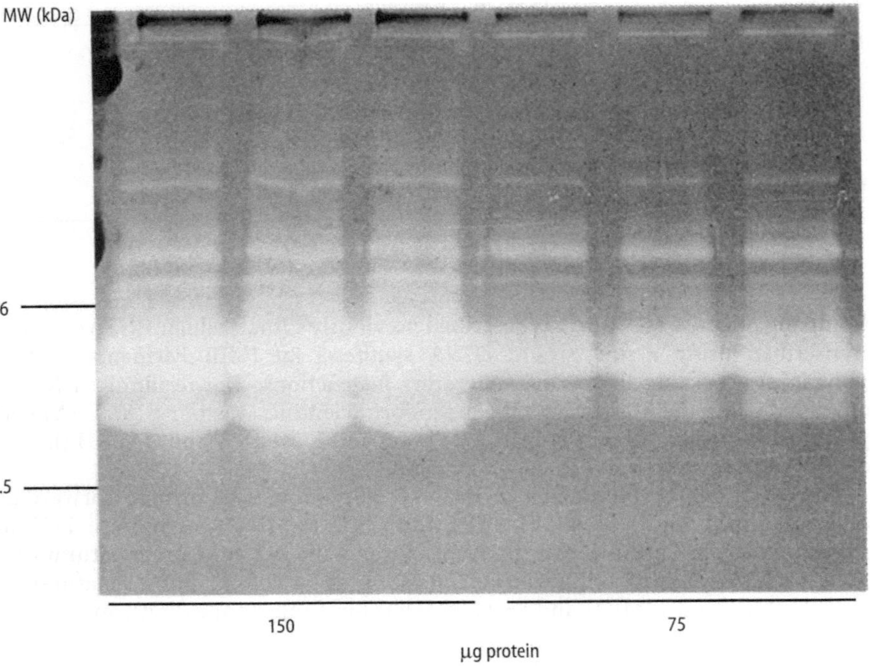

a

Figure 17.3. Expression of matrix metalloproteinases (MMPs) and their inhibitors (TIMPs) in pancreatic stellate cells. **a** Zymography of PSC secretions (75 and 150 μg protein) revealed the presence of numerous lytic bands indicating the presence of MMPs in the samples; most of the activity was found in the region of the gel corresponding to a molecular weight range of 65–80 kD. **b** Western blotting of PSC secretions using a monoclonal anti-MMP2 antibody revealed the presence of a single band corresponding to the known molecular weight of MMP2 i.e. 72 kD. Recombinant MMP2 was used as the positive control. **c** Expression of MMP9 in five separate PSC preparations was demonstrated using RT-PCR techniques. **d** RT-PCR was also used to demonstrate the expression of TIMP1 and TIMP2 in 5 separate PSC preparations. **e** TGFβ1 at concentrations of 0.5 and 1 ng/ml significantly increased MMP2 expression in PSCs as assessed by western blotting (a representative immunoblot is shown above the graph). **f** IL6 at concentrations of 0.1 and 10 ng/ml significantly increased MMP2 secretion by PSCs as assessed by western blotting (a representative immunoblot is shown above the graph). **g** Both ethanol (at concentrations of 10 mM and 50 mM) and its metabolite acetaldehyde (150 μM and 200 μM) significantly increased the secretion of MMP2 by PSCs. A representative western blot for five separate PSC preparations is depicted.

the cells secrete increased amounts of specific MMPs such as MMP2 which leads to increased degradation of normal basement membrane collagen (type IV) and facilitates the deposition of abnormal fibrillar collagens, thereby potentiating fibrosis within the gland. Further work is required to examine the complement and process of activation of latent MMPs secreted by stellate cells, the role of TIMPs in MMP inactivation and the influence of paracrine factors such as acinar cell secretions on MMP production. This work will help to characterise the capacity of PSCs for ECM degradation/remodelling.

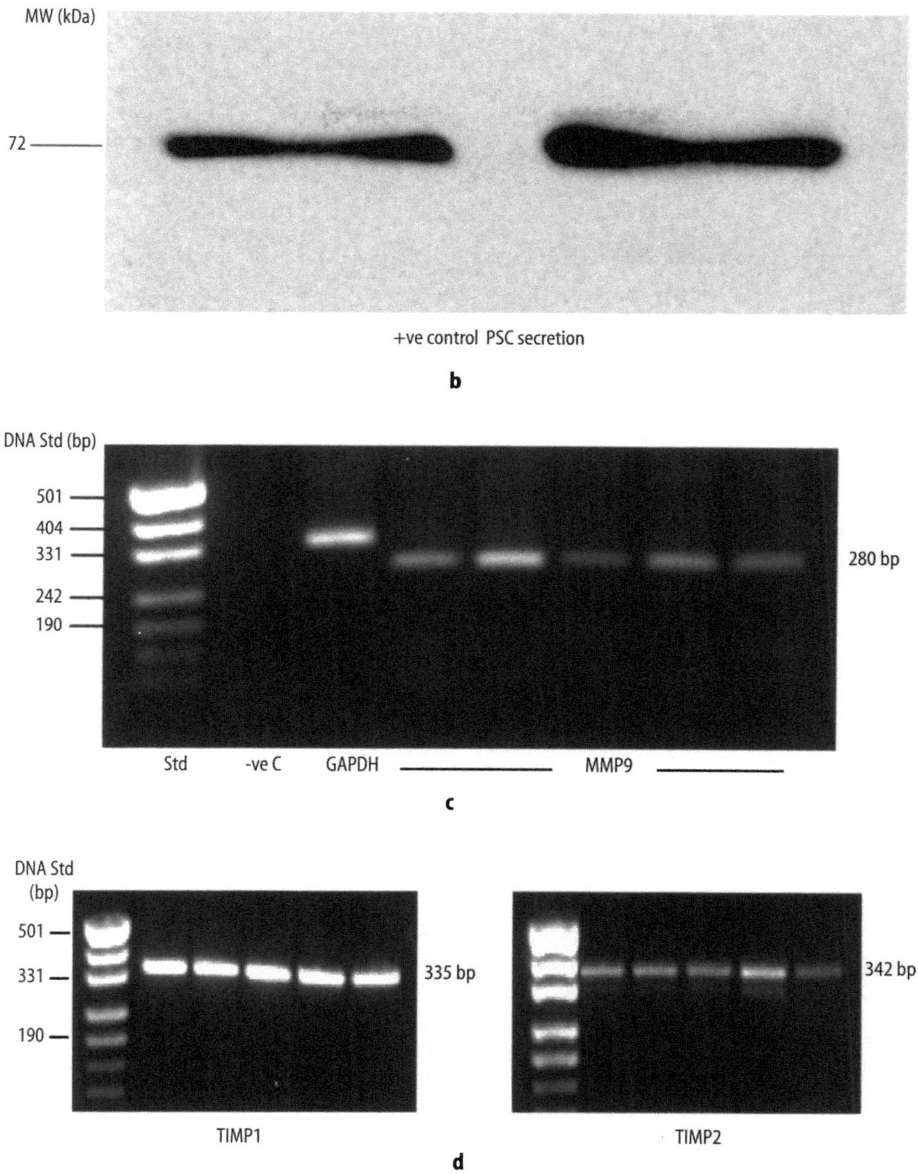

Figure 17.3. (*Continued*)

Endogenous Cytokine Expression

The effects of a number of exogenously added cytokines on PSC activation has been well described in the literature (the main findings to date are summarised in Table 17.3). These cytokines act via cell surface receptors, which have also been

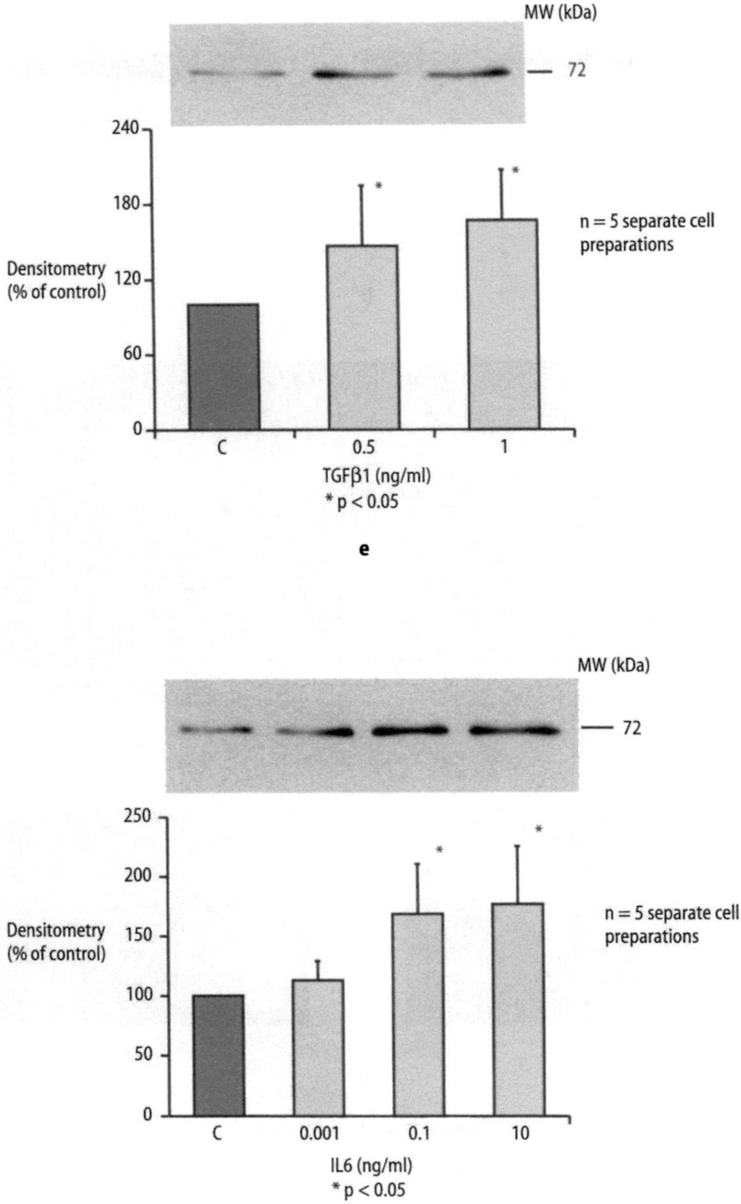

Figure 17.3. (*Continued*)

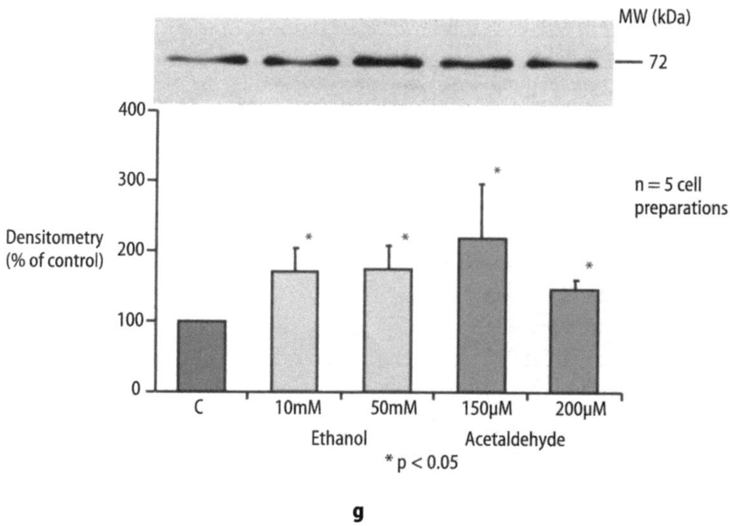

Figure 17.3. (*Continued*)

demonstrated on PSCs.[9,10] The data suggest that PSCs are responsive to paracrine influences during tissue injury. The possibility that PSCs may express cytokines endogenously was explored because of the potential for the existence of an autocrine loop that would lead to perpetuation of cell activation. To address this issue we used RT-PCR techniques to assess the expression of TGFβ1 and IL1α in PSCs. In addition, we examined the effect of extraneous activating factors such as ethanol and acetaldehyde on endogenous expression of the above cytokines in PSCs using a quantitative real time PCR assay.

Expression of TGFβ1, IL1 and GAPDH (internal control) by PSCs was examined by RT-PCR. The primers used were as follows:[46,47]

TGFβ1 Forward primer 5' TGA GTG GCT GTC TTT TGA CG 3',
Reverse primer 5' TGG GAC TGA TCC CAT TGA TT 3';

IL1α Forward primer 5' CAG GAT GAG GAC ATG AGC ACC 3',
Reverse primer 5' CTC TGC AGA CTC AAA CTC CAC 3';

GAPDH Forward primer 5' AAT CCC ATC ACC ATC TTC CA 3',
Reverse primer 5' GGC AGT GAT GGC ATG GAC TG 3';

The reaction mix contained 4 μl of cDNA, 50 pmol of each primer (forward and reverse), 2 mM $MgCl_2$, 0.2 mM dNTPs, and 2.5 U Taq DNA polymerase. PCR was performed on a Perkin–Elmer thermal cycler with a 2 min predenaturation at 94°C, and 35 cycles of amplification consisting of 94°C for 1 min (denaturation), 55°C for 1 min (annealing), 72°C for 2 min 30 sec (extension) and 72°C for a further 8 min. Amplified products were separated on a 1% agarose gel and visualised by ethidium bromide staining.

Table 17.3. Effect of cytokines on pancreatic stellate cells

Cytokine	Effect on PSCs
PDGF[4]	↑ cell proliferation
$TGF_{\beta}1$[4,10]	↑ αSMA expression ↑ ECM protein synthesis ↑ PDGF receptor ß expression ↑ MMP2 secretion
TNF_{α}[59]	↑ cell proliferation ↑ αSMA expression ↑ ECM protein synthesis
IL1[59]	↑ αSMA expression
IL6[59]	↑ αSMA expression ↑ MMP2 secretion

In order to determine whether known PSC activating factors such as ethanol and acetaldehyde influence the expression of TGFβ1 and IL1α in the cells, real time PCR was used. Pancreatic stellate cells were treated in serum free culture medium for 24 h with either ethanol (10 or 50 mM) or acetaldehyde (150 or 200 μM). Total RNA was then extracted as described above using Tri Reagent. Primers and probes specific for the two cytokines and for the internal control 18S (ribosomal RNA) were obtained from Applied Biosystems (USA). The manufacturers instructions were followed using Pre-Developed Taqman© Assay Reagents for TGFβ1, IL1α and 18S. Briefly, RNA was reverse transcribed and the cDNA was diluted 1:10 before addition into the PCR reaction. Multiplex reactions (target + control reactions) were performed in a 96 well reaction plate using the ABI PRISM© 7700 Sequence Detection System. All PCR reactions were prepared in duplicate. The amplification conditions were as follows – 2 min at 50°C followed by 10 min at 95°C and then 40 cycles at a melting temperature of 95°C (15 seconds) and annealing extension temperature of 60°C (1 min). Data are expressed as a fraction of cytokine expression in control cells (i.e. cells not treated with ethanol or acetaldehyde).

RT-PCR demonstrated that PSCs express both TGFβ1 and IL1α as evident from amplification products with the expected sizes of 146bp and 447bp respectively (Figures 17.4a and b). IL1 expression in PSCs was significantly induced by 50 mM ethanol and 150 μM acetaldehyde (Fig. 174c). TGFβ1 expression in PSCs was not influenced by 10 mM or 50 mM ethanol or by 150 μM acetaldehyde but was significantly reduced by 200 μM acetaldehyde (Fig. 17.4d). The latter finding was unexpected and the reasons for this effect are unclear. Toxicity of acetaldehyde at this concentration is an unlikely explanation because we have previously demonstrated that the synthesis of other proteins such as collagen and αSMA in PSCs exposed to 200 μM acetaldehyde is significantly increased compared to control cells.[5]

The above studies have thus demonstrated that PSCs are capable of endogenous production of cytokines and that this production can be increased in response to factors known to activate the cells. These findings suggest that, during pancreatic injury, PSCs may not only be activated by exogenous factors via paracrine pathways, but may also be activated via autocrine pathways, thereby resulting in the perpetuation of the activated state and potentiation of fibrosis. Future work in this area will include studies to determine the full complement of cytokines and their receptors expressed by PSCs and to identify the factors that influence such expression, so that strategies to interrupt the perpetuation of PSC activation may be devised.

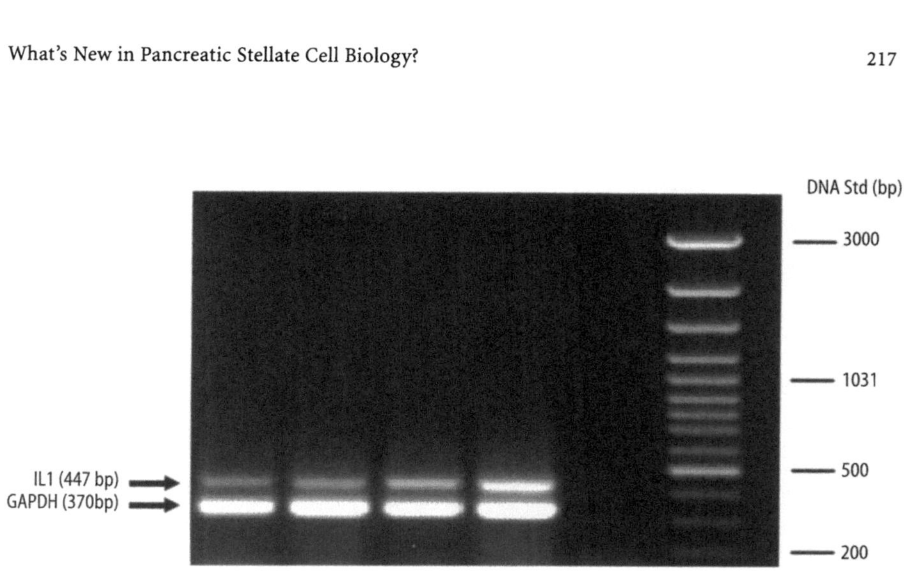

a

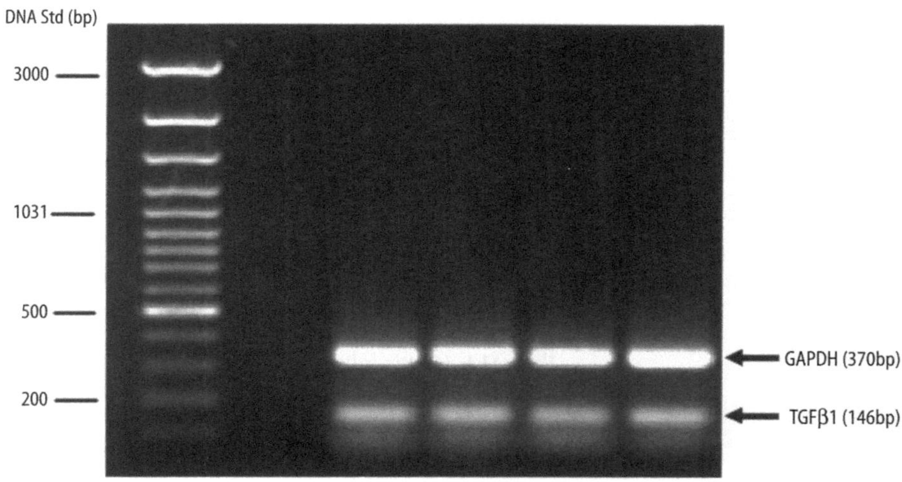

b

Figure 17.4. Endogenous expression of cytokines by PSCs. **a** RT-PCR analysis of RNA extracted from PSCs demonstrated the expression of IL1 and GAPDH (internal control) in PSCs. **b** RT-PCR analysis of RNA extracted from PSCs demonstrated the expression of the TGFβ1 and GAPDH (internal control) in PSCs. **c** The effect of ethanol (10 and 50 mM; E10 and E50 respectively) and acetaldehyde (150 and 200 μM; A150 and A200 respectively) on the mRNA levels for IL1 in PSCs was examined by real time PCR. Ethanol at a concentration of 50 mM significantly increased IL1 expression in PSCs compared to control cells (C) incubated with culture medium alone. Acetaldehyde did not influence IL1 expression in PSCs. **d** The effect of ethanol (10 and 50 mM; E10 and E50 respectively) and acetaldehyde (150 and 200 μM; A150 and A200 respectively) on the mRNA levels for TGFβ1 in PSCs was examined by real time PCR. Ethanol (10 and 50 mM) and acetaldehyde (150 μM) did not change TGFβ1 mRNA levels in PSCs compared to controls (C). Acetaldehyde (200 μM) significantly decreased TGFβ1 mRNA levels in PSCs.

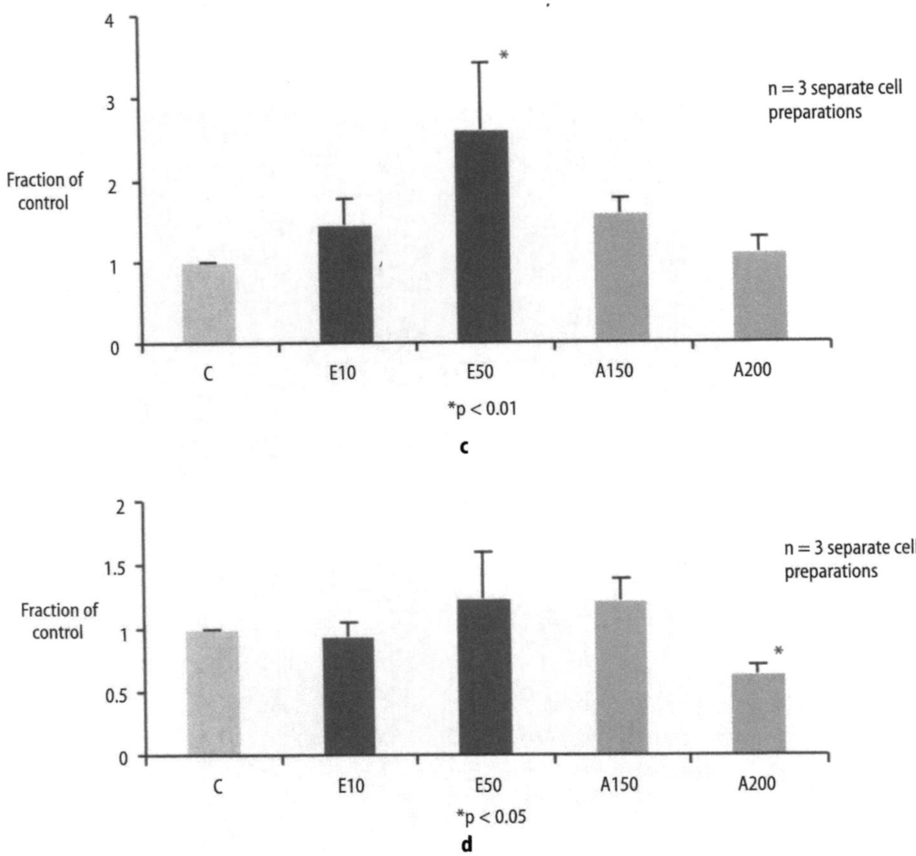

Figure 17.4. *(Continued)*

Signalling Pathways Mediating Cell Activation

It is well documented that most cellular functions including cell metabolism, protein synthesis, cell proliferation and differentiation are regulated by signal transduction pathways induced by a variety of hormones, growth factors and cytokines and by cellular stressors such as toxins, irradiation, heat shock, osmotic imbalance and oxidant stress.[48] In general, interaction of ligands with cell surface receptors, or direct effects of cellular stressors, stimulate a cascade of phosphorylation of intracellular protein kinases, which in turn influence the nuclear factors that regulate a variety of cell functions.[49] An understanding of the signalling pathways that mediate the response of PSCs to various activating factors released during pancreatic injury is an important step because it may eventually enable modulation of specific signalling events in order to prevent or reverse the adverse effects of stellate cell activation.

One of the major pathways mediating cellular responses to extracellular signals is the mitogen activated protein (MAP) kinase pathway.[49] MAP kinases are classified into three subfamilies including extracellular signal regulated kinases (ERK1 and 2), stress activated protein kinases [SAPK, also called c-jun NH_2 kinase (JNK)] and p38 kinase.[50] Activation of the MAPK pathway results in activation of nuclear transcription factors leading to altered gene expression in cells.[50] Our initial experiments were aimed at examining the signalling pathways influenced by exposure of PSCs to ethanol or acetaldehyde. There is no available published literature to date regarding this area, but studies with ethanol and acetaldehyde on signalling in other cell systems have been reported.[51, 52] Acetaldehyde has been shown to induce c-jun and c-fos protooncogenes (downstream mediators of the MAPK pathway) via activation of protein kinase C in hepatic stellate cells.[53] It has also been reported to activate the transcription factors NF-κB and AP-1 in hepatocyte cell lines.[54] Ethanol has been reported to induce ERK 1 and ERK 2 activity in embryonic liver cells and vascular smooth muscle cells.[55]

Activity of ERK1 and 2 in PSCs exposed to ethanol (50 mM) or its metabolite acetaldehyde (200μM) at 37°C was assessed as follows:

Cultured PSCs (passages 1–3) were incubated with ethanol (50 mM) or acetaldehyde (200 μM) in serum free culture medium for periods of 15 min, 30 min, 60 min and 24 h in airtight culture plates. At the end of the incubation periods, medium was removed and cells lysed. 100–150 μg of total cellular protein was then subjected to immunoprecipitation using a monoclonal antibody to ERK1/2 (p44/p42) (Cell signalling Technology, Beverly, MA) to selectively immunoprecipitate active ERK1/2. The immunoprecipitate was washed and then incubated for 30 min with ELK-1 (a fusion protein that is phosphorylated by active ERK1/2 in the presence of ATP and kinase buffer). The reaction was stopped by the addition of 3 Œ SDS sample buffer to the reaction mix. Samples were then separated by SDS-PAGE, transferred to nitrocellulose and probed with an antibody to phosphorylated ELK-1 (Cell Signalling Technology, Beverly, MA). Western blots were autoradiographed and bands were analysed by densitometry.

The effect of both ethanol and acetaldehyde on ERK1/2 activity in PSCs was biphasic (Figures 17.5a and b). A significant increase in ERK1/2 activity over controls was evident early in the incubation period (at 15 min of incubation) after exposure to both compounds. ERK1/2 activity returned to control levels at 30 and 60 min and was followed by another increase over controls at 24 h.

The above results indicate that ethanol and acetaldehyde influence a major signalling pathway in PSCs early after exposure. Work is underway in our laboratory to assess other MAP kinases as well as other signalling pathways, to fully characterise the signalling molecules that mediate the activation of PSCs after exposure to ethanol and acetaldehyde. Studies are also underway to delineate the pathways responsible for PSC activation in response to other factors such as cytokines and oxidant stress.

Role of PSC in Pancreatic Cancer

Pancreatic cancer is a leading cause of cancer death in the world.[56] The disease has an extremely poor prognosis because of the high propensity of these tumours for local invasion and distant metastasis. Most research into the pathobiology of this disease has focused on the molecular genetics of the tumour cells themselves.[57, 58] However, to date, almost no attention has been paid to the

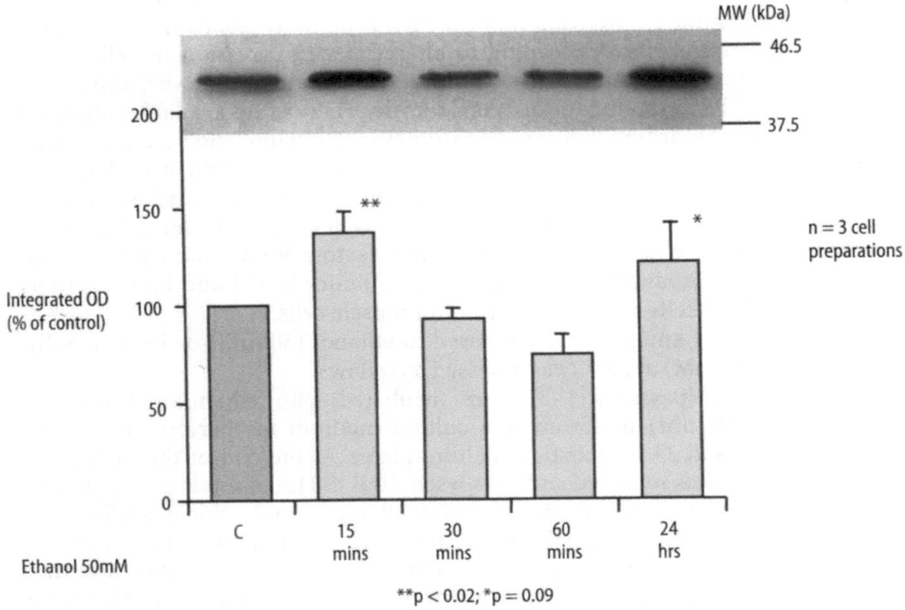
MW (kDa)
46.5
37.5
200
150
100
50
0
Integrated OD
(% of control)
**
*
n = 3 cell
preparations
C
15
mins
30
mins
60
mins
24
hrs
Ethanol 50mM
**p < 0.02; *p = 0.09

a

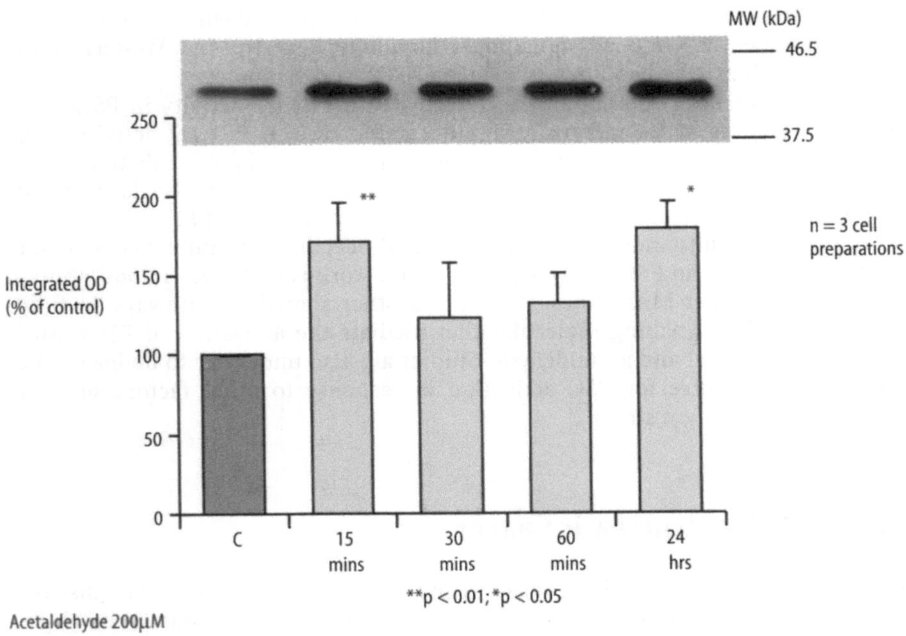
MW (kDa)
46.5
37.5
250
200
150
100
50
0
Integrated OD
(% of control)
**
*
n = 3 cell
preparations
C
15
mins
30
mins
60
mins
24
hrs
**p < 0.01; *p < 0.05
Acetaldehyde 200μM

b

striking stromal (desmoplastic) reaction around the tumour, a characteristic feature of a majority of pancreatic cancers.[2] We hypothesise that a) the cells responsible for the production of the desmoplastic reaction around pancreatic cancers are pancreatic stellate cells and b) pancreatic stellate cells play a role in local spread and distant metastasis of pancreatic cancer by producing matrix degrading enzymes and angiogenic factors that promote tumour invasion, and by interacting with factors produced by the tumour cells themselves. The above hypothesis is based on our recent studies (using dual staining methodology i.e. immunostaining combined with in situ hybridisation) which have demonstrated that the stroma around pancreatic cancers contains stellate shaped cells that stain positive for both α smooth muscle actin (suggesting an activated phenotype of stellate cells) and collagen messenger RNA (suggesting that these cells are the source of the collagen in the stroma) (Fig. 17.6a). The hypothesis is further supported by the findings (described earlier in this chapter) that PSCs can secrete matrix degrading enzymes (MMPs), suggesting a possible mechanism by which these cells may facilitate local tumour invasion.

Studies are currently underway in our laboratory to define the role of PSCs in the pathobiology of pancreatic cancer, using two approaches i) *in vivo* studies (using tissue from patients with pancreatic cancer and/or from animal models of the disease); and ii) *in vitro* studies examining the interaction of PSCs and pancreatic cancer cells in culture.

Archival pancreatic cancer samples as well as prospectively collected pancreatic resection specimens have been obtained by our laboratory. Serial sections of these samples are being examined histologically following H and E staining, Sirius red staining for collagen, immunostaining for αSMA and for stellate cell selective markers such as desmin (Fig. 17.6b) and glial fibrillary acidic protein, and in situ hybridisation to identify the source of collagen in the stromal reaction. Studies are also underway to determine the expression of angiogenic growth factors and of matrix degrading enzymes and their inhibitors in stromal areas and to correlate the expression of these proteins with PSC activation. In vitro studies are being undertaken to examine the interaction of pancreatic cancer cell lines (Pancl and MiaPaCa2) with PSCs.

In summary, the studies discussed in this Chapter provide new insights into a number of features of pancreatic stellate cell biology and strengthen the concept that activation of PSCs is a key step in the fibrogenic process in the pancreas. Characterisation of this activation process and its consequence (i.e. the production of fibrosis) are areas of study that are currently being pursued by a number of research groups around the world. However, there is another equally important issue with respect to PSC activation that needs attention, namely the post-activation events that may result in the resolution of fibrosis via the reversal of PSCs to quiescence and/or apoptosis of activated PSCs. Elucidation of these aspects of PSC biology will enable identification of the molecular mechanisms that may be candidates for therapeutic modulation so as to prevent/retard the development or aid the resolution of pathological fibrosis within the gland.

◀ **Figure 17.5.** Effects of ethanol and acetaldehyde on the MAP kinase pathway in PSCs. ERK1/2 activity was assessed in PSCs incubated with (**a**) 50 mM ethanol or (**b**) 200 μM acetaldehyde by in vitro activity assays. ERK 1/2 activity in PSCs exhibited a biphasic response to both ethanol and acetaldehyde exposure, with a significant increase in activity early in the incubation period (at 15 min), a return of activity to control levels at 30 and 60 min of incubation and a second increase in activity over control levels at 24 h of incubation.

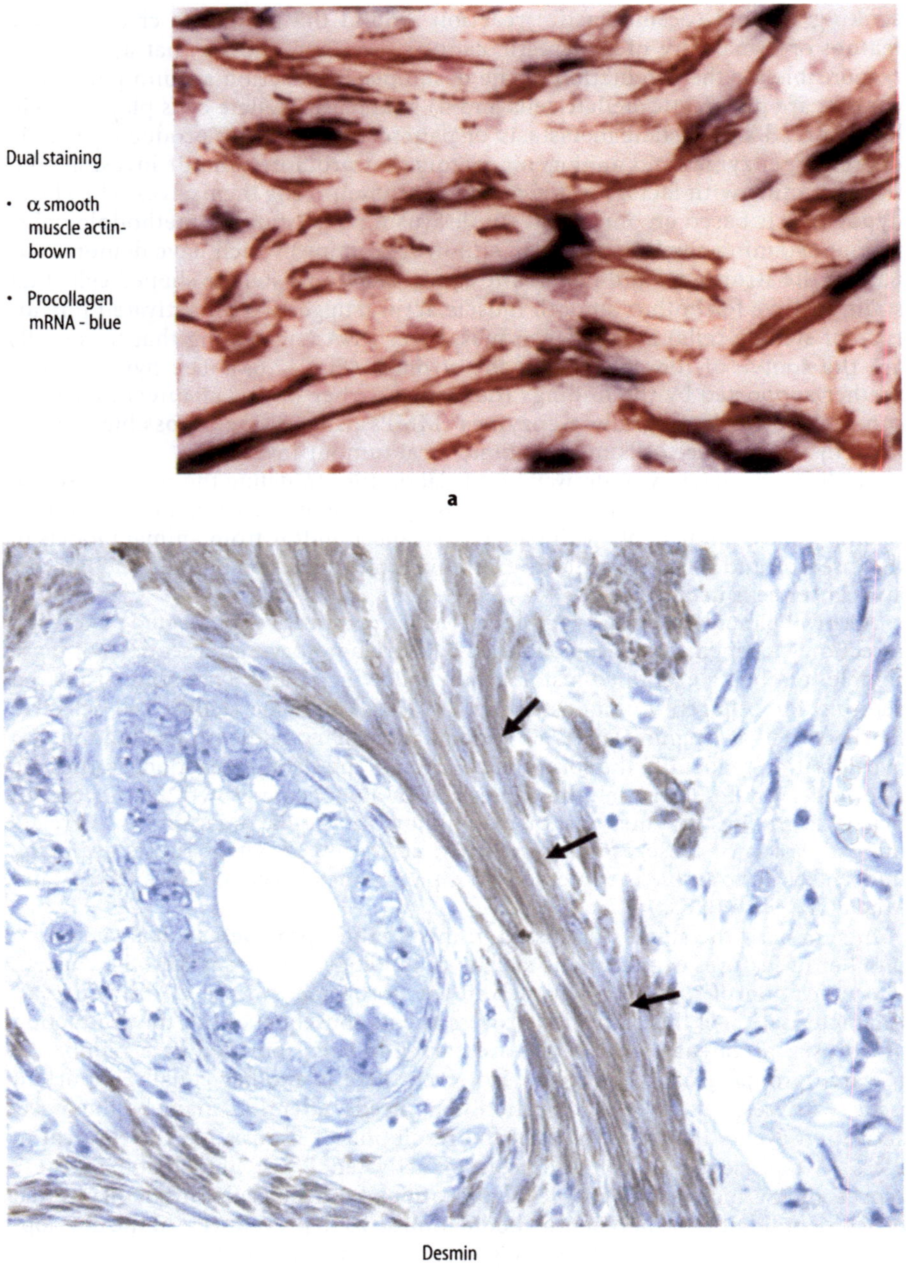

Figure 17.6. Role of pancreatic stellate cells in pancreatic cancer. **a** Human pancreatic cancer sections were subjected to immunostaining for α smooth muscle actin and in situ hybridisation for procollagen mRNA. The Figure depicts an area of the stroma showing that αSMA positive (brown staining) stromal cells also exhibit positive staining (blue) for procollagen mRNA, suggesting that activated PSCs are the predominant source of collagen in the desmoplastic reaction around pancreatic cancers. **b** Human pancreatic cancer sections immunostained for desmin. Stromal cells exhibit positive staining for the cytoskeletal marker desmin (arrows).

Acknowledgments

Studies described in this manuscript were supported by grants from the National Health and Medical Research Council of Australia and the Australian Brewers' Foundation.

References

1. DiMagno EP, Layer P, Clain JE. Chronic pancreatitis. In: Go VLW, DiMagno EP, Gardner JD, et al., editors. The pancreas : Biology, pathobiology and disease. New York: Raven Press; 1993; pp. 665–706.
2. Kloppel G. Pathology of non-endocrine pancreas. In: Go VLW, DiMagno EP, Gardner JD, et al., editors. The pancreas : Biology, pathobiology and disease. New York: Raven Press; 1993; pp. 871–897.
3. Apte MV, Haber PS, Applegate TL, et al. Periacinar stellate shaped cells in rat pancreas-identification, isolation, and culture. Gut 1998; 43 (1):128–133.
4. Apte MV, Haber PS, Darby SJ, et al. Pancreatic stellate cells are activated by proinflammatory cytokines: Implications for pancreatic fibrogenesis. Gut 1999; 44 (4):534–541.
5. Apte MV, Phillips PA, Fahmy RG, et al. Does alcohol directly stimulate pancreatic fibrogenesis? Studies with rat pancreatic stellate cells. Gastroenterology 2000; 118 (4):780–794.
6. Bachem MG, Schneider E, Gross H, et al. Identification, culture, and characterization of pancreatic stellate cells in rats and humans. Gastroenterology 1998; 115 (2):421–432.
7. Casini A, Galli A, Pignalosa P, et al. Collagen type i synthesized by pancreatic periacinar stellate cells (PSC) co-localizes with lipid peroxidation-derived aldehydes in chronic alcoholic pancreatitis. J Pathol 2000; 192 (1):81–89.
8. Emmrich J, Weber I, Nausch M, et al. Immunohistochemical characterization of the pancreatic cellular infiltrate in normal pancreas, chronic pancreatitis and pancreatic carcinoma. Digestion 1998; 59 (3):192–198.
9. Haber PS, Keogh GW, Apte MV, et al. Activation of pancreatic stellate cells in human and experimental pancreatic fibrosis. Am J Pathol 1999; 155 (4):1087–1095.
10. Schneider E, Schmid-Kotsas A, Zhao J, et al. Identification of mediators stimulating proliferation and matrix synthesis of rat pancreatic stellate cells. Am J Physiol: Cell Physiology 2001; 281 (2):C532–543.
11. Friedman SL. The virtuosity of hepatic stellate cells. Gastroenterology 1999; 117 (5):1244–1246.
12. Niki T, De Bleser PJ, Xu G, et al. Comparison of glial fibrillary acidic protein and desmin staining in normal and CCl4-induced fibrotic rat livers. Hepatology 1996; 23 (6):1538–1545.
13. Niki T, Pekny M, Hellemans K, et al. Class VI intermediate filament protein nestin is induced during activation of rat hepatic stellate cells. Hepatology 1999; 29 (2):520–527.
14. Nakatani K, Seki S, Kawada N, et al. Expression of neural cell adhesion molecule (N-CAM) in perisinusoidal stellate cells of the human liver. Cell & Tissue Research 1996; 283 (1):159–165.
15. Knittel T, Aurisch S, Neubauer K, et al. Cell-type-specific expression of neural cell adhesion molecule (N-CAM) in ito cells of rat liver. Up-regulation during in vitro activation and in hepatic tissue repair. Am J Pathol 1996; 149 (2):449–462.
16. Cassiman D, Denef C, Desmet VJ, et al. Human and rat hepatic stellate cells express neurotrophins and neurotrophin receptors. Hepatology 2001; 33 (1):148–158.
17. Emmrich J, Weber I, Sparmann GH, et al. Activation of pancreatic stellate cells in experimental chronic pancreatitis in rats. Gastroenterology 2000; 118:A166.
18. Bothwell M. Functional interactions of neurotrophins and neurotrophin receptors. Ann Rev in Neuro 1995; 18:223–253.
19. Lindsay RM, Wiegand SJ, Altar CA, et al. Neurotrophic factors: From molecule to man. Trends in Neuroscience 1994; 17 (5):182–190.
20. Barbacid M. Structural and functional properties of the TRK family of neurotrophin receptors. Ann of the New York Acad of Sci 1995; 766:442–458.
21. Friess H, Zhu ZW, di Mola FF, et al. Nerve growth factor and its high-affinity receptor in chronic pancreatitis. Ann of Surg 1999; 230 (5):615–624.
22. Trim N, Morgan S, Evans M, et al. Hepatic stellate cells express the low affinity nerve growth factor receptor p75 and undergo apoptosis in response to nerve growth factor stimulation. Am J Pathol 2000; 156 (4):1235–1243.
23. Dacie JV, Lewis SM, editors. Practical haematology. 6th Edition ed: Churchill Livingstone; 1984.
24. Ikeda K, Wakahara T, Wang YQ, et al. In vitro migratory potential of rat quiescent hepatic stellate cells and its augmentation by cell activation. Hepatology 1999; 29 (6):1760–1767.
25. Birkedal-Hansen H, Moore WG, Bodden MK, et al. Matrix metalloproteinases: A review. Critical Reviews in Oral Biology & Medicine 1993; 4 (2):197–250.

26. Woessner JF, Jr. Matrix metalloproteinases and their inhibitors in connective tissue remodeling. FASEB Journal 1991; 5:2145–2154.
27. Woessner JF. Role of matrix proteases in processing enamel proteins. Connective Tissue Research 1998; 39 (1-3):373–377.
28. Murphy G, Cawston TE, Reynolds JJ. An inhibitor of collagenase from human amniotic fluid. Purification, characterization and action on metalloproteinases. Bio J 1981; 195 (1):167–170.
29. Stetler-Stevenson WG, Krutzsch HC, Liotta LA. Tissue inhibitor of metalloproteinase (TIMP-2). A new member of the metalloproteinase inhibitor family. J Bio Chem 1989; 264 (29):17374–17378.
30. Pavloff N, Staskus PW, Kishnani NS, et al. A new inhibitor of metalloproteinases from chicken: CHIMP-3. A third member of the timp family. J Bio Chem 1992; 267 (24):17321–17326.
31. Leco KJ, Apte SS, Taniguchi GT, et al. Murine tissue inhibitor of metalloproteinases-4 (TIMP-4): Cdna isolation and expression in adult mouse tissues. FEBS Letters 1997; 401 (2-3):213–217.
32. Corcoran M, Hewitt R, Kleiner DJ, et al. MMP-2: Expression, activation and inhibition. Enzyme Protein 1996; 49:7–19.
33. Friedman SL. Molecular regulation of hepatic fibrosis, an integrated cellular response to tissue injury. J Bio Chem 2000; 275 (4):2247–2250.
34. Herron G, Werb Z, Dwyer K, et al. Secretion of metalloproteinases by stimulated capillary endothelial cells. J Bio Chem 1986; 261:2810–2813.
35. Lowry O, Rosebrough N, Farr A, et al. Protein measurement with the Folin phenol reagent. J Bio Chem 1951; 193:265–275.
36. Chomczynski P, Sacchi N. Single-step method of rna isolation by acid guanidinium thiocyanate-phenol-chloroform extraction. Anal Bio 1987; 162:156–159.
37. Okada A, Garnier JM, Vicaire S, et al. Cloning of the cdna encoding rat tissue inhibitor of metalloproteinase 1 (TIMP-1), amino acid comparison with other timps, and gene expression in rat tissues. Gene 1994; 147:301–302.
38. Okada A, Santavicca M, Basset P. The cDNA cloning and expression of the gene encoding rat gelatinase B. Gene 1995; 164:317–321.
39. Cook TF, Burke JS, Bergman K, et al. Cloning and regulation of rat tissue inhibitor of metalloproteinase-2 in osteoblastic cells. Archives of Biochemistry and Biophysics 1994; 311:313–320.
40. Iredale JP, Murphy G, Hembry RM, et al. Human hepatic lipocytes synthesize tissue inhibitor of metalloproteinases-1. Implications for regulation of matrix degradation in liver. The J Clin Invest 1992; 90 (1):282–287.
41. Benyon RC, Iredale JP, Goddard S, et al. Expression of tissue inhibitor of metalloproteinases 1 and 2 is increased in fibrotic human liver. Gastroenterology 1996; 110 (3):821–831.
42. Knittel T, Mehde M, Kobold D, et al. Expression patterns of matrix metalloproteinases and their inhibitors in parenchymal and non-parenchymal cells of rat liver: Regulation by TNF-alpha and TGF-beta 1. Journal of Hepatology 1999; 30 (1):48–60.
43. Norman J, Franz M, Riker A. Rapid elevation of pro-inflammatory cytokines during acute pancreatitis and their origination within the pancreas. Surgical Forum 1994; 45:148–160.
44. Slater SD, Williamson RC, Foster CS. Expression of transforming growth factor-beta 1 in chronic pancreatitis. Digestion 1995; 56 (3):237–241.
45. Van Laethem JL, Deviere J, Resibois A, et al. Localization of transforming growth factor beta 1 and its latent binding protein in human chronic pancreatitis. Gastroenterology 1995; 108 (6):1873–1881.
46. Norman JG, Fink GW, Denham W, et al. Tissue-specific cytokine production during experimental acute pancreatitis. A probable mechanism for distant organ dysfunction. Digestive Diseases and Sciences 1997; 42 (8):1783–1788.
47. Faouzi S, Lepreux S, Bedin C, et al. Activation of cultured rat hepatic stellate cells by tumoral hepatocytes. Laboratory Investigation 1999; 79 (4):485–493.
48. Kyriakis JM, Avruch J. Mammalian mitogen-activated protein kinase signal transduction pathways activated by stress and inflammation. Physiology Reviews 2001; 81 (2):807–869.
49. Lopez-Ilasaca M. Signaling from g-protein-coupled receptors to mitogen-activated protein (map)-kinase cascades. Biochemical Pharmacology 1998; 56 (3):269–277.
50. Tibbles LA, Woodgett JR. The stress-activated protein kinase pathways. Cell and Molecular Life Sciences 1999; 55 (10):1230–1254.
51. Sachinidis A, Gouni-Berthold I, Seul C, et al. Early intracellular signalling pathway of ethanol in vascular smooth muscle cells. Bri J Pharmacology 1999; 128 (8):1761–1771.
52. Svegliati-Baroni G, Ridolfi F, Di Sario A, et al. Intracellular signaling pathways involved in acetaldehyde-induced collagen and fibronectin gene expression in human hepatic stellate cells. Hepatology 2001; 33:1130–1140.

53. Casini A, Galli G, Salzano R, et al. Acetaldehyde induces c-fos and c-jun proto-oncogenes in fat-storing cell cultures through protein kinase c activation. Alcohol and Alcoholism 1994; 29 (3):303–314.
54. Roman J, Colell A, Blasco C, et al. Differential role of ethanol and acetaldehyde in the induction of oxidative stress in hep g2 cells: Effect on transcription factors AP-1 and NF-kappaB. Hepatology 1999; 30 (6):1473–1480.
55. Reddy MA, Shukla SD. Potentiation of mitogen-activated protein kinase by ethanol in embryonic liver cells. Biochemical Pharmacology 1996; 51 (5):661–668.
56. Ahlgren JD. Epidemiology and risk factors in pancreatic cancer. Seminars in Oncology 1996; 23 (2):241–250.
57. Lemoine NR. Molecular advances in pancreatic cancer. Digestion 1997; 58 (6):550-556.
58. Kern SE. Advances from genetic clues in pancreatic cancer. Current Opinion in Oncology 1998; 10 (1):74–80.
59. Mews P, Phillips P, Fahmy R, et al. Pancreatic stellate cells respond to inflammatory cytokines: Potential role in chronic pancreatitis. Gut 2001; 2002; 50 (4):535–541.

18 Pancreatic Stellate Cells and Their Role in Fibrogenesis

Max G. Bachem, Alexandra Schmid-Kotsas, Marco Siech, Hans G. Beger,
Thomas Gress and Guido Adler

Pancreas fibrosis is a result of an increased deposition and a reduced degradation of extracellular matrix.[1,2] Until recently the molecular mechanisms and cell-cell interactions resulting in pancreas fibrosis were largely unknown. Years ago the presence of retinoid containing fat-storing cells was demonstrated in panceas of mice,[3] rats and humans.[4] While a potential role of these cells in pancreas remodelling and fibrosis was already discussed by Ikejiri et al.,[4] it took another 8 years to isolate and characterize these cells.[5,6] In 1998 we reoprted the isolation of retinoid-containing fat-storing cells from pancreas of humans, rats, and mice.[6] Because these cells show similarities in their retinoid metabolism and morphology to hepatic stellate cells e.g. numerous retinoid-containing perinuclear fat droplets, cytoplasmic extensions, stellate shape morphology, expression of the cytoskeletal filaments vimentin, desmin, and α-smooth muscle actin, we named them pancreatic stellate cells (PSC).[6]

Characterization of Pancreatic Stellate Cells – Differences from Pancreas Fibroblasts

In earlier reports fibroblasts or 'fibroblast-like' cells were suggested to be responsible for the increased extracellular matrix synthesis resulting in pancreas fibrosis.[2,7–9] However, in contrast to fibroblasts, these cells expressed smooth-muscle-α-actin and formed dense bodies (microfilaments) like myofibroblast-like cells.[8,9] In order to answer the question whether PSC and pancreas fibroblasts (PFB) are the same, or different cell types, and to identify the effector cell of pancreas fibrosis, we isolated PSC and pancreas fibroblasts (PFB) from human and rat pancreas, and characterized the cells by immunofluorescence stainings, collagen I and fibronectin measurements and quantitative RT-PCR.

Compared to cultured PSC, which had a stellate shape morphology (some were also triangular or spindle shaped) cultured PFB were spindle-shaped (Fig.1). Cultured PFB were much smaller compared to PSC (Fig. 18.1). Immunofluorescence stainings demonstrated, that 20–40% of PSC were desmin positive and >90% were smooth-muscle-α-actin positive while PFB were desmin and smooth msucle α actin negative (Fig.2). Both cell types stained positively with anti-vimentin (Fig. 18.2), anti-collagen I (Fig. 18.3 A and B), anti-

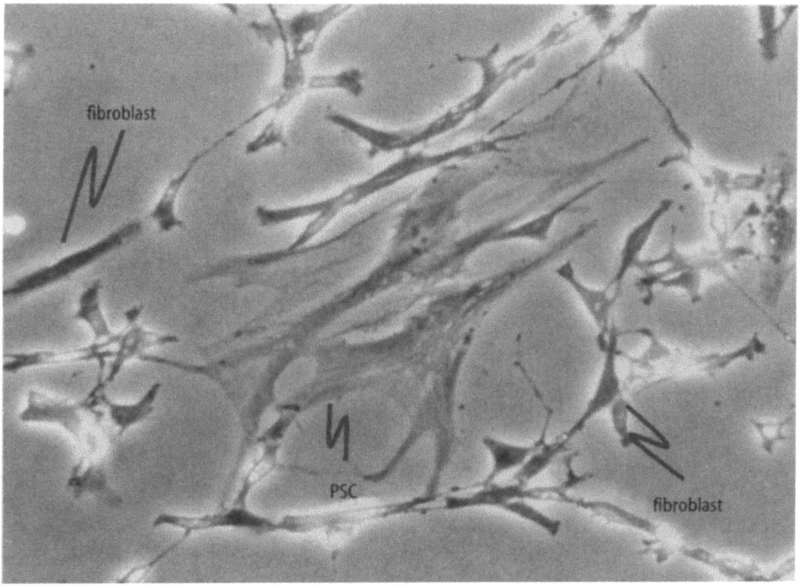

Figure 18.1. Morphology of cultured human pancreatic stellate cells and pancreas fibroblasts. Phase contrast micrograph showing a coculture of human pancreatic stellate cells (4th passage) and pancreas fibroblasts (6th passage). The cells were grown in 6-well plates in the presence of 10% fetal calf serum. Two days after passage photographs were taken. PSC are stellate shaped and PFB appear spindle shaped and much smaller than PSC. Original magnification ×200.

collagen III (Fig. 18.3 C and D) and anti-fibronectin (Fig. 18.3 E and F). However extracellular matrix synthesis was more pronounced in cultured PSC (Fig. 18.3 A,C and E) compared with PFB (Fig. 18.3 B,D and F). In addition the steady state mRNA-concentrations of collagen I, collagen III and fibronectin were higher in PSC compared to PFB (Fig. 18.4). Gene expression profiling (gene microarray analysis) demonstrated that PSC are related to hepatic stellate cells and fibroblasts. A significant difference between hepatic stellate cells and PSC was detected in 29 of 2500 tested genes (data not shown).

In-vitro and In-vivo Activation of Pancreatic Stellate Cells

On untreated plastics, cultured PSC are activated, their retinoid content decreases and the cells acquire a highly proliferative and ´synthetic´ phenotype.[6] Furthermore, within 4–8 days after seeding, the number and size of the fat-droplets decrease, the diameter of the cells increases, the cells develop a prominent endoplasmic reticulum, and the cells express α-smooth muscle actin in increasing amounts. Smooth muscle α-actin immunofluorescence stainings demonstrate that PSC activation is accelerated by the polypeptide growth factors transforming growth factor ß1 (TGFß1) and tumor necrosis factor alpha (TNFα) (Fig. 18.5). The 'myofibroblast-like' phenotype of PSC produces and secretes significant amounts of collagen types I and III and fibronectin.

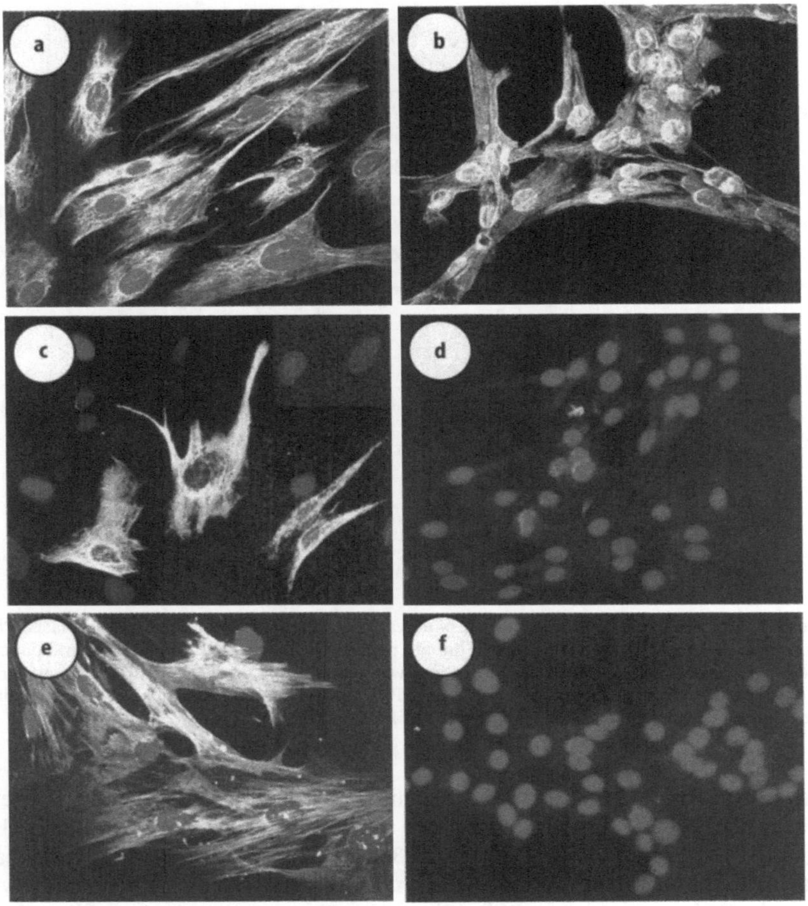

Figure 18.2. Difference between PSC and pancreas fibroblasts demonstrated by immunostaining of cytofilaments. Fluorescence micrographs showing the immunoreactivity of vimentin (A,B), desmin (C,D,) and sm-α-actin (E,F) were taken using cultured human PSC (A,C,E) and human pancreas fibroblasts (B;D,F). Cells were grown in 75 cm^2 flasks. After passage cells were cultured on glass coverslips. 24 h after passage fetal calf serum was reduced from 10% to 0.1%. 24 h later cultures were washed, fixed in acetone and immunostainings were performed. To compare staining intensities all micrographs were taken using the same exposure time. Original magnification ×400.

Measurement of retinoids by HPLC demonstrated that with the change in the phenotype, the cellular content of retinol and retinyl-palmitate decreased significantly.[6] The characteristics of the 'fat-storing' and the 'myofibroblast-like' phenotype of PSC are summarized in Fig. 18.6.

Identification of Fibrogenic Mediators

To identify the fibrogenic mediators, we added the polypeptide growth factors basic fibroblast growth factor (bFGF), transforming growth factor α (TGFα),

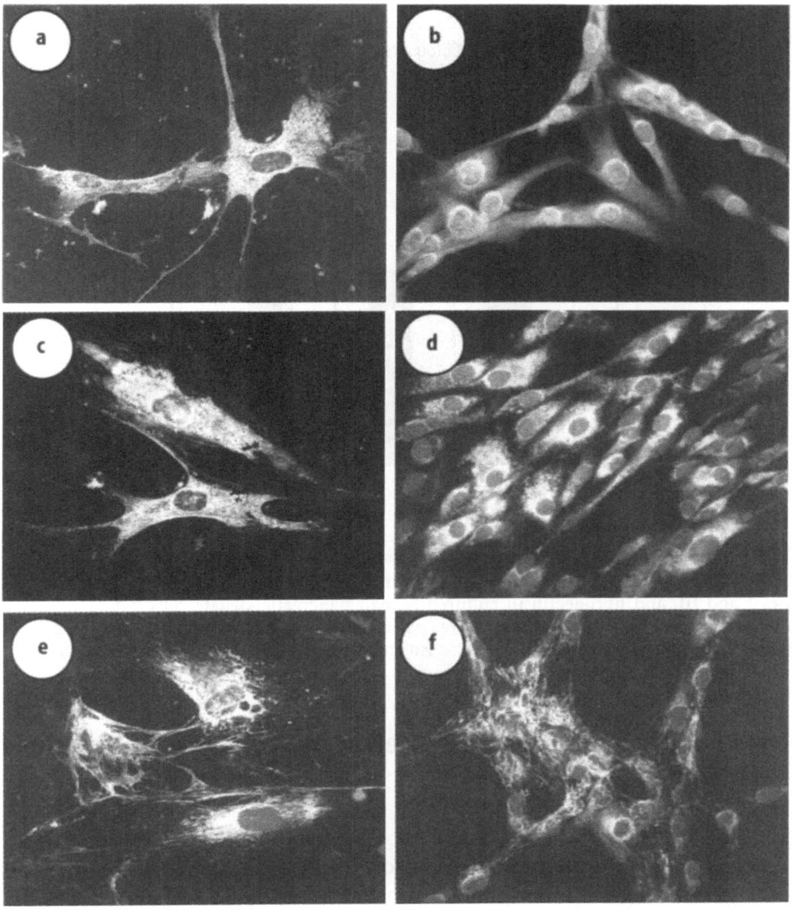

Figure 18.3. Difference between PSC and pancreas fibroblasts demonstrated by immunostaining of collagen types I and III, and fibronectin. Fluorescence micrographs showing the immunoreactivity of collagen type I (A,B), collagen type III (C,D,) and fibronectin (E,F) were taken using cultured human PSC (A,C,E) and human pancreas fibroblasts (B;D,F). Cells were grown in 75 cm^2 flasks. After passage cells were cultured on glass coverslips. 24 h after passage fetal calf serum was reduced from 10% to 0.1%. 24 h later cultures were washed, fixed in acetone and immunostainings were performed. To compare staining intensities all micrographs were taken using the same exposure time. Original magnification ×400.

TGFß1, platelet derived growth factor (PDGF), insulin-like growth factor 1 (IGF1), IGF2, and tumor necrosis factor α (TNFα), respectively, to cultured PSC and measured proliferation and matrix synthesis.[10] PDGF represented the most effective mitogen both in human and rat PSC (Fig. 18.7A). TGFα, TGFß1, PDGF and bFGF, respectively, stimulate extracellular matrix synthesis of cultured rat PSC (Fig. 18.7B). Matrix synthesis of human PSC was best stimulated by TGFß1.[6] In addition to these growth factors ethanol,[11] acetaldehyde[11] and modified lipoproteins e.g. oxidized LDL and VLDL and enzymatically degraded VLDL stimulate proliferation and extracellular matrix synthesis of PSC (data not shown).

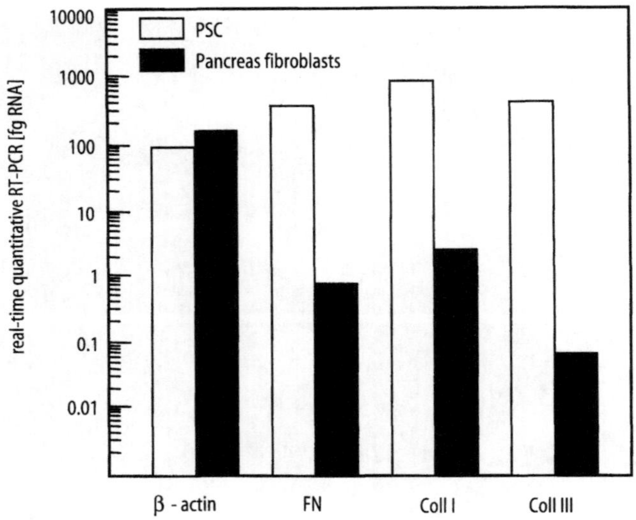

Figure 18.4. Difference between PSC and pancreas fibroblasts demonstrated by real-time quantitative RT-PCR of ß-actin, collagen types I and III, and fibronectin. Real-time quantitative RT-PCR for ß-actin, collagen types I and III, and fibronectin in cultured human pancreatic stellate cells (white columns) and human pancreas fibroblasts (black columns) was performed using specific primers with the Light-Cycler technology (Roche, Basel Swizerland). RNA was isolated from the cells 12 h after medium change.

Paracrine Stimulation of PSC by Injured Acinar Cells, Macrophages and Platelets

Because pancreatic fibrosis is commonly associated with acinar cell injury and inflammation,[12] we studied the effects of injured acinar cells (AC), activated macrophages and aggregating platelets on PSC (Fig. 18.8). AC were isolated from normal rat pancreas by density gradient centrifugation after collagenase digestion. By addition of ethanol together with fat (VLDL, very low density lipoproteins) oxidative stress and acinar cell injury were induced (data not shown). Low concentrations of the supernatants obtained from these injured AC 6 h after addition of VLDL (50 μg/ml protein) in the presence of ethanol (0.2–0.5%, v/v) stimulated proliferation (data not shown) and the synthesis and deposition of fibronectin and collagen types I and III in cultured PSC (Figures 18.9 and 18.10). Preliminary data indicate that modified fatty acids, e.g. fatty acid ethyl esters and hydroxylated fatty acids, might represent the fibrogenic activity in these AC supernatants.

Mononuclear cells infiltrating injured pancretic tissue release cytokines and growth factors.[13,14] To study paracrine stimulation of PSC by activated macrophages we isolated mononuclear cells from buffy coat. During the next 10–12 days in culture, monocytes transformed to macrophages. Using these macrophages, medium was conditioned for 24–48 h in the presence and absence of LPS. After addition of the macrophage conditioned media to cultured PSC, proliferation and extracellular matrix synthesis were measured. Immunofluorescence staining of cell associated collagen types I and III, Northern-blot and immunoassay for collagen type I and c-fibronectin in cell culture supernatants

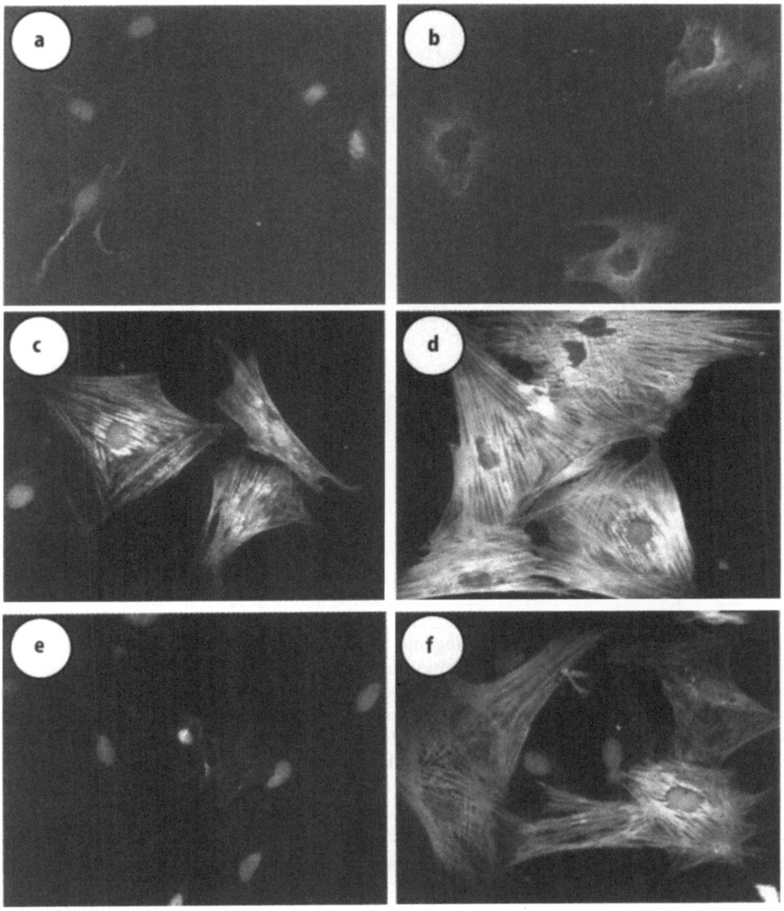

Figure 18.5. Effect of TGFß1 and TNFα on PSC activation during primary culture demonstrated by immunofluorescence microscopy of smooth-muscle-α-actin. Cells were isolated from normal Wistar rats by density gradient centrifugation and seeded with a density of 0.5×10^4 cells/cm^2 on glass cover-slips. Cells were cultured in the presence of 0.1% fetal calf serum. TGFß1 (2ng/ml) and TNFα (8 ng/ml) were added 24 h and 72 h after seeding. 3 and 5 days after seeding cultures were stopped and indirect immunofluorescence stainings using anti-smooth-muscle-α-actin were performed. A,C,E fixation 72 h after seeding; B,D,F fixation 120 h after seeding; A,B control (without growth factors); C,D 2 ng/ml TGFß1; E,F 8 ng/ml TNFα. Original magnification ×400.

demonstrated upregulation of extracellular matrix synthesis of cultured human PSC.[15] Highest stimulation was obtained by transiently acidified supernatants of LPS-stimulated macrophages.[15] By pre-incubating the supernatants with TGFß1 neutralizing antibodies it was demonstrated that in particular TGFß1 represents the fibrogenic mediator present in macrophage supernatants.

Furthermore, because platelet aggregates have been detected in capillaries of pancreas tissue from patients with pancreatitis,[16] we studied the effects of platelet derived growth factors on proliferation and matrix synthesis of cultured human PSC. Native platelet lysate (nPL) and to an even higher extent acidified platelet

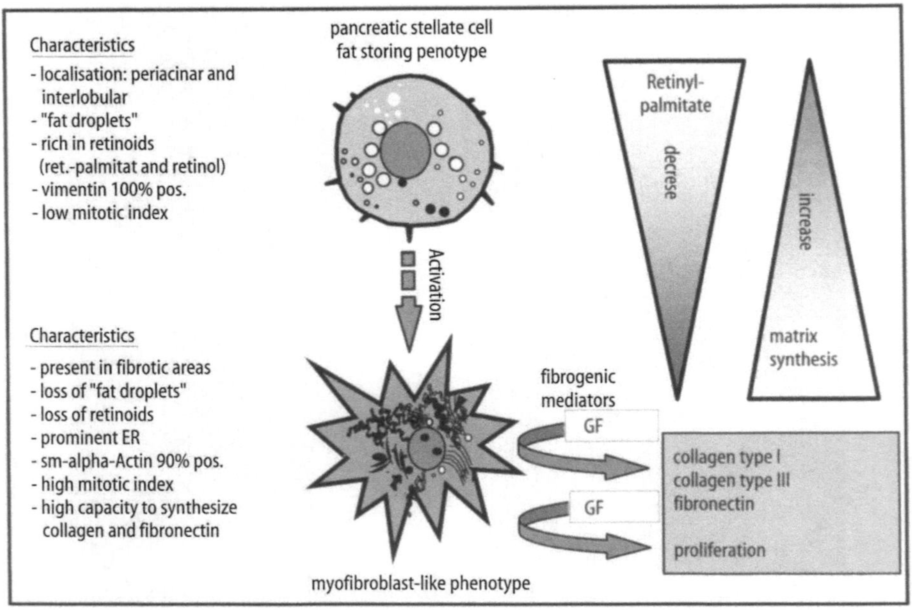

Figure 18.6. Characterization of the *fat-storing* and *myofibroblast-like* phenotype of pancreatic stellate cells. During pancreatitis and also in primary culture the number and size of retinoid containing fat-droplets decrease in parallel to the increase in sm-α-actin-expression and extracellular matrix synthesis. The *myofibroblast-like* phenotype of PSC synthesizes and secretes high amounts of collagen types I and III and fibronectin. The fibrogenic mediators TGFß1, bFGF and PDGF, respectively, stimulate extracellular matrix synthesis and PDGF represents the most important mitogen stimulating PSC proliferation.

lysate (aPL) significantly stimulated cell proliferation.[16] Furthermore, platelet lysate significantly stimulated the synthesis of collagen type I and fibronectin.[16] By preincubation of aPL with TGFß1 and PDGF-neutralizing antibodies and the TGFß-latency associated peptide, respectively, TGFß1 was identified as the main mediator stimulating matrix synthesis and PDGF as the reponsible mitogen. From these data we suggest that platelets and PSC co-operate in the development of human pancreas fibrosis.

Autocrine Stimulation of PSC

The observations that (i) PSC express TGFß-receptors (Fig. 11A), (ii) PSC respond to added TGFß1 by an increased matrix synthesis and (iii) PSC synthesize TGFß1 (Fig. 18.11B), suggested the activation of autocrine stimulatory mechanisms. To investigate this hypothesis, alpha-2-macroglobulin, a scavenger of growth factors, TGFß-neutralizing antibodies, and the TGFß-latency associated peptide, respectively, were added to PSC growing in dense culture in the absence of serum. Alpha-2-macroglobulin dose dependently reduced fibronectin synthesis and proliferation of cultured PSC (data not shown). TGFß-neutralizing antibodies and the TGFß-latency associated peptide also reduced extracellular matrix synthesis by 20–30% (Fig. 18.11C) but did not influence proliferation. Because alpha-2-macroglobulin

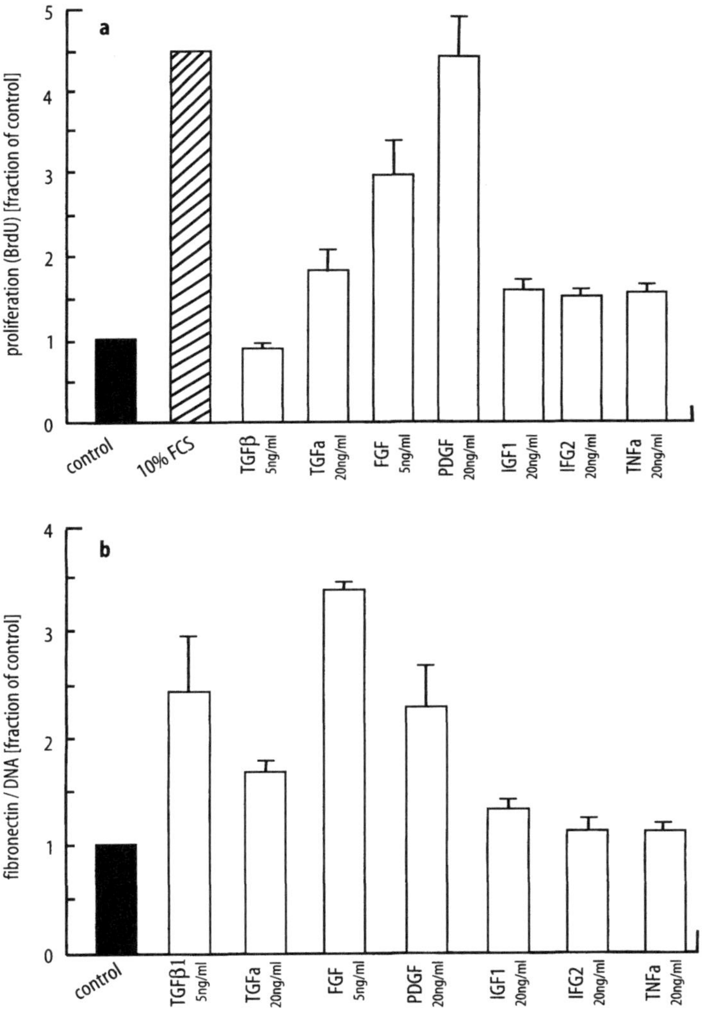

Figure 18.7. Effect of growth factors on proliferation (A) and fibronectin synthesis (B) of cultured rat PSC. **(A):** Two days after passage growth factors (TGFß1 5 ng/ml, TGFα 20 ng/ml, bFGF 50 ng/ml, PDGF(AB) 50 ng/ml, IGF-1 50 ng/ml, IGF-2 50 ng/ml, TNFα 8 ng/ml per ml medium) were added to PSC (after 2nd or 3rd passage) in the presence of 0.5% fetal calf serum. Six hours later BrdU (final concentration 5×10^{-5} M) was added for another 18 hours. Thereafter cultures were stopped and BrdU incorporation was measured by time-resolved immunofluorescence using an Europium chelate. The results are expressed as fraction of control (cells grown in DMEM with 0.5% fetal calf serum) and represent the mean +/- SD of three experiments (each condition performed in triplicate wells). *, denotes a statistically significant difference ($p < 0.05$) compared to control. **(B):** Two days after passage growth factors (TGFß1 5 ng/ml, TGFα 20 ng/ml, bFGF 50 ng/ml, PDGF(AB) 50 ng/ml, IGF-1 50 ng/ml, IGF-2 50 ng/ml, TNFα 8 ng/ml per ml medium) were added to PSC (after 2nd–4th passage) grown in Dulbecco's modification of Eagles medium with 0.5% fetal calf serum. After 24 hours cultures were stopped and fibronectin was measured in cell supernatants; DNA was measured in the cell layer. Values are expressed as means ± SEM of three independent experiments, each condition performed in triplicate culture wells.

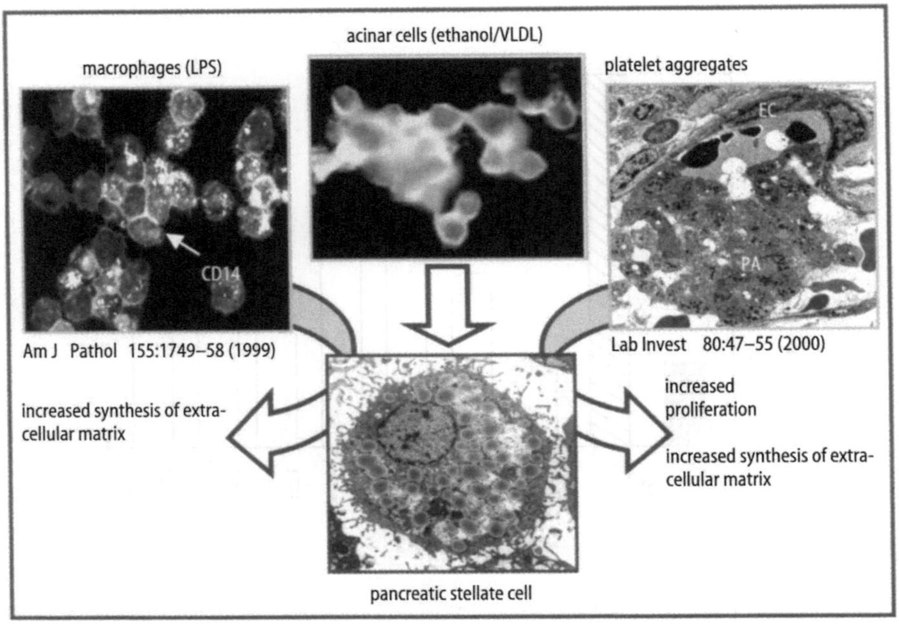

Figure 18.8. Present knowledge regarding paracrine stimulation of pancreatic stellate cells by supernatants of activated macrophages, injured acinar cells and platelet lysate.

also binds mitogens in addition to TGFß1 we suggest that autocrine stimulation of matrix synthesis via TGFß1 and autocrine stimulation of PSC proliferation may occur via presently unidentified mitogen(s). To confirm autocrine stimulation we transfected highly active PSC in culture with a TGFß1-antisense oligonucleotide using the transfection reagent DOSPER (Roche, BASEL Swiss). In contrast to sense- and scrambled-oligonucleotides TGFß1-antisense oligonucleotides reduced collagen type synthesis by 70–80% (Fig. 18.11D). These data strongly support the conclusion of an autocrine loop in PSC whereby extracellular matrix synthesis is stimulated by TGFß1.

Summary and Conclusion

Fibrogenesis in pancreatitis is the result of a dynamic cascade of mechanisms beginning with acinar cell injury and necrosis and followed by inflammation, activation of macrophages,[12,15] aggregation of platelets,[16] release of growth factors and reactive oxygen species, activation of pancreatic stellate cells (PSC), stimulated synthesis of connective tissue and matrix acumulation (Fig. 18.11). Pancreatic stellate cells represent the main cellular source of extracellular matrix in chronic pancreatitis.[11,17,18,19] PSC share homologies to hepatic stellate cells including storage of retinyl palmitate, retinol esterification, expression of the cytofilaments vimentin and desmin and phenotypic transition to an active matrix producing myofibroblast-like cell.[6] The change in the cells phenotype includes the disappearance of fat droplets and retinyl-esters, the development of a prominent endoplasmatic reticulum, the expression of smooth muscle-α-actin, an increased cell proliferation, and a stimulated production of collagen types I and III and fibronectin.[6]

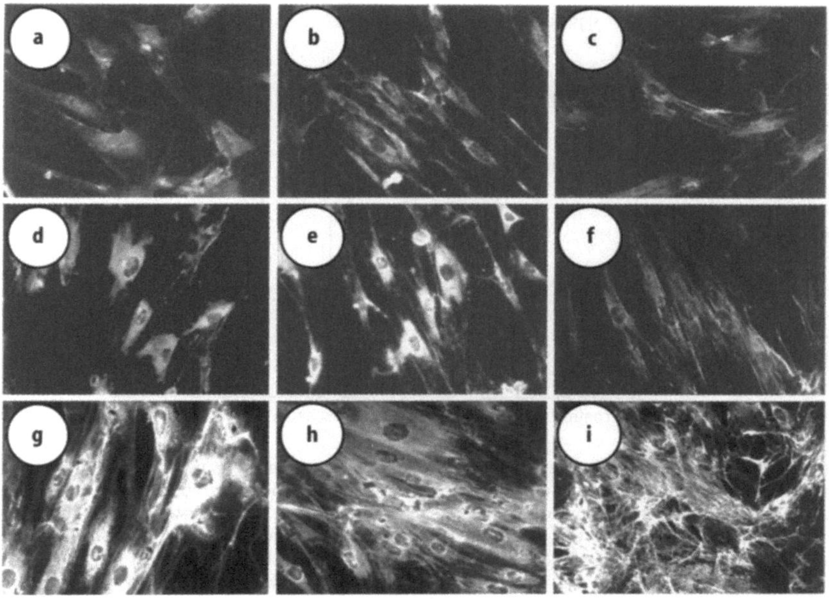

Figure 18.9. Fluorescence micrographs showing the immunoreactivity of collagen type I, collagen type III and fibronectin in cultured rat PSC stimulated with acinar cell supernatans. Acinar cells were isolated from normal rat pancreas by density gradient centrifugation after collagenase digestion and cultured for 1 h in 10% fetal calf serum. Thereafter fetal calf serum was reduced to 0.1% and ethanol together with VLDL was added. 6h later supernatants were collected and added to cultured human PSC (6th passage) grown on glass coverslips in the presence of 0.5% fetal calf serum. PSC were stimulated for 48 h with acinar cell supernatants. Thereafter cultures were washed, fixed in acetone and immunostaining was performed. A,D,G collagen type I; B,E,H collagen type III; C,F,I fibronectin; A,B,C control 0.5% fetal calf serum; D,E,F native acinar cell supernatant; G,H,I, supernatant of acinar cells receiving 0.2% ethanol and 50 µg/ml VLDL. To compare staining intensities all micrographs were taken using the same exposure time. Original magnification x400.

Preliminary data obtained after addition of cultured acinar cell supernatants to cultured PSC suggest paracrine stimulation of PSC by injured acinar cells. This is consitent with are recently published data demonstrating the sequence of acinar cell induced lipid-peroxidation phenomena in chronic ethanol-induced pancreatitis and active collagen synthesis by activated PSC.[17] In human and experimental chronic pancreatitis high numbers of iso-α-smooth muscle actin positive PSC are located in and around fibrotic areas (in the neighborhood of injured acinar cells). Supernatants of activated macrophages, and platelet lysates stimulate extracellular matrix synthesis and proliferation of cultured PSC. The growth factors TGFß, bFGF, PDGF, and TGFα (which are released by activated macrophages and aggregating platelets) were identified to stimulate extracellular matrix synthesis of PSC. In particular PDGF acts as a mitogen for PSC. Furthermore, cultured PSC has the ability to stimulate their own matrix synthesis via production of TGFß1. Therefore we suggest that pancreas fibrosis might accelerate also in the absence of further injury and inflammation if the number of activated PSC is high enough to undergo paracrine and autocrine stimulation. A simplified model demonstrating cell-cell

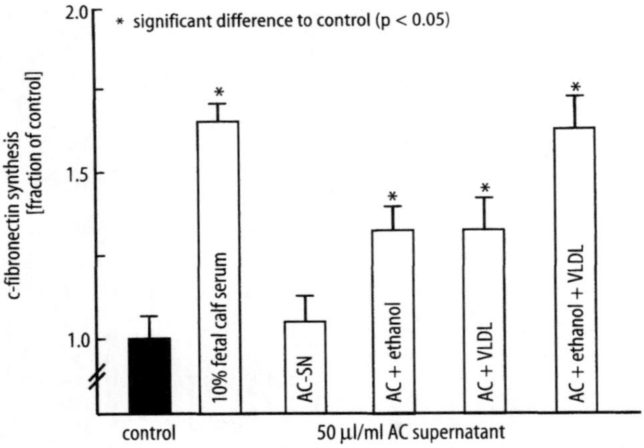

Figure 18.10. Stimulation of fibronectin synthesis in cultured human PSC by supernatants of injured acinar cells. Acinar cells were isolated from normal rat pancreas and cultured for 1 h in 10% fetal calf serum. Thereafter fetal calf serum was reduced to 0.1% and ethanol together with VLDL was added. 6h later supernatants were collected and added to cultured human PSC (4th–6th passage) grown in 24-well-plates in the presence of 0.1% fetal calf serum. PSC were stimulated for 24 h with acinar cell supernatants. Thereafter PSC supernatants were collected and fibronectin was measured by time-resolved immunoassay. DNA was measured in the cell layer. Values are expressed as means ± SD of three independent experiments, each condition performed in triplicate culture wells. (*significant difference fro the control value.)

interaction via polypeptide growth factors in acute and chronic pancreatitis (and pancreas cancer) is presented in Fig. 18.12.

Taken together, valuable insights into th pathogenesis of pancreas fibrogenesis have been obtained in recent years. Future studies will further analyze the cell-cell interactions and molecular mechanisms leading to pancreatic fibrogenesis. *In vivo* and *in vitro* data have demonstrated that PSC play a central role in fibrogenesis but the highly complicated cascade of interacting cell types and molecular mediators requires an experimental design which provides better images of the *in situ* situation. Only if our knowledge of these mechanisms increases, will adaequate therapies be developed to reduce the enhanced extracellular matrix deposition in chronic pancreatitis.

Acknowledgements

The authors were supported by a grant from the Deutsche Forschungsgemeinschaft (SFB 518, Project A7 to M.G.B.).

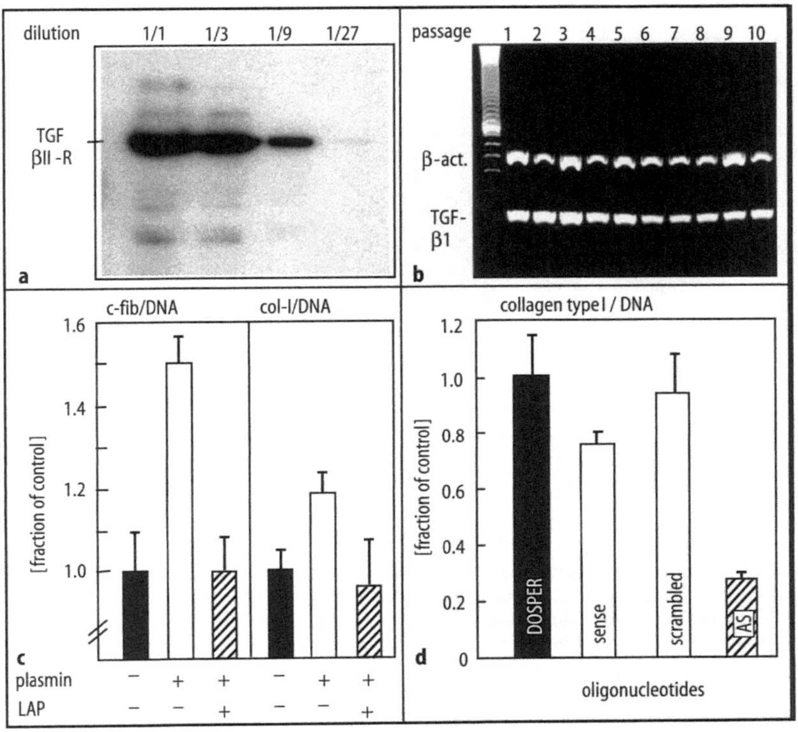

Figure 18.11. Autocrine stimulation of pancreatic stellate cells. **a** Demonstration of TFGß-receptor type II in cultured human PSC. PSC (4th passage) were cultured in 25 cm^2 flasks in the presence of 10% fetal calf serum. 24 h prior to cell lysis PSC were serum starved. Cultures were stopped 5 days after seeding by solubilizing cellular proteins using RIPA-buffer. Western-blot with chemiluminescence detection was performed using different dilutions of cell lysate. PSC constitutively express TGFß-receptor type II. **b** PSC synthesize TGFß1. Reverse transcriptase polymerase chain reaction (RT-PCR) of TGFß1. RNA was isolated from cultured human PSC 24 h after passage 1–10. 12 h prior RNA isolation fetal calf serum was reduced to 0.1%. Equal amounts of RNA were reverse transcribed and amplified during 32 cycles. Lanes 1–10: RNA isolated from PSC of passage 1–10. Left lane represents the base pair ladder. **c** Reduction of autocrine stimulated extracellular matrix synthesis by the TGFß-latency associated peptide (LAP). PSC (4th–6th passage) were cultured in 6 well-plates with 10% fetal calf serum. After reaching confluence fetal calf serum was reduced to 0.1%. Low concentration of plasmin (2 mU/ml) was added to activate latent-TGFß1; TGFß-LAP (200 ng/ml) was added to inactivate TGFß1. 48 h later supernatants were collected to measure c-fibronectin and collagen type I. DNA was measured using the cell monolayer. Values are expressed as means ± SD of three independent experiments, each condition performed in triplicate culture wells. **d** Reduction of collagen type I synthesis in cultured hPSC by an antisense oligonucleotide binding to the TGFß1-mRNA. PSC (4th–6th passage) were cultured in 6well-plates with 10% fetal calf serum. After reaching confluency fetal calf serum was reduced to 0.1%. TGFß1-sense and -antisense oligonucleotides and a scrambled oligonucleotide were added in the presence of the transfection reagent DOSPER. 48 h later supernatants were collected to measure collagen type I. DNA was measured using the cell monolayer. Values are expressed as means ± SD of one experiment, each condition performed in triplicate culture wells.

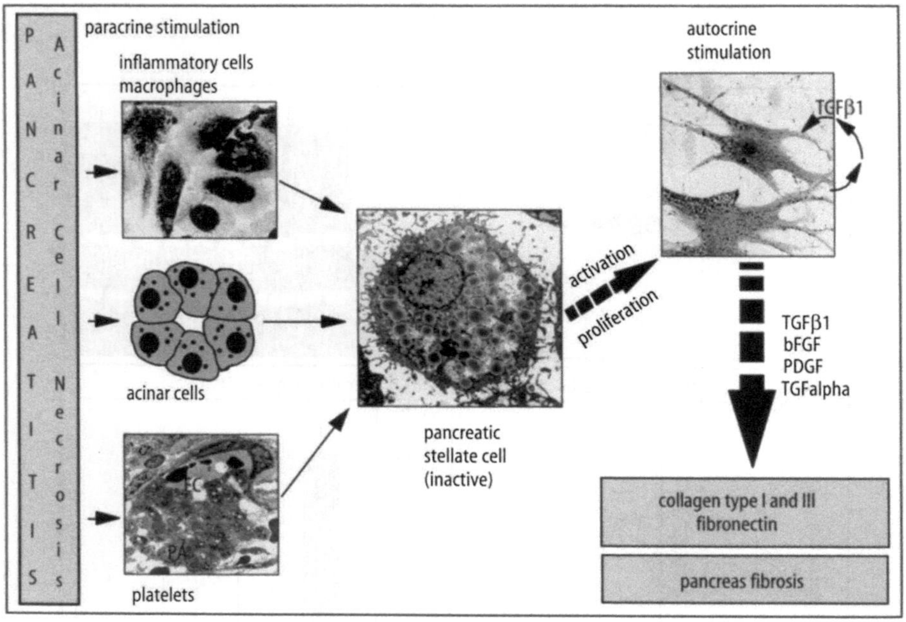

Figure 18.12. Simplified model demonstrating cell-cell interactions via soluble mediators in pancreatic fibrogenesis. Injured acinar cells, activated macrophages and aggregating platelets release fibrogenic mediators stimulating proliferation of pancreatic stellate cells and a change in the cell phenotype to a *myofibroblast-like cell.* The *myofibroblast-like phenotype* synthesizes high amounts of extracellular matrix including collagen types I and III and fibronectin. Activated PSC is also able to stimulate itself by production of TGFß1 (and probably other growth factors). The result of these mechanisms is an increased matrix synthesis leading to pancreatic fibrosis.

References

1. Uscanga L, Kennedy RH, Choux R, et al. Sequential connective matrix changes in experimental acute pancreatitis. An immunohistochemical and biochemical assessment in the rat. Int J Pancreatol 1987; 2:33–45.
2. Gress TM, Menke A, Bachem M, et al. Role of extracellular matrix in pancreatic diseases. Digestion 1998; 59:625–637.
3. Watari N, Hotta Y, Mabuchi Y. Morphological studies on a vitamin A-storing cell and ist complex with macrophage observed in mouse pancreatic tissues following excess vitamin A administration. Okajimas Folia Anat Jpn 1982; 58:837–858.
4. Ikejiri N. The vitamin A-storing cells in the human and rat pancreas. Kurume Med J 1990; 37:67–81.
5. Apte MV, Haber PS, Applegate TL, et al. Periacinar stellate shaped cells in rat pancreas: identification, isolation, and culture. Gut 1998; 43:128–33.
6. Bachem MG, Schneider E, Gross H, et al. Identification, culture, and characterization of pancreatic stellate cells in rats and humans. Gastroenterology 1998; 115:421–32.
7. Saotome T, Inoue H, Fujimiya M, et al. Morphological and immunocytochemical identification of periacinar fibroblast-like cells derived from human pancreatic acini. Pancreas 1997; 14:373–82.
8. Kato Y, Inoue H, Fujiyama Y, et al. Morphological identification and collagen synthesis by periacinar fibroblastoid cells cultured from isolated rat pancreatic acini. J Gastroenterol. 1996; 31:565–71.
9. Okumura Y, Shintani Y, Kato Y, et al. Proliferative effect of phospholipase A2 on rat periacinar fibroblastoid cells of the pancreas. Pancreas. 1998; 16:505–10.

10. Schneider E, Schmid-Kotsas A, Weidenbach H, et al. Identification of mediators stimulating proliferation and matrix synthesis of cultured rat pancreatic cells. Am J Physiol - Cell Physiol 2001; 281:532–543.
11. Apte MV, Phillips PA, Fahmy RG, et al. Does alcohol directly stimulate pancreatic fibrogenesis? Studies with rat pancreatic stellate cells. Gastroenterology 2000; 118:780–794.
12. Emmerich J, Weber I, Nausch M, et al. Immunohistochemical characterization of the pancreatic cellular infiltrate in normal pancreas, chronic pancreatitis and pancreatic carcinoma. Digestion 1998; 59:192–198.
13. Bockmann DE, Büchler M, Beger HG. Ultrastructure of human acute pancreatitis: Int J Pancreatol 1986; 1:141–153.
14. Wahl SM, McCartney-Francis N, Mergenhagen SE. Inflammatory and immunoregulatory roles of TGFß. Immunol Today 1989; 10:258–261.
15. Schmid-Kotsas A, Gross J, Menke A, et al. LPS-activated macrophages stimulate the synthesis of collagen type I and c-fibronectin in cultured pancreatic stellate cells. Am J Pathol 1999; 155:1749–1758.
16. Luttenberger T, Schmid-Kotsas A, Menke A, et al. Platelet-derived growth factors stimulate proliferation and extracellular matrix synthesis of pancreatic stellate cells: implications in pathogenesis of pancreas fibrosis. Lab Invest 2000; 80:47–55.
17. Casini A, Galli A, Pignalosa P, et al. Collagen type I synthesized by pancreatic periacinar stellate cells (PSC) co-localizes with lipid peroxidation-derived aldehydes in chronic alcoholic pancreatitis. J Pathol 2000; 192:81–89.
18. Haber PS, Keogh GW, Apte MV, et al. Activation of pancreatic stellate cells in human and experimental pancreatic fibrosis. Am J Pathol. 1999; 155:1087–1095.
19. Neuschwander-Tetri BA, Burton FR, Presti ME, et al. Repetitive self-limited acute pancreatitis induces pancreatic fibrogenesis in the mouse. Dig Dis Sci 2000; 45:665–674.

19 Factors Influencing Pancreatic Stellate Cell Phenotype and Cell Turnover

David R. Fine and Fanny Shek

To the clinician, the fibrosis of chronic pancreatic pancreatitis appears relentless and unregulated. To an extent this is a feature of the natural history of the disease. Although the presentations of our patients vary, some with episodes of acute pancreatitis; some with chronic pain and others with exocrine and endocrine failure; however, all present with established fibrosis. Whilst we may witness the progression of this disease over many years we do not see the early stages. The reasons for this are both anatomical and physiological; by comparison with the liver or kidney, the pancreas is relatively difficult to image and biopsy, and there are no routine blood tests to mark the early stages of dysfunction. As a result our understanding of the processes initiating and driving fibrosis in the pancreas is relatively poor. However, there are some clues.

First, both acute and chronic pancreatitis occur in the genetic disorder hereditary pancreatitis. The demonstration of the R117H cationic trypsinogen mutation in this condition[1] suggests that the initiating factor in both manifestations of the disease is abnormal intracellular trypsin activation. Second, we know that despite its fearsome reputation the pancreas repairs itself well. Even after severe acute pancreatitis, scans frequently show normal appearances within a few months. Third, the cancers arising in chronic pancreatitis are adenocarcinomas and not fibrosarcomas: this suggests that the cells mediating fibrosis are under normal cellular regulation. Put together this suggests that pancreatic fibrosis is, at the cellular level, a regulated process and at least initially it is driven by events in the acinar cells.

It is now accepted that pancreatic fibrosis is mediated by pancreatic stellate cells (PSC).[2;3] These cells have a quiescent and an activated phenotype. The activated phenotype is capable of secreting collagen,[4] its degrading enzymes the matrix metalloproteinases (MMPs)[(5;6] and their antagonists the tissue inhibitors of metalloproteinases (TIMPs). It seems likely that if pancreatic fibrosis is regulated, there should be evidence of regulation of PSC numbers, phenotype and collagen secretion.

Proliferation and Apoptosis

Almost without exception, cell populations are dynamic and the number of cells present is a result of the balance between cellular proliferation and removal. In recent years it has been recognised that apoptosis, programmed cell death, is the major pathway by which cells are removed from a population.[7] If the PSC in an area of pancreatic fibrosis are dynamic, rather than sitting inertly in a mass of collagen, we would expect to see evidence of both proliferation and apoptosis. We have examined this by staining resection specimens of chronic pancreatitis using MIB 1, a proliferation marker and TUNEL, a marker of apoptosis. Using dual-staining for the PSC activation marker alpha-smooth muscle actin, we demonstrated that 0.74% of PSC nuclei were positive for MIB 1 and 0.34% of nuclei were both TUNEL positive and showed features of apoptosis. Of course, that these figures are a 'snapshot' of two dynamic processes so a balance cannot be assessed by simple arithmetic. We believe that they do, however, provide proof of the concept that even in mature pancreatic fibrosis the PSC population is dynamic.

Effect of Growth Factors

If PSC populations are dynamic, they should be susceptible to environmental factors such as growth factors and cytokines. We therefore studied the effects of manipulating growth factors on PSC in tissue culture. Passage 3–4 rat PSC were studied in parallel in 24-well plates. Apoptosis was quantified using the vital stain Acridine Orange. Control cells were incubated for 8 h in our standard 16% FCS and compared to serum deprived cells incubated in 1% BSA alone. As shown in Fig. 19.1, this resulted in an increase in apoptosis from 4.0 to 23.9%. A further study group was incubated in 1% BSA but with the addition of 10 nM recombinant Insulin-like Growth Factor 1 (IGF-1). This resulted in a significant reduction in apoptosis to 20.6%. In a separate inestigation shown in Fig. 19.2 addition of 10 nG/ml Nerve Growth Factor (NGF), the ligand of the death-domain receptor P75 expressed on both hepatic and pancreatic stellate cells,[8] resulted in a further

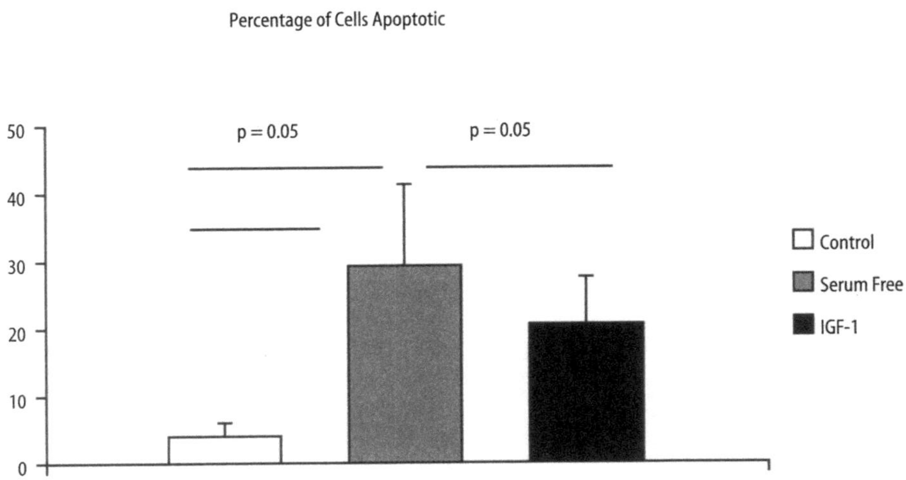

Figure 19.1. The effects of serum deprivation and IGF-1 on Apoptosis

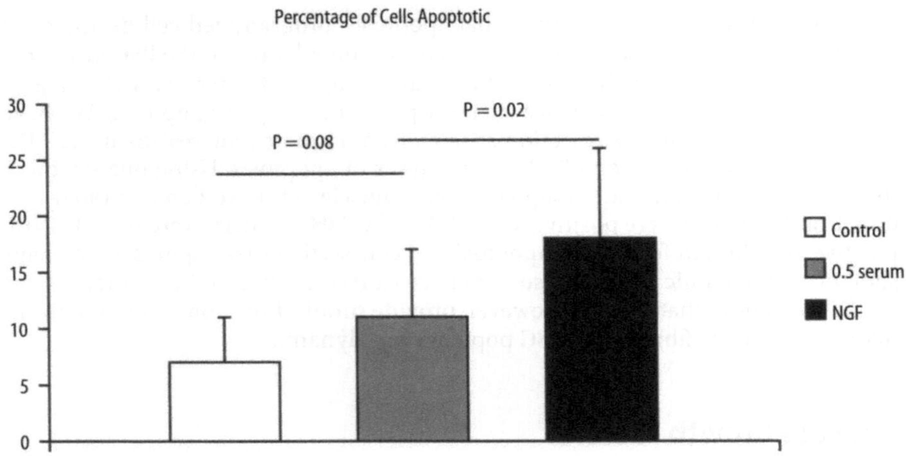

Figure 19.2. Effects of serum deprivation and NGF on PSC Apoptosis

significant increase in apoptosis. We concluded that cultured PSC respond to local changes in growth factors and a death-domain ligand.

The response of these cells to NGF is particularly interesting as it has been shown to be over-expressed in acinar areas within chronic pancreatitis.[9] This would suggest that NGF should have little influence within fibrotic bands but might inhibit PSC invasion into surviving acinar tissue.

TGF-β is known to be a potent modulator of fibroblast and myofibroblast activity. In fibroblasts TGF-β1 is a pro-fibrotic molecule which increases collagen secretion but reduces proliferation. PSC conform to this paradigm in terms of proliferation-rate. Fig. 19.3 shows the effect of three different concentrations of TGF-β1 on the incorporation of tritiated thymidine into PSC incubated in serum-free conditions as described above. All three concentrations significantly inhibit proliferation as compared to controls.

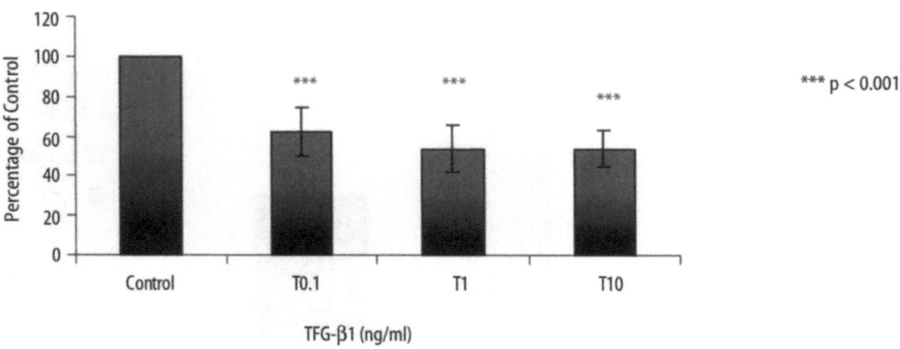

Figure 19.3. The effects of TGF-ß1 on PSC proliferation in tissue culture.

Role of Matrix

The findings described above show that PSC populations *in vivo* show markers of proliferation and apoptosis, and that in tissue culture they respond to growth factors, cytokines and death-domain ligands. During an acute episode of pancreatic injury it is self-evident that there will be a flux of cytokines and growth-factors from injured native cells and recruited leukocytes which will contribute to PSC activation. It seems likely that in a self-limiting episode of pancreatitis, activated PSC participate in the initial inflammatory process by breaking down matrix and replacing it with scar collagen. In the regeneration phase we further hypothesise that they re-model the scar tissue as normal cell populations are re-established. This poses the question of what happens to activated PSC at the end of a healing episode of pancreatitis. Our in vitro data suggest that as the local growth factor concentration declines apoptosis will increase: this in itself may be sufficient to reverse the process of fibrogenesis. Another process which might contribute to this reversal is transdifferation of PSC to the quiescent form. Hepatic stellate cells are known to respond to matrix changes in this way. We have therefore investigated the effects of matrix changes on PSC phenotype.

For these experiments passage 3–5 rat PSC were passaged in parallel into plain plastic flasks and flasks coated with growth factor depleted Matrigel® a proprietary basement membrane derivative. The cells were grown to confluence under standard conditions and lysed for RNA extraction. As shown in Fig. 19.4, these cells undergo a phenotypic change and revert towards a quiescent appearance. The left hand panel shows an activated phenotype with the cells forming extended processes which you will recognise from the previous talks as being typical of activated PSC. In the right hand panel the cells are globular and clumped. Whilst this change looks impressive, it is possible that it is a simple change of shape resulting from the transfer from a hard surface on which the PSC can only form a monolayer to a gel in which they can adopt a more globular appearance. We therefore looked at the expression of two PSC activation markers, TIMP 1 and Alpha-1 Procollagen by Northern analysis (Fig. 19.5). The expression of Procollagen is clearly reduced on the blot and this is confirmed for both markers on densitometry (Fig. 19.6).

These data suggest that activated PSC retain phenotypic plasticity and the ability to transdifferentiate back towards a quiescent phenotype. This has two important consequences. First, it suggests that even in established severe fibrosis the PSC will retain the ability to revert towards quiescence if appropriate signals are received. Second, activated cells encountering normal matrix may meet a pressure towards quiescence which may limit fibrogenesis in healthy areas of tissue.

Autocrine Stimulation

If PSC remain plastic why do they remain activated in chronic pancreatitis? In the early stages at least, activation is probably driven by acinar cell injury and the associated immune response. Looking at resection specimens of severe chronic pancreatitis we were struck however at how far removed many PSC must be from any external influences, embedded as they are in broad swathes of fibrous tissue. We therefore studied the effects of TGF-β and in particular whether an autocrine loop could be perpetuating fibrogenesis in this circumstance.

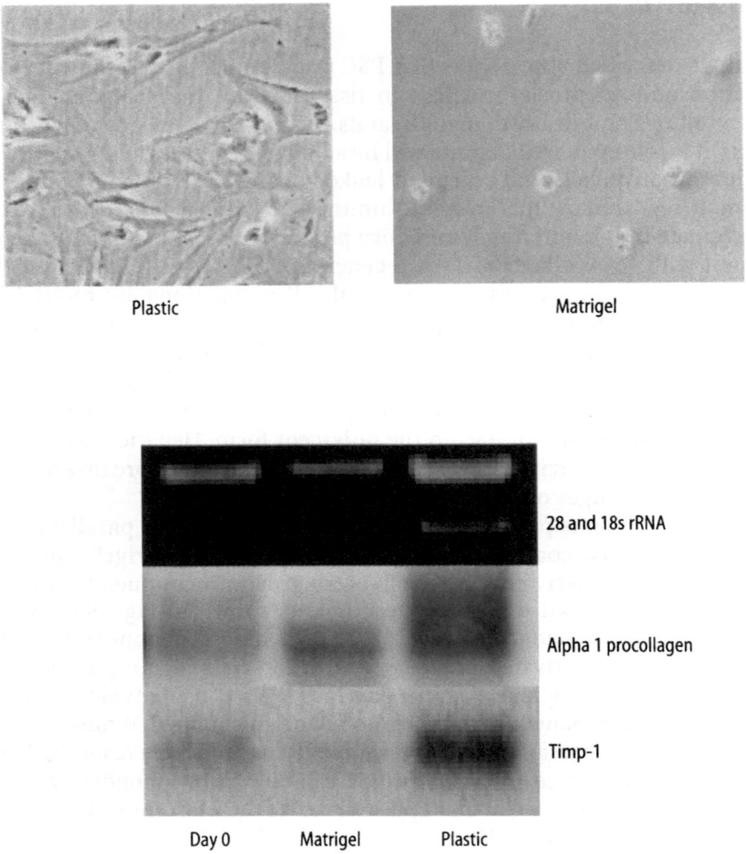

Figure 19.4. Activated Passage PSC were passaged in duplicate into plastic and Matrigel® coated flasks. Note the change in phenotype after 5 days culture on Matrigel

Fig. 19.7 shows the effects of TGF-β1 and also of neutralising antibodies to TGF-β1 and pan-TGF-β on proline incorporation into collagen. The addition of TGF-β1 increases collagen formation whereas the antibodies have the reverse effect. This suggests that PSC are secreting TGF-β and responding to it in an autocrine fashion.

Furthermore, as shown in Fig. 19.8, conditioned media from pre-washed cells contain active TGF-β1. The concentration and the percentage activated are the same at 24 and 48 hours, suggesting a regulated process of secretion and thatactivation is occurring.

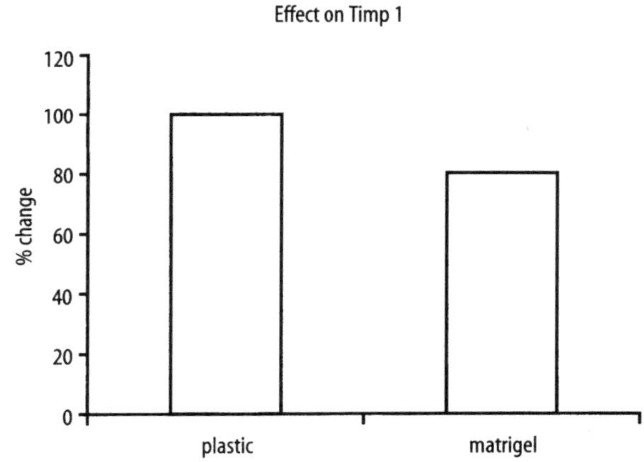

Figure 19.5. Northern blots showing the response of Timp-1 and Alpha-1 Procollagen expression by Passage 3–4 PSC (Day 0) passaged onto plastic or Matrigel for five days

Finally, Western blot analysis shows that PSC express both TGF-β receptors 1&2, indicating that PSC possess the receptors necessary for a TGF-β response (Fig. 19.9).

Conclusion

Taken overall these experiments suggest that PSC exhibit a TGF-β autocrine loop. We suggest that *in vivo* this might tend to perpetuate the fibrogenic process within large masses of fibrous tissue in chronic pancreatitis even though our other experiments suggest that activated PSC *in vitro* retain the ability to undergo apoptosis or revert to a quiescent phenotype.

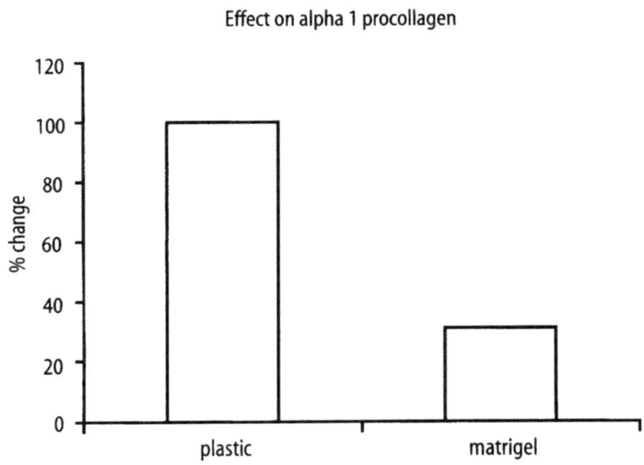

Figures 19.6. Effects of passage onto Matrigel on **a)** TIMP-1 and **b)** Alpha-1 Procollagen mRNA expression.

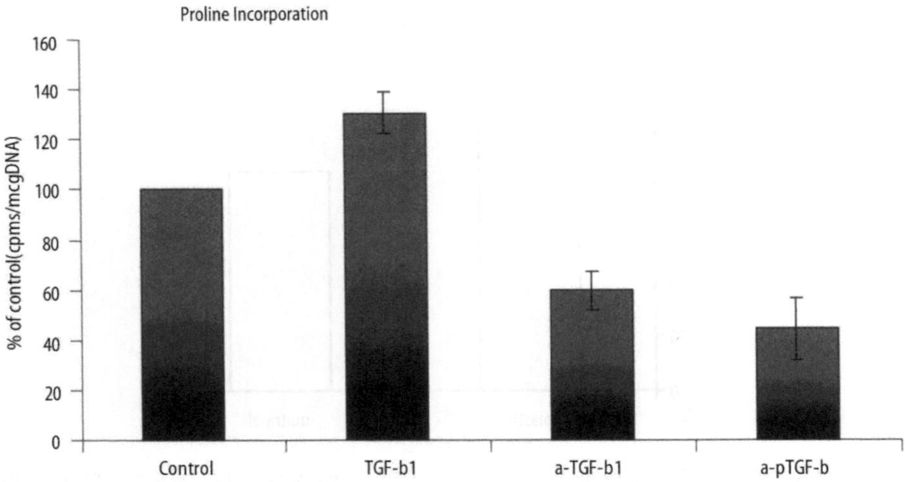

Figure 19.7. Effects of TGF-ß1 and of blocking antibodies to TGF-ß1 (a-TGF-ß1) and pan- TGF-ß (a-p TGF-ß) on proline incorporation into activated PSC.

Dynamic features of PSC include:

- Regulation of cell turnover
- Regulation of phenotype
- Reversibility of active phenotype by matrix manipulation
- Autocrine regulation of proliferation and collagen synthesis via TGF-β

All these features indicate a high level of regulation of phenotype and synthesis. We conclude that PSC are likely to play an active rather that a passive role in the dysregulation of inflammation and repair occurring in chronic pancreatitis.

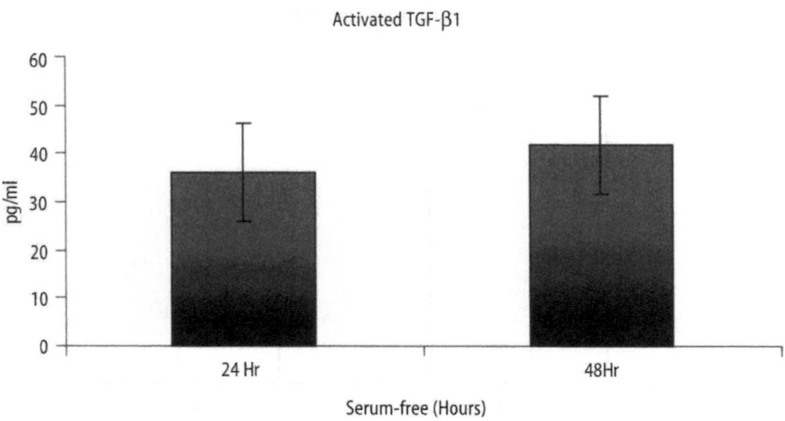

Figure 19.8. Activated TGF-ß1 concentration in conditioned media from activated PSC is similar at 24 and 48 h.

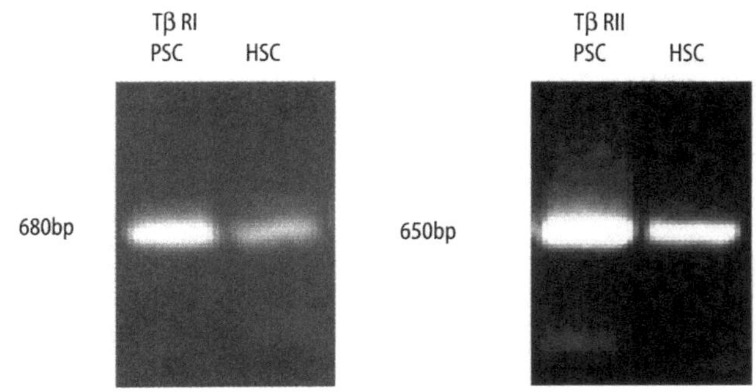

Figure 19.9. Western blots demonstrating the presence of TGF-ß receptors 1&11. Hepatic stellate cells (HSC) have been used as positive controls.

Acknowledgements

In addition to the workers mentioned in the text I am grateful to Professor John Iredale who has allowed this work to be conducted in his department and has encouraged and supported the project from its inception. Dr Adrian Bateman has supervised all the histopathological studies and provided invaluable advice on the interpretation of histochemistry. Penny Johnson has supervised the immunohistochemical staining.

Some of the work was performed by Paul Davies and Abigail Oyetade and Fiona Walker.

Fanny Shek is an Amelie Waring Fellow of the Digestive Disorders Foundation. The support of Hope, The Mason Medical Foundation and The Peel Trust is also gratefully acknowleged.

References

1. Whitcomb DC, Gorry MC, Preston RA, et al. Hereditary pancreatitis is caused by a mutation in the cationic trypsinogen gene. Nat Genet 1996; 14 (2):141–5.
2. Apte MV, Haber PS, Applegate TL, et al. Periacinar stellate shaped cells in rat pancreas: identification, isolation, and culture. Gut 1998; 43 (1):128–33.
3. Bachem MG, Schneider E, Gross H, et al. Identification, culture, and characterization of pancreatic stellate cells in rats and humans. Gastroenterology 1998; 115 (2):421–32.
4. Casini A, Galli A, Pignalosa P, et al. Collagen type I synthesized by pancreatic periacinar stellate cells (PSC) co-localizes with lipid peroxidation-derived aldehydes in chronic alcoholic pancreatitis. J Pathol 2000; 192 (1):81–9.
5. Phillips PA, McCarroll JA, Park S, et al. Rat pancreatic stellate cells secrete matrix metalloproteinases: implications for extracellular matrix turnover. Gut 2003; 52 (2):275–82.
6. Shek FW, Benyon RC, Walker FM, et al. Expression of transforming growth factor-beta 1 by pancreatic stellate cells and its implications for matrix secretion and turnover in chronic pancreatitis. Am J Pathol 2002; 160 (5):1787–98.
7. Kerr, JFR. Apoptosis: a basic biological phenomenon with wide-ranging implications in tissue kinetics. Wyllie, AH, Currie AH. Br J Cancer 1972; 26:239–257.
8. Trim N, Morgan S, Evans M, et al. Hepatic stellate cells express the low affinity nerve growth factor receptor p. 75 and undergo apoptosis in response to nerve growth factor stimulation. Am J Pathol 2000; 156 (4):1235–43.
9. Friess H, Zhu ZW, di Mola FF, et al. Nerve growth factor and its high-affinity receptor in chronic pancreatitis. Ann Surg 1999; 230 (5):615–24.

Diabetes and Chronic Pancreatitis

20 Acinar–Islet Cell Interactions: Diabetes Mellitus in Chronic Pancreatitis

David Malka and Philippe Lévy

The Marseille–Rome classification of 1988 has defined chronic pancreatitis as "a continuing inflammatory disease of the pancreas characterised by the irreversible destruction of exocrine parenchyma and fibrosis and at least in the later stages, the destruction of the endocrine parenchyma".[1]

Chronic pancreatitis remains an important source of morbidity in Western countries. Acute exacerbations leading to repeated and often prolonged hospital admissions, and chronic, intractable pain usually prevail in the early course of the disease, often recur despite medical, endoscopic and/or surgical therapeutic attempts, and may lead to chronic (ab)use of narcotics. Patients with long-standing chronic pancreatitis are also at increased risk of developing pancreatic cancer. Besides this catastrophic but rather rare complication, the vast majority of patients with advanced chronic pancreatitis, with the exception of the obstructive form of the disease when obstruction is removed, ultimately develop exocrine pancreatic insufficiency, endocrine pancreatic insufficiency, or both.[2]

Diabetes mellitus is the major late sequel of chronic pancreatitis.[2–5] In contrast to exocrine pancreatic insufficiency, endocrine pancreatic insufficiency may lead to life-threatening complications such as severe hypoglycemia or to chronic microvascular and macrovascular complications.[6,7] A study of quality of life after pancreatic resections found that diabetes and its complications had the greatest negative influence on everyday well-being.[8] Diabetes may affect long-term mortality in patients with chronic pancreatitis.[9–11]

Epidemiology of Diabetes in Chronic Pancreatitis

Reliable data on the incidence and prevalence of diabetes secondary to chronic pancreatitis are difficult to obtain, mostly because corresponding data for chronic pancreatitis itself are scarce. The incidence of chronic pancreatitis varies geographically from 1.6 to 23 new cases per year among 100 000 inhabitants.[12–15] This wide range may be explained by differences in morphological, functional, and clinical diagnostic criteria for chronic pancreatitis.[2,16] However, the mean prevalence of chronic pancreatitis might be as high as 13% in non-selected autopsies.[17,18] Pancreatic diseases (including chronic pancreatitis, haemochromatosis, pancreatic resections and cystic fibrosis) could thus be responsible for many more cases of

Table 20.1. Cumulative rates of appearance of diabetes and insulin requirement in chronic pancreatitis. From Malka et al.[5]

	Diabetes (%)	Insulin requirement (%)
At the onset of chronic pancreatitis	10	2
At 10 years	50 ± 3	26 ± 3
At 25 years	83 ± 4	53 ± 6

diabetes than the low figure of about 0.15% to 1.15%, as commonly believed.[17,19] This may explain why reduced exocrine pancreatic function[20] and pancreatographic abnormalities suggestive of chronic pancreatitis have been observed in a high percentage of patients with type 1 or type 2 diabetes.[21,22]

Differences in diagnostic criteria not only for chronic pancreatitis, but also for disturbances in glucose metabolism, along with variations in the definition of the onset of chronic pancreatitis, in the duration of follow-up, and in the clinical setting (medical, surgical, or mixed recruitment of the patients) account for the wide variation in the prevalence of diabetes in large series of patients with chronic pancreatitis, with reported values ranging between 40% and 90%.[3,4,19,23–27]

Diabetes, which can be insulin-dependent, may already be present at the clinical onset of chronic pancreatitis.[5,16] However, diabetes usually occurs later in the course of the disease, at a mean of approximately 5 years after the onset of chronic pancreatitis.[5] In fact, data from large medical–surgical prospective studies of patients with chronic pancreatitis followed up a long time indicate that the cumulative incidence of diabetes is a linear function of time (Table 20.1). Annual rates of diabetes and insulin requirement were estimated by linear regression to be 3.5% and 2.2%, respectively.[5] Hence, about 80–90% of patients with chronic pancreatitis eventually develop diabetes after 25 years (Table 20.1).

Pathophysiology of Diabetes in Chronic Pancreatitis

In chronic pancreatitis, islet cells are often well preserved despite extensive acinar cell damage.[28] The mechanism for the loss of exocrine parenchyma and the relative preservation of endocrine epithelial cells in chronic pancreatitis is unclear, but could be due to an increase in apoptotic index within acinar cells but not islet cells, possibly because the latter possess mechanisms for inhibiting apoptosis, in particular Fas/Fas ligand triggered apoptosis by Fas ligand bearing cytotoxic T-lymphocytes infiltrating the pancreas,[29] as believed in the development of autoimmune diabetes mellitus.[30]

Autoimmune (type 1A) diabetes mellitus is caused by loss of insulin-secreting capacity due to selective autoimmune destruction of the pancreatic beta cells.[31] Insulitis (i.e., mononuclear-cell infiltration of the pancreatic islets) is the direct result of the autoimmune process. Antibodies to the cytoplasm of islet cells, glutamic acid decarboxylase, insulin, and tyrosine phosphatase–like protein (IA-2 or IA-2ß), which appear before the clinical onset of diabetes, are good markers of the autoimmune process.[31] Such autoantibodies are rare in type 2 diabetes, lipoatrophic diabetes, and in diabetes secondary to chronic pancreatitis.[32–35] Systemic immune cellular dysregulation may participate in the pathogenesis of chronic pancreatitis, but data supporting a direct role of such abnormalities in islet cell loss are lacking. An immune-mediated reaction to pancreatic structures has been postulated for the pathogenesis of chronic pancreatitis, according to several reports which have demonstrated the presence of autoantibodies to the pancreatic ductal epithelium (e.g. autoantibodies to carbonic anhydrase I and II) in some patients suffering from chronic pancreatitis. However, such autoantibodies have been detected mostly in patients with idiopathic chronic pancreatitis and Sjögren's syndrome, and no consistent correlation with diabetes has been found.[32,36,37] Islet cell destruction occurring during chronic pancreatitis does not seem to trigger islet autoimmunity, even in the presence of HLA-DR 3 and/or DR 4 diabetes susceptibility genes,[38] which have been generally found in patients with chronic pancreatitis at the same frequency than in the general non-diabetic population.[33] The absence of insulitis and autoantibodies to islet cells may contribute to the slower destruction of the beta cells in chronic pancreatitis than in type 1 diabetes, and may explain at least in part why beta-cell function is preserved to a greater extent and glucoregulation is better in patients with insulin-dependent diabetes secondary to chronic pancreatitis than in comparable type 1 diabetic patients. In fact, corticosteroid-responsive diabetes mellitus associated with autoimmune chronic pancreatitis probably represents the only condition in which diabetes secondary to chronic pancreatitis is caused by an autoimmune destruction of pancreatic beta$_{\text{cells}}$.[39] Histopathological changes include intra- and peri-insular mononuclear cell-mainly CD8+ T cell infiltration as well as mononuclear cell infiltration around the ductal cells, islet beta cell destruction, and beta-cell differentiation from pancreatic ductal cells.[39,40]

Type 1 diabetes mellitus is now classified as autoimmune (type 1A) or idiopathic (type 1B). In this latter type, in which type 1A diabetes-associated autoantibodies (e.g., autoantibodies to glutamic acid decarboxylase, islet cells, IA-2, and insulin) are absent, diabetes may present as a fulminant disorder characterized by the absence of insulitis, and high serum pancreatic enzyme concentrations. However, no histologic evidence of chronic pancreatitis has been found in such cases.[41]

Genes predisposing to chronic pancreatitis (e.g., PRSS1, CFTR, and SPINK1 genes) have not been consistently associated with an increased risk of diabetes in patients with chronic pancreatitis.[42] Tropical pancreatitis, a distinct type of early-onset chronic pancreatitis endemic in parts of Asia and Africa including tropical calcific pancreatitis and fibrocalculous pancreatic diabetes, has recently been found to be associated with the N34S variant of the SPINK1 trypsin inhibitor gene.[43,44] The frequency of the N34S variant was higher in patients with fibrocalculous pancreatic diabetes in one report;[43] however, it was similar among patients with or without diabetes in another.[44] Thus, evidence of genetic factors modulating the risk of diabetes in patients with chronic pancreatitis is still lacking. The recent identification of two highly significant quantitative trait loci for chronic pancreatitis and diabetes mellitus on completely different chromosomal regions from those of PRSS1, CFTR, and SPINK1 genes in the WBN/Kob rat model of spontaneous chronic pancreatitis might help to further elucidate this issue.[45]

Risk Factors for Diabetes

Aetiology of the Pancreatitis

Although alcoholism represents the most important cause of chronic pancreatitis in Western countries, a constellation of predisposing risk factors, categorized as either toxic-metabolic causes, genetic predispositions, vascular/ischemic diseases, obstructive causes, or isolated or syndromic autoimmune conditions, may cause chronic pancreatitis, which thus must be considered as a syndrome that encompasses the many sequelae of long-standing pancreatic injury. Furthermore, no causal agent is identified in a significant proportion of cases of chronic pancreatitis, which are therefore unsatisfyingly classified as 'idiopathic'. Indeed, the current classification systems of chronic pancreatitis focus on generalized effects of the destructive process rather than aetiology.[46–48] Moreover, not only the diagnosis of chronic pancreatitis, but also the proper staging of pancreatic injury, function, and fibrosis relies on somewhat controversial classifications and stratifications. Hence, many uncertainties remain concerning the clinical and natural history of chronic pancreatitis developing in the context of these various risk factors. In particular, it is not known whether different subsets of chronic pancreatitis carry different risks of diabetes.

Progressive deterioration of exocrine and endocrine function is observed in both alcoholic and idiopathic (nonalcoholic) chronic pancreatitis. However, in alcoholic chronic pancreatitis the rate of progression of exocrine dysfunction after diagnosis is more rapid and more closely associated with the onset of pancreatic calcifications, and the incidence of diabetes in relation to marked exocrine insufficiency is higher than in nonalcoholic chronic pancreatitis. Steatorrhoea precedes diabetes in about 50% of cases of alcoholic chronic pancreatitis and 80% of cases of nonalcoholic chronic pancreatitis, respectively.[49] Patients with early-onset idiopathic chronic pancreatitis have initially and thereafter a long course of severe pain but slowly develop morphological and functional pancreatic damage, whereas patients with late-onset idiopathic chronic pancreatitis have a mild and often a painless course. In early-onset idiopathic chronic pancreatitis, calcification and exocrine and endocrine insufficiency develop more slowly than in late-onset idiopathic and alcoholic chronic pancreatitis.[18,25–27,49–51] We found, in a multivariate analysis of risk factors for diabetes in 453 patients with chronic pancreatitis, that alcohol-related chronic pancreatitis was significantly associated with the risk of diabetes (risk ratio, 1.7; 95% confidence interval, 1.0-2.7; $p = 0.04$), but not with the risk of insulin requirement.[5]

It has been suggested that the inexorable natural path of chronic pancreatitis toward progressive exocrine and endocrine insufficiency and calcification generally coincides tightly with the eventual 'burnout' of the gland and spontaneous remission of pain. However, Layer *et al.* found that the remission of pain occurred independently of pancreatic calcification and the appearance of exocrine or endocrine insufficiency.[27] Lankisch *et al.* found that more than 50% of patients followed for a median of 9 years still had significant pain after 10 years of observation. Although alcoholics were slightly more likely to experience pain relief than nonalcoholics with the appearance of exocrine failure, 54% of alcoholics and 73% of nonalcoholics still experienced attacks of pain despite exocrine insufficiency requiring enzyme replacement, and there was no pain reduction with the development of severe endocrine insufficiency.[52] These two groups stressed that the different subsets of chronic pancreatitis (alcoholic vs. nonalcoholic; early vs. late onset) may harbour differences in natural history, including endocrine insufficiency.

Alcohol Withdrawal

The effect of cessation of alcohol use on the course of pancreatic dysfunction in alcoholic chronic pancreatitis is not clear. Pancreatic functional changes caused by alcoholic chronic pancreatitis may progress even after cessation of alcohol use; however, the progression may be slower and less severe when alcohol intake is stopped.[53]

Complications of Chronic Pancreatitis

Diabetes mellitus may develop less frequently in patients with alcoholic chronic pancreatitis who have experienced bouts of acute pancreatitis than in their counterparts who never have had such acute exacerbations of their disease. This apparently paradoxical finding may be explained by the fact that experiencing recurrent attacks of acute pancreatitis may favour alcohol withdrawal.[54] Nevertheless, we subsequently found that the only independent clinical factor significantly associated with the risk of diabetes was the early onset of pancreatic calcifications; once they appeared, the risk of diabetes and insulin requirement increased by more than 3-fold.[5] Because we took into account the time-dependent pattern of the onset of pancreatic calcifications, we can conclude that the earlier they appear in the course of chronic pancreatitis, the greater the risk of diabetes and insulin requirement. This observation suggests that the onset of diabetes in patients with chronic pancreatitis is mainly caused by progression of the disease. Complications of chronic pancreatitis (e.g. attacks of acute pancreatitis, pseudocysts, duodenal stenosis, splenic or portal vein occlusion, common bile duct obstruction) and associated liver disease were not associated with an increased risk of diabetes in our series.[5] However, as the complication 'acute pancreatitis' was entered as a categorical variable (yes/no) in our multivariate analysis, we cannot exclude that the repetition of attacks of acute pancreatitis may hasten the progression of chronic pancreatitis, and hence the onset of pancreatic endocrine dysfunction.

Pancreatic Surgery

Pancreatoduodenectomy

The influence of pancreatoduodenectomy on the risk of postoperative diabetes is unclear. It has been shown that pancreatoduodenectomy results in decreased insulin secretion after surgery. In 16 series including a total of 1143 patients with chronic pancreatitis followed up between 1.5 and 8.3 years after pancreatoduodenectomy, the rate of new-onset postoperative diabetes ranged from 7 to 50%.[10,55–69] However, most surgical series included patients with chronic pancreatitis and those with other pancreatic diseases, or lacked a nonsurgical control group. In contrast with these studies, we found that pancreatoduodenectomy did not significantly increase the risk of diabetes compared with the natural history of chronic pancreatitis in patients treated medically.[5] The lack of a statistically significant difference between pancreatoduodenectomy (n = 37, 36% ± 18%) and nonpancreatic drainage procedures (n = 86, 24% ± 7%), which may be considered as positive surgical controls, with respect to the risk of diabetes is consistent with this finding.[5] Glucose tolerance improved more often and postoperative diabetes developed less frequently after pancreatoduodenectomy in patients operated on for malignant, focal disease than in patients with chronic pancreatitis.[70] We[5] and others[10] have observed that the appearance of diabetes after pancreatoduodenectomy performed for chronic pancreatitis was almost always delayed for a minimum of 1 year after surgery, suggesting that disease progression prevails in the risk of diabetes.

Duodenum-preserving Resection of the Pancreatic Head

Duodenum-preserving resection of the pancreatic head may result in less postoperative endocrine pancreatic dysfunction than pancreatoduodenectomy in patients with chronic pancreatitis. New-onset diabetes has been reported to develop in 0 to 21% of patients with chronic pancreatitis after Beger or Frey duodenum-preserving resection of the pancreatic head.[71–77] In the most extensive single-center experience including a total of 504 patients with chronic pancreatitis, the rate of insulin-dependent diabetes increased from 25% preoperatively to 44% after a median of 5.7 years after duodenum-preserving resection of the pancreatic head; the rate of late postoperative new-onset insulin-dependent diabetes was 21%, whereas an improvement of glucose metabolism was noted in 11% of patients, resulting in a drop of normal glucose tolerance from 49% before surgery to 39% after surgery.[77] A randomized trial showed that patients had a significantly better glucose tolerance (mean fasting blood glucose levels, 88 vs. 130 mg/dl, $p \leqslant 0.01$) and a higher insulin secretion capacity 6 months after duodenum-preserving pancreatic head resection (n = 20) than after pylorus-preserving pancreatoduodenectomy (n = 20).[74] In another prospective randomized trial in 43 patients with chronic pancreatitis, six of 21 patients (29%) who have undergone Whipple pancreatoduodenectomy and two of 22 patients (9%) who have undergone duodenum-preserving resection of the head of the pancreas developed diabetes within a postoperative follow-up ranging from 36 months to 5.5 years.[75] This favorable effect is thought to be due to preservation of the enteroinsular axis and reduced unstimulated levels of the antiinsulin hormones glucagon and somatostatin, although mere differences in lost body mass between duodenum-preserving resection of the pancreatic head and pancreatoduodenectomy (30–40% vs. 40–60%, respectively[74]) cannot be excluded.[69,71,77] Indeed, the actual benefit, if any, of duodenum-preserving resection of the pancreatic head is unlikely to be related to the prevention of functional decline in patients with chronic pancreatitis (the rates of new-onset diabetes after duodenum-preserving resection of the pancreatic head being close to those reported after pancreatoduodenectomy, nonpancreatic drainage procedures, or even to in patients with chronic pancreatitis treated medically [although no direct comparison is available to date]); rather, the originator of duodenum-preserving resection of the pancreatic head stressed that endocrine function may improve (e.g., transition from insulin dependency to indepedency) transiently or permanently in the early or late postoperative period in a small but clinically significant percentage of patients.[77] However, duodenum-preserving resection of the pancreatic head is devoted to patients in whom an inflammatory mass in the pancreatic head has developed (about 30% of patients with chronic pancreatitis), which are not necessarily representative of the whole population of patients with chronic pancreatitis.

Distal Pancreatectomy

In seven studies including a total of 255 patients with chronic pancreatitis followed up for a mean of 1.7 to 7.0 years after a 40%–80% distal pancreatectomy, the rate of new-onset postoperative diabetes ranged from 15% to 48%.[50,60,78–82] In one study, 75% of patients who developed postoperative diabetes underwent a 60% or greater distal pancreatectomy.[60] Increasing the extent of distal pancreatectomy to 80%–95% led to a postoperative rate of diabetes of 44%–100% and increased late mortality.[55,78,83,84] However, most of these studies did not compare distal pancreatectomy with other elective pancreatic surgical procedures, or lacked a control group. In our prospective, medical–surgical, single-center cohort study of 453 patients with chronic pancreatitis (mean follow-up, 7 years; range, 0–35 years), we found that the prevalence of diabetes was significantly higher 5 years after distal pancreatectomy (n = 62, 57%) than after pancreatoduodenectomy (n = 37, 36%), pancreatic drainage (n = 46, 36%), or cystic, biliary, or digestive drainage (n = 86, 24%) (p = 0.005).[5] Time-dependent multivariate analysis showed that distal pancreatectomy was the only elective pancreatic surgical procedure increasing the risk of diabetes (risk ratio, 2.4; 95% confidence interval, 1.6–3.8; $p \leqslant 0.0001$).[5] Efforts should thus be made to avoid distal pancreatectomy when other surgical (or endoscopic) procedures are feasible.

In an attempt to lessen the risk of diabetes after subtotal or total pancreatectomy (with or without duodenectomy), autotransplantation of either part of the organ[84] or of islet tissue[78,85,86] has been described. Late postoperative insulin independence was obtained in 12% to 83% of patients (average, about 40%[86,87]) who have undergone islet autotransplantation following either total or subtotal pancreatectomy.[78,85–89] Although more than 200 patiens with chronic pancreatitis have undergone pancreatic resection with islet autotransplantation,[88] and insulin independence has been documented in some cases for more than 10 years, the technical problems of this procedure, mainly the reduced number of islets that can be isolated from fibrotic pancreata,[86,87] and postoperative complications (e.g. splenic or portal vein thrombosis) have not been sufficiently solved to consider it more than experimental. However, all centers undertaking total or subtotal pancreatectomy for chronic pancreatitis should examine the possibility of islet autotransplantation, since even a background level of glucose responsiveness is likely to facilitate postoperative management considerably in this difficult group of patients.

Pancreatic Drainage

Whether pancreatic drainage preserves or even improves pancreatic function by releasing obstructed pancreatic juice remains controversial. In nine studies including a total of 378 patients with chronic pancreatitis followed up for a mean of 1.0 to 8.1 years after pancreatic drainage, the rate of new-onset postoperative diabetes ranged from 0% to 35%.[60,78,90–96] The first suggestion of a significant delay in pancreatic dysfunction by surgical pancreatic drainage was provided by Nealon *et al.*.[97] In a partially randomized prospective study including 143 patients followed up for a mean of 47.3 months, they showed that eight of the 56 patients (14%) with 'mild/moderate' disease (according to authors' composite grading system) who underwent pancreatic drainage had 'progressive loss of their functional status' (without further explanation) compared with 34 of the 44 comparable patients (77%) conservatively treated. No patient in either the operated (n = 40) or non-operated (n = 20) group who were originally designated as 'severe' disease had sufficient improvement in function in follow-up to achieve a designation of 'mild/moderate' disease.[98] However, the principal criterion to determine candidacy for duct drainage in this series was the presence of a dilated pancreatic duct. Thus, what the study actually reported was the outcome of pancreatic drainage in patients with dilated ducts compared to the natural history of patients with chronic pancreatitis and no ductal dilation. It is therefore uncertain whether the slower deterioration of pancreatic endocrine function in patients who underwent surgery was actually caused by the surgical drainage procedure. Other series did not report long-term favorable results of pancreatic drainage procedures despite radiologic evidence of anastomotic patency.[78,90,94,96] A recent study showed that duct drainage achieved after endoscopic therapy and extracorporeal shockwave lithotripsy did not correlate with an improvement in pancreatic endocrine function.[99] We found that the prevalence of diabetes 5 years after pancreatic drainage (n = 46, 36%) was not statistically different from that after pancreatoduodenectomy (n = 37, 36%), or cystic, biliary, or digestive drainage (n = 86, 24%), and that pancreatic drainage did not prevent the eventual appearance of diabetes, as assessed by time-dependent multivariate analysis.[5] These findings suggest that pancreatic duct obstruction plays a minor role in the appearance of diabetes compared with parenchymal destruction and does not support a policy of prophylactic pancreatic drainage procedures performed early in the course of chronic pancreatitis as a means of preventing the progression of endocrine pancreatic insufficiency.

Complications of Diabetes in Chronic Pancreatitis

Acute Metabolic Complications

Hypoglycemia

Pancreatic alpha-cell function generally persists in patients with chronic pancreatitis, including those with complete disappearance of endogenous insulin production.[34,100] However, glucagon levels are generally low, and in contrast to patients with type 1 diabetes, insulin-induced hypoglycemia does not stimulate glucagon secretion in patients with diabetes secondary to chronic pancreatitis; this may explain the increased susceptibility to severe and potentially life-threatening hypoglycemia in these patients, often further aggravated by blunted epinephrine responses to insulin-induced hypoglycemia.[34,100,101] Diminished oral intake during pain episodes, malabsorption due to pancreatic exocrine insufficiency, alcohol- or biliary-induced liver disease, and persistent excessive acute and chronic alcohol intake may further increase the risk of hypoglycemia.[34,100] Nevertheless, no study has compared the risk of hypoglycemia in patients with diabetes secondary to chronic pancreatitis and patients with type 1 diabetes.

Ketoacidosis

The absence of increased glucagon secretion following insulin dissipation may also explain the reduced tendency to development of ketoacidosis.[34,101-103] However, ketoacidosis may occur in patients with diabetes secondary to chronic pancreatitis, particularly in case of attack of acute pancreatitis, infection, or abrupt increase in nutrient or pancreatic enzyme intake.[104]

Long-term Complications

Patients with diabetes secondary to chronic pancreatitis have been considered for a long time to be relatively spared from long-term microvascular and macrovascular complications,[100] as compared to type 1 diabetic patients.[105] However, microvascular and macrovascular complications may occur in patients with diabetes secondary to chronic pancreatitis at a similar rate than type 1 diabetics, and may be expected to be seen more frequently as these patients survive longer.[6] Macrovascular complications seem to be more frequent in patients with alcoholic chronic pancreatitis, probably in part because of the very high proportion of smokers in this population.[7,25]

Retinopathy

The reported prevalences of diabetic retinopathy in diabetes secondary to chronic pancreatitis ranged between 7% and 48%,[6,25,105-108] depending on the duration of diabetes.[106-108] The prevalence exceeded 40% after 8 years of diabetes duration, a figure similar to that observed in patients with type 1 diabetes of equal duration in most studies.[106,107] The spectrum of retinopathy was not different from that in type 1 diabetes,[6] but severe forms with visual impairment seemed to be rarer.[106,108]

Nephropathy

Diabetic nephropathy rarely occurs during the first 10 years after the onset of diabetes, whether primary or secondary to chronic pancreatitis.[34] Glomerular hyperfiltration, a risk factor for diabetic nephropathy, has been detected among all types of diabetics, including patients with pancreatic diabetes.[109] Microalbuminuria has been detected in 29% of patients with diabetes secondary to chronic pancreatitis and in up to 60% of those with associated diabetic retinopathy.[110] Nephropathy was detected in 21% of cases in a series of 649 patients with chronic pancreatitis.[25] These percentages are similar to those observed in patients with type 1 diabetes of equal duration.[6] Diabetic nephropathy correlated with retinopathy in several studies.[6,110]

Neuropathy

Data about diabetic neuropathy in chronic pancreatitis are scarce, and are difficult to interpret owing to the prevalence of coexisting risk factors for this complication (e.g. alcoholism and malnutrition). The prevalence of diabetic neuropathy was reported to be 36% in a large series of patients with chronic pancreatitis,[25] and was similar to that observed in type 1 diabetics. In a recent study, autonomic neuropathy was found in 67% of patients with alcoholic chronic pancreatitis and associated diabetes, as compared to 30% of patients with chronic pancreatitis without evidence of diabetes and 29% of patients with insulin-dependent diabetes without evidence of chronic pancreatitis.[111]

Arteriopathy

Lower-extremity arteriopathy, assessed by non-invasive tests, has the same distribution and a prevalence similar or even somewhat higher in patients with diabetes secondary to chronic pancreatitis as compared to patients with primary diabetes matched for sex, age, diabetes duration and treatment. This emphasizes the role of chronic hyperglycaemia and its duration in the pathogenesis of macroangiopathy in diabetic patients.[7]

Other complications

Diabetes secondary to chronic pancreatitis may favour perturbations of the vitamin A, vitamin E, magnesium, copper, selenium, and zinc metabolism.[112–115]

Latent or overt intestinal bacterial overgrowth is not uncommon in patients with chronic pancreatitis, particularly in older patients,[116] and in those with persistent alcoholism, associated pancreatic exocrine insufficiency, or a history of gastroduodenal surgery.[117,118] Diabetes may favor intestinal bacterial overgrowth, which may in turn worsen malabsorption and glycemic control.[118]

Diabetes and chronic pancreatitis have both been associated with an increased risk of pancreatic cancer in the general population. However, diabetes does not seem to further increase the risk of pancreatic cancer in patients with chronic pancreatitis.[119]

Treatment goals

The treatment of diabetes secondary to chronic pancreatitis is not codified. Following are some suggestions of treatment principles and goals, taking into account the specific aspects of diabetes secondary to chronic pancreatitis detailed in this review:

Appropriate diet (carbohydrates: 50–60%; proteins: 20%; fat: 20–30%) is advised. However, priority should be placed on the correction of malnutrition and weight loss.[120] Vitamin and trace element deficiencies should be searched for and corrected.[115]

Pancreatic exocrine insufficiency should be corrected. Oral pancreatic enzymes should be administered before every meal and snack. The initiation of, as well as the compliance to pancreatic enzyme substitution should be closely monitored, in order to avoid ketoacidosis and hypoglycemia, respectively.[104]

Pain episodes usually lead to reduced nutrient intake, and thus favour hypoglycemia. Pain relief (or at least pain control by non-opiate analgesics) should thus be obtained. If surgery is advocated, distal pancreatectomy should be avoided whenever possible.[5,55,60,78–82] Efforts to enhance the long-term benefits of pancreatic islet autotransplantation following either subtotal or total pancreatectomy should be encouraged in specialized centers.[78,85–89] Duodenum-preserving resection of the head of the pancreas might be less diabetogenic than pancreatoduodenectomy, perhaps by sparing the enteroinsular axis.[71–77] Pancreatic drainage, whether surgical or endoscopic, should be performed when indicated, but a policy of systematic, prophylactic drainage to delay or even prevent the onset of diabetes cannot be warranted at yet.[5,60,78,90–98]

Pancreatogenic diabetes responds only for a short period, if at all, to oral antidiabetics.[121] Insulin therapy is thus required in almost every case when diet becomes ineffective. Owing to the risk of severe hypoglycemia, the approach should be conservative in regard to intensive insulin therapy and tight blood glucose control. Realistic glycemic goals (after weight gain) should range between 7.2 mmol/l (130 mg/dl) and 10.0 mmol/l (180 mg/dl). However, more intensive insulin therapy is possible in compliant patients. In every case, a stable insulin requirement should be obtained. Diabetic education should be provided, ideally in specialised centers. Special attention should be paid at the time of hospital discharge and return to the 'real world', where increased physical activity, recurrent alcoholism, inappropriate diet, non-compliance with pancreatic enzyme substitution, and inadequate monitoring and adaptation of insulin therapy, along with intrinsic glucagon deficiency, expose patients to life-threatening hypoglycemia.

Complete alcohol withdrawal is mandatory. Besides the disastrous extrapancreatic effects of alcohol (accounting, along with smoking, for the majority of deaths in patients with alcoholic chronic pancreatitis[11]), persistent alcoholism may hasten the onset of diabetes.[5,19,25-27,49-51] A multidisciplinary approach is often needed in patients with chronic pancreatitis, in whom multiple addictions often coexist. Smoking cessation should be encouraged, to reduce the risk of macroangiopathic complications in patients with diabetes secondary to chronic pancreatitis.[7]

In the particular case of diabetes secondary to autoimmune chronic pancreatitis, corticosteroid therapy improves insulin secretion and glycaemic control.[39]

References

1. Sarles H, Bernard JP, Gullo L. Pathogenesis of chronic pancreatitis. Gut 1990; 31:629–32.
2. Mergener K, Baillie J. Chronic pancreatitis. Lancet 1997; 340:1379–85.
3. Ammann RW, Muellhaupt B, Group ZPS. The natural history of pain in alcoholic chronic pancreatitis. Gastroenterology 1999; 116:1132–40.
4. Bernades P, Belghiti J, Athouel M, et al. Histoire naturelle de la pancréatite chronique: étude de 120 cas. Gastroenterol Clin Biol 1983; 7:8–13.
5. Malka D, Hammel P, Sauvanet A, et al. Risk factors for diabetes mellitus in chronic pancreatitis. Gastroenterology 2000; 119:1324–32.

6. Levitt NS, Adams G, Salmon J, et al. The prevalence and severity of microvascular complications in pancreatic diabetes and IDDM. Diabetes Care 1995; 18:971–4.
7. Ziegler O, Candiloros H, Guerci B, et al. Lower-extremity arterial disease in diabetes mellitus due to chronic pancreatitis. Diabetes Metab 1994; 20:540–5.
8. Petrin P, Andreoli A, Antoniutti M, et al. Surgery for chronic pancreatitis: what quality of life ahead? World J Surg 1995; 19:398–402.
9. Miyake H, Harada H, Ochi K, et al. Prognosis and prognostic factors in chronic pancreatitis. Dig Dis Sci 1989; 34:449–55.
10. Traverso LW, Kozarek RA. Pancreatoduodenectomy for chronic pancreatitis. Anatomic selection criteria and subsequent long-term outcome analysis. Ann Surg 1997; 226:429–38.
11. Lévy P, Milan C, Pignon JP, et al. Mortality factors associated with chronic pancreatitis. Unidimensional and multi-dimensional analysis of a medical-surgical series of 240 patients. Gastroenterology 1989; 96:1165–72.
12. The Copenhagen Pancreatitis Study Group. Copenhagen pancreatitis study. An interim report from a prospective epidemiological multicentre study. Scand J Gastroenterol 1981; 16:305–12.
13. Lin Y, Tamakoshi A, Matsuno S, et al. Nationwide epidemiological survey of chronic pancreatitis in Japan. J Gastroenterol 2000; 35:136–41.
14. Dite P, Stary K, Novotny I, et al. Incidence of chronic pancreatitis in the Czech Republic. Eur J Gastroenterol Hepatol 2001; 13:749–50.
15. Secknus R, Mossner J. Incidenz- und Pravalenzveranderungen der akuten und chronischeN Pankreatitis in Deutschland. Chirurg 2000; 71:249–52.
16. DiMagno E, Layer P, Clain J. Chronic pancreatitis. In: Go VLW, Scheele GA, DiMagno EP, et al., eds. The pancreas: biology, pathobiology, and disease. New York: Lippincott-Raven, 1993; 665–706.
17. Hardt PD, Kloer HU. Diabetes mellitus and exocrine pancreatic disease. In: Johnson CD, Imrie CW, eds. Pancreatic disease. Towards the year 2000. London: Springer-Verlag, 1999; 235–41.
18. Olsen TS. The incidence and clinical relevance of chronic inflammation in the pancreas in autopsy material. Acta Pathol Microbiol Scand [A] 1978; 86A:361–5.
19. Koizumi M, Yoshida Y, Abe N, et al. Pancreatic diabetes in Japan. Pancreas 1998; 16:385–91.
20. Hardt PD, Krauss A, Bretz L, et al. Pancreatic exocrine function in patients with type 1 and type 2 diabetes mellitus. Acta Diabetol 2000; 37:105–10.
21. Hardt PD, Killinger A, Nalop J, et al. Chronic pancreatitis and diabetes mellitus. A retrospective analysis of 156 ERCP investigations in patients with insulin-dependent and non-insulin-dependent diabetes mellitus. Pancreatology 2002; 2:30–3.
22. Nakanishi K, Kobayashi T, Miyashita H, et al. Exocrine pancreatic ductograms in insulin-dependent diabetes mellitus. Am J Gastroenterol 1994; 89:762–6.
23. Lankisch PG, Lohr-Happe A, Otto J, et al. Natural course in chronic pancreatitis. Pain, exocrine and endocrine pancreatic insufficiency and prognosis of the disease. Digestion 1993; 54:148–55.
24. Cavallini G, Frulloni L, Pederzoli P, et al. Long-term follow-up of patients with chronic pancreatitis in Italy. Scand J Gastroenterol 1998; 33:880–9.
25. Okuno G, Oki A, Kawakami F, et al. Prevalence and clinical features of diabetes mellitus secondary to chronic pancreatitis in Japan; a study by questionnaire. Diabetes Res Clin Pract 1990; 10:65–71.
26. Dancour A, Lévy P, Milan C, et al. Histoire naturelle de la pancréatite chronique non alcoolique. Etude de 37 cas et comparaison avec 319 cas de pancréatite chronique alcoolique. Gastroenterol Clin Biol 1993; 17:915–24.
27. Layer P, Yamamoto H, Kalthoff L, et al. The different courses of early- and late-onset idiopathic and alcoholic chronic pancreatitis. Gastroenterology 1994; 107:1481–7.
28. Yeo CJ, Bastidas JA, Schmieg RE Jr, et al. Pancreatic structure and glucose tolerance in a longitudinal study of experimental pancreatitis-induced diabetes. Ann Surg 1989; 210:150–8.
29. Bateman AC, Turner SM, Thomas KSA, et al. Apoptosis and proliferation of acinar and islet cells in chronic pancreatitis: evidence for differential cell loss mediating preservation of islet function Gut 2002; 50:542–8.
30. Kreuwel HT, Morgan DJ, Krahl T, et al. Comparing the relative role of perforin/granzyme versus Fas/Fas ligand cytotoxic pathways in CD8+ T cell-mediated insulin-dependent diabetes mellitus. J Immunol 1999; 163:4335–41.
31. Bach JF. Insulin-dependent diabetes mellitus as an autoimmune disease. Endocr Rev 1994; 15:516–42.
32. Rumessen JJ, Marner B, Pedersen NT, et al. Autoantibodies in chronic pancreatitis. Scand J Gastroenterol 1985; 20:966–70.

33. Larsen S, Hilsted J, Jakobsen BK, et al. Insulin-dependent diabetes mellitus secondary to chronic pancreatitis is not associated with HLA or the occurrence of islet-cell antibodies. J Immunogenet 1990; 17:189–93.
34. Larsen S. Diabetes mellitus secondary to chronic pancreatitis. Dan Med Bull 1993; 40:153–62.
35. Panz VR, Kalk WJ, Zouvanis M, et al. Distribution of autoantibodies to glutamic acid decarboxylase across the spectrum of diabetes mellitus seen in South Africa. Diabet Med 2000; 17:524–7.
36. Onodera M, Okazaki K, Morita M, et al. Immune complex specific for the pancreatic duct antigen in patients with idiopathic chronic pancreatitis and Sjogren syndrome. Autoimmunity 1994; 19:23–9.
37. Frulloni L, Bovo P, Brunelli S, et al. Elevated serum levels of antibodies to carbonic anhydrase I and II in patients with chronic pancreatitis. Pancreas 2000; 20:382–8.
38. Lampeter EF, Seifert I, Lohmann D, et al. Inflammatory islet damage in patients bearing HLA-DR 3 and/or DR 4 haplotypes does not lead to islet autoimmunity. Diabetologia 1994; 37:471–5.
39. Tanaka S, Kobayashi T, Nakanishi K, et al. Corticosteroid-responsive diabetes mellitus associated with autoimmune pancreatitis. Lancet 2000; 356:910–1.
40. Tanaka S, Kobayashi T, Nakanishi K, et al. Evidence of primary beta-cell destruction by T-cells and beta-cell differentiation from pancreatic ductal cells in diabetes associated with active autoimmune chronic pancreatitis. Diabetes Care 2001; 24:1661–7.
41. Imagawa A, Hanafusa T, Miyagawa J, et al. A novel subtype of type 1 diabetes mellitus characterized by a rapid onset and an absence of diabetes-related antibodies. Osaka IDDM Study Group. N Engl J Med 2000; 342:301–7.
42. Keim V, Bauer N, Teich N, et al. Clinical characterization of patients with hereditary pancreatitis and mutations in the cationic trypsinogen gene. Am J Med 2001; 111:622–6.
43. Schneider A, Suman A, Rossi L, et al. SPINK1/PSTI mutations are associated with tropical pancreatitis and type II diabetes mellitus in Bangladesh. Gastroenterology 2002; 123:1026–30.
44. Bhatia E, Choudhuri G, Sikora SS, et al. Tropical calcific pancreatitis: strong association with SPINK1 trypsin inhibitor mutations. Gastroenterology 2002; 123:1020–5.
45. Tsuji A, Nishikawa T, Mori M, et al. Quantitative trait locus analysis for chronic pancreatitis and diabetes mellitus in the WBN/Kob rat. Genomics 2001; 74:365–9.
46. Sarles H, Adler G, Dani R, et al. The pancreatitis classification of Marseilles, Rome 1988. Scand J Gastroenterol 1989; 24:641–2.
47. Sarner M, Cotton PB. Classification of pancreatitis. Gut 1984; 25:756–9.
48. Ammann RW. A clinically based classification system for alcoholic chronic pancreatitis: summary of an international workshop on chronic pancreatitis. Pancreas 1997; 14:215–21.
49. Ammann RW, Buehler H, Muench R, et al. Differences in the natural history of idiopathic (nonalcoholic) and alcoholic chronic pancreatitis. A comparative long-term study of 287 patients. Pancreas 1987; 2:368–77.
50. Hayakawa T, Kondo T, Shibata T, et al. Chronic alcoholism and evolution of pain and prognosis in chronic pancreatitis. Dig Dis Sci 1989; 34:33–8.
51. Robles-Diaz G, Vargas F, Uscanga L, et al. Chronic pancreatitis in Mexico City. Pancreas 1990; 5:479–83.
52. Lankisch PG, Seidensticker F, Lohr-Happe A, et al. The course of pain is the same in alcohol- and nonalcohol-induced chronic pancreatitis. Pancreas 1995; 10:338–41.
53. Gullo L, Barbara L, Labo G. Effect of cessation of alcohol use on the course of pancreatic dysfunction in alcoholic pancreatitis. Gastroenterology 1988; 95:1063–8.
54. Fourdan O, Lévy P, Lévy-Bellaïche S, et al. Taux d'abstinence alcoolique chez les malades ayant une pancréatite chronique alcoolique. Gastroenterol Clin Biol 1994; 18:852–8.
55. Frey CF, Child CG III, Fry W. Pancreatectomy for chronic pancreatitis. Ann Surg 1976; 184:403–14.
56. Rossi RL, Rothschild J, Braasch JW, et al. Pancreatoduodenectomy in the management of chronic pancreatitis. Arch Surg 1987; 122:416–20.
57. Schneider MU, Meister R, Domschke S, et al. Whipple's procedure plus intraoperative pancreatic duct occlusion for severe chronic pancreatitis: clinical, exocrine, and endocrine consequences during a 3-year follow-up. Pancreas 1987; 2:715–26.
58. Stone WM, Sarr MG, Nagorney DM, et al. Chronic pancreatitis: results of Whipple's resection and total pancreatectomy. Arch Surg 1988; 123:815–9.
59. Gall FP, Zirngibl H, Gebhardt C, et al. Duodenal pancreatectomy with occlusion of the pancreatic duct. Hepatogastroenterology 1990; 37:290–4.
60. Jalleh RP, Williamson RCN. Pancreatic exocrine and endocrine function after operations for chronic pancreatitis. Ann Surg 1992; 216:656–62.

61. Saeger HD, Schwall G, Trede M. Standard Whipple in chronic pancreatitis. In: Beger HG, Buechler M, Malfertheiner P, eds. Standards in pancreatic surgery. Berlin Heidelberg New York: Springer, 1993; 385–91.
62. Markowitz JS, Rattner DW, Warshaw AL. Failure of symptomatic relief after pancreaticojejunal decompression for chronic pancreatitis. Strategies for salvage. Arch Surg 1994; 129:374–80.
63. Watanapa P, Williamson RCN. Resection of the pancreatic head with or without gastrectomy. World J Surg 1995; 19:403–9.
64. Martin RF, Rossi RL, Leslie KA. Long-term results of pylorus-preserving pancreatoduodenectomy for chronic pancreatitis. Arch Surg 1996; 131:247–52.
65. Stapleton GN, Williamson RC. Proximal pancreatoduodenectomy for chronic pancreatitis. Br J Surg 1996; 83:1433–40.
66. Rumstadt B, Forssmann K, Singer MV, et al. The Whipple partial duodenopancreatectomy for the treatment of chronic pancreatitis. Hepatogastroenterology 1997; 44:1554–9.
67. Vickers SM, Chan C, Heslin MJ, et al. The role of pancreaticoduodenectomy in the treatment of severe chronic pancreatitis. Am Surg 1999; 65:1108–12.
68. Sakorafas GH, Farnell MB, Nagorney DM, et al. Pancreatoduodenectomy for chronic pancreatitis: long-term results in 105 patients. Arch Surg 2000; 135:517–24.
69. Jimenez RE, Fernandez-del Castillo C, Rattner DW, et al. Outcome of pancreaticoduodenectomy with pylorus preservation or with antrectomy in the treatment of chronic pancreatitis. Ann Surg 2000; 231:293–302.
70. Sato N, Yamaguchi K, Yokohata K, et al. Changes in pancreatic function after pancreatoduodenectomy. Am J Surg 1998; 176:59–61.
71. Beger HG, Büchler M, Bittner RR, et al. Duodenum-preserving resection of the head of the pancreas in severe chronic pancreatitis. Early and late results. Ann Surg 1989; 209:273–8.
72. Frey CF, Amikura K. Local resection of the head of the pancreas combined with longitudinal pancreaticojejunostomy in the management of patients with chronic pancreatitis. Ann Surg 1994; 220:492–507.
73. Izbicki JR, Bloechle C, Knoefel WT, et al. Duodenum-preserving resection of the head of the pancreas in chronic pancreatitis. A prospective, randomized trial. Ann Surg 1995; 221:350–8.
74. Büchler MW, Friess H, Muller MW, et al. Randomized trial of duodenum-preserving pancreatic head resection versus pylorus-preserving Whipple in chronic pancreatitis. Am J Surg 1995; 169:65–70.
75. Klempa I, Spatny M, Menzel J, et al. Pankreasfunktion und Lebensqualitat nach Pankreaskopfresektion bei der chronischen Pankreatitis. Eine prospektive, randomisierte Vergleichsstudie nach duodenumerhaltender Pankreaskopfresektion versus Whipple'scher Operation. Chirurg 1995; 66:350–9.
76. Izbicki JR, Bloechle C, Broering DC, et al. Extended drainage versus resection in surgery for chronic pancreatitis: a prospective randomized trial comparing the longitudinal pancreaticojejunostomy combined with local pancreatic head excision with the pylorus-preserving pancreatoduodenectomy. Ann Surg 1998; 228:771–9.
77. Beger HG, Schlosser W, Friess HM, et al. Duodenum-preserving head resection in chronic pancreatitis changes the natural course of the disease: a single-center 26-year experience. Ann Surg 1999; 230:512–23.
78. Morrow CE, Cohen JI, Sutherland DER, et al. Chronic pancreatitis: long-term surgical results of pancreatic duct drainage, pancreatic resection, and near-total pancreatectomy and islet autotransplantation. Surgery 1984; 96:608–16.
79. Warshaw AL. Conservation of pancreatic tissue by combined gastric, biliary, and pancreatic duct drainage for pain from chronic pancreatitis. Am J Surg 1985; 149:563–9.
80. Sawyer R, Frey CF. Is there still a role for distal pancreatectomy in surgery for chronic pancreatitis? Am J Surg 1994; 168:6–9.
81. Govil S, Imrie CW. Value of splenic preservation during distal pancreatectomy for chronic pancreatitis. Br J Surg 1999; 86:895–8.
82. Schoenberg MH, Schlosser W, Ruck W, et al. Distal pancreatectomy in chronic pancreatitis. Dig Surg 1999; 16:130–6.
83. Keith RG, Saibil FG, Sheppard RH. Treatment of chronic alcoholic pancreatitis by pancreatic resection. Am J Surg 1989; 157:156–62.
84. Rossi RL, Soeldner JS, Braasch JW, et al. Long-term results of pancreatic resection and segmental pancreatic autotransplantation for chronic pancreatitis. Am J Surg 1990; 159:51–8.
85. Farney AC, Najarian JS, Nakhleh RE, et al. Autotransplantation of dispersed pancreatic islet tissue combined with total or near-total pancreatectomy for treatment of chronic pancreatitis. Surgery 1991; 110:427–39.

86. Wahoff DC, Papalois BE, Najarian JS, et al. Autologous islet transplantation to prevent diabetes after pancreatic resection. Ann Surg 1995; 222:562–79.
87. Robertson GS, Dennison AR, Johnson PR, et al. A review of pancreatic islet autotransplantation. Hepatogastroenterology 1998; 45:226–35.
88. White SA, Robertson GS, London NJ, et al. Human islet autotransplantation to prevent diabetes after pancreas resection. Dig Surg 2000; 17:439–50.
89. White SA, Davies JE, Pollard C, et al. Pancreas resection and islet autotransplantation for end-stage chronic pancreatitis. Ann Surg 2001; 233:423–31.
90. Warshaw AL, Popp JW Jr, Schapiro RH. Long-term patency, pancreatic function, and pain relief after lateral pancreaticojejunostomy for chronic pancreatitis. Gastroenterology 1980; 79:289–93.
91. Prinz RA, Greenlee HB. Pancreatic duct drainage in 100 patients with chronic pancreatitis. Ann Surg 1981; 194:313–20.
92. Cooper MJ, Williamson RC. Drainage operations in chronic pancreatitis. Br J Surg 1984; 71:761–6.
93. Pain JA, Knight MJ. Pancreaticogastrostomy: the preferred operation for pain relief in chronic pancreatitis. Br J Surg 1988; 75:220–2.
94. Ebbehøj N, Klaaborg K-E, Kronborg O, et al. Pancreaticogastrostomy for chronic pancreatitis. Am J Surg 1989; 157:315–7.
95. Delcore R, Rodriguez FJ, Thomas JH, et al. The role of pancreaticojejunostomy in patients without dilated pancreatic ducts. Am J Surg 1994; 168:598–602.
96. Adams DB, Ford MC, Anderson MC. Outcome after lateral pancreaticojejunostomy for chronic pancreatitis. Ann Surg 1994; 219:481–9.
97. Nealon WH, Townsend CM Jr, Thompson JC. Operative drainage of the pancreatic duct delays functional impairment in patients with chronic pancreatitis. A prospective analysis. Ann Surg 1988; 208:321–9.
98. Nealon WH, Thompson JC. Progressive loss of pancreatic function in chronic pancreatitis is delayed by main pancreatic duct decompression. A longitudinal prospective analysis of the modified puestow procedure. Ann Surg 1993; 217:458–68.
99. Adamek HE, Jakobs R, Buttmann A, et al. Long term follow up of patients with chronic pancreatitis and pancreatic stones treated with extracorporeal shock wave lithotripsy. Gut 1999; 45:402–5.
100. Bank S, Marks IN, Vinik AI. Clinical and hormonal aspects of pancreatic diabetes. Am J Gastroenterol 1975; 64:13–22.
101. Keller U, Szollosy E, Varga L, et al. Pancreatic glucagon secretion and exocrine function (BT-PABA test) in chronic pancreatitis. Dig Dis Sci 1984; 29:853–7.
102. Larsen S, Hilsted J, Philipsen EK, et al. The effect of insulin withdrawal on intermediary metabolism in patients with diabetes secondary to chronic pancreatitis. Acta Endocrinol (Copenh) 1991; 124:510–5.
103. Barnes AJ, Bloom SR, Goerge K, et al. Ketoacidosis in pancreatectomized man. N Engl J Med 1977; 296:1250–3.
104. O'Keefe SJ, Cariem AK, Levy M. The exacerbation of pancreatic endocrine dysfunction by potent pancreatic exocrine supplements in patients with chronic pancreatitis. J Clin Gastroenterol 2001; 32:319–23.
105. Maekawa N, Ohneda A, Kai Y, et al. Secondary diabetic retinopathy in chronic pancreatitis. Am J Ophthalmol 1978; 85:835–40.
106. Gullo L, Parenti M, Monti L, et al. Diabetic retinopathy in chronic pancreatitis. Gastroenterology 1990; 98:1577–81.
107. Couet C, Genton P, Pointel JP, et al. The prevalence of retinopathy is similar in diabetes mellitus secondary to chronic pancreatitis with or without pancreatectomy and in idiopathic diabetes mellitus. Diabetes Care 1985; 8:323–8.
108. Tiengo A, Segato T, Briani G, et al. The presence of retinopathy in patients with secondary diabetes following pancreatectomy or chronic pancreatitis. Diabetes Care 1983; 6:570–4.
109. Marre M, Hallab M, Roy J, et al. Glomerular hyperfiltration in type I, type II, and secondary diabetes. J Diabet Complications 1992; 6:19–24.
110. Briani G, Riva F, Midena E, et al. Prevalence of microangiopathic complications in hyperglycemia secondary to pancreatic disease. J Diabet Complications 1988; 2:50–2.
111. Rosa-e-Silva L, Oliveira RB, Troncon LE, et al. Autonomic nervous function in alcohol-related chronic pancreatitis. Pancreas 2000; 20:361–6.
112. Yokota T, Tsuchiya K, Furukawa T, et al. Vitamin E deficiency in acquired fat malabsorption. J Neurol 1990; 237:103–6.

113. Van Gossum A, Closset P, Noel E, et al. Deficiency in antioxidant factors in patients with alcohol-related chronic pancreatitis. Dig Dis Sci 1996; 41:1225–31.
114. Papazachariou IM, Martinez-Isla A, Efthimiou E, et al. Magnesium deficiency in patients with chronic pancreatitis identified by an intravenous loading test. Clin Chim Acta 2000; 302:145–54.
115. Quilliot D, Dousset B, Guerci B, et al. Evidence that diabetes mellitus favors impaired metabolism of zinc, copper, and selenium in chronic pancreatitis. Pancreas 2001; 22:299–306.
116. McEvoy A, Dutton J, James OF. Bacterial contamination of the small intestine is an important cause of occult malabsorption in the elderly. Br Med J (Clin Res Ed) 1983; 287:789–93.
117. Casellas F, Guarner L, Vaquero E, et al. Hydrogen breath test with glucose in exocrine pancreatic insufficiency. Pancreas 1998; 16:481–6.
118. Trespi E, Ferrieri A. Intestinal bacterial overgrowth during chronic pancreatitis. Curr Med Res Opin 1999; 15:47–52.
119. Talamini G, Falconi M, Bassi C, et al. Previous cholecystectomy, gastrectomy, and diabetes mellitus are not crucial risk factors for pancreatic cancer in patients with chronic pancreatitis. Pancreas 2001; 23:364–7.
120. Wakasugi H, Funakoshi A, Iguchi H. Clinical assessment of pancreatic diabetes caused by chronic pancreatitis. J Gastroenterol 1998; 33:254–9.
121. Lankisch PG. Conservative treatment of chronic pancreatitis. Digestion 1987; 37 (Suppl 1):47–55.

21 Acinar–Islet Interactions: Pancreatic Exocrine Insufficiency in Diabetes Mellitus

Jutta Keller and Peter Layer

In a considerable proportion of patients with diabetes mellitus not only endocrine but also exocrine function of the pancreas is impaired.[1-10] Moreover, marked morphological alterations of the exocrine pancreas are observed in diabetic patients.[11-17] The pathophysiological mechanisms leading to pancreatic exocrine insufficiency are not fully elucidated but disturbance of acinar–islet interactions with imbalance of stimulatory and inhibitory islet hormones is probably one of the main reasons. In addition, pancreatic fibrosis due to angiopathy, autoimmune mechanisms and autonomic neuropathy may contribute to pancreatic exocrine insufficiency in diabetes mellitus.

Most studies revealed mild to moderate pancreatic exocrine insufficiency in diabetic patients,[1;4-10] whereas severe pancreatic exocrine insufficiency causing clinically overt steatorhoea[9;18] is rare. Therefore, the clinical relevance of pancreatic exocrine insufficiency associated with diabetes mellitus remains unclear. However, a distal shift of nutrient digestion and absorption caused by decreased enzyme output[19;20] induces regulatory and motor disturbances[21-24] which may contribute to abdominal symptoms frequently observed in diabetes mellitus.[25;26] Consequently, clinical studies of enzyme supplementation are warranted.

The aim of this chapter is to discuss our current knowledge of morphological and functional alterations of the exocrine pancreas in diabetes mellitus, potential pathophysiological mechanisms, clinical relevance and therapeutic implications of pancreatic exocrine insufficiency in diabetes mellitus.

Morphological Changes of the Exocrine Pancreas in Diabetes Mellitus

Compared with healthy controls, the pancreas of patients with diabetes is smaller,[27] mainly caused by involution of the exocrine tissue.[13] Atrophy particularly affects the pancreatic body[13] and is more pronounced in insulin dependent diabetes mellitus patients (IDDM) compared with non-insulin dependent diabetics (NIDDM).[12-14] Diabetics treated with but not dependent on insulin show intermediate reductions in pancreatic size.[13] It is controversial, whether morphological alterations correlate with the duration or the age at onset of the disease.[14;17;27]

An abnormal pancreatogram is observed in 40% of patients with IDDM, in 59% of patients with islet cell antibody (ICA)-positive NIDDM, but only in 9% of ICA-negative NIDDM patients.[28]

Histopathological alterations are more pronounced in IDDM as well and include pancreatic fibrosis,[17;29;30] fatty infiltration,[17] and intra- and peri-insular inflammatory infiltrates in IDDM.[15–17;31] Lymphocytic insulitis, a predominant characteristic of IDDM, disappears after the β-cells have been totally destroyed.[31]

However, even within the group of IDDM patients, pathological findings vary. According to pathological examinations and clinical characteristics, Imagawa *et al.* proposed 3 distinct subtypes of type 1 diabetes:[15] about 60% of patients showed no insulitis, over-expression of class I MHC molecules in the islet cells, a high prevalence of diabetes-related autoantibodies and a progressive loss of β-cell function after onset of disease ('autoimmune type'), 30% showed neither insulitis nor over-expression of class I MHC molecules, had a low prevalence of autoantibodies and a slow β-cell loss ('non-autoimmune non-fulminant type'), about 10% showed no insulitis, normal expression of class I MHC molecules and no autoantibodies, but lymphocytic infiltration in the exocrine tissue, elevated serum pancreatic enzyme levels and an aggressive course of the disease ('nonautoimmune fulminant type').[15;32]

Autopsy findings in recent-onset IDDM patients demonstrated that the acinar tissue around insulin-containing islets was normal whereas severe acinar cell atrophy was present around insulin-deficient islets.[33] These findings underline the importance of the *insulo-acinar portal system*, in general, and the loss of the trophic effect of insulin, in particular, for the morphology and function of peri-insular acinar cells (see below).

Pancreatic Exocrine Function in Diabetes Mellitus

Most studies investigating pancreatic exocrine function in diabetes mellitus show mild to moderate impairment of bicarbonate and enzyme secretion in a subset of patients. Prevalence of pancreatic insufficiency is particularly high in IDDM and ranges between about 40–80% in these patients.[1;2;4–9] Our own study in 12 IDDM patients confirmed that overall pancreatic enzyme secretion was decreased, however, the degree of impairment varied among different enzymes (Fig. 21.1): Amylase output was normal in the interdigestive state, during moderate endogenous and maximal exogenous stimulation. Diminished fasting lipase output increased regularly in response to endogenous but not to exogenous stimulation. Chymotrypsin output apparently was most susceptible and was decreased under all experimental conditions. Consequently, pancreatic enzyme pattern appears to be altered in response to different stimuli in IDDM.[8]

In NIDDM patients, the prevalence of pancreatic exocrine insufficiency is somewhat lower and ranges between 15 and 73%.[3–5;9] In the subgroup of patients with diarrhea and peripheral neuropathy, however, all patients showed impaired exocrine function with amylase and bicarbonate secretion amounting to about 40% of healthy controls in response to endogenous and exogenous stimulation.[10]

Pathophysiology of pancreatic exocrine insufficiency in diabetes mellitus

The pathophysiological mechanisms leading to pancreatic exocrine insufficiency are not fully elucidated but probably include an imbalance of stimulatory and

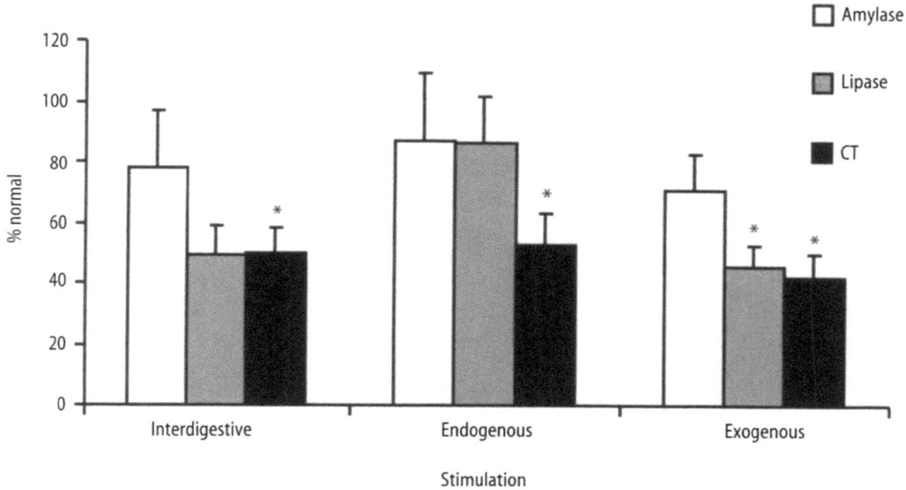

Figure 21.1. Pancreatic enzyme output in 12 IDDM patients during the fasting state, during endogenous stimulation by duodenal perfusion of essential amino acids (EAA, 450 μmol/min) and during exogenous stimulation with secretin (1 U/kg/h) and cerulein (75 ng/kg/h). Amylase output is normal in the interdigestive state, during moderate endogenous and maximal exogenous stimulation. Diminished fasting lipase output increases regularly in response to endogenous but not to exogenous stimulation. Chymotrypsin (CT) output is decreased under all experimental conditions. Data are given as mean±SE (modified according to Ref. 8).

inhibitory islet hormones, pancreatic fibrosis due to angiopathy, autoimmune mechanisms, autonomic neuropathy and altered release of gastrointestinal regulatory mediators (Table 21.1, Fig. 21.2).

Imbalance of Stimulatory and Inhibitory Islet Hormones

Insulo-acinar portal system. The blood flow within the pancreas is directed from the islets to the exocrine tissue. This *insulo-acinar portal system* consists of afferent vessels that first reach the islets, form an intra-islet glomerulus and leave the islets as efferent capillaries which subsequently perfuse the exocrine tissue.[34;35] Therefore, under physiological circumstances, the concentrations of islet hormones, including insulin, to which the exocrine pancreas is exposed are much higher than in the general circulation. The morphological distribution of islets throughout the exocrine tissue and the specific blood flow pattern of the

Table 21.1. Pathophysiological mechanisms potentially leading to pancreatic exocrine insufficiency in diabetes mellitus

- imbalance of stimulatory and inhibitory islet hormones (insulin ↓, glucagon & somatostatin ↑, *insulo-acinar axis*)
- pancreatic fibrosis due to angiopathy
- autoimmune mechanisms
- autonomic neuropathy
- altered release of gastrointestinal regulatory mediators (*entero-insular axis*).

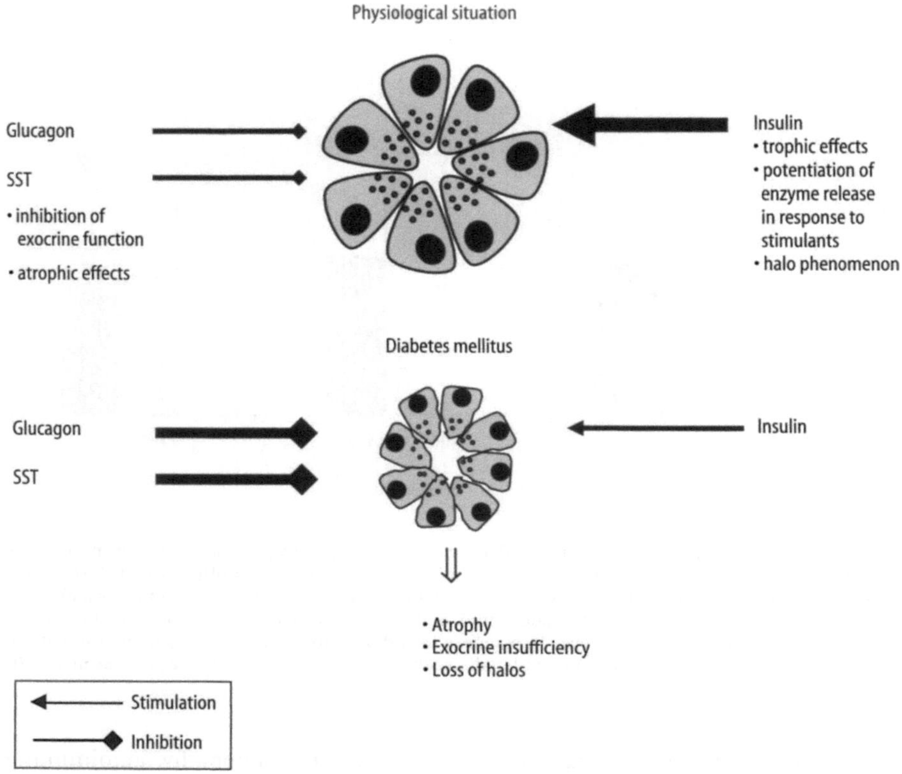

Figure 21.2. Imbalance of stimulatory and inhibitory islet hormones in diabetes mellitus.

insulo–acinar portal system suggest functional interactions between the endocrine and exocrine tissue, i.e. regulation of pancreatic exocrine secretion by stimulatory and inhibitory islet hormones.

Insulin has various effects on pancreatic acinar cells and pancreatic exocrine function (Fig. 21.2): Insulin stimulates acinar cell growth via the IGF-1 receptor,[36] i.e. insulin exerts trophic effects on the exocrine pancreas. Insulin potentiates enzyme release, specifically amylase secretion, in response to secretin and CCK, acetylcholine and electrical field stimulation in isolated acini and in the isolated pancreas from the rat.[37–40] Recent studies suggest that the stimulatory effect of insulin depends on the presence of viable islets of Langerhans.[38;41] Accordingly, in IDDM patients with residual insulin secretion, C-peptide levels correlated with amylase and bicarbonate output.[42] These trophic and stimulatory insulin effects are reflected by particularly large peri-insular acinar cells packed with zymogen granules, the so called halo phenomenon.[43] The halo phenomenon is lost in diabetes mellitus and is not restored by exogenous insulin administration, probably because the physiologically high insulin concentrations in the insulo–acinar portal system and particularly in the peri-insular region cannot be re-established.

In vivo, however, insulin may also have inhibitory effects on pancreatic exocrine function. In rats, insulin administration reduced pancreatic lipase synthesis on a pre-translational level.[44] Inhibition of basal amylase and lipase activities occurred with physiological insulin doses.[45]

In healthy humans, experimental hyperinsulinemia inhibited basal but not CCK-stimulated enzyme output during euglycemia. Apart from that, hyperglycemia had insulin-independent inhibitory effects on pancreatic exocrine function.[46] In patients with poorly controlled diabetes, amylase activity in pure pancreatic juice was decreased by about 30% compared with healthy controls.[47] Changes in lipase activity, protein and bicarbonate concentration were negligible in this study. Strict glycemic control for one to three months significantly but only slightly increased amylase activity in diabetics. According to recent studies in IDDM and NIDDM patient, the observed decrease in fecal elastase 1 concentrations in diabetics was associated with poor glycemic control.[2;3] By contrast, we did not observe differences in pancreatic exocrine function in IDDM patients with good or poor glycemic control (unpublished results). Accordingly, short-term effects of hyperglycemia do not account for the total reduction in enzyme activity and secretion observed in diabetes patients.

On the other hand, we observed significantly lower pancreatic enzyme output in short term IDDM diabetics compared with long term patients (unpublished results). Because progressive loss of residual β-cells occurs during the course of the disease, short-term diabetics probably have higher intra-pancreatic insulin concentrations compared with long-term patients. Therefore, the degree of insulin privation does not fully explain pancreatic exocrine dysfunction in diabetics, either.

Taken together, these divergent findings suggest that the effects of endogenous insulin release and of exogenous insulin administration on pancreatic growth and exocrine function may differ in healthy humans and in diabetics, respectively. Moreover, the net effects of the loss of insulin secretion in diabetics on pancreatic enzyme secretion still remain to be fully elucidated.

There is evidence that increased levels of inhibitory islet hormones may further contribute to pancreatic exocrine insufficiency in diabetes mellitus. In particular, glucagon and somatostatin release was increased in diabetes patients.[48–50] Glucagon decreased rat basal trypsin and lipase release at low doses, and amylase release only at higher doses[45] and inhibited pancreatic exocrine function in man.[51] Moreover, it has been suggested that glucagon may contribute to pancreatic atrophy.[52] Somatostatin decreased basal human inter-digestive enzyme output by 50% at physiological doses[53] and inhibited meal stimulated exocrine secretion.[54] This appears to be due to direct inhibition as well as to reduction of CCK release.[54]

These findings allow the conclusion that disturbance of acinar-islet interactions with imbalance of stimulatory and inhibitory islet hormones (Fig. 21.2) is probably one of the main reasons for pancreatic exocrine dysfunction in diabetes mellitus but does not explain it sufficiently.

Pancreatic Fibrosis due to Angiopathy

It has been hypothesized that diabetic angiopathy can induce arterial lesions which may further contribute to pancreatic fibrosis in a subgroup of patients.[5;30] However, the available data is scarce.

Autoimmune Mechanisms

Loss of β-cells in IDDM has been attributed to autoimmune mechanisms that may affect the exocrine pancreas, as well. Autoimmunity may be triggered by a multitude of factors, particularly genetic predisposition in connection with environmental factors, e.g. viruses.[31] In IDDM patients, circulating autoantibodies against pancreatic lipase have been identified in about 75% of patients, in more than 30% of first-degree relatives but only in about 10% or less in healthy controls and control patients with other pancreatic or autoimmune diseases.[55] Moreover, the presence of these autoantibodies was relatively low in NIDDM patients (17%). The authors of this study suggest, on the one hand, that these antibodies may originate from lysis of acinar cells surrounding the islets, as a result of macrophage and lymphocytic infiltration. On the other hand, high circulating glucose concentrations might affect acinar cell metabolism and lead to immunogenic protein glycosylation products.[55] Furthermore, additional autoantibodies against exocrine components such as anti-cytokeratin-autoantibodies have been observed in diabetics and some well-known islet autoantigens in diabetes mellitus appear to be not islet-specific but were also expressed in the exocrine tissue. Consequently, autoimmune reactions against these autoantigens would probably also affect the exocrine pancreas.[56]

These findings agree with the data of Semakula *et al.*[57] who showed that, in IDDM patients at the clinical onset of the disease, circulating pancreatic enzyme activities were frequently abnormal. In about 10% of patients increased lipase or amylase levels were observed and these were associated with higher titers of islet cell and glucagon autoantibodies. In about 20% of patients, circulating activities of lipase or pancreatic amylase were decreased. The authors suggested that increased enzyme levels may reflect acute acinar cell damage, whereas decreased enzyme levels may be due to reduced peri-insular acinar cell function.[57]

By contrast, Imagawa *et al.* recently described a novel subtype of IDDM characterized by rapid onset and absence of diabetes-related antibodies.[15;32] This subtype occurred in about 10% of patients who showed no insulitis, normal expression of class I MHC molecules and no autoantibodies, but lymphocytic infiltration in the exocrine tissue, elevated serum pancreatic enzyme levels and an aggressive course of the disease ('nonautoimmune fulminant type', see above).[32] These findings suggest that mechanisms other than autoimmune may induce inflammatory destruction of pancreatic exocrine tissue in diabetes mellitus.

Moreover, lymphocytic insulitis, a predominant characteristic of IDDM, disappeared after the β-cells had been totally destroyed[31] suggesting that the impairment of pancreatic exocrine function by autoimmune and inflammatory mechanisms might be more important for the early compared with the late course of the disease. Accordingly, we found in a prospective study that pancreatic exocrine function was disturbed more severely in IDDM patients with a shorter duration of diabetes (less than 10 years) compared with long-lasting diabetes (unpublished results).

In conclusion, the role of autoimmune and inflammatory mechanisms in diabetes mellitus remains unclear. Possibly, common autoimmune or inflammatory mechanisms might affect the whole gland simultaneously, inflammatory destruction might start in the islets with secondary involvement of the exocrine tissue or, *vice versa*, inflammation might start in the exocrine tissue and lead to secondary destruction of the islets.

Autonomic Neuropathy and Altered Release of Gastrointestinal Hormones

Autonomic neuropathy is a rather frequent complication of long-standing diabetes mellitus and may lead to gastroparesis in a subset of patients.[58] In a smaller proportion of diabetics, accelerated gastric emptying was observed.[58] In addition, we have shown impairment of intestinal motility in long-term IDDM patients.[59] These alterations of gastrointestinal motility may impair secretory–motor-coupling and lead to reduced pancreatic exocrine response to endogenous stimulation. Moreover, human pancreatic enzyme secretion is predominantly dependent on the cholinergic tone which is modulated by activation of CCK-receptors located on cholinergic nerves.[60] This means that not only endogenous but also exogenous stimulation of pancreatic exocrine secretion by CCK or CCK-analogues may be impaired in patients with autonomic neuropathy. Accordingly, decreased enzyme release in response to amino acids and CCK was observed in all patients in a small group of NIDDM patients with diarrhoea and neuropathy.[10]

Pancreatic polypeptide (PP) release has been shown to be a sensitive marker of autonomic neuropathy.[61;62] Impairment of PP response to a test meal appears to be correlated to the degree of autonomic neuropathy[63;64] in diabetes patients. In our group of IDDM patients, mean basal PP plasma levels, PP plasma levels during the early and late cephalic phase of sham feeding as well as during the gastric phase (water distension) were significantly reduced compared with healthy controls (unpublished results) despite the fact that only a minority of patients showed clinical evidence of neuropathy. This may suggest that sub-clinical autonomic neuropathy may impair pancreatic exocrine function in diabetes patients before other symptoms of diabetic neuropathy occur. On the other hand, it cannot be ruled out that reduction of PP release in diabetics may reflect dysfunction of the PP secreting islet cells.[65]

Apart from that, disturbances of gut hormone release with potential influence on pancreatic exocrine function have been observed in diabetes mellitus. These include increased basal and post-prandial plasma motilin concentrations[66;67] and increased post-prandial CCK release[63] in patients with autonomic neuropathy. By contrast, NIDDM patients showed reduced post-prandial CCK secretion.[68] Moreover, we observed slightly decreased GLP-1 and PYY plasma levels in IDDM during endogenous or exogenous stimulation (unpublished results), whereas in NIDDM basal GLP-1 levels and GLP-1 release after an oral glucose tolerance test were increased.[69] Both, GLP-1 and PYY are distal intestinal hormones and inhibit upper gastrointestinal functions[70;71] including pancreatic exocrine function in healthy humans.[72–74]

In summary, disturbances of gut hormone release probably differ in IDDM and NIDDM and their influence on pancreatic exocrine function in diabetes mellitus is not understood, to date.

Clinical Relevance and Therapeutic Implications

Despite the rather high prevalence rates of pancreatic exocrine dysfunction observed in diabetics ranging from 15–100%, we assume that the degree of pancreatic insufficiency is usually only mild to moderate. In these patients, clinically overt steatorhoea does not occur[18] and it is therefore questionable, whether minor impairment of pancreatic exocrine function is of major clinical relevance.

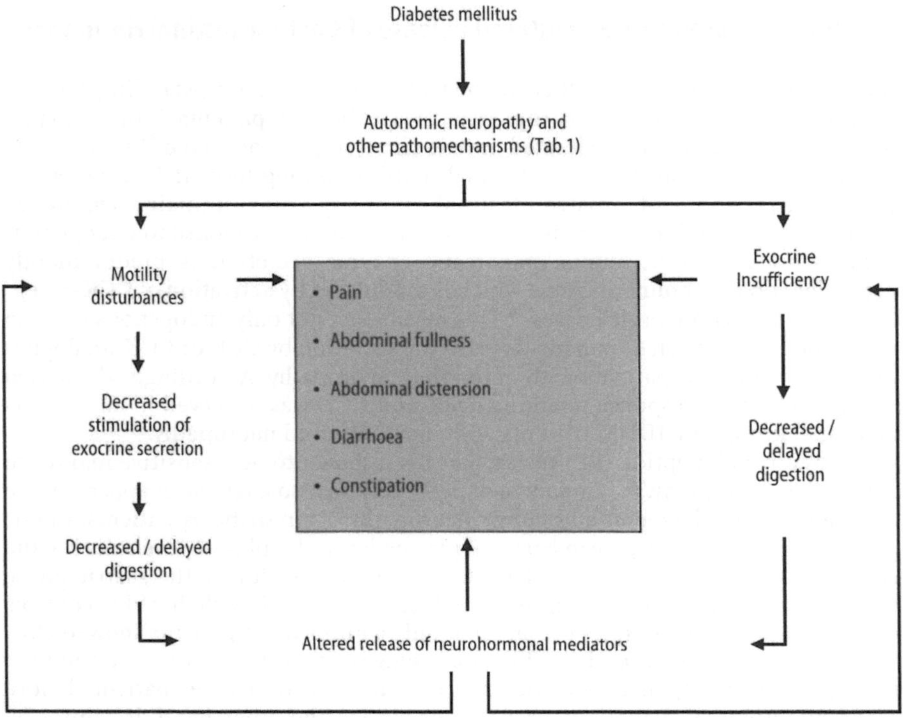

Figure 21.3. Pathophysiology of abdominal symptoms in diabetes mellitus: Regulatory pathways.

Under physiological circumstances, up to 80% of nutrients, particularly lipids, are absorbed proximal to the ligament of Treitz.[20;75;76] A complex interplay between gastric and small intestinal motility, on the one hand, and secretion of pancreatic and biliary juice, on the other hand ensures rapid and effective absorption: The stomach delivers only small portions of nutrients (2–3 kcal/min) to the duodenum in a regulated fashion. These are mixed thoroughly with pancreatic and biliary secretions and brought into contact with the absorptive epithelium by segmenting contractions of the small intestine. In mild-to-moderate pancreatic insufficiency, enzymatic activity is sufficient to achieve digestion and absorption of normal amounts of nutrients, overall. However, the site of main digestion is shifted to more distal segments of the small intestine. In response to increased nutrient exposure, release of distal intestinal (mostly inhibitory) mediators is enhanced.[20] This, in turn, causes regulatory disturbances of motor and secretory functions which, we can speculate, may contribute to abdominal symptoms (Fig. 21.3) and could be corrected by enzyme treatment.[20;77] Accordingly, restoration of regulatory disturbances may explain the favorable effect of enzyme therapy on pain in patients with chronic pancreatitis even in the absence of steatorrhoea.[78]

Patients with diabetes mellitus frequently suffer from a wide range of abdominal symptoms which markedly contribute to impairment of quality of life.[25;26] At least some of these symptoms such as pain and diarrhoea may be attributable in part to (compensated) pancreatic exocrine insufficiency (Fig. 21.2) and might respond to enzyme treatment. It has been shown that enzyme supplementation may decrease dyspeptic symptoms in healthy subjects following a high-fat meal,[79] but no studies have been reported of the effect of enzyme treatment on abdominal symptoms in diabetics. However, it has to be taken in mind that enzyme supplementation may exacerbate endocrine dysfunction as shown in patients with chronic pancreatitis and secondary diabetes mellitus.[80]

Consequently, potential beneficial effects of enzyme supplementation on abdominal symptoms in diabetes mellitus warrant clinical studies. On the other hand, potential adverse effects of enzyme supplementation on glucose homeostasis need to be carefully monitored.

References

1. Pollard H, Miller L, Brewer W. External secretion of the pancreas and diabetes (study of secretin test). Am J Dig Dis 1943; 10:20.
2. Icks A, Haastert B, Giani G, et al. Low fecal elastase-1 in type I diabetes mellitus. Z Gastroenterol 2001; 39:823–830.
3. Rathmann W, Haastert B, Icks A, et al. Low faecal elastase 1 concentrations in type 2 diabetes mellitus. Scand J Gastroenterol 2001; 36:1056–1061.
4. Chey WY, Shay H, Shuman CR. External pancreatic secretion in diabetes mellitus. Ann Intern Med 1963; 812–821.
5. Vacca JB, Henke WJ, Knight WA. The exocrine pancreas in diabetes mellitus. Ann Intern Med 1964; 61:242–247.
6. Frier BM, Saunders JH, Wormsley KG, et al. Exocrine pancreatic function in juvenile-onset diabetes mellitus. Gut 1976; 17:685–691.
7. Lankisch PG, Manthey G, Otto J, et al. Exocrine pancreatic function in insulin-dependent diabetes mellitus. Digestion 1982; 25:211–216.
8. Gröger G, Keller J, Bertram C, et al. Pancreatic enzyme responses are altered in patients with insulin dependent diabetes mellitus. Digestion 1999; 60:378(Abstract).
9. Hardt PD, Krauss A, Bretz L, et al. Pancreatic exocrine function in patients with type 1 and type 2 diabetes mellitus. Acta Diabetol 2000; 37:105–110.
10. El Newihi H, Dooley CP, Saad C, et al. Impaired exocrine pancreatic function in diabetics with diarrhea and peripheral neuropathy. Dig Dis Sci 1988; 33:705–710.
11. Lohr M, Kloppel G. Pathology of the pancreas in chronic type 1 diabetes mellitus: B-cell content, exocrine atrophy and angiopathy. Verh Dtsch Ges Pathol 1987; 71:114–119.
12. Alzaid A, Aideyan O, Nawaz S. The size of the pancreas in diabetes mellitus. Diabet Med 1993; 10:759–763.
13. Gilbeau JP, Poncelet V, Libon E, et al. The density, contour, and thickness of the pancreas in diabetics: CT findings in 57 patients. AJR Am J Roentgenol 1992; 159:527–531.
14. Silva ME, Vezozzo DP, Ursich MJ, et al. Ultrasonographic abnormalities of the pancreas in IDDM and NIDDM patients. Diabetes Care 1993; 16:1296–1297.
15. Imagawa A, Hanafusa T, Miyagawa J, et al. A proposal of three distinct subtypes of type 1 diabetes mellitus based on clinical and pathological evidence. Ann Med 2000; 32:539–543.
16. Imagawa A, Hanafusa T, Tamura S, et al. Pancreatic biopsy as a procedure for detecting in situ autoimmune phenomena in type 1 diabetes: close correlation between serological markers and histological evidence of cellular autoimmunity. Diabetes 2001; 50:1269–1273.
17. Gepts W. Pathology of the pancreas in juvenile diabetes. Diabetes 1965; 14:619–633(Abstract).
18. DiMagno EP, Go WL, Summerskill WH. Impaired cholecystokinin-pancreozymin secretion, intraluminal dilution, and maldigestion of fat in sprue. Gastroenterology 1972; 63:25–32.
19. Layer P, Ohe M, Groeger G, et al. Luminal availability and digestive efficacy of substituted enzymes in pancreatic insufficiency. Pancreas 1992; 7:745(Abstract).
20. Layer P, von der O, Holst JJ, et al. Altered postprandial motility in chronic pancreatitis: role of malabsorption. Gastroenterology 1997; 112:1624–1634.
21. Layer P, Peschel S, Schlesinger T, et al. Human pancreatic secretion and intestinal motility: effects of ileal nutrient perfusion. Am J Physiol 1990; 258:G196–G201.
22. Keller J, Conrads H, Goebell H, et al. Differential responses of human pancreatic and biliary secretion to graded ileal lipid perfusion. Digestion 1998; 59:206(Abstract).

23. Keller J, Conrads H, Holst JJ, et al. The ratios between pancreatic secretory enzymes are modulated by physiologic ileal lipid concentrations. Pancreas 1998; 17:442(Abstract).
24. Keller J, VanKrieken A, Goebell H, et al. Differential responses of pancreatic secretion and intestinal motility to graded ileal nutrient perfusion. Gastroenterology 1997; 112:452(Abstract).
25. Bytzer P, Talley NJ, Leemon M, et al. Prevalence of gastrointestinal symptoms associated with diabetes mellitus: a population-based survey of 15,000 adults. Arch Intern Med 2001; 161:1989–1996.
26. Talley SJ, Bytzer P, Hammer J, et al. Psychological distress is linked to gastrointestinal symptoms in diabetes mellitus. Am J Gastroenterol 2001; 96:1033–1038.
27. Lohr M, Kloppel G. Residual insulin positivity and pancreatic atrophy in relation to duration of chronic type 1 (insulin-dependent) diabetes mellitus and microangiopathy. Diabetologia 1987; 30:757–762.
28. Nakanishi K, Kobayashi T, Miyashita H, et al. Exocrine pancreatic ductograms in insulin-dependent diabetes mellitus. Am J Gastroenterol 1994; 89:762–766.
29. Lazarus SS, Volk BW. The effect of protracted glucagon administration on blood glucose and pancreatic morphology. Endocrinology 1958; 63:359–371.
30. Warren S, LeCompte PM. The pathology of diabetes mellitus. Philadelphia: Lea and Febiger, 1952.
31. Kloppel G, Clemens A. Insulin-dependent diabetes mellitus. Current aspects of morphology, etiology and pathogenesis. Pathologe 1996; 17:269–275.
32. Imagawa A, Hanafusa T, Miyagawa J, et al. A novel subtype of type 1 diabetes mellitus characterized by a rapid onset and an absence of diabetes-related antibodies. Osaka IDDM Study Group. N Engl J Med 2000; 342:301–307.
33. Foulis AK. Histology of the islet in insulin-dependent diabetes mellitus: a possible sequence of events. In: Pickup JC, Williams G, eds. Textbook of diabetes, 2 ed. Oxford: Blackwell Science, 1997: 15:24–29.
34. Fujita T, Murakami T. Microcirculation of monkey pancreas with special reference to the insulo-acinar portal system. A scanning electron microscope study of vascular casts. Arch Histol Jpn 1973; 35:255–263.
35. Groger G, Layer P. Exocrine pancreatic function in diabetes mellitus. Eur J Gastroenterol Hepatol 1995; 7:740–746.
36. Logsdon CD. Stimulation of pancreatic acinar cell growth by CCK, epidermal growth factor, and insulin in vitro. Am J Physiol 1986; 251:G487–G494.
37. Singh J. Mechanism of action of insulin on acetylcholine-evoked amylase secretion in the mouse pancreas. J Physiol 1985; 358:469–482.
38. Singh J, Adeghate E, Salido GM, et al. Interaction of islet hormones with cholecystokinin octapeptide-evoked secretory responses in the isolated pancreas of normal and diabetic rats. Exp Physiol 1999; 84:299–318.
39. Matsushita K, Okabayashi Y, Koide M, et al. Potentiating effect of insulin on exocrine secretory function in isolated rat pancreatic acini. Gastroenterology 1994; 106:200–206.
40. Kanno T, Saito A. The potentiating influences of insulin on pancreozymin-induced hyperpolarization and amylase release in the pancreatic acinar cell. J Physiol 1976; 261:505–521.
41. Singh J, Adeghate E. Effects of islet hormones on nerve-mediated and acetylcholine-evoked secretory responses in the isolated pancreas of normal and diabetic rats. Int J Mol Med 1998; 1:627–634.
42. Frier BM, Faber OK, Binder C, et al. The effect of residual insulin secretion on exocrine pancreatic function in juvenile-onset diabetes mellitus. Diabetologia 1978; 14:301–304.
43. Kramer MF, Tan HT. The peri-insular acini of the pancreas of the rat. Z Zellforsch Mikrosk Anat 1968; 86:163–170.
44. Duan RD, Wicker C, Erlanson-Albertsson C. Effect of insulin administration on contents, secretion, and synthesis of pancreatic lipase and colipase in rats. Pancreas 1991; 6:595–602.
45. Ferrer R, Medrano J, Diego M, et al. Effect of exogenous insulin and glucagon on exocrine pancreatic secretion in rats in vivo. Int J Pancreatol 2000; 28:67–75.
46. Lam WF, Gielkens HA, Coenraad M, et al. Effect of insulin and glucose on basal and cholecystokinin-stimulated exocrine pancreatic secretion in humans. Pancreas 1999; 18:252–258.
47. Kawamori R, Katsura M, Ishida S, et al. Subclinical exocrine pancreatic derangement in human diabetic patients evaluated from pure pancreatic juice. J Diabetes Complications 1995; 9:69–73.
48. Muller WA, Faloona GR, Aguilar-Parada E, et al. Abnormal alpha-cell function in diabetes. Response to carbohydrate and protein ingestion. N Engl J Med 1970; 283:109–115.
49. Unger RH, Aguilar-Parada E, Muller WA, et al. Studies of pancreatic alpha cell function in normal and diabetic subjects. J Clin Invest 1970; 49:837–848.
50. Ertan A, Arimura A, Akdamar K, et al. Pancreatic immunoreactive somatostatin and diabetes mellitus. Dig Dis Sci 1984; 29:625–630.

51. Dyck WP, Texter ECJ, Lasater JM, et al. Influence of glucagon on pancreatic exocrine secretion in man. Gastroenterology 1970; 58:532–539.
52. Konturek SJ, Tasler J, Obtulowicz W. Characteristics of inhibition of pancreatic secretion by glucagon. Digestion 1974; 10:138–149.
53. von der O, Layer P, Wollny C, et al. Somatostatin 28 and coupling of human interdigestive intestinal motility and pancreatic secretion. Gastroenterology 1992; 103:974–981.
54. Emoto T, Miyata M, Izukura M, et al. Simultaneous observation of endocrine and exocrine functions of the pancreas responding to somatostatin in man. Regul Pept 1997; 68:1–8.
55. Panicot L, Mas E, Thivolet C, et al. Circulating antibodies against an exocrine pancreatic enzyme in type 1 diabetes. Diabetes 1999; 48:2316–2323.
56. Mally MI, Cirulli V, Hayek A, et al. ICA69 is expressed equally in the human endocrine and exocrine pancreas. Diabetologia 1996; 39:474–480.
57. Semakula C, Vandewalle CL, Van Schravendijk CF, et al. Abnormal circulating pancreatic enzyme activities in more than twenty-five percent of recent-onset insulin-dependent diabetic patients: association of hyperlipasemia with high-titer islet cell antibodies. Belgian Diabetes Registry. Pancreas 1996; 12:321–333.
58. Lipp RW, Schnedl WJ, Hammer HF, et al. Effects of postprandial walking on delayed gastric emptying and intragastric meal distribution in longstanding diabetics. Am J Gastroenterol 2000; 95:419–424.
59. Gröger G, Kenter M, Schweflinghaus C, et al. Changes in small intestinal motility during the long-term course of insulin-dependent diabetes mellitus. Gastroenterology 1998; 118:A382(Abstract).
60. Adler G, Beglinger C, Braun U, et al. Interaction of the cholinergic system and cholecystokinin in the regulation of endogenous and exogenous stimulation of pancreatic secretion in humans. Gastroenterology 1991; 100:537–543.
61. Schwartz TW. Pancreatic polypeptide: a hormone under vagal control. Gastroenterology 1983; 85:1411–1425.
62. Schwartz TW, Stenquist B, Olbe L, et al. Synchronous oscillations in the basal secretion of pancreatic-polypeptide and gastric acid. Depression by cholinergic blockade of pancreatic-polypeptide concentrations in plasma. Gastroenterology 1979; 76:14–19.
63. Glasbrenner B, Dominguez-Munoz E, Riepl RL, et al. Cholecystokinin and pancreatic polypeptide release in diabetic patients with and without autonomic neuropathy. Dig Dis Sci 1995; 40:406–411.
64. Loba JM, Saryusz-Wolska M, Czupryniak L, et al. Pancreatic polypeptide secretion in diabetic patients with delayed gastric emptying and autonomic neuropathy. J Diabetes Complications 1997; 11:328–333.
65. Rasmussen MH, Carstensen H, List S, et al. Impaired pancreatic polypeptide response to a meal in type 1 diabetic patients: vagal neuropathy or islet cell dysfunction? Acta Endocrinol (Copenh) 1993; 128:221–224.
66. Nilsson H, Bergstrom B, Lilja B, et al. Prospective study of autonomic nerve function in type 1 and type 2 diabetic patients: 24 hour heart rate variation and plasma motilin levels disturbed in parasympathetic neuropathy. Diabet Med 1995; 12:1015–1021.
67. Achem-Karam SR, Funakoshi A, Vinik AI, et al. Plasma motilin concentration and interdigestive migrating motor complex in diabetic gastroparesis: effect of metoclopramide. Gastroenterology 1985; 88:492–499.
68. Rushakoff RA, Goldfine ID, Beccaria LJ, et al. Reduced postprandial cholecystokinin (CCK) secretion in patients with noninsulin-dependent diabetes mellitus: evidence for a role for CCK in regulating postprandial hyperglycemia. J Clin Endocrinol Metab 1993; 76:489–493.
69. Hirota M, Hashimoto M, Hiratsuka M, et al. Alterations of plasma immunoreactive glucagon-like peptide-1 behavior in non-insulin-dependent diabetics. Diabetes Res Clin Pract 1990; 9:179–185.
70. Layer P, Holst JJ, Grandt D, et al. Ileal release of glucagon-like peptide-1 (GLP-1). Association with inhibition of gastric acid secretion in humans. Dig Dis Sci 1995; 40:1074–1082.
71. Keller J, Franke A, Rippel K, et al. Termination of digestive pancreatic secretory and intestinal motor responses: importance of GLP-1 and PYY. Digestion 1999; 60:383(Abstract).
72. Franke A, Keller J, Holst JJ, et al. Glucagon-like peptide-1 decreases human endogenously stimulated exocrine pancreatic secretion. Pancreas 1996; 13:436–436(Abstract).
73. Grandt D, Bein S, Beglinger C, et al. Peptide YY inhibits interdigestive pancreatic enzyme secretion in humans. Pancreas 1995; 11:430(Abstract).
74. Grandt D, Gschossmann JM, Schimiczek M, et al. Peptide YY inhibits low-dose but not high-dose CCK-stimulated enzyme secretion in humans. Gastroenterology 1995; 108:972(Abstract).
75. Keller J, Runzi M, Goebell H, et al. Duodenal and ileal nutrient deliveries regulate human intestinal motor and pancreatic responses to a meal. Am J Physiol 1997; 272:G632–G637.

76. Holtmann G, Kelly DG, Sternby B, et al. Survival of human pancreatic enzymes during small bowel transit: effect of nutrients, bile acids, and enzymes. Am J Physiol 1997; 273:G553–G558.
77. Layer P, Keller J. Pancreatic enzymes: secretion and luminal nutrient digestion in health and disease. J Clin Gastroenterol 1999; 28:3–10.
78. Slaff J, Jacobson D, Tillman CR, et al. Protease-specific suppression of pancreatic exocrine secretion. Gastroenterology 1984; 87:44–52.
79. Suarez F, Levitt MD, Adshead J, et al. Pancreatic supplements reduce symptomatic response of healthy subjects to a high fat meal. Dig Dis Sci 1999; 44:1317–1321.
80. O'Keefe SJ, Cariem AK, Levy M. The exacerbation of pancreatic endocrine dysfunction by potent pancreatic exocrine supplements in patients with chronic pancreatitis. J Clin Gastroenterol 2001; 32:319–323.

Part 3

Hereditary Pancreatitis and Genetic Predispositions

22 Genetic Basis of Hereditary and Sporadic Pancreatitis

Jane E. Creighton and Richard M. Charnley

The clinical syndromes of hereditary pancreatitis and cystic fibrosis have been recognised for many years but it is only recently that there has been interest in establishing whether there is a genetic basis in some patients with sporadic pancreatitis. A proportion of patients, particularly those with 'idiopathic' disease, has a family history of pancreatitis and the increasing sophistication of molecular biology techniques has allowed this to be studied more fully.

Interest has focused on three genes in which mutations causing pancreatitis have been found. Mutations in the cationic trypsinogen gene (*PRSS1*), the cystic fibrosis transmembrane conductance regulator gene (*CFTR*), and the pancreas secreted trypsinogen inhibitor gene (*SPINK1*) have been shown to be associated with pancreatitis. However the mechanism by which they predispose to pancreatitis differs in each case.

Hereditary Pancreatitis

Mutations in the cationic trypsinogen gene (known as *PRSS1* in genetic nomenclature) have been shown to cause hereditary pancreatitis[1–3] Hereditary pancreatitis is an autosomal dominant condition with 80% penetrance. It is characterised by recurrent attacks of acute pancreatitis, which progress to the development of chronic pancreatitis over a variable period of time. Symptoms usually begin in childhood or adolescence, although onset at a more advanced age is not unusual.[4] With time, exocrine and/or endocrine insufficiency may develop. The clinical condition of hereditary pancreatitis was first reported in 1952,[5] and since then, many families have been described around the world.

Genetics of Hereditary Pancreatitis

The gene causing hereditary pancreatitis was mapped to chromosome 7q35 in 1996.[6;7] A mutation in the third exon of the cationic trypsinogen gene (*PRSS1*) was demonstrated by Whitcomb *et al* in the same year and was shown to cause hereditary pancreatitis.[8] This mutation is a guanine (G) to adenine (A) transition, which substitutes histidine (CAC) for arganine (CGC) at codon 117 (using the then accepted chymotrypsin numbering system). It was originally known as R117H. However, since the discovery of the cationic trypsinogen gene mutations, a new nomenclature system for human gene mutations has been devised and accepted. This has changed the name of this mutation from R117H to R122H.[9;10] This first mutation creates a novel recognition site for the restriction endonuclease *Afl*III, making it simple to identify in the laboratory. It has been shown recently that a neutral polymorphism within this enzyme recognition site may produce a false negative result.[11]

A second mutation in the cationic trypsinogen gene was subsequently discovered, which was found to be a single A to thiamine (T) transition in exon 2 resulting in an asparagine (ACC) to isoleucine (ATC) substitution at amino acid 29.[2] Again, earlier literature used the chymotrypsin numbering system, and this mutation was reported as N21I, rather than the currently accepted N29I.

These two mutations (R122H and N29I) have now been identified in families with hereditary pancreatitis from many countries including France,[3] Germany,[12] United Kingdom,[13] Japan[14] and the USA.[2;8] A further mutation, which appears to be much less common, is the A16V mutation, which was originally identified in three patients with idiopathic pancreatitis and in one patient with hereditary pancreatitis.[15] Other mutations have subsequently been described, but their relative importance in the aetiology of hereditary pancreatitis is unclear.[3;16;17]

There is also evidence that mutations in genes other than the cationic trypsinogen gene might be associated with hereditary pancreatitis.[18]

Pathophysiology

Understanding the mechanisms by which mutations in the cationic trypsinogen gene cause hereditary pancreatitis is important for several reasons. First, the cellular mechanisms of acute pancreatitis and progression to chronic pancreatitis in non-hereditary pancreatitis are poorly understood. Second, it is not known why the pancreas of one individual is susceptible to alcohol whilst the pancreas of another is not. Third, focusing on the link between genetics and pancreatitis might provide a clue to the aetiology of pancreatic cancer, which can occur as a complication in sporadic and hereditary pancreatitis.

Trypsinogen is secreted by the pancreatic acinar cell.[19] In the human pancreas, approximately two thirds is cationic trypsinogen and the remaining third is anionic trypsinogen. Trypsinogen is activated to trypsin within the duodenum by enterokinase, which cleaves an 8-aminoacid N-terminal peptide (trypsinogen activation peptide [TAP]). Trypsin then activates a cascade of digestive enzyme precursors. A number of mechanisms exist to prevent inappropriate activation of trypsin within the pancreas before its secretion into the duodenum. The pancreas produces pancreatic secretory trypsin inhibitor (PSTI), which is a protein, which competitively binds to and inactivates trypsin within the pancreas. It is theoretically able to deactivate up to 80% of trypsin activated in the pancreas. A second 'fail-safe' mechanism exists which involves the breakdown of trypsin by a number of enzymes, including trypsin itself. It is hypothesised that the R122H mutation alters a trypsin recognition site, which prevents deactivation of trypsin within the pancreas by this second mechanism. This prolongs the existence of inappropriately activated trypsin within the pancreas.[1] Studies on recombinant trypsins with and without the R122H substitution have demonstrated this prolongation of action in-vitro.[20–22]

The mechanism whereby the N29I mutation causes pancreatitis is unclear. It has been suggested, however, that the N29I mutation may impair trypsin inactivation by altering the accessibility of the initial hydrolysis site to trypsin. It may also enhance autoactivation of trypsinogen,[23] stabilise activated trypsin[24] or alter the binding of pancreatic secretory trypsin inhibitor (PSTI).[2] Predicted molecular conformational changes in the structure of trypsin support this.[1]

The pathogenic mechanism whereby the A16V mutation causes pancreatitis is speculative but it is thought to alter the cleavage site of the signal peptide.[15] There appears little doubt, however, that inappropriate prevention of the deactivation of trypsin within the pancreas is responsible for hereditary pancreatitis in the majority of cases.

The penetrance of cationic trypsinogen gene mutations remains at approximately 80% in the majority of studies. To investigate factors contributing to this, a study was carried out of monozygotic twins with hereditary pancreatitis.[25] Of 11 sets of twins, seven were suitable for this study. Whereas four of these seven sets were concordant for pancreatitis, three of the seven sets of twins (43%) were discordant for phenotypic expression of pancreatitis. The overall penetrance in the seven pairs of twins was 78%. The conclusion from this study was that genetic and/or environmental factors contribute to the expression and age of onset of hereditary pancreatitis. As yet the mechanism of non-penetrance remains unclear.

Clinical Presentation in Hereditary Pancreatitis

The clinical presentation of hereditary pancreatitis is variable, but in most cases, attacks of acute pancreatitis begin in childhood and progress to chronic pancreatitis with time.[5;26] The age of onset is highly variable, even within the same family.[4] The presentation during an acute attack is identical to an attack of gallstone-induced, alcoholic or idiopathic acute pancreatitis. The presentation of chronic pancreatitis in these patients is likewise indistinguishable from alcoholic, idiopathic or other forms of chronic pancreatitis.[26–28] Paediatric patients with hereditary pancreatitis have a similar presentation to idiopathic juvenile chronic pancreatitis.[29] It is, however, very common for these patients to remain undiagnosed for many years; they have often suffered from chronic symptoms since childhood.[30] We have found that recognition of the disease within a family may lead to several relatives being newly diagnosed with pancreatitis whereas previously they had been labelled as 'gallstones', 'peptic ulcer' or 'chronic abdominal pain'.

In Newcastle upon Tyne, UK, the pancreatic clinic now has individuals belonging to 14 families with hereditary pancreatitis. Data on nine of these families has been previously published.[13] The R122H (R117H) mutation was identified in three families and the N29I (N21I) mutation was demonstrated in a further five families. In a remaining family, no mutations were demonstrated in any of the five exons of the *PRSS1* gene. The families and patients belonging to the R122H group were compared with those belonging to the N29I group. Comparison of clinical details including complications of pancreatitis was carried out. The mean age at onset of symptoms of pancreatitis was lower in the R122H group at 8.4 vs 6.5 years, (p = 0.007) and more patients with the R122H mutation had developed symptoms by the age of 20 years (89% *vs* 64%). More patients with the R122H mutation required surgical intervention (8 of 12 vs 4 of 17, p = 0.029) and this tended to occur at an earlier age (not statistically significant). There was also a tendency for more patients with the R122H mutation to develop exocrine failure (NS) but the incidence and age of onset of endocrine failure (as measured by the development of insulin dependent diabetes mellitus) was similar in both groups. Patients in both groups identified alcohol as a provoking factor for the symptoms. These observations were also noted in the original description of the N29I mutation in 1997[2] and have also been reported by the European Registry of Hereditary Pancreatitis and Pancreatic Cancer (EUROPAC).[31] As an incidental finding, female patients also noted that menstruation or pregnancy provoked attacks. This has since been confirmed by other groups.[32]

It is also clear that as well as hereditary pancreatitis being identical to other forms of pancreatitis in terms of the mode of clinical presentation, the associated radiological and histopathological features are also identical.[33] Apart from earlier onset and delay in diagnosis, hereditary pancreatitis has been found to have a natural history similar to that of chronic alcoholic pancreatitis in terms of a similar prevalence of pancreatic calcification, and a similar amount of pancreatic insufficiency both endocrine and exocrine. However, the hereditary form has a higher prevalence of pseudocysts.[30]

Risk of Cancer in Hereditary Pancreatitis

Sporadic chronic pancreatitis carries a significantly increased risk of pancreatic cancer. This has been clearly demonstrated by a multi-centre historical cohort study of over 2000 patients.[38] The standardised incidence ratio, i.e. the ratio of observed to expected pancreatic cancers was 16.5. This study may have been subject to detection bias, in that increased surveillance of chronic pancreatitis patients may have increased the number of cancers diagnosed, compared with the general population. A study of Swedish patients, however, confirmed an increased risk of pancreatic cancer in sporadic chronic pancreatitis but with a standardised incidence ratio of 3.8.[39] Patients with hereditary pancreatitis have not been included in either of these studies but have since been examined for the risk of developing pancreatic cancer by the International Hereditary Pancreatitis Study Group. A cohort of 246 patients with hereditary pancreatitis was identified from ten countries with a mean follow-up period of over 14 years.[40] Eight patients with pancreatic adenocarcinoma were identified yielding a standardised incidence ratio of 53.3. The estimated cumulative risk of pancreatic cancer developing in these patients was nearly 40% and was greater for patients with a paternal inheritance pattern. These figures have been confirmed by the Midwest Multicentre Pancreatic Study Group.[41] The conclusions from these cancer studies are that, first chronic pancreatitis is a risk factor for pancreatic cancer, and second hereditary pancreatitis puts patients at an even higher risk of developing cancer than the sporadic disease. It is not known whether the risk of cancer is due to prolonged inflammatory change, or whether it is related to the presence of a cationic trypsinogen mutation per se. The evidence available at present, however, indicates that those patients with hereditary pancreatitis who develop cancer are those with a prolonged history of chronic pancreatitis.[41] The small number of cancers which have been documented in hereditary pancreatitis patients have so far not allowed an investigation into which mutation(s) might predispose to cancer more than another. This data, however, will be available with time. A study of pancreatic tissue from 34 patients with sporadic ductal adenocarcinoma has shown no specific relationship between the R122H mutation and pancreatic cancer.[42] Further such studies are expected, as tissue from patients with hereditary pancreatitis becomes available for analysis.

Management Dilemmas in Hereditary Pancreatitis

When faced with a patient or a family with a possible diagnosis of hereditary pancreatitis, three questions are commonly asked. First, what can be done about the patient with pancreatitis? Second, are other relatives likely to be affected? Third, what can be done to reduce the risk of cancer?

Management of the Pancreatitis

There are no specific medical therapies recommended in patients with hereditary pancreatitis. The management of acute attacks of pancreatitis is the same as for the sporadic disease that is, rehydration, analgesia and careful monitoring. Severe necrotising pancreatitis is rare in hereditary pancreatitis but pseudocysts seem to be relatively common. It has been suggested that antioxidant therapy may be helpful to prevent acute attacks but there is no evidence to support this and it is not currently recommended. Chronic pancreatitis should be treated as in any other patient. Enzyme supplements are likely to be required and analgesics as necessary. If diabetes mellitus occurs it is likely to require insulin therapy. Surgical treatment may be needed for complications such as pseudocyst, biliary obstruction or duodenal obstruction. In older patients requiring surgery a total pancreatectomy should be considered in order to abolish the cancer risk (see below).

Genetic Counselling of Relatives

Relatives should be told that although the majority of cases of hereditary pancreatitis are revealed by the age of 18, the disease might not manifest itself until the age of 30 or older. In these unaffected individuals, genetic testing confers no advantage and should be discouraged. Since unaffected (non-carrier) individuals and unaffected carriers do not have pancreatitis, evidence suggests that they carry no increased risk of developing cancer.

Screening of Hereditary Pancreatitis Patients for Cancer

Since patients with this disease exhibit a 53-fold increased risk of pancreatic cancer with a cumulative risk of 40% by the age of 70, an attempt at screening would appear to be essential. Unfortunately, no adequate screening test exists. The measurement of tumour markers, endoscopic techniques and radiological imaging lack the sensitivity and specificity for early diagnosis. Tumours are particularly difficult to detect on a background of chronic pancreatitis. It is thought therefore that molecular based strategies are likely to offer the best opportunities for the screening of these high risk patients for pancreatic ductal adenocarcinoma.[43] It has been suggested that the banking of blood and pancreatic juice samples should be mandatory in any screening protocol and that imaging of the pancreas should be carried out by endoscopic ultrasound.[44] One such protocol for the secondary screening of patients with hereditary pancreatitis has been established by EUROPAC (European Registry of Hereditary Pancreatitis and Pancreatic Cancer). As part of a research programme only, affected individuals over the age of 30 are offered imaging by CT and endoscopic ultrasound (EUS), followed, after genetic counselling, by genetic analysis of pancreatic juice obtained at ERCP for K-ras mutations. Patients negative for K-ras continue with repeat screening at 3 yearly intervals by CT, EUS and K-ras analysis of pancreatic juice. Patients who are K-ras positive undergo further genetic analysis looking for abnormalities in p53, p16 and aberrant methylation. If positive, these patients may be at risk of pancreatic ductal carcinoma and an attempt should be made to obtain cells for cytology by ERCP brushing of the pancreatic duct. The ultimate preventative measure in these patients would be a total pancreatectomy but this is a relatively high morbidity operation with the certainty of becoming diabetic. Certainly any patient with hereditary pancreatitis aged 30 or over, who requires surgery for relief of symptoms should undergo a total pancreatectomy rather than a lesser procedure, in order to abolish the cancer risk. This is not, however, appropriate in patients who are well unless there is clear evidence that they possess cellular atypia or a focal abnormality suspicious of cancer.

Hereditary pancreatitis is a fascinating condition which has provided new insights into the pathophysiology of pancreatitis. There are however many unanswered questions particularly in relation to the ways in which these mutations relate to pancreatitis and cancer. Management of these patients should be carried out by a team of experienced pancreatic specialists who are also able to provide genetic counselling. Registration of patients with one of the large Hereditary Pancreatitis Registries is essential if management strategies are to be improved and genetic research to be continued.

Cationic Trypsinogen Gene Mutations in Non-hereditary Pancreatitis

Taking a family history is very important in all patients with pancreatitis because the majority of patients with cationic trypsinogen gene mutations have a clear-cut family history of pancreatitis. It is, however, common for patients to be referred to a pancreatic specialist with so-called idiopathic pancreatitis without a reliable family history having been obtained.[34] It has also been considered whether idiopathic chronic pancreatitis might be due to *PRSS1* gene mutations. An investigation of patients with chronic alcoholic pancreatitis showed no evidence of the R122H or N29I mutation in 21 patients,[35] but a much larger and important study investigated 221 patients with idiopathic chronic pancreatitis and no family history. The entire *PRSS1* gene was sequenced in these patients. Only three patients had mutations, one with R122H and two patients with A16V.[16] A genetic background has also been investigated in patients with idiopathic juvenile chronic pancreatitis, a disease which closely mimics the clinical pattern of hereditary pancreatitis.[36] The R122H mutation was detected in one patient with idiopathic juvenile chronic pancreatitis and the A16V mutation was also found in one patient.

Table 22.1. *CFTR* mutations

Class I: Mutations affecting biosynthesis (preventing synthesis of full length, normal *CFTR* polypeptide);
Class II: Mutations affecting protein maturation (blocking processing and preventing *CFTR* reaching the apical membrane);
Class III: Mutations affecting Cl^- channel regulation (preventing function as a chloride channel);
Class IV: Mutations affecting Cl^- conductance or channel gating (reducing function);
Class V: Mutations causing reduced synthesis.

It is clear from these studies that new mutations do occur and that screening of individuals with idiopathic pancreatitis for cationic trypsinogen gene mutations is worthwhile. It is, therefore, our policy in patients with idiopathic pancreatitis, after exclusion of other causes, to perform genetic counselling and genetic testing. Many patients are keen to know their genetic status in relation to this disease.[37]

Cystic Fibrosis

Cystic fibrosis is recognised as being the most common recessive genetic disorder in Caucasian populations. It was shown to be caused by mutations in the cystic fibrosis transmembrane conductance regulator gene (*CFTR*) in 1989,[45] the most important of these being the △F508 mutation which causes classical cystic fibrosis and accounts for between 70 and 80% of all mutations in *CFTR*. Since the identification of the gene, cystic fibrosis has been shown to be a spectrum of syndromes rather than a single disease.[46–48] The clinical presentation can be correlated to the mutation causing the disease in some cases, although the relationship between the genotype and pancreatic disease is much closer than that between the genotype and lung disease.[49–51] To date, around 200 mutations and almost 1000 polymorphisms (alterations in the DNA which are either neutral or do not cause disease) have been recognized.[52] *CFTR* protein is a chloride channel protein, concerned with chloride transport across the cell membrane. Mutations in *CFTR* are classified into five groups according to the amount of functioning *CFTR* protein they cause to be present on the apical membrane of epithelial cells (Table 22.1).

When considering effects on the pancreas, the simplest classification is whether the mutation causes mild (pancreas sufficient) cystic fibrosis or severe (pancreas insufficient) disease. In Classes I, II and III, there is no or only minimal (typically <1% normal) *CFTR* protein on the cell surface, generally causing pancreas insufficient disease. In Classes IV and V, there is generally enough *CFTR* protein present to preserve pancreatic exocrine function. This picture is made more complicated by the presence of compound heterozygotes. These are individuals who carry two different *CFTR* mutations. In these cases, the more mild mutation acts dominantly, and a patient with a 'severe' and a 'mild' mutation will demonstrate mild cystic fibrosis (ie. will retain pancreatic exocrine function).

Cystic Fibrosis and Pancreatitis

Since its first description, cystic fibrosis has been associated with pancreatic dysfunction. Its relationship to pancreatitis is less clear. Acute pancreatitis has been reported as a rare complication of cystic fibrosis in a few cases.[53–55] It has also been reported as the presenting feature of cystic fibrosis in some young adults.[53;56–58] Studies on some patients with idiopathic pancreatitis have shown similar sweat electrolyte abnormalities to those seen in cystic fibrosis patients, although this has not always been supported by mutation analysis.[56] It is therefore not unexpected that mutations in *CFTR* have been shown to be associated with pancreatitis in some patients, but the mechanism by which mutations cause pancreatitis is not yet well understood, although pancreatitis appears to be associated with 'mild' *CFTR* mutations.

Studies of CFTR in Pancreatitis

Two important studies looking for *CFTR* mutations in patients with pancreatitis were published in 1998.[59;60] Cohn *et al* screened 27 patients with idiopathic chronic pancreatitis for 18 mutations in *CFTR*. Ten patients (37%) were found to have a mutation of one allele, and of these three had mutations of both alleles. Sharer *et al* studied a group of 134 patients, of whom 60 had idiopathic pancreatitis. Screening for 22 mutations was carried out and 18 patients (13.4%), of whom 12 had non-alcoholic pancreatitis, were shown to have a mutation of one allele. In both cases, there was a statistically significant difference from a control group. None of the patients studied had clinical evidence of cystic fibrosis lung disease, although further investigations in both groups did show some abnormalities in lung function tests and of nasal cyclic AMP mediated chloride transport. Cohn *et al* found one patient who was a compound heterozygote. This patient had both the ΔF508 (severe) and R117H (mild) mutations in *CFTR*.

In Newcastle-upon-Tyne, we studied a group of 48 patients with idiopathic pancreatitis. Mutation rich exons of the *CFTR* gene[50] were screened in these patients and the results compared to those in a control population. A significantly higher proportion of pancreatitis patients carried mutations, compared to the control group. Of particular interest was a patient who was found to be a compound heterozygote, who was subsequently found to have a family history of classical cystic fibrosis. This patient carried both the ΔF508 and P67L (mild) mutations.

Many more recent studies have demonstrated that patients with idiopathic pancreatitis are more likely to carry mutations in *CFTR* than a control population, including studies of non-caucasian populations.[61–71] It has also been shown that the majority of patients with pancreatitis assumed to be caused by *CFTR* mutations are compound heterozygotes.[72–74] In these patients there is sufficient functioning *CFTR* protein present on the cell surface to prevent the development of lung disease, but they have increased susceptibility to the development of pancreatitis. More complete mutational screening of *CFTR* is likely to demonstrate more mutations and in particular is likely to identify more compound heterozygotes.

Idiopathic pancreatitis is now formally recognised as part of the spectrum of *CFTR* associated diseases. However, it is clear that most individuals with *CFTR* mutations do not go on to develop pancreatitis. Screening for *CFTR* mutations is not recommended at present. Most of the pancreatitis associated mutations are not readily detected by the widely available screening methods, and a positive identification has no implications for clinical management.[75–78]

SPINK1

The identification of mutations in *PRSS1* and *CFTR* led to the screening of other candidate genes in order to investigate, more extensively, the intricacies of the inheritance of a susceptibility to pancreatitis. *SPINK1*, which codes for serine protease inhibitor Kazal type 1 (pancreatic secretory trypsin inhibitor or PSTI), has been studied in this context. The PSTI protein competitively inhibits inappropriately activated trypsin within the pancreas, and so mutations causing loss of function may be expected to predispose an individual to pancreatitis. A German study in 1999 investigated 96 children and adolescents with idiopathic pancreatitis. Mutations were found in 18 patients, of whom six were homozygous. The most common mutation was identified as N34S,[15] and this has also been shown in further studies.[79;80] A Japanese study also showed *SPINK1* mutations in a paediatric population, but another mutation (-215G'A) was found to be most prevalent.[81] More recently, it has been shown that the N34S mutation appears to be relatively common in patients with idiopathic pancreatitis, particularly of the juvenile onset type. Studies have reported mutation rates of between 4–12% in these patients.[82–84] Evidence is increasing that it does not in itself cause pancreatitis, but instead can be used as a marker and probably acts as a modifier on another gene, possibly *CFTR*.[85]

SPINK1 and CFTR

A number of studies have investigated this modifier function of *SPINK1* mutations by studying them in combination with mutations in *PRSS1* and *CFTR*. They have shown that the N34S mutation in *SPINK1* increases the risk of developing pancreatitis between 14 and 20 times as compared to a control population, and a mutation in *CFTR* increases the risk 40 times. The combination of mutations appears to act synergistically, increasing the risk between 600 and 900 times.[74;86] There is also some evidence that this combination predicts more severe disease in terms of an earlier onset of symptoms than a *CFTR* mutation alone. *SPINK1* is increasingly being viewed as a disease modifying rather than disease causing gene, and may also interact with mutations in *PRSS1*.[83;87]

Genetic Testing for CFTR and SPINK1 Mutations

Although the presence of mutations in *CFTR* and *SPINK1* increases the risk of developing pancreatitis, the majority of people with these mutations will remain asymptomatic, even if there is a family history of pancreatitis. In the case of *CFTR*, thorough mutation screening is difficult and commercial kits screening for the mutations more commonly associated with pancreatitis are not available. The presence of these mutations has not been shown to be associated with an increased risk of cancer, unlike *PRSS1* mutations in symptomatic patients. Identification of mutations does not help with the clinical management of these patients, and therefore at the present time screening is not recommended outside of a research protocol. An analysis of the arguments for and against genetic testing in idiopathic chronic pancreatitis has been previously cited.[76;78]

Conclusion

The last few years has seen a vast increase in our knowledge of the genetics of pancreatitis. In the majority of patients with hereditary pancreatitis, the mutation can now be identified but for this disease, preventing the development of pancreatic cancer remains the greatest challenge. Future research is also likely to improve our understanding of the genetics of pancreatic cancer. In addition, the identification of a genetic link between pancreatitis and CFTR and SPINK1 mutations has meant that now at least 30% of patients with idiopathic pancreatitis can be shown to have a genetic basis to their disease.

References

1. Whitcomb DC. Hereditary pancreatitis: new insights into acute and chronic pancreatitis. Gut 1999; 45:317–22.
2. Gorry MC, Gabbaizedeh D, Furey W, et al. Mutations in the cationic trypsinogen gene are associated with recurrent acute and chronic pancreatitis. Gastroenterology 1997; 113:1063–8.
3. Ferec C, Raguenes O, Salomon R, et al. Mutations in the cationic trypsinogen gene and evidence for genetic heterogeneity in hereditary pancreatitis. J Med Genet 1999; 36:228–32.
4. Sibert JR. Pancreatitis in children. A study in the North of England. Arch Dis Child 1975; 50:443–8.
5. Comfort MW, Steinberg AG. Pedigree of a family with hereditary chronic relapsing pancreatitis. Gastroenterology 1952; 21:54–63.
6. Whitcomb DC, Preston RA, Aston CE, et al. A gene for hereditary pancreatitis maps to chromosome 7q35. Gastroenterology 1996; 110:1975–80.
7. Pandya A, Blanton SH, Landa B, et al. Linkage studies in a large kindred with hereditary pancreatitis confirms mapping of the gene to a 16-cM region on 7q. Genomics 1996; 38:227–30.
8. Whitcomb DC, Gorry MC, Preston RA, et al. Hereditary pancreatitis is caused by a mutation in the cationic trypsinogen gene. Nat Genet 1996; 14:141–5.
9. Antonarakis SE. Recommendations for a nomenclature system for human gene mutations. Nomenclature Working Group. Hum Mutat 1998; 11:1–3.
10. Teich N, Hoffmeister A, Keim V. Nomenclature of trypsinogen mutations in hereditary pancreatitis. Hum Mutat 2000; 15:197–8.
11. Howes N, Greenhalf W, Rutherford S, et al. A new polymorphism for the RI22H mutation in hereditary pancreatitis. Gut 2001; 48:247–50.
12. Teich N, Mossner J, Keim V. Mutations of the cationic trypsinogen in hereditary pancreatitis. Hum Mutat 1998; 12:39–43.
13. Creighton JE, Lyall R, Wilson DI, et al. Mutations of the cationic trypsinogen gene in patients with hereditary pancreatitis. Br J Surg 2000; 87:170–5.
14. Nishimori I, Kamakura M, Fujikawa-Adachi K, et al. Mutations in exons 2 and 3 of the cationic trypsinogen gene in Japanese families with hereditary pancreatitis. Gut 1999; 44:259–63.
15. Witt H, Luck W, Becker M. A signal peptide cleavage site mutation in the cationic trypsinogen gene is strongly associated with chronic pancreatitis. Gastroenterology 1999; 117:7–10.
16. Chen JM, Piepoli BA, Le Bodic L, et al. Mutational screening of the cationic trypsinogen gene in a large cohort of subjects with idiopathic chronic pancreatitis. Clin Genet 2001; 59:189–93.
17. Le Marechal C, Bretagne JF, Raguenes O, et al. Identification of a novel pancreatitis-associated missense mutation, R116C, in the human cationic trypsinogen gene (PRSS1). Mol Genet Metab 2001; 74:342–4.
18. Bartness MA, Duerr RH, Ford MA, et al. Potential linkage of a pancreatitis related gene to chromosome 12. Pancreas 1998; 17:426.
19. Scheele G, Kern H. The Exocrine Pancreas. In Desnuelle P, Sjöström H, Norén O, eds. Molecular and Cellular Basis of Digestion, pp. 173–94. Amsterdam: Elsevier, 1986.
20. Kukor Z, Toth M, Pal G, et al. Human cationic trypsinogen. Arg(117) is the reactive site of an inhibitory surface loop that controls spontaneous zymogen activation. J Biol Chem 2002; 277:6111–7.
21. Sahin-Toth M. The pathobiochemistry of hereditary pancreatitis: studies on recombinant human cationic trypsinogen. Pancreatology 2001; 1:461–5.

22. Sahin-Toth M, Graf L, Toth M. Trypsinogen stabilization by mutation Arg117 -> His: a unifying pathomechanism for hereditary pancreatitis? Biochem Biophys Res Commun 1999; 264:505–8.
23. Sahin-Toth M, Toth M. Gain-of-function mutations associated with hereditary pancreatitis enhance autoactivation of human cationic trypsinogen. Biochem Biophys Res Commun 2000; 278:286–9.
24. Sahin-Toth M. Hereditary pancreatitis-associated mutation asn(21) -> ile stabilizes rat trypsinogen in vitro. J Biol Chem 1999; 274:29699–704.
25. Amann ST, Gates LK, Aston CE, et al. Expression and penetrance of the hereditary pancreatitis phenotype in monozygotic twins. Gut 2001; 48:542–7.
26. Perrault J. Hereditary pancreatitis. Gastroenterol Clin North Am 1994; 23:743–52.
27. Konzen KM, Perrault J, Moir C, et al. Long-term follow-up of young patients with chronic hereditary or idiopathic pancreatitis. Mayo Clin Proc 1993; 68:449–53.
28. Kattwinkel J, Lapey A, Di Sant'Agnese PA, et al. Hereditary pancreatitis: three new kindreds and a critical review of the literature. Pediatrics 1973; 51:55–69.
29. DuBay D, Sandler A, Kimura K, et al. The modified Puestow procedure for complicated hereditary pancreatitis in children. J Pediatr Surg 2000; 35:343–8.
30. Paolini O, Hastier P, Buckley M, et al. The natural history of hereditary chronic pancreatitis: a study of 12 cases compared to chronic alcoholic pancreatitis. Pancreas 1998; 17:266–71.
31. Howes N, Rutherford S, McRonald F, et al. Trypsinogen mutations in families with hereditary pancreatitis in the UK and Ireland. International Journal of Pancreatology 1999; 25:237.
32. Heinig J, Simon P, Weiss FU, et al. Treatment of menstruation-associated recurrence of hereditary pancreatitis with pharmacologic ovarian suppression. Am J Med 2002; 113:164.
33. Sossenheimer MJ, Aston CE, Preston RA, et al. Clinical characteristics of hereditary pancreatitis in a large family, based on high-risk haplotype. The Midwest Multicenter Pancreatic Study Group (MMPSG). Am J Gastroenterol 1997; 92:1113–6.
34. Creighton J, Lyall R, Wilson DI, et al. Mutations of the cationic trypsinogen gene in patients with chronic pancreatitis. Lancet 1999; 354:42–3.
35. Teich N, Mossner J, Keim V. Screening for mutations of the cationic trypsinogen gene: are they of relevance in chronic alcoholic pancreatitis? Gut 1999; 44:413–6.
36. Truninger K, Kock J, Wirth HP, et al. Trypsinogen gene mutations in patients with chronic or recurrent acute pancreatitis. Pancreas 2001; 22:18–23.
37. Applebaum-Shapiro SE, Peters JA, O'Connell JA, et al. Motivations and concerns of patients with access to genetic testing for hereditary pancreatitis. Am J Gastroenterol 2001; 96:1610–7.
38. Lowenfels AB, Maisonneuve P, Cavallini G, et al. Pancreatitis and the risk of pancreatic cancer. International Pancreatitis Study Group. N Engl J Med 1993; 328:1433–7.
39. Ekbom A, McLaughlin JK, Karlsson BM, et al. Pancreatitis and pancreatic cancer: a population-based study. J Natl Cancer Inst 1994; 86:625–7.
40. Lowenfels AB, Maisonneuve P, DiMagno EP, et al. Hereditary pancreatitis and the risk of pancreatic cancer. International Hereditary Pancreatitis Study Group. J Natl Cancer Inst 1997; 89:442–6.
41. Whitcomb DC, Applebaum S, Martin SP. Hereditary pancreatitis and pancreatic carcinoma. Ann NY Acad Sci 1999; 880:201–9.
42. Hengstler JG, Bauer A, Wolf HK, et al. Mutation analysis of the cationic trypsinogen gene in patients with pancreatic cancer. Anticancer Research 2000; 20:2967–74.
43. Howes N, Greenhalf W, Neoptolemos J. Screening for early pancreatic ductal adenocarcinoma in hereditary pancreatitis. Med Clin North Am 2000; 84:719–38, xii.
44. Martin SP, Ulrich CD. Pancreatic cancer surveillance in a high-risk cohort. Is it worth the cost? Med Clin North Am 2000; 84:739–xiii.
45. Riordan JR, Rommens JM, Kere B-S, et al. Identification of the Cystic Fibrosis Gene: Cloning and Characterisation of Complementary DNA. Science 1989; 245:1066–73.
46. Boyle MP. The spectrum of CFTR-related disease. Intern Med 2001; 40:522–5.
47. Castellani C, Quinzii C, Altieri S, et al. A pilot survey of cystic fibrosis clinical manifestations in CFTR mutation heterozygotes. Genet Test 2001; 5:249–54.
48. Noone PG, Knowles MR. 'CFTR-opathies': disease phenotypes associated with cystic fibrosis transmembrane regulator gene mutations. Respir Res 2001; 2:328–32.
49. Hamosh A, Corey M. Correlation between genotype and phenotype in patients with cystic fibrosis. The cystic fibrosis genotype-phenotype consortium. N Engl J Med 1993; 329:1308–13.
50. Zielenski J, Tsui L-C. Cystic Fibrosis: Genotypic and Phenotypic Variations. Annual Review of Genetics 1995; 29:777–807.
51. Zielenski J. Genotype and phenotype in cystic fibrosis. Respiration 2000; 67:117–33.
52. Naruse S, Kitagawa M, Ishiguro H, et al. Cystic fibrosis and related diseases of the pancreas. Best Pract Res Clin Gastroenterol 2002; 16:511–26.

53. Shwachman H, Lebenthal E, Khaw KT. Recurrent acute pancreatitis in patients with cystic fibrosis with normal pancreatic enzymes. Pediatrics 1975; 55:86–95.
54. Blythe SA, Farrell PM. Advances in the diagnosis and management of cystic fibrosis. Clinical Biochemistry 1984; 17:277–83.
55. Atlas AB, Orenstein SR, Orenstein DM. Pancreatitis in young children with cystic fibrosis. J Pediatr 1992; 120:756–9.
56. Bluestein PK, Gaskin K, Filler R, et al. Endoscopic retrograde cholangiopancreatography in pancreatitis in children and adults. Pediatrics 1981; 68:387–93.
57. Masaryk TJ, Achkar E. pancreatitis as the initial presentation of cystic fibrosis in young adults. Dig Dis Sci 1983; 28:874–8.
58. Conway SP, Peckham DG, Chu CE, et al. Cystic fibrosis presenting as acute pancreatitis and obstructive azoospermia in a young adult male with a novel mutation in the CFTR gene. Pediatr Pulmonol 2002; 34:491–5.
59. Cohn JA, Friedman KJ, Noone PG, et al. Relation between mutations of the cystic fibrosis gene and idiopathic pancreatitis. N Engl J Med 1998; 339:653–8.
60. Sharer N, Schwarz M, Malone G, et al. Mutations of the cystic fibrosis gene in patients with chronic pancreatitis. N Engl J Med 1998; 339:645–52.
61. Durie PR. Pancreatitis and mutations of the cystic fibrosis gene. N Engl J Med 1998; 339:687–8.
62. Arduino C, Gallo M, Brusco A, et al. Polyvariant mutant CFTR genes in patients with chronic pancreatitis. Clin Genet 1999; 56:400–4.
63. Bornstein JD, Cohn JA. Cystic fibrosis in the pancreas: recent advances provide new insights. Curr Gastroenterol Rep 1999; 1:161–5.
64. Castellani C, Bonizzato A, Rolfini R, et al. Increased prevalence of mutations of the cystic fibrosis gene in idiopathic chronic and recurrent pancreatitis. Am J Gastroenterol 1999; 94:1993–5.
65. Choudari CP, Lehman GA, Sherman S. Pancreatitis and cystic fibrosis gene mutations. Gastroenterol Clin North Am 1999; 28:543–viii.
66. Cohn JA, Jowell PS. Are mutations in the cystic fibrosis gene important in chronic pancreatitis? Surg Clin North Am 1999; 79:723–31, viii.
67. Malats N, Casals T, Porta M, et al. Cystic fibrosis transmembrane regulator (CFTR) DeltaF508 mutation and 5T allele in patients with chronic pancreatitis and exocrine pancreatic cancer. PANKRAS II Study Group Gut 2001; 48:70–4.
68. Arduino C, Gaia E. Genetics of chronic pancreatitis. Biomed Pharmacother 2000; 54:394–9.
69. Kimura S, Okabayashi Y, Inushima K, et al. Polymorphism of cystic fibrosis gene in Japanese patients with chronic pancreatitis. Dig Dis Sci 2000; 45:2007–12.
70. Ockenga J, Stuhrmann M, Ballmann M, et al. Mutations of the cystic fibrosis gene, but not cationic trypsinogen gene, are associated with recurrent or chronic idiopathic pancreatitis. Am J Gastroenterol 2000; 95:2061–7.
71. Truninger K, Malik N, Ammann RW, et al. Mutations of the cystic fibrosis gene in patients with chronic pancreatitis. Am J Gastroenterol 2001; 96:2657–61.
72. Castellani C, Gomez LM, Frulloni L, et al. Analysis of the entire coding region of the cystic fibrosis transmembrane regulator gene in idiopathic pancreatitis. Hum Mutat 2001; 18:166.
73. Cohn JA, Bornstein JD, Jowell PS. Cystic fibrosis mutations and genetic predisposition to idiopathic chronic pancreatitis. Med Clin North Am 2000; 84:621–31, ix.
74. Cohn JA, Noone PG, Jowell PS. Idiopathic pancreatitis related to CFTR: complex inheritance and identification of a modifier gene. J Investig Med 2002; 50:247S–55S.
75. DiMagno EP. Gene mutations and idiopathic chronic pancreatitis: clinical implications and testing. Gastroenterology 2001; 121:1508–12.
76. Cohn JA. Motion – Genetic testing is useful in the diagnosis of nonhereditary pancreatic conditions: Arguments against the motion. Can J Gastroenterol 2003; 17:53–5.
77. Rolston RK, Kant JA. Genetic testing in acute and chronic pancreatitis. Curr Gastroenterol Rep 2001; 3:115–20.
78. Whitcomb DC. Motion – Genetic testing is useful in the diagnosis of nonhereditary pancreatic conditions: Arguments for the motion. Can J Gastroenterol 2003; 17:47–52.
79. Witt H, Luck W, Hennies HC, et al. Mutations in the gene encoding the serine protease inhibitor, Kazal type 1 are associated with chronic pancreatitis. Nat Genet 2000; 25:213–6.
80. Witt H. Gene mutations in children with chronic pancreatitis. Pancreatology 2001; 1:432–8.
81. Kaneko K, Nagasaki Y, Furukawa T, et al. Analysis of the human pancreatic secretory trypsin inhibitor (PSTI) gene mutations in Japanese patients with chronic pancreatitis. J Hum Genet 2001; 46:293–7.
82. Gaia E, Salacone P, Gallo M, et al. Germline mutations in CFTR and PSTI genes in chronic pancreatitis patients. Dig Dis Sci 2002; 47:2416–21.

83. Audrezet MP, Chen JM, Le Marechal C, et al. Determination of the relative contribution of three genes-the cystic fibrosis transmembrane conductance regulator gene, the cationic trypsinogen gene, and the pancreatic secretory trypsin inhibitor gene-to the etiology of idiopathic chronic pancreatitis. Eur J Hum Genet 2002; 10:100–6.
84. Drenth JP, te MR, Jansen JB. Mutations in serine protease inhibitor Kazal type 1 are strongly associated with chronic pancreatitis. Gut 2002; 50:687–92.
85. Threadgold J, Greenhalf W, Ellis I, et al. The N34S mutation of SPINK1 (PSTI) is associated with a familial pattern of idiopathic chronic pancreatitis but does not cause the disease. Gut 2002; 50:675–81.
86. Noone PG, Zhou Z, Silverman LM, et al. Cystic fibrosis gene mutations and pancreatitis risk: relation to epithelial ion transport and trypsin inhibitor gene mutations. Gastroenterology 2001; 121:1310–9.
87. Truninger K, Ammann RW, Blum HE, et al. Genetic aspects of chronic pancreatitis: insights into aetiopathogenesis and clinical implications. Swiss Med Wkly 2001; 131:565–74.

23 Cytokines in Chronic Pancreatitis

Mark Cartmell and Andrew Kingsnorth

A role for genetics in the predisposition to chronic pancreatitis (CP) has been suggested for many years. Evidence is accumulating although none is conclusive.

Alcohol-induced pancreatitis occurs in approximately 5% of alcoholics[1] and alcoholic cirrhosis in around 10% and hepatitis in 10–35%,[2] whilst no, or minimal, pancreatic fibrosis is found in 32% of alcoholics.[3] The heterogeneity of the response to alcohol implicates genetic factors especially in pancreatic disease, whilst in liver disease and psychosis a genetic component beyond disposition to excessive alcohol use has been questioned.[4]

In the idiopathic form of the disease (ICP) two subtypes are sometimes recognised based on a bimodal distribution of age of onset;[5] early onset/juvenile and late onset ICP.[6] Aetiological factors remain to be identified.

Tropical chronic pancreatitis has long been known to have a familial tendency ever since the publications of Geevarghese and Pitchumoni.[7,8] More recent investigations in Southern India have again shown familial aggregation of cases.[9,10]

Whilst the pathogenesis is far from fully understood, chronic pancreatitis is multi-factorial in origin, with alcohol as a major 'factor'. The role of genetics may underpin many of the molecular and cellular effects already implicated in the disease process.

Cytokines

Cytokines are small peptides involved in cell-cell signalling in both a predominantly paracrine but also autocrine manner. They are secreted by leukocytes and other cell types and act through specific receptors. They are integral to the inflammatory and post-inflammatory cascades. They are sometimes regarded as being grouped by the cellular subtypes which secrete them, such as T-helper 1 *versus* T-helper 2 cells, there is however a great deal of overlap in their actions and some which remain to be fully elucidated.

Cytokines are a disparate group and individual cytokines are often pleiotropic (having multiple actions). They signal a number of 'messages' ranging from chemotaxis (the 'chemokines'), to cellular activation/proliferation to fibrosis. Not all are pro-inflammatory (e.g. interleukin(IL)-10), and a balance between for example a secreted receptor antagonist and agonist (IL-1a, IL-1b and IL-1 receptor antagonist) further enables regulation.

A Component of Genetic Predisposition Attributable to Cytokines

In any condition with an inflammatory or fibrotic basis, or even a component, this process will be subject to genetic predisposition. This response may predispose the individual to a more pro-inflammatory/fibrotic response, or an imbalanced response to a given (relevant) stimulus. The various hypotheses on the pathogenesis of CP involve inflammatory changes and then fibrosis. As such, the influence of the genetic variability of either the inflammatory response or fibrosis may affect predisposition to disease or progression of disease and therefore its clinical presentation. Cytokines are key mediators in both pathways.

Pathology and Cellular Involvement in CP

The pathology of chronic pancreatitis is typified by fibrotic changes, typically patchy in the early stages, with infiltration of leukocytes.[11]

Macrophage and T-cell infiltrates predominate and are found at increased levels in CP.[12–14] Lymphocytes are found at the margins of parenchyma and fibrosis and increase in greater numbers than do macrophages,[12] with a lesser proportion of memory cells than normal tissue or tissue adjacent to tumour.

Systemic increases in T-cells (both $CD4^+$ and $CD8^+$ subtypes) have been found in CP, apparently returning to normal after resection of an inflammatory mass in the pancreatic head.[13] In a study of peripheral leukocytes in CP,[14] an increased ratio of $CD4^+$:$CD8^+$ cells was found although there was no increase in total number of leukocytes or lymphocytes. This is in contrast to, but not incompatible with the findings of Emmerlich *et al.*[12] in pancreatic tissue, where $CD8^+$ cells just predominated. However, further studies of pancreatic tissue in CP did find a predominance of $CD4^+$ over $CD8^+$ cells in the pancreas in CP.[15,16]

According to the necrosis-fibrosis theory of chronic pancreatitis circulating leukocytes responding to cytokine chemotaxis infiltrate the pancreas and become resident cytotoxic T-cells. This is also compatible with other theories of pathogenesis. Recurrent acinar cell injury is caused by cytokine release from activated cytotoxic T-cells and macrophages, which also release TGF beta. TGF beta (a group of five cytokines) increases infiltration, differentiation and proliferation of stellate cells. In genetically susceptible individuals the environmental or toxic agent would trigger a greater inflammatory response causing an increase in cytokine mediators, which activate T-cells. The perpetuation of the antigenic stimulus and cytokine production results in destruction of pancreatic parenchyma and fibrosis, the magnitude of which is thus genetically determined.

Evidence for Cytokines in Chronic Pancreatitis

Cytokines involved in the T-cell and macrophage responses, such as TNFalpha, IFN-gamma and IL-1alpha and beta and IL-6 warrant consideration in CP as T-cells and macrophages are major cell types involved as discussed above.

In a study by Bamba *et al*[17]in 1994 serum levels of both IL-1beta and IL-6 were found to be elevated in patients with CP. Il-1b was confirmed as elevated in serum in CP.[18] The same authors found TNF-alpha at increased serum levels.[18]

Interestingly this study did not show increased levels of either IL-10 or TGF-beta (see below). In addition, mRNA (in peripheral blood mononuclear cells) of TNF-alpha and both soluble TNF-Receptors (p55 and p75) are significantly elevated in CP compared to healthy controls.[19] From these observations it is clear that the T-cell response in the pancreas is of the Th-1 type with a predominance of cells secreting TNF and related mediators.

Pancreatic cell lines have been shown to produce IL-6 and the chemokine IL-8 in response to TNF-alpha and to endotoxin,[20] implicating the pathway further. Chemokines IL-8 and MCP-1 are also secreted by human periacinar myofibroblasts in response to IL-1beta and TNF-alpha and RANTES in response to TNF-alpha, although a further chemokine (MIP-1alpha) was not elevated in this study.[21] Chemokines are also found in the pancreas of patients with CP, which are not found in normal pancreas.[22]

Apparently conflicting results with the above findings, in a study of the pancreatic juice of patients with CP did not detect IL-6, IL-10 or TNF alpha, although TGF-beta was found in a greater number of patients than controls.[23] TGF-beta has, on account of its role in the induction of fibrosis, been one of the most studied cytokines in chronic pancreatitis, although as stated above serum levels were not increased in one study.[18]

TGF-beta1 mRNA expression is increased in alcoholic CP, with transcripts found in several cell types including pancreatic stellate cells, acinar, and ductal cells.[24] An immunohistochemistry study showed TGF-beta maximal in ductal and acinar cells[25] and perifibrotic acinar cells and spindle cells,[26] with similar findings in human CP and a rat model. In a further study TGF-beta1 was found in CP throughout the ducts, rather than isolated acinar and distal ductular cells in normal controls.[27] Analogous findings were shown with enhanced mRNA expression of TGF beta1, TGF beta Receptor-II, connective tissue growth factor (which is regulated by TGF beta), and collagen type I in CP compared with normal controls.[28]

Functional animal studies investigating TGFbeta also suggest a role in CP. A rat model indicated a peak of TGFbeta 1 activity occurring before the peak of fibrosis.[29] The pancreas morphology of transgenic mice that overexpress transforming growth factor-beta1 (TGF-beta1) in the pancreas partially resembles morphological features of chronic pancreatitis, (such as progressive accumulation of extracellular matrix). Also increased mRNA levels of TGF-beta1 occur early and coincidentally with collagen types I and III and later with increasing numbers of pancreatic stellate cells.[30] Another study of a transgenic mouse overexpressing TGF beta1 in pancreatic beta cells revealed massive fibrosis of the pancreas; in adult mice, most of the acini were replaced by fibrotic and adipose tissues.[31] In a series of studies by van Laetham *et al.* TGFbeta was not only being secreted in ductal cells and mononuclear cells[32] in humans, but was shown to promote fibrosis following repeated bouts of experimental acute pancreatitis.[33]

Evidence for a Genetic Component to Cytokine Responses in CP

With the study of cytokines in chronic, as opposed to acute, pancreatitis in its infancy, the evidence regarding a genetic component in the responses of different cytokines is also early in its development. The 'Th1 cytokines' involved with recruitment and activation of T cells and macrophages are implicated by the evidence above and are the first to have been studied with regard to genetic predisposition.

In a study by our group, an association between CP and genetic variation in the IFN gamma gene (a micro-satellite in intron 1) was found in a study of 54 patients with CP and 104 controls. Increased frequencies of the 12 (high production) and 14 alleles were associated with CP.[34] This is in keeping with a Th-1 response in the pancreas.

Preliminary studies from two groups have looked at a possible role for genetic predisposition in relation to TNF alpha. A difficulty, as with any genetic study, is with the surrounding area of the chromosome, for example, the TNFalpha gene lies within the MHC (class III) region. This is proposed as the reason for an apparent functional association of TNF levels associated with the TNF alpha –238 polymorphism in anti-phospholipid syndrome.[35]

Examining the polymorphisms at the -238 and -308 positions in the promoter region of the TNF-alpha gene; the frequency of the variant allele at -308 is associated with increased transcription (in a reporter gene study)[36] and increased production of TNFalpha.[37] The variant allele was found at significantly higher frequency in patients with AICP; whilst for the -238 polymorphism, there was no difference in the frequency.[38]

Data from our group also indicates a possible genetic role in TNF alpha studied with regard to microsatellite haplotypes. However, in this study those haplotypes associated with intermediate function, notably the TNFa6b5 c1d3e3 haplotype, were found significantly more frequently in CP than normal controls, with a suggestion of an association of the higher secreting haplotypes with alcoholic liver disease.[39]

In a previous study, in acute pancreatitis, of an IL-1alpha (intron 6, di-nucleotide repeat) polymorphism we have associated the 2,4 genotype with alcoholic acute pancreatitis and worse organ failure score with the 1,2 genotype.[40] In a study of this polymorphism in 52 patients with CP and 150 controls we could not identify an analogous association either with the 2,4 genotype and AICP, the 1,2 genotype with CP as a whole or any other genotypes or alleles; thus genetic variation in IL-1a does not appear to affect disposition to CP (unpublished data).

In a further unpublished study (D.A. O'Reilly, personal communication) looking at an NFkB micro-satellite polymorphism (a transcription factor playing a pivotal role in cytokines transcription) also found no significant associations were found with CP.

The data presented above would make examination of a genetic component in TGF beta production in CP an interesting avenue of investigation. This is especially true with functional polymorphism of TGFbeta 1 having been described.[41]

What Does all this Mean?

Although difficult to interpret with such sparse data it seems that some of the cytokines responsible for the cellular processes seen in CP may well have a genetic component to their response. This association may simply be with increased production, or be more complicated with involvement and disruption of the delicate balance of pro- and anti-inflammatory and pro- or anti-fibrotic pathways.

References

1. Dreiling DA. The Natural History of Alcoholic Pancreatitis: Update 1985. Mount Sinai J of Medicine 1985; 52:340–342.
2. Grant BF, Dufour MC, Harford TC. Epidemiology of alcoholic liver disease. Semin Liver Dis 1988; 8:12–25.
3. Pitchumoni CS, Glasser M, Saran RM, et al. Pancreatic fibrosis in chronic alcoholics and non-alcoholics without clinical pancreatitis. Am J Gastroenterol 1984; 79:382–388.
4. Reed T, Page WF, Viken RJ, et al. Genetic Predisposition to Organ-Specific Endpoints of Alcoholism. Alcoholism, Clin and Exp Res 1996; 20:1528–1533.
5. Chari ST, Singer MV. Idiopathic Chronic Pancreatitis. Chapter 68 In 'The Pancreas' Eds Beger HG, et al. pp. 683–687. Blackwell Science Ltd., 1998.
6. Layer P, Yamamoto H, Kalthoff L, et al. The different courses of early- and late-onset idiopathic and alcoholic chronic pancreatitis. Gastroenterology 1994; 107:1481–1487.
7. Pitchumoni CS, Geevarghese PJ. Familial Pancreatitis and Diabetes Mellitus, 1966.
8. Pitchumoni CS. Familial Pancreatitis. In 'Pancreatic Diseases' Eds Pai KN, Soman CR, Varghese R pp. 46–48. Geo Printers, Trivandrum, 1970.
9. Mohan V, Chari ST, Hitman GA, et al. Familial Aggregation in Tropical Fibrocalculus Pancreatic Diabetes. Pancreas 1989; 4:690–693.
10. Thomas PG, Augustine P, Ramesh H, et al. Observations and Surgical Management of Tropical Pancreatitis in Kerala and Southern India. World J of Surg 1990; 14:32–42.
11. Kloppel G, Maillet B. Pathology of Chronic Pancreatitis. Chapter 73 In 'The Pancreas' Eds Beger HG, et al. pp. 720–723. Blackwell Science Ltd., 1998.
12. Emmrich J, Weber I, Nausch M, et al. Immunohistochemical Characterization of the Pancreatic Cellular Infiltrate in Normal Pancreas, Chronic Pancreatitis and Pancreatic Carcinoma. Digestion 1998; 59:192–198.
13. Gansauge F, Gansauge S, Eh M, et al. Distributional and functional alterations of immuno-competent peripheral blood lymphocytes in patients with chronic pancreatitis. Ann Surg 2001; 233:365–370.
14. Ockenga J, Jacobs R, Kemper A, et al. Lymphocyte subsets and cellular immunity in patients with chronic pancreatitis. Digestion 2000; 62:14–21.
15. Ebert MP, Ademmer K, Muller-Ostermeyer F, et al. CD8+CD103+ T cells analogous to intestinal intraepithelial lymphocytes infiltrate the pancreas in chronic pancreatitis. Am J Gastroenterol 1998; 93:2141–2147.
16. Hunger RE, Mueller C, Z'Graggen K, et al. Cytotoxic Cells are Activated in Cellular Infiltrates of Alcoholic Pancreatitis. Gastroenterology 1997; 112:1656–1663.
17. Bamba T, Yoshioka U, Inoue H, et al. Serum levels of interleukin-1 beta and interleukin-6 in patients with chronic pancreatitis. J Gastroenterol 1994; 29:314–319.
18. Szuster-Ciesielska A, Daniluk J, Kandefer-Zerszen M. Serum levels of cytokines in alcoholic liver cirrhosis and pancreatitis. Arch Immunol Ther Exp (Warsz) 2000; 48:301–307.
19. Hanck C, Rossol S, Hartmann A, et al. Cytokine gene expression in peripheral blood mononuclear cells reflects a systemic immune response in alcoholic chronic pancreatitis. Int J Pancreatol 1999; 26:137–145.
20. Blanchard JA, Barve S, Joshi-Barve S, et al. Cytokine production by CAPAN-1 and CAPAN-2 cell lines. Dig Dis Sci 2000; 45:927–932.
21. Andoh A, Takaya H, Saotome T, et al. Cytokine regulation of chemokine (IL-8, MCP-1, and RANTES) gene expression in human pancreatic periacinar myofibroblasts. Gastroenterology 2000; 119:211–219.
22. Saurer L, Reber P, Schaffner T, et al. Differential expression of chemokines in normal pancreas and in chronic pancreatitis. Gastroenterology 2000; 118:356–367.
23. Kazbay K, Tarnasky PR, Hawes RH, et al. Increased transforming growth factor beta in pure pancreatic juice in pancreatitis. Pancreas 2001; 22:193–195.
24. Casini A, Galli A, Pignalosa P, et al. Collagen type I synthesized by pancreatic periacinar stellate cells (PSC) co-localizes with lipid peroxidation-derived aldehydes in chronic alcoholic pancreatitis. J Pathol 2000; 192:81–89.
25. Korc M, Friess H, Yamanaka Y, et al. Chronic pancreatitis is associated with increased concentrations of epidermal growth factor receptor, transforming growth factor alpha, and phospholipase C gamma. Gut 1994; 35:1468–1473.
26. Haber PS, Keogh GW, Apte MV, et al. Activation of pancreatic stellate cells in human and experimental pancreatic fibrosis. Am J Pathol 1999; 155:1087–1095.

27. Slater SD, Williamson RC, Foster CS. Expression of transforming growth factor-beta 1 in chronic pancreatitis. Digestion 1995; 56:237–241.
28. di Mola FF, Friess H, Martignoni ME, et al. Connective tissue growth factor is a regulator for fibrosis in human chronic pancreatitis. Ann Surg 1999; 230:63–71.
29. Su SB, Motoo Y, Xie MJ, et al. Expression of transforming growth factor-beta in spontaneous chronic pancreatitis in the WBN/Kob rat. Dig Dis Sci 2000; 45:151–159.
30. Vogelmann R, Ruf D, Wagner M, et al. Effects of fibrogenic mediators on the development of pancreatic fibrosis in a TGF-beta1 transgenic mouse model. Am J Physiol Gastrointest Liver Physiol 2001; 280:G164–G172.
31. Sanvito F, Nichols A, Herrera PL, et al. TGF-beta 1 overexpression in murine pancreas induces chronic pancreatitis and, together with TNF-alpha, triggers insulin-dependent diabetes. Biochem Biophys Res Commun 1995; 217:1279–1286.
32. Van Laethem JL, Deviere J, Resibois A, et al. Localization of Transforming Growth Factor beta 1 and its latent binding protein in human chronic pancreatitis. Gastroenterology 1995; 108:1873–1881.
33. Van Laethem JL, Robberecht P, Resibois A, et al. Transforming Growth Factor beta promotes development of fibrosis after repeated courses of acute pancreatitis in mice. Gastroenterology 1996; 110:576–582.
34. O'Reilly DA, Jahromi M, Cartmell MT, et al. Association of Interferon gamma Genetic Polynorphisms with Susceptibility to Chronic Pancreatitis (abstract). Digestion 2000; 61:A111.
35. Bertolaccini ML, Atsumi T, Lanchbury JS, et al. Plasma tumor necrosis factor alpha levels and the -238*A promoter polymorphism in patients with antiphospholipid syndrome. Thrombosis and Haemostasis 2001; 85:198–203.
36. Wilson AG, Symons JA, McDowell TL, et al. Effects of a Polymorphism in the Human Tumor Necrosis Factor Promoter on Transcriptional Activation. Proc Natl Acad Sci USA 1997; 94:3195–3199.
37. Louis E, Franchimont D, Piron A, et al. Tumour necrosis factor (TNF) gene polymorphism influences TNF-alpha production in lipopolysaccharide (LPS)-stimulated whole blood cell culture in healthy humans. Clin Exp Immunol 1998; 113:401–406.
38. Abdulrazeg E-SM, Alfirevic A, Gilmore IT, et al. TNFalpha Promoter Region Polymorphisms In Patients with Alcohol-Induced Chronic Pancreatitis (abstract). Gastroenterology 2000; A167.
39. O'Reilly DA, Dunlop S, Sargen K, et al. Different Tumour Necrosis Factor Haplotypes are Associated with Alcoholic Pancreatitis than with Alcoholic Liver Disease (abstract). Int J of Pancreatology 2000; 28:141.
40. AM. Cytokine Gene Polymorphisms and Acute Pancreatitis. PhD Thesis University of Plymouth Smithies, 2001.
41. Awad MR, El Gamel A, Hasleton P, et al. Genotypic variation in the transforming growth factor-beta1 gene: association with transforming growth factor-beta1 production, fibrotic lung disease, and graft fibrosis after lung transplantation. Transplantation 1998; 66:1014–1020.

24 Cytokine Gene Polymorphisms in Acute Pancreatitis

Colin J. McKay and Anton Buter

Acute pancreatitis is increasing in incidence but overall mortality has remained steady in the past decade at approximately 8%.[1] Death from acute pancreatitis is usually the result of multiple organ dysfunction syndrome (MODS). Like other acute inflammatory conditions, MODS in acute pancreatitis is associated with the release of cytokines, chemokines and other inflammatory mediators.[2–5] Increased expression of a wide variety of mediators has been reported in patients with severe acute pancreatitis although the association between the dynamics of the cytokine response and the development of MODS or death is less clear.[2] It seems that the persistence of an inflammatory response is the important factor in the pathophysiology of MODS. In a recent study of 121 patients with predicted severe acute pancreatitis,[6] more than 60% of cases met the criteria for the systemic inflammatory response syndrome (SIRS). Forty-four of these patients developed MODS and this was strongly associated with persistence of SIRS for more than 48 h. Mortality overall was 11% and was confined to the small subgroup of patients with *deteriorating* MODS. Previous studies, based on the original Atlanta criteria,[7] have grouped all patients with MODS as having 'severe' pancreatitis (including patients with both transient and persisting MODS) and compared these with the larger group of patients with uncomplicated attacks. These recent clinical data suggest that it is only the small subgroup of patients with deteriorating MODS in whom the inflammatory response should be considered pathological. In the remainder of patients, homeostasis is rapidly restored.[6]

If deteriorating MODS is a consequence of the persistence of an inflammatory response, this may be a consequence of an imbalance between pro-inflammatory cytokines (such as TNF, IL-8, and IL-1ß)and anti-inflammatory cytokines (including IL-10 and IL-1RA). This failure of self-regulation of the inflammatory response may be due to an on-going pro-inflammatory stimulus (perhaps driven by pancreatic necrosis) or to a failure of key regulatory cytokines to control the inflammatory response. There is a great deal of genetic variability in the cytokine response to injury and it is unclear to what degree the severity of any given attack is due to the magnitude of the insult to the pancreas or to genetic control of the innate inflammatory response.

Genetic Influence on TNF Expression

There is evidence that both the humoral and cellular response are subject to polymorphic genetic control and that cytokines play a major role in this.[8] In keeping with this hypothesis, there are large and stable inter-individual differences in the capacity of monocytes to produce TNF[9] and IL-10.[10] A study of monozygotic twins allowed the inherited component of differences in TNF and IL-10 production to be estimated at 60 per cent and 75 per cent respectively.[11]

TNF Gene Variability

The diversity in TNF production ability was initially correlated with class II HLA genotype.[12] However, the location of the TNF gene within the major histocompatibility complex raised the possibility that genetic differences in the TNF locus may be directly involved.[9] The TNF locus is 12 kilobases in length and contains several polymorphic areas including five micro satellites.[13] Of the five microsatellites (TNFa to e), the TNFa microsatellite has the greatest level of variation, with 14 recorded alleles (named TNFa1 to TNFa14) in the population.[13] It has been shown that the TNFa2 microsatellite allele is associated with high TNF secretion, whereas the TNFa6 allele is associated with lower TNF production from lipopolysaccharide (LPS) activated monocytes.[14] In addition to the microsatellite polymorphisms, several single nucleotide polymorphisms of TNF have been identified within the promoter region of the gene. Of these, a polymorphism affecting TNF production has been identified at the –308 position. Substitution of A (TNF1) for G (TNF2) at this position is associated with increased TNF transcription.[15] Finally, cleavage within the TNF locus by the restriction enzyme Nco1identifies a bi-allelic restriction fragment length polymorphism, TNFB. Individuals who are homozygous for TNFB2 have higher levels of TNF production than heterozygous individuals or those homozygous for TNFB1,[14]

TNF Gene Polymorphisms in Acute Illness

TNF is a central mediator of the systemic manifestations of severe sepsis and multiple organ dysfunction associated with major trauma, burn injury and other acute illness. Several studies have examined the possible influence of TNF gene polymorphisms on outcome in these conditions. In 40 patients with severe sepsis, Stuber and colleagues examined the relationship between the Nco1 polymorphism and outcome.[16] Patients homozygous for TNFB2 (associated with high TNF production) had increased mortality compared to heterozygous patients. These patients also had higher circulating levels of TNF. The same TNF polymorphism was studied in a cohort of 110 patients with severe blunt trauma.[17] Once again, patients homozygous for TNFB2 were at increased risk of developing severe sepsis and had higher circulating TNF levels.

Similar results have been reported when the –308 single nucleotide polymorphism was studied in severe sepsis. In a multi-centre study from France,[18] Mira and colleagues reported significantly greater mortality in patients homozygous or heterozygous for TNF2. After correction for age and severity of illness, patients with TNF2 had a 3.7-fold increased risk of death. Tang and colleagues also reported increased mortality in patients with TNF2 who developed septic shock following surgery.[19] Conflicting results were reported by Stuber's group who found no association with the –308 polymorphism and outcome,[20] in contrast to their findings with the Ncol polymorphism.[16] Taken together, these studies suggest that carrying a TNF polymorphism associated with increased TNF production is associated with a poor outcome following the development of severe sepsis.

TNF Polymorphisms in Acute Pancreatitis

Two studies have assessed the relationship between TNF gene polymorphisms and outcome. In a study from Edinburgh,[21] both the Ncol polymorphism and the −308 SNP were studied in 113 patients with mild attacks and 77 severe cases. Neither polymorphism was related to the severity of acute pancreatitis. The frequency of the polymorphisms studied was also similar in patients with acute pancreatitis and healthy controls. Kingsnorth and colleagues studied the TNF −308 SNP in 135 patients with acute pancreatitis.[22] TNF1 was present in 16% of patients compared with 22% of controls, with no significant difference between mild and severe cases. The same group analysed the frequencies of the TNF microsatellite polymorphisms and reported no significant difference in TNFa2 between mild and severe acute pancreatitis or between acute pancreatitis patients and healthy controls. Our group in Glasgow carried out a similar study in 104 patients with predicted severe acute pancreatitis. One hundred and four patients with acute pancreatitis were included. The aetiology of pancreatitis was gallstones (67%), alcohol (17%), induced by endoscopic retrograde cholangiopancreatography (ERCP) (3%) and unknown (13%). We analysed the frequencies of the TNF microsatellite polymorphisms in relation to the development of MODS and in comparison to a group of healthy blood donors. The microsatellite associated with high TNF production, TNFa2, was present in 36% of patients compared with 20% of controls. In the published studies in patients with severe sepsis, polymorphisms associated with high TNF production are associated with a poor outcome. We therefore analysed the frequency of TNFa2 in those patients who developed MODS in order to determine if the same pattern was seen in acute pancreatitis. Twelve patients with early organ dysfunction who died were compared with the 36 patients with MODS who survived. There was no difference in the frequency of the TNFa2 allele (25 per cent *vs.* 39 per cent; $p = 0.32$, $OR = 0.52$, $CI = 0.19–1.48$). Therefore, unlike in the published studies in sepsis, the polymorphism associated with high TNF production was if anything less common in non-survivors than survivors. It is therefore difficult to determine the clinical importance of the initial observation, as patients with TNFa2 had no increase in mortality or of severe systemic complications. A further difficulty in interpreting these data is the natural variation in allele frequency between populations, particularly when such small numbers of patients are studied. In the Plymouth study[22] for example, the frequency of TNFa2 in the healthy control population was 36%, identical to that seen in the Glasgow patient group. Indeed, in that study, patients with acute pancreatitis actually had a lower frequency of TNFa2 than the control group.

Interleukin 10 Gene Variability

The promoter region of the IL-10 gene contains several single nucleotide polymorphisms that are related to differences in IL-10 production.[23] Two IL-10 microsatellite polymorphisms, IL10.R and IL-10.G are also related to IL-10 production with IL10.R3/G7 haplotypes being associated with low IL-10 production and IL10.R2/G14 with high IL-10 production in a stimulated whole blood assay.[10] Kingsnorth's group has reported the frequencies of three single nucleotide polymorphisms of the IL-10 promoter in patients with acute pancreatitis. No difference was observed between IL-10 SNP frequencies and severity of disease. Allele frequencies in patients with acute pancreatitis were similar to healthy controls. Our group reported the early results of a study in which the low IL-10 secreting haplotype, IL10.R3, was compared in patients with severe and mild acute pancreatitis. There was no difference in the frequency of the IL10.R3 allele when patients with acute pancreatitis were compared with controls (40 per cent vs. 31%, $p = 0.07$, odds ratio = 0.69, confidence interval = 0.45–1.04). Fatal acute pancreatitis was associated with an increase in the frequency of IL-10.R3 from 24% to 50% ($p = 0.02$, OR = 3.24, CI = 1.23–8.51). These results suggested that polymorphisms other than IL10.R3 may protect against the most severe manifestations of acute pancreatitis but this observation will need to be tested against a much larger patient group before any meaningful conclusions can be drawn.

Interleukin 1 Gene Variability

The genes encoding interleukin 1 (IL-1a and IL-1b) and interleukin 1 receptor antagonist (IL-1ra) are located within the same region on chromosome 2 and these genes are also highly polymorphic. A bi-allelic restriction fragment length polymorphism exists in the IL-1b gene, and allele 2 is associated with increased mortality in patients with sepsis.[24] Two studies have analysed the association between IL-1b gene polymorphisms and outcome in acute pancreatitis[21,25] but in both, the frequency of allele 2 was similar in healthy controls and in patients with acute pancreatitis, regardless of severity.

A polymorphism of the IL-1ra gene has also been described and, in severe sepsis, patients homozygous for allele 2 were reported to have an increased mortality rate.[24,26] Mononuclear cells from patients homozygous for allele 2 also have lower IL-1ra production.[26] Results from two studies in acute pancreatitis are contradictory: Smithies and colleagues described increased frequency of allele 1 in patients with severe attacks.[25] They suggested that this allele may be associated with reduced IL-1ra production, thereby exposing patients to unregulated effects of IL-1. Unfortunately, this intriguing hypothesis is directly contradicted by the available evidence on the effect of the IL-1ra polymorphism on secretion[26] and a study from Edinburgh found frequency of allele 1 to be identical in the mild and severe groups.[21]

Summary and Conclusions

Acute pancreatitis is associated with wide variability in clinical behaviour. Our understanding of the cellular events underlying the systemic complications of acute pancreatitis has advanced in recent years but we are still no nearer explaining these differing clinical manifestations. The genetic variation in cytokine responses offers the possibility of an attractive unifying hypothesis. Initial studies in patients with severe sepsis would appear to confirm the suggestion that a pro-inflammatory genotype is associated with increased mortality rate. Unfortunately the results from studies in acute pancreatitis are less promising. Three studies in TNF immunogenetics failed to show an association between high-secretory genotypes and disease severity. One IL-10 gene polymorphism has been reported to be associated with a fatal outcome in patients with acute pancreatitis complicated by MODS, but this small study needs confirmation in a larger group and preferably in different populations. IL-1b polymorphisms have shown no association with disease severity and the two studies examining IL-1ra polymorphisms are contradictory. At present there is no evidence that cytokine gene polymorphisms can satisfactorily explain the diverse clinical behaviour that typifies acute pancreatitis.

References

1. McKay CJ, Evans S, Sinclair M, et al. High early mortality rate from acute pancreatitis in Scotland, 1984–1995. Br J Surg 1999; 86 (10):1302–5.
2. Brivet FG, Emilie D, Galanaud P. Pro- and anti-inflammatory cytokines during acute severe pancreatitis: an early and sustained response, although unpredictable of death. Parisian Study Group on Acute Pancreatitis. Crit Care Med 1999; 27 (4):749–55.
3. Hirota M, Nozawa F, Okabe A, et al. Relationship between plasma cytokine concentration and multiple organ failure in patients with acute pancreatitis. Pancreas 2000; 21 (2):141–6.
4. McKay CJ, Gallagher G, Brooks B, et al. Increased monocyte cytokine production in association with systemic complications in acute pancreatitis. Br J Surg 1996; 83 (7):919–23.
5. Norman J. The role of cytokines in the pathogenesis of acute pancreatitis. Amer J of Surg 1998; 175 (1):76–83.
6. Buter A, Imrie CW, Carter CR, et al. Dynamic nature of early organ dysfunction determines outcome in acute pancreatitis. Br J Surg 2002; 89 (3):298–302.
7. Bradley EL. A clinically based classification system for acute pancreatitis. Summary of the International Symposium on Acute Pancreatitis, Atlanta, Ga, September 11 through 13, 1992. Arch of Surg 1993; 128 (5):586–90.
8. Bidwell J, Keen L, Gallagher G, et al. Cytokine gene polymorphism in human disease: on-line databases. Genes & Immunity 1999; 1 (1):3–19.
9. Molvig J, Baek L, Christensen P, et al. Endotoxin-stimulated human monocyte secretion of interleukin 1, tumour necrosis factor alpha, and prostaglandin E2 shows stable interindividual differences. Scand J of Immun 1988; 27 (6):705–16.
10. Eskdale J, Gallagher G, Verweij CL, et al. Interleukin 10 secretion in relation to human IL-10 locus haplotypes. Proc National Acad Sci USA 1998; 95 (16):9465–70.
11. Westendorp RG, Langermans JA, Huizinga TW, et al. Genetic influence on cytokine production and fatal meningococcal disease. Lancet 1997; 349 (9046):170–3.
12. Jacob CO, Fronek Z, Lewis GD, et al. Heritable major histocompatibility complex class II-associated differences in production of tumor necrosis factor alpha: relevance to genetic predisposition to systemic lupus erythematosus. Proc National Acad Sci 1990; 87 (3):1233–7.
13. Nedospasov SA, Udalova IA, Kuprash DV, et al. DNA sequence polymorphism at the human tumor necrosis factor (TNF) locus. Numerous TNF/lymphotoxin alleles tagged by two closely linked microsatellites in the upstream region of the lymphotoxin (TNF-beta) gene. J of Immun 1991; 147 (3):1053–9.
14. Pociot F, Molvig J, Wogensen L, et al. A tumour necrosis factor beta gene polymorphism in relation to monokine secretion and insulin-dependent diabetes mellitus. Scand J of Immun 1991; 33 (1):37–49.
15. Wilson AG, Symons JA, McDowell TL, et al. Effects of a polymorphism in the human tumor necrosis factor alpha promoter on transcriptional activation. Proc National Acad Sci 1997; 94 (7):3195–9.
16. Stuber F, Petersen M, Bokelmann F, et al. A genomic polymorphism within the tumor necrosis factor locus influences plasma tumor necrosis factor-alpha concentrations and outcome of patients with severe sepsis. Crit Care Med 1996; 24 (3):381–4.

17. Majetschak M, Flohe S, Obertacke U, et al. Relation of a TNF gene polymorphism to severe sepsis in trauma patients. Ann of Surg 1999; 230 (2):207–14.
18. Mira JP, Cariou A, Grall F, et al. Association of TNF2, a TNF-alpha promoter polymorphism, with septic shock susceptibility and mortality: a multicenter study. JAMA 1999; 282 (6):561–8.
19. Tang GJ, Huang SL, Yien HW, et al. Tumor necrosis factor gene polymorphism and septic shock in surgical infection. Crit Care Med 2000; 28 (8):2733–6.
20. Stuber F, Udalova IA, Book M, et al. -308 tumor necrosis factor (TNF) polymorphism is not associated with survival in severe sepsis and is unrelated to lipopolysaccharide inducibility of the human TNF promoter. J of Inflammation 1995; 46 (1):42–50.
21. Powell JJ, Fearon KC, Siriwardena AK, et al. Evidence against a role for polymorphisms at tumor necrosis factor, interleukin-1 and interleukin-1 receptor antagonist gene loci in the regulation of disease severity in acute pancreatitis. Surgery 2001; 129 (5):633–40.
22. Sargen K, Demaine AG, Kingsnorth AN. Cytokine gene polymorphisms in acute pancreatitis. JOP: Journal of the Pancreas 2000; 1 (2):24–35.
23. Turner DM, Williams DM, Sankaran D, et al. An investigation of polymorphism in the interleukin-10 gene promoter. Eur J of Immun 1997; 24 (1):1–8.
24. Ma P, Chen D, Pan J, et al. Genomic polymorphism within interleukin-1 family cytokines influences the outcome of septic patients. Crit Care Med 2002; 30 (5):1046–50.
25. Smithies AM, Sargen K, Demaine AG, et al. Investigation of the interleukin 1 gene cluster and its association with acute pancreatitis. Pancreas 2000; 20 (3):234–40.
26. Arnalich F, Lopez-Maderuelo D, Codoceo R, et al. Interleukin-1 receptor antagonist gene polymorphism and mortality in patients with severe sepsis. Clin & Exp Immun 2002; 127 (2):331–6.

25 Genetic Polymorphism, the Immune Response and Chronic Pancreatitis

Adrian C. Bateman and W. Martin Howell

Chronic pancreatitis is characterised clinically by severe abdominal pain together with malabsorption and, in advanced disease, diabetes mellitus. The triggering event cannot be determined in every case. However, chronic excess alcohol consumption is the most common aetiological factor with other cases occurring due to chronic pancreatic duct occlusion, an inherited genetic predisposition (hereditary pancreatitis) or autoimmune pancreatitis.

The clinical features of chronic pancreatitis are mirrored pathologically by destruction of pancreatic epithelium with gradual replacement of the organ by fibrous scar tissue. Fibrosis is first visible as bands of collagen surrounding islands of acinar tissue ('nodular pancreatitis') and as delicate collagen strands surrounding individual acini. As the disease becomes more advanced and acinar destruction more marked, the bands of fibrosis coalesce to form sheets of scar tissue. The exocrine (i.e. acinar) tissue is lost first while islets of Langerhans are preserved until late in the disease process and are often visible in moderately advanced cases within a sea of fibrous tissue. Macrophage and lymphocytic infiltration is invariably present with the latter predominantly comprising a diffuse population of T-lymphocytes within both the fibrous tissue and in intimate association with the acinar epithelium (but not islets) together with scattered aggregates of B-lymphocytes usually within the fibrous tissue. The exocrine pancreatic ducts often appear dilated and may contain concretions of inspissated secretion. It has been suggested that the aetiology of the process can be inferred from the histopathological appearances of the pancreas[1] but we believe that significant overlap in pathological features occurs between cases of differing aetiology and that this precludes confident determination of the underlying cause in this way.

T-lymphocytes and Disease Pathogenesis

Several histopathological features suggest that specific interactions between T-lymphocytes and pancreatic epithelium may play an important role in the pathogenesis of chronic pancreatitis. In particular, these are the intimate spatial association between T-lymphocytes and pancreatic acinar epithelium[2] and the up-regulation of Human Leukocyte Antigen (HLA) class II molecules by the epithelium in chronic pancreatitis[3]. The presence of T-lymphocytes and HLA class II up-regulation within chronic pancreatitis strongly suggests, whatever the 'trigger' for initiating the inflammatory process, that these cells and molecules are important in the development and progression of this disease, representing an additional mechanism for disease pathogenesis that is separate from the role played by the cationic trypsinogen gene in hereditary pancreatitis[4]. Furthermore, T-lymphocyte infiltration is present almost entirely in association with the acinar epithelium, which is characteristically destroyed early in the disease process. In contrast, very few T-lymphocytes are present within islets, even in relatively advanced cases.[2] This observation provides additional evidence supporting the hypothesis that T-lymphocyte-mediated cellular damage is important in the pathogenesis of chronic pancreatitis.

HLA Molecules and T-lymphocyte Activation

HLA molecules are required for antigen presentation to T-lymphocytes, with the antigenic peptide held within a groove in the HLA molecule for interaction with the T-cell receptor. HLA class I molecules present intracellularly processed peptides largely derived from endogenous antigens such as viral antigens, to CD8+ T-lymphocytes, the majority of which are of cytotoxic phenotype. HLA class II molecules present processed peptides largely derived from exogenous antigens to CD4+ T-lymphocytes, which are mainly of 'helper' phenotype. While HLA class I molecules are expressed on virtually all nucleated cells and platelets, HLA class II expression is more limited, being restricted to B cells, professional antigen presenting cells and activated T-lymphocytes. Expression is also interferon-γ inducible, and up-regulated HLA class II expression is often observed in inflammatory and autoimmune diseases.

The genes encoding the HLA molecules, within the Major Histocompatibility Complex (MHC), are the most polymorphic within the human genome, with 225 HLA-A, 444 HLA-B, 111 HLA-C 2 DRA, 350 DRB, 22 DQA1, 47 DQB1, 20 DPA1 and 96 DPB1 alleles currently recognised.[5] The antigen binding groove of class I molecules is encoded by exons 2 and 3 of the gene while the class II antigen binding groove is encoded by exon 2 of the respective A and B genes for that sub-region of the MHC. The vast majority of coding polymorphisms are contained within these exons. In addition, polymorphism is clustered within a limited number of hypervariable regions within each exon (e.g. typically six hypervariable regions for exon 2 of an HLA class II gene such as DPB1). Polymorphic differences in the hypervariable regions of these exons are rarely allele-specific. Rather, hypervariable sequence motifs are often shared between a number of alleles and so a unique allele sequence is comprised of a unique combination of sequence motifs at these hypervariable regions. The situation with respect to HLA class I genes is more complex, not only because polymorphism is spread over two exons, but because sequence motifs at the hypervariable regions are not only shared between different alleles of the same locus, but also can be shared between alleles of more than one class I gene or pseudogene. This genetic polymorphism affects the shape of the antigen-binding groove and therefore the efficiency with which antigens are presented to T-lymphocytes. In this way, genetic polymorphism within the HLA-encoding genes can modulate the immune response to a vast range of antigens. Due to this extreme polymorphism and its central role in the immune response, characterisation of this polymorphism within the HLA genes and encoded molecules forms the basis of 'tissue typing' used prior to bone marrow[6] and solid organ transplantation[7] and HLA-disease association studies. Characterisation of this polymorphism also has proven utility in the determination of individual identity during the investigation of potentially contaminated or mislabelled surgical biopsy specimens.[8–11]

Characterisation of Polymorphism Within the HLA System

Early methods for HLA typing were based on the detection of expressed HLA molecules on the surface of separated T cells (HLA class I products) and B cells (HLA class II products) using panels of antisera, usually obtained from multiparous women in a complement-dependent cytotoxicity test.[12] This technique has limited powers of resolution, especially for HLA class II alleles.

For the past decade, DNA-based methods have been the principal tools for HLA typing in both research and clinical laboratories. The first comprehensive DNA-based HLA class II DR/DQ typing system was based on restriction fragment length polymorphism (DNA-RFLP).[13] DNA-RFLP typing has now been almost entirely superseded by the more rapid polymerase chain reaction (PCR)-based methods. When combined with initial PCR amplification of the gene or exon in question, restriction enzyme cutting sites can be identified within PCR amplicons (PCR-RFLP).[14] The principle of the widely used PCR-sequence-specific oligonucleotide probe (PCR-SSOP) typing approach is that individual alleles or allele groups can be discriminated by hybridization of immobilized PCR product containing the hypervariable regions to be typed with appropriately labeled SSOPs.[15] PCR-sequence-specific primer (PCR-SSP) methods are based upon the specificity of a PCR being dependent upon precise matching of the terminal 3′ end of a PCR primer and its target DNA sequence.[16] PCR-sequence-specific conformation polymorphism (PCR-SSCP) relies on single-stranded form PCR products containing different sequence polymorphisms that will adopt different conformations and will therefore differ in mobility in electrophoresis.[17] Heteroduplex analysis is another conformation-based technique that relies on the formation of mismatched heteroduplexes between closely similar but non-identical complementary DNA strands during PCR.[18]

Despite their tremendous utility, PCR-SSOP and PCR-SSP-based methods can only test for known HLA polymorphisms, although aberrant typing results may provide preliminary evidence for potential new alleles.[19] Direct DNA sequencing is needed to identify and characterize such alleles.

HLA Genetic Polymorphism and Disease

Inter-individual differences in HLA-encoding genes have been related to the development of a growing number of diseases. The first conditions found to be HLA-associated were inflammatory and in particular, autoimmune diseases (Table 25.1).[20] Some HLA-disease associations occur with only a single or related group of HLA alleles within a particular HLA gene (e.g. ankylosing spondylitis and variants of the HLA-B27 locus)[21] while others are rather complex (e.g. type 1 diabetes mellitus

Table 25.1. 'HLA-associated' non-neoplastic diseases (reviewed in Thorsby[20])

Disease	Associated HLA locus / allele	Relative risk†
Ankylosing spondylitis	B27	>150
Reiter's disease	B27	>40
Anterior uveitis	B27	>20
Narcolepsy	DQ6	>38
Grave's disease	DR3	4
Myasthenia gravis	DR3	2
Addison's disease	DR3	5
Rheumatoid arthritis	DR4	9
Juvenile rheumatoid arthritis	DR8	8
Coeliac disease‡	DQ2	250
Multiple sclerosis	DR2, DQ6	12
Type I diabetes mellitus§	DQ8	14
	DQ6	0.02

Key: † = the relative risk is a measure of how much more frequently the disease in question occurs in individuals possessing the particular HLA locus allele, compared to those not carrying the allele; ‡ = the most common HLA association with coeliac disease is with the DQ(α1*0501, ß1*0201); § = complex HLA associations exist with type I diabetes mellitus.

which is associated with a certain combination of HLA-DQB1 alleles inherited either on the same or on different chromosomes).[20] These associations are believed to occur due to inter-individual differences in the efficiency of presentation of antigens important in the disease pathogenesis, to T-lymphocytes.

The link between HLA genetic polymorphism and the precise three dimensional structure of the antigen-binding groove on the encoded HLA molecules suggests that it should not be impossible to determine the antigen, or group of antigens, associated with the aberrant immune response that may represent a key event in the development of this group of diseases. Despite this, the antigens that may be 'responsible' for initiating autoimmune and other HLA-associated inflammatory diseases are not known for the majority of diseases. In a minority of diseases, the molecular mechanism responsible for the HLA-disease association has been elucidated. For example, the variants of the HLA-DRB1*04 allele that are associated with rheumatoid arthritis contain identical nucleotide sequences at residues 67–74 (with the exception of a single amino acid substitution in one allele) within an otherwise extremely polymorphic area of the DRB1 locus. These observations suggest that this region of the disease-associated alleles may perform an important role in generating susceptibility to rheumatoid arthritis (the 'shared epitope hypothesis').[22] The amino acids encoded by this highly conserved nucleotide sequence form two of the pockets in the peptide binding cleft of the DR molecules, and therefore may favour binding and presentation of certain 'arthritogenic' peptides, which have yet to be identified. The susceptibility-conferring HLA-DR molecules contain an amino acid sequence that also occurs in glycoprotein B of the Epstein-Barr virus and of the heat shock protein DnaJ of *Escherichia coli*. Therefore, it is possible that infections with these organisms may lead to the development of antibodies that recognise these 'self' MHC molecules. This mechanism of induction of autoimmune disease has been termed 'molecular mimicry'.[23]

In coeliac disease, the molecular mechanism underlying the very strong association between HLA-DQA1*0501, DQB1*0201 association with this wheat gluten sensitive enteropathy is particularly well established. Elegant experiments have shown that the pathological intestinal T-lymphocyte response to α-gliadin in adult celiac disease is focused on two immunodominant, DQA1*0501, DQB1*0201

Table 25.2. 'HLA-associated' neoplastic diseases (reviewed in Howell 1995 [25])

Disease	Associated HLA locus / allele
Hodgkin's disease†	DPB1*0301, DPB1*0401, DPB1*0901
Acute lymphoblastic leukaemia	DPB1*02, DPB1*05
Cervical intraepithelial neoplasia	DQB1*03, DQB1*0602
Cervical squamous cell carcinoma	DQB1*0301, 0303, 0602
Kaposi's sarcoma	DR5
Burkitt's lymphoma	A1, B12, DR7
Colorectal carcinoma‡	DQB1*0301
EATL§	DQB1*03, DQA1*0501, 0201
Cutaneous malignant melanoma	DQB1*0301, 0303 [26]

Key: † = DPB1*0401 is associated with a protective effect for Hodgkin's disease in Orientals, while DPB1*0901 is associated with a shorter duration of disease remission in Japanese patients; ‡ = DQB1*0301 may be associated with *less* advanced tumours; § = enteropathy-associated T-cell lymphoma.

restricted peptides that overlap by a seven-residue fragment of gliadin. These peptides contain a glutamic acid residue (produced by the action of tissue transglutaminase on native antigen) which is critical for HLA-DQA1*0501, DQB1*0201 binding and T-cell recognition. These peptides cannot bind to HLA-DQ molecules expressed by individuals of other HLA-DQ genotypes, who are therefore tolerant of gluten in their diet.[24]

More recently, HLA associations have also been found to be important in determining susceptibility to a range of neoplastic conditions (Table 25.2).[25] Some of these associations relate to the risk of disease development (e.g. cutaneous malignant melanoma and the HLA-DQB1*0301 allele)[26] while others relate to clinical outcome once the disease is present (e.g. adverse prognosis in colorectal cancer and the HLA-DQB1*0301 allele).[27] The mechanisms for these HLA-disease associations have not been fully elucidated. However, many of the malignancies in which HLA associations have been identified either directly involve the lymphoreticular system (e.g. Hodgkin's disease, enteropathy-associated T-cell lymphoma) or may be associated with an inflammatory cell infiltrate (e.g. cutaneous malignant melanoma, colorectal carcinoma).

The precise role of inflammatory cell infiltrates occurring in non-lymphoreticular malignancy is unclear and any such association is likely to be complex. For example, an inflammatory cell infiltrate may represent an immune response against the tumour, as may be seen in cases of tumour 'regression' in cutaneous malignant melanoma.[26] Alternatively, inflammatory cells may promote or inhibit tumour growth via secondary effects on other molecular processes such as angiogenesis.[28] The latter hypothesis provides a potential link between HLA molecules and cytokines in the control of the immune response in both inflammatory and neoplastic diseases.

HLA Polymorphism and Chronic Pancreatitis

Despite the sound scientific reasons supporting the hypothesis that specific T-lymphocyte-antigen interactions occur during the pathogenesis of chronic pancreatitis, there has been relatively little investigation of HLA associations with chronic pancreatitis. The majority of published data have been derived from serological studies i.e. characterising HLA polymorphism at the molecular rather than

Table 25.3. Serological HLA associations with chronic pancreatitis

Study	Ethnicity	N.	HLA association	
Fauchet *et al.* 1979[30]		90	Alcohol	B40
Lankish *et al.* 1980[31]	Caucasian	65	All cases	A10*, B40*
Homma *et al.* 1981[32]	Japanese	18	Idiopathic	B5
		28	Alcohol	none detected
Homma *et al.* 1981[33]	Japanese	47	Idiopathic	B5†
		81	Alcohol	B13†
Forbes *et al.* 1987[34]	Caucasian	50	All cases	B44, Cw5
		28	Idiopathic	A25, Cw1, *negative* B7‡
		22	Alcohol	B44, Cw5, DR4
Anderson *et al.* 1988[35]	Caucasian	36	Idiopathic	A1
		52	Alcohol	B21

Key: N = number of patients within each group or study. * = these trends were shown but did not achieve significance at the 5% level. † = these associations were found in Eastern but not western Japan. ‡ = the frequency of HLA-B7 was decreased in idiopathic chronic pancreatitis compared to controls.

the genetic level (Table 25.3). Interestingly, chronic alcoholism may be an HLA-associated disease in its own right[29] and the major role of chronic excess alcohol consumption in the aetiology of chronic pancreatitis therefore represents a potential confounding factor for studies of HLA associations with the latter condition. Previous studies have allowed for this by separating alcohol and non-alcohol-related chronic pancreatitis into separate groups prior to analysis. Using this approach, HLA class I B13 and B5 associations have been described for alcohol and non-alcohol-related chronic pancreatitis in Japanese patients, with some suggestion of geographic variation in HLA association within Japan.[32,33] Two serological studies in Caucasian patients have revealed variable associations between chronic pancreatitis and HLA-A and -B antigens with no clear cut and consistent trend between the studies.[34,35] Limited analysis of HLA class II associations in chronic pancreatitis has been undertaken,[34] with little work performed since the advent of accurate, improved resolution DNA-based genotypes.

Cytokine Genetic Polymorphism and Disease

Cytokines are generally small molecules secreted by one cell to alter the behaviour of itself or another cell, generally within the haematopoietic system. Cytokines act on target cells by binding to specific receptor ligands, initiating signal transduction and second messenger pathways within the target cell. Cytokines function as players in a highly complex, co-ordinated network in which they induce or repress their own synthesis as well as that of other cytokines and cytokine receptors. This complexity is compounded by the fact that there is often considerable overlap and redundancy between the functions of individual cytokines. Production of numerous cytokines by the cells of the immune system, in response to both antigen-specific and non-specific stimuli, plays a critical role in the generation of both pro- and anti-inflammatory immune responses. For example, cytokines such as interleukin (IL)-1 are usually regarded as key pro-inflammatory cytokines, while cytokines such as IL-10 are anti-inflammatory, with strong immunosuppressive properties.

A considerable body of research undertaken in recent years (reviewed by Bidwell *et al*)[36] has shown that polymorphisms occur in the upstream regulatory ('promoter') regions of many cytokine genes, which may be functionally relevant in that these polymorphisms may influence the level of expression of these genes. Many studies support this hypothesis for several cytokine genes e.g. tumour necrosis factor (TNF)-α[37] IL-10,[38] although *in vivo* the situation is almost certainly more complex, and genotype-expression correlations may be influenced both by stimulus and cell type.[39] Due to the documented role of up-regulation or dys-regulation of expression of key pro- and anti-inflammatory cytokines in inflammatory lesions and often in the serum of patients with a large number of autoimmune diseases and malignancies, there has been considerable interest in determining whether the cytokine genetic profile of an individual results in qualitative or quantitative programming of his or her inflammatory response, such that cytokine gene polymorphisms may predispose to particular immunologically mediated diseases, or influence their clinical course. For example, claimed associations between TNF-α -238, -308 and -376 promoter polymorphisms and rheumatoid arthritis,[40] cerebral malaria,[41] asthma,[42] and cardiac and renal transplant rejection[43,44] have been reported. Likewise, associations between IL-10 promoter polymorphisms and systemic lupus erythematosus,[45] rheumatoid arthritis[46] and asthma [47] have been described. Other studies have reported associations between TNF-α and/or TNF-β polymorphisms and a number of cancers, including chronic lymphocytic leukaemia,[48] non-Hodgkin's lymphoma and breast cancer.[49] Work from our group has suggested that IL-10 promoter polymorphisms may play a role in both susceptibility to and prognosis in cutaneous malignant melanoma, with 'low expression' genotypes associated with disease susceptibility and with markers of more advanced, poorer prognosis disease, while 'high expression' genotypes are protective. This may be mediated by high levels of IL-10 inhibiting expression of vascular endothelial growth factor, a potent mediator of tumour angiogenesis.[50]

Characterisation of Cytokine Genetic Polymorphism

Unlike HLA polymorphisms, which are comprised of multiple polymorphic sites within a single gene, with clusters of hypervariable sequence motifs resulting in multiple expressed alleles, most cytokine coding and non-coding coding sequence polymorphisms are single nucleotide polymorphisms (SNPs), usually bi-allelic in nature. Despite this fundamental difference, many of the methods used to type for HLA polymorphisms can also be used to type for cytokine SNPs. Screening for novel cytokine promoter SNPs is often undertaken using the PCR-SSCP approach,[51] with subsequent confirmation by DNA sequencing. Genotyping for known polymorphisms can then be performed by a number of approaches, principally PCR-RFLP, PCR-SSOP and amplification refractory mutation system (ARMS)-PCR, the latter being synonymous with PCR-SSP.

Certain cytokine SNPs lead to substitutions in the recognition sites of particular restriction endonucleases e.g. the TNF-β (LT-α) +252 intron polymorphism results in 2 alleles, the DNA of one allele being sensitive to digestion by the *Nco* I restriction enzyme, while DNA from the second allele is not.[52] Polymorphisms such as these are detectable by the PCR-RFLP approach. Further examples of such polymorphisms are TNF-α -308 (*Bsm*F I) and IL-6 -174 (*Nco* I). Numerous other cytokine SNPs correspond to restriction endonuclease cutting sites (see review by Bidwell *et al*).[53]

In principle, all cytokine SNPs are detectable using PCR-SSOP, using separate oligonucleotide probes for each SNP.[53] ARMS-PCR approaches have also been developed for numerous cytokine SNPs.[50,54,55] While standard ARMS-PCR techniques for bi-allelic SNPs utilise 2 PCRs per SNP i.e. one for each allele, it is possible to modify the methodology such that both alleles are typable in a single PCR, using the so-called 'tetraprimer approach'.[56,57]

Cytokine Genetic Polymorphism and Chronic Pancreatitis

Chronic pancreatitis is associated with increased levels of several cytokines within serum (interleukin-1β),[58] pancreatic juice (transforming growth factor [TGF]-β)[59] and involved pancreatic tissue. *In situ* hybridization, northern blotting and immunohistochemical methods have revealed increases in connective tissue growth factor (CTGF)[60] and TGF-β1 mRNAs and proteins,[60–62] the pro-inflammatory cytokines interleukin-8 mRNA and protein[63,64] and the pro-inflammatory cytokines MCP-1 and ENA-78 mRNAs[64] in human chronic pancreatitis tissue. In particular, the central role of TGF-β in modulating fibrosis in chronic pancreatitis is becoming well established. Similar tissue increases in the pro-inflammatory cytokines TNF-α, interleukin 6 and interferon gamma mRNAs and the pro-fibrotic TGF-β1 mRNA have been identified using reverse transcriptase PCR, *in situ* hybridisation and immunohistochemistry within rat models of chronic pancreatitis.[65,66] These studies provide evidence to support the hypothesis that genetic factors influencing cytokine expression may be important in determining the development and progression of chronic pancreatitis. However, despite this work and growing evidence that genetic modulation of cytokine expression influences susceptibility and prognosis in a number of inflammatory and neoplastic diseases, the potential role of genetic polymorphisms influencing levels of cytokine expression has not yet been investigated extensively in chronic pancreatitis. A single study has found an increased frequency of TNF-α haplotypes associated with an intermediate level of TNF-α expression in both alcohol and non-alcohol-associated chronic pancreatitis patients compared to controls.[67]

Conclusion

The T-lymphocyte infiltrate and upregulation of HLA class II molecules observed in chronic pancreatitis suggest that the disease may occur and progress at least partly due to a specific T-lymphocyte-mediated immune response leading to destruction of acinar epithelium and later of islet cells, with replacement of the normal pancreatic parenchyma by fibrous tissue. Previous studies have demonstrated that genetic modulation of the immune response, both via changes in the efficiency of antigen presentation to T-lymphocytes and alterations in the level of expression of several cytokines, is important in the development of many diseases. Early low-resolution serological studies of HLA associations with chronic pancreatitis have produced conflicting results, with associations apparently differing according to underlying aetiological factors. A small number of more recent studies have also identified alterations in pro-inflammatory and pro-fibrotic cytokine levels in chronic pancreatitis, suggesting that genetic modulation of cytokine expression may also be important in the determination of disease progression. We are currently investigating the effect of genetic polymorphism, both within the HLA system and within several cytokine genes (or their promoter regions), on susceptibility to chronic pancreatitis, in order more fully to assess the potential importance of these genetic factors in the development of this disease.

References

1. Suda K, Takase M, Takei K, et al. Histopathologic study of coexistent pathologic states in pancreatic fibrosis in patients with chronic alcohol abuse: two distinct pathologic fibrosis entities with different mechanisms. Pancreas 1996; 12:369–372.
2. Bateman AC, Turner SM, Thomas KSA, et al. Apoptosis and proliferation of acinar and islet cells in chronic pancreatitis: evidence for differential cell loss mediating preservation of islet cell function. Gut 2002; 50:542–548.
3. Bedossa P, Bacci J, Lemaigre G, et al. Lymphocyte subsets and HLA-DR expression in normal pancreas and chronic pancreatitis. Pancreas 1990; 5:415–420.
4. Whitcomb DC. Hereditary pancreatitis: new insights into acute and chronic pancreatitis. Gut 1999; 45:317–322.
5. Robinson J, Waller MJ, Parham P, et al. IMGT/HLA Database – a sequence database for the human major histocompatibility complex. Nucleic Acids Res 2001; 29:210–213.
6. Davies SM, Ramsay NKC, Haake RJ, et al. Comparison of engraftment in recipients of matched sibling or unrelated donor marrow allografts. Bone Marrow Transplant 1994; 13:51–57.
7. Takemoto S, Terasaki PI, Cecka JM, et al. Survival of nationally shared, HLA-matched kidney transplants from cadaveric donors. N Engl J Med 1992; 24:2342–2355.
8. Bateman AC, Leung ST, Howell WM, et al. Detection of specimen contamination in routine histopathology by HLA class II typing using the polymerase chain reaction and sequence specific oligonucleotide probing. J Pathol 1994; 173:243–248.
9. Bateman AC, Sage DA, Al-Talib RK, et al. Investigation of specimen mislabelling in paraffin-embedded tissue using a rapid, allele-specific, PCR-based HLA class II typing method. Histopathology 1996; 28:169–174.
10. Bateman AC, Hemmatpour SK, Theaker JM, et al. Nested polymerase chain reaction-based HLA class II typing for the unique identfication of formalin-fixed and paraffin-embedded tissue. J Pathol 1997; 181:228–234.
11. Bateman AC, Turner SJ, Theaker JM, et al. Polymerase chain reaction-based human leukocyte antigen genotyping for the investigation of suspected gastrointestinal biopsy contamination. Gut 1999; 45:259–263.
12. Mittal KK, Mickey MR, Singal DP, et al. Serotyping for homotransplantation: refinement of microdroplet lymphocyte cytotoxicity test. Transplantation 1968; 6:913–927.
13. Bidwell JL, Bidwell EA, Savage DA, et al. A DNA-RFLP typing system that positively identifies serologically well-defined and ill-defined HLA-DR and DQ alleles, including DRw10. Transplantation 1989; 45:640–646.
14. Uryu N, Maeda M, Ota M, et al. A simple and rapid method for HLA-DRB and -DQB typing by digestion of PCR-amplified DNA with allele specific restriction endonucleases. Tissue Antigens 1990; 35:20–31.
15. Krausa P, Browning M. Detection of HLA gene polymorphism. In: Browning M, McMichael A (eds). HLA and MHC: genes, molecules and function. BIOS Scientific Publishers Ltd, Oxford, 1996; pp. 113–137.
16. Olerup O, Zetterquist H. HLA-DR typing by PCR amplification with sequence-specific primers (PCR-SSP) in 2 hours: An alternative to serological DR typing in clinical practice including donor-recipient matching in cadaveric transplantation. Tissue Antigens 1992; 39:225–235.
17. Shintaku S, Fukuda Y, Kimura A, et al. DNA conformation polymorphism analysis of DR52 associated HLA-DR antigens by polymerase chain reaction: a simple, economical and rapid examination for HLA matching in transplantation. Jpn J Med Sci Biol 1993; 46:165–181.

18. Savage DA, Tang JP, Wood NA, et al. A rapid HLA-DRB1*04 subtyping method using PCR and heteroduplex generators. Tissue Antigens 1996; 47:284–292.
19. Hemmatpour SK, Dunn PPJ, Evans PR, et al. Functional characterization and exon 2-intron 2-exon 3 gene sequence of HLA-B*2712 as found in a British family. Eur J Immunogenet 1998; 25:395–402.
20. Thorsby E. HLA-associated disease susceptibility – which genes are primarily involved? Immunologist 1995; 3:51–58.
21. Sorrentino R, Tosi R. HLA-B27 subtypes: ankylosing spondylitis association versus peptide binding specificity. In: López-Larrea C (ed) HLA-B27 in the development of spondyloarthropathies. Springer, Heidelberg 1997; pp. 135–144.
22. Ollier B. Shock revelations about HLA-DR4 – a shortcut to rheumatoid arthritis? Nature Med 1996; 2:279–280.
23. Baum H, Davies H, Peakman M. Molecular mimickry in the MHC: hidden clues to autoimmunity? Immunol Today 1996; 17:64–70.
24. Arentz-Hansen H, Korner R, Molberg O, et al. The intestinal T cell response to a-gliadin in adult celiac disease is focused on a single deamidated glutamine targeted by tissue transglutaminase. J Exp Med 2000; 191:603–612.
25. Howell WM, Jones DB. The role of human leukocyte antigen genes in the development of malignant disease. J Clin Pathol Mol Pathol 1995; 48:M302–M306.
26. Bateman AC, Turner SJ, Theaker JM, et al. HLA-DQB1*0303 and *0301 alleles influence susceptibility to and prognosis in cutaneous malignant melanoma in the British caucasian population. Tissue Antigens 1998; 52:67–73.
27. Fossum B, Breivik J, Meling GI, et al. A K-ras 13Gly-Asp mutation is recognised by HLA-DQ7 restricted T cells in a patient with colorectal cancer. Modifying effect of DQ7 on established cancers harbouring this mutation? Int J Cancer 1994; 58:506–511.
28. Leek RD, Lewis CE, Whitehouse R, et al. Association of macrophage infiltration with angiogenesis and prognosis in invasive breast carcinoma. Cancer Res 1996; 56:4625–4629.
29. List S, Gluud C. A meta-analysis of HLA-antigen prevalences in alcoholics and alcoholic liver disease. Alcohol Alcohol 1994; 29:757–764.
30. Fauchet R, Genetet B, Gosselin M, et al. HLA antigens in chronic pancreatitis. Tissue Antigens 1979; 13:163–166.
31. Lankish PG, Hierholzer E, Koop H, et al. HLA-antigens in acute and chronic pancreatitis. Z Gastroenterol 1980; 18:524–526.
32. Homma T, Aizawa T, Nagata A, et al. HLA antigens in chronic idiopathic pancreatitis compared with chronic alcoholic pancreatitis. Dig Dis Sci 1981; 26:449–452.
33. Homma T, Kubo K, Sato T. HLA antigen and chronic pancreatitis in Japan. Digestion 1981; 21:267–272.
34. Forbes A, Schwarz G, Mirakian R, et al. HLA antigens in chronic pancreatitis. Tissue Antigens 1987; 30:176–183.
35. Anderson RJ, Dyer PA, Donnai D, et al. Chronic pancreatitis, HLA and autoimmunity. Int J Pancreatol 1988; 3:83–90.
36. Bidwell J, Keen L, Gallagher G, et al. Cytokine gene polymorphism in human disease: on-line databases. Genes and Immunity 1999; 1:3–19.
37. Allen RD. Polymorphism of the human TNF-a promoter – random variation or functional diversity? Molecular Immunology 1999; 36:1017–1027.
38. Turner DM, Williams DM, Sankaran D, et al. An investigation of polymorphism in the interleukin-10 gene promoter. Eur J Immunogenet 1997; 24:1–8.
39. Kroeger KM, Steer JH, Joyce DA, et al. Effects of stimulus and cell type on the expression of the -308 tumour necrosis factor promoter polymorphism. Cytokine 2000; 12:110–119.
40. Brinkman BM, Huizinga TW, Kurban SS, et al. Tumour necrosis factor alpha gene polymorphisms in rheumatoid arthritis: association with susceptibility to, or severity of, disease? Br J Rheumatol 1997; 36:516–521.
41. Knight JC, Udalova I, Hill AVS, et al. A polymorphism that affects OCT-1 binding to the TNF promoter region is associated with severe malaria. Nature Genetics 1999; 22:145–150.
42. Moffatt MF, Cookson WO. Tumour necrosis factor Haplotypes and asthma. Hum Mol Genet 1997; 6:551–554.
43. Turner D, Grant S, Yonan N, et al. Cytokine gene polymorphism and heart transplant rejection. Transplantation 1997; 64:776–779.

44. Sankaran D, Ashraf S, Martin S, et al. High interleukin 10 producer genotype is not protective against renal allograft rejection in high TNFa producers. Eur J Immunogenet 1998; 25:68 (abstract).
45. Lazarus M, Hajeer AH, Turner D, et al. Genetic variation in the interleukin 10 gene promoter and systemic lupus erythematosus. J Rheumatol 1997; 24:2314–2317.
46. Hajeer AH, Lazarus M, Turner D, et al. IL-10 gene promoter polymorphisms in rheumatoid arthritis. Sacand J Rheumatol 1998; 27:142–145.
47. Lim S, Crawley E, Woo P, et al. Haplotype associated with low interleukin-10 production in patients with severe asthma. Lancet 1998; 352:113 (letter).
48. Demeter J, Porzsolt F, Ramisch S, et al. Polymorphism of the tumour necrosis factor-alpha and Lymphotoxin-alpha genes in chronic lymphocytic leukaemia. Br J Haematol 1997; 97:107–112.
49. Chouchane L, Ben Ahmed S, Baccouche S, et al. Polymorphism in the tumour necrosis factor-α promotor region and in the heat shock protein 70 genes associated with malignant tumours. Cancer 1997; 80:1489–1496.
50. Howell WM, Turner SJ, Bateman AC, et al. Il-10 promoter polymorphisms influence prognosis in cutaneous malignant melanoma. Genes and Immunity 2001; 2:25–31.
51. Fishman D, Faulds G, Jeffery R, et al. The effect of novel polymorphisms in the interleukin-6 (IL-6) gene on IL-6 transcription and plasma IL-6 levels, and an association with systemic-onset juvenile chronic arthritis. J Clin Invest 1998; 102:1369–1376.
52. Messer G, Spengler U, Jung MC, et al. Polymorphic structure of the tumor necrosis factor (TNF) locus: an NcoI polymorphism in the first intron of the human TNF-β gene correlates with a variant amino acid in position 26 and a reduced level of TNF-β production. J Exp Med 1991; 173:209–219.
53. Perrey C, Pravica V, Sinnott PJ, et al. Genotyping for polymorphisms in interferon-γ, interleukin-10, transforming growth factor-β1 and tumour necrosis factor-a genes: a technical report. Transplant Immunology 1998; 6:193–197.
54. Perrey C, Turner SJ, Pravica V, et al. ARMS-PCR methodologies to determine IL-10, TNF-α, TNF-β and TGFβ-1 gene polymorphisms. Transplant Immunology 1999; 7:127–128.
55. Howell WM, Turner SJ, Collins A, et al. Influence of TNFa and LTa single nucleotide polymorphisms on susceptibility to and prognosis in cutaneous malignant melanoma in the British population. Eur J Immunogenet 2002; 29:17–23.
56. Karhukorpi J, Karttunen R. Genotyping interleukin-10 high and low producers with single-tube bi-directional allele-specific amplification. Exp Clin Immunogenet 2001; 18:67–70.
57. Ye S, Dillon S, Ke X, et al. An efficient procedure for genotyping single nucleotide polymorphisms. Nucleic Acids Res 2001; 29:e88.
58. Bamba T, Yoshioka U, Inoue H, et al. Serum levels of interleukin-1b and interleukin-6 in patients with chronic pancreatitis. J Gastroenterol 1994; 29:314–319.
59. Kazbay K, Tarnasky PR, Hawes RH, et al. Increased transforming growth factor beta in pure pancreatic juice in pancreatitis. Pancreas 2001; 22:193–195.
60. di Mola FF, Friess H, Martignoni ME, et al. Connective tissue growth factor is a regulator for fibrosis in chronic pancreatitis. Ann Surg 1999; 230:63–71.
61. Satoh K, Shimosegawa T, Hirota M, et al. Expression of transforming growth factor beta 1(TGF-β1) and its receptors in pancreatic duct cell carcinoma and in chronic pancreatitis. Pancreas 1998; 16:468–474.
62. Slater SD, Williamson RC, Foster CS. Expression of transforming growth factor beta-1 in chronic pncreatitis. Digestion 1995; 56:237–241.
63. Di Sebastiano P, di Mola FF, Di Febbo C, et al. Expression of interleukin 8 (IL-8) and substance P in human chronic pancreatitis. Gut 2000; 47:423–428.
64. Saurer L, Reber P, Schaffner T, et al. Differential expression of chemokines in normal pancreas and in chronic pancreatitis. Gastroenterology 2000; 118:358–367.
65. Xie MJ, Motoo Y, Su SB, et al. Expression of tumour necrosis factor-alpha, interleukin-6 and interferon-gamma in spontaneous chronic pancreatitis in the WBN/Kob rat. Pancreas 2001; 22:400–408.

66. Su SB, Motoo Y, Xie MJ, et al. Expression of transforming growth factor-beta in spontaneous chronic pancreatitis in the WBN/Kob rat. Dig Dis Sci 2000; 45:151–159.
67. O'Reilly DA, Sargen KD, Dunlop S, et al. Association of tumour necrosis factor microsatellite haplotypes with chronic pancreatitis. Br J Surg 2000; 87:362–373.

26 Xenobiotic Metabolising Enzymes in Pancreatitis

Helena Tabry, K. Palmer and Colin D. Johnson

Acute pancreatitis is a severe disease with a mortality rate of up to 9%. Forty percent of these deaths occur in the first 48 h, irrespective of age.[1] Although improved supportive treatment has become available over the past decade, there is no specific effective therapy for the disease. It is hoped that by gaining a greater understanding into the aetiology of acute pancreatitis, specific therapies can be developed which target known points in the evolution of the disease.

Xenobiotics such as cigarette smoke, ethanol and hydrocarbons in the working environment have all been implicated in the aetiology of pancreatitis.[1] Thus, the efficiency of the body's xenobiotic metabolising enzymes (XMEs) may be relevant to the incidence of pancreatitis. Several XMEs are known to be polymorphic, i.e. some individuals produce enzymes whose activities differ from the rest of the population. This is genetically determined.

Fat-soluble toxins entering the liver are metabolised in two stages, phase I and phase II metabolism, which renders the toxins water-soluble and usually less toxic. They are then excreted in the bile or the urine. Polymorphisms may increase or decrease XME activity, leading to more or less rapid metabolism of xenobiotics. If a mutation affecting a Phase 1 enzyme leads to reduced metabolism of xenobiotics, these may accumulate with toxic effects. However, as the xenobiotics are metabolised in two stages, imbalance of the two phases may lead to accumulation of toxic metabolites. For example, if the second phase enzymes are metabolising at a normal rate and the first phase enzymes are metabolising more quickly, or if second phase metabolism is reduced, even when Phase 1 is normal, intermediate metabolites can build up. In some cases these intermediate metabolites are toxic. Thus a decreased metabolism in Phase II could increase the toxin load, whereas an increased metabolism in phase I may increase the production of toxic intermediate metabolites.

Phase I metabolising enzymes consist of several (mainly microsomal) enzymes and families of enzymes, an important example being the cytochrome p450 group of enzymes (CYP). Several of the CYP group are known to be polymorphic. Phase II metabolising enzymes include microsomal UDP (uridine diphosphate)-glucuronosyltransferases, which are the most common phase II conjugating enzymes. They also include N acetyltransferases (NATs) and several other groups of enzymes. There are two types of NATs, NAT1 and NAT2, which are both known to be polymorphic. They are produced close together on chromosome 8 at band 8p22.[2] The two acetyltransferases vary in their substrate specificity. It was NAT2 which was found to acetylate, and thus detoxify, isoniazid in 1953.[3]

Table 26.1. XME genes studied, their human functions and the effects of polymorphisms recorded

Enzyme	Function	Polymorphism
CYP1A1	Activates environmental aromatic hydrocarbons	10% have highly inducible variety
CYP2D6	Metabolises cigarette smoke	5–10% are poor metabolisers
CYP2E1	Metabolises ethanol	1–5% have a gene with 10x more transcription (-1019bp C-T)
NAT1	Metabolises heterocyclic & aromatic amines	20–50% are slow acetylators
NAT2	Similar, but not identical substrates to NAT1	55–70% are slow acetylators

The frequency of 5 polymorphic XMEs has been examined in patients with pancreatitis and in controls. Polymorphisms in XMEs vary with ethnic group[4] and the frequencies of polymorphisms relating to the Caucasian population are shown in Table 26.1. The present study thus concerns patients of Caucasian origin, with age and sex-matched Caucasian controls.

Frequencies of Polymorphic Xenobiotic Metabolising Enzymes

The DNA from 85 Caucasian patients with pancreatitis has been analysed for XMEs and compared with a control population from the same genetic background. In 30 of the patients pancreatitis was due to gall stones, 22 patients had alcohol-related pancreatitis, 27 had idiopathic pancreatitis and six had pancreatitis due to other causes. The last group was too small for independent analysis, so it was analysed with the idiopathic group.

DNA was extracted from leukocytes and amplified by the polymerase chain reaction (PCR). Restriction endonuclease assays were used to determine the genotype for each enzyme. The two-tailed Chi square test was used to compare distributions in the groups.

When all the acute pancreatitis patients were included as one group, there were no significant differences from the control subjects (Table 26.2). There were also no differences for any of the CYP polymorphisms nor for NAT1, when the subgroups were analysed separately.

However, when subgroups of different aetiologies of acute pancreatitis were analysed with respect to NAT2 polymorphisms, all 22 (100%) of the alcohol related pancreatitis patients were slow acetylators for NAT2, compared with 57 (67%) of controls (Chi squared test, $p = 0.0059$). The proportions of slow acetylators in the two non-alcohol related pancreatitis groups were similar to the controls, being 68% (67% gallstone, 70% other causes). The observed association between NAT2 slow acetylator status and alcohol related acute pancreatitis may be related to the known role of NAT2 as a phase II detoxification enzyme within the liver.[4] Phase II

Table 26.2. Polymorphisms in pancreatitis patients, compared with controls

Enzyme	Phenotype	Pancreatitis %	Control %
CYP1A1	Highly inducible	8	10
CYP2D6	Poor metabolisers	7	6
CYP2E1	↑ transcription	4	5
NAT1	Slow acetylators	52	46
NAT2	Slow acetylators	76	67

metabolism at a reduced level in the pancreas may lead to a reduced clearance of toxic metabolites.

N acetyltransferases (NATs) are important phase II metabolising enzymes. They metabolise heterocyclic and aromatic amines entering the liver, thus reducing their toxicity and allowing them to be excreted in the bile or urine. Individuals who are slow acetylators have decreased NAT2 activity, leading to less rapid metabolism of xenobiotics. A decreased metabolism of NAT2 could therefore increase the toxin load. The metabolism of ethanol to acetaldehyde is known to occur in pancreatic acinar cells as well as in the liver,[5] but acetaldehyde does not achieve sufficient concentration in the pancreas to cause acinar cell injury.[6] Furthermore, the enzyme responsible for conversion of ethanol to acetaldehyde is alcohol dehydrogenase and NAT2 is not involved in the metabolism of either ethanol or acetaldehyde. Fatty acid ethyl esters are ethanol metabolites that may be implicated in the pathogenesis of alcohol related pancreatitis.[7] It is difficult to postulate a mechanism that relates these metabolites to changes in NAT2 function.

An alternative role for NAT2 could relate to its contribution to the generation of antioxidants, which are known to play an important role in modulating the severity of pancreatitis. NAT2 may also be involved in the regeneration of antioxidant defences through the production of N-acetyl cysteine (NAC). This possibility seems a more likely explanation of our observation.

Oxidative Stress

The role of reactive oxygen species in acute pancreatitis has been demonstrated in 53 patients admitted with acute pancreatitis. Blood was taken to determine markers of oxidative stress. Superoxide radicals, lipid peroxides and oxidised ascorbic acid (dehydroascorbic acid) were all significantly increased; moreover, the levels of these markers of oxidative stress were all significantly greater in patients with severe acute pancreatitis compared with milder disease.[8]

Excessive free radical activity has also been shown in a rat model of acute pancreatitis. Following L-arginine administration, there was a significant increase within the pancreas in lipid peroxidation and in the level of glutathione peroxidase.[9] Glutathione peroxidase is an enzyme that detoxifies lipid peroxides.[10] Furthermore, the intraductal delivery of hydrogen peroxide to the pancreas experimentally causes severe acute pancreatitis.[11]

Glutathione as an Antioxidant

Glutathione (GSH) is an important antioxidant produced in several organs, including the kidney, liver and pancreas.[12] It is also thought to play a role in the delivery of digestive enzymes.[13] It is depleted to 17% of its initial value four hours after the induction of pancreatitis by cerulein in mice. The pancreatitis was ameliorated by the addition of glutathione monoethyl ester. GSH itself does not easily cross cell membranes, but its ester does and is then converted to GSH within the cell.[12]

The enzyme essential for the synthesis of GSH, ϒ-glutamylcysteine synthetase, is induced in mice by ethanol and corn oil. However the concentration of GSH does not change. This suggests that the GSH is being used up as quickly as it is produced. GSH probably protects the pancreas from oxidative stress.[14] Ethanol is known to deplete hepatic glutathione[15] and perhaps has a similar effect in the pancreas.

Other Antioxidants

Blood levels of antioxidants are significantly lower in patients with chronic pancreatitis.[16] Decreased availability of antioxidants in the diet of people living in impoverished communities may explain the significantly lower blood levels of antioxidants found in healthy people in Johannesburg, compared with controls in Manchester.[17] In clinical studies, supplementation of dietary antioxidants (methionine, ascorbate, α-tocopherol, β-carotene and selenium) may reduce the pain of chronic pancreatitis.[18] In three patients with type I hyperlipidaemia, similar supplementation reduced the frequency of attacks of recurrent pancreatitis by 83%, 97% and 100% respectively.[19]

It is likely that patients who consume large quantities of alcohol also have a poor diet thus furthering the potential for pancreatic damage.[10] Most patients with pancreatitis smoke[17] and the many toxic constituents of cigarette smoke may increase the oxidative stress within the pancreas. These observations suggest that oxidative stress is an important feature of acute pancreatitis. The role of NAT2 as a possible source of antioxidant activity requires examination.

N-acetylcysteine as an Antioxidant

NAC is an antioxidant which is widely used in experimental models of oxidative stress. It decreases the severity of acute pancreatitis when given prophylactically to mice with either cerulein- or CDE (choline-deficient, DL-ethionine-supplemented) diet-induced pancreatitis.[20]

The mechanism by which NAC could act has been studied in cellular and animal models of pancreatitis. In one study, cytokines were produced from rat pancreatic acinar cells by activated neutrophils. This cytokine production was mediated by the transcription factor NFκB (Nuclear Factor κB). The presence of either NAC or superoxide dismutase (SOD) inhibited the production of cytokines by inhibiting NFκB.[21] In another study, pancreatitis was induced in rats by the intraductal administration of taurocholate. This increased the activation of NFκB by more than 5-fold. In rats given prophylactic NAC, the activation of NFkB was greatly reduced, as was the inflammatory response.[22]

NAC has two possible alternative roles.[23] Studies of the action of NAC as a therapeutic agent in paracetamol toxicity have shown that it may act as a sulphate donor (thus detoxifying the paracetamol), but also that it may prevent glutathione depletion.

N Acetyltransferase and N Acetylcysteine

NAT2 may be an important enzyme in the synthesis of N acetylcysteine. A variety of NAT found on microsomal membranes in the opossum kidney acetylates cysteine S-conjugates.[24] There is also a variety of NAT which acetylates S-acetyldextran polymer derivatives of cysteine in the rat liver and kidney.[25] To date, the NAT corresponding to human NAT2 has been found in the pancreas of congenic rats[26] although NAT2 has not been demonstrated in the human pancreas. NAT2 is known to be present in human liver and intestine.[3] It is therefore possible that hepatic, gut or even pancreatic NAT2 may have a role to play in the acetylation of cysteine to NAC. This could represent a possible role for endogenous NAC as an antioxidant. Such a role would explain why NAT2 polymorphisms that equate to slow acetylation are associated with alcohol related acute pancreatitis.

Further Studies

The frequency of slow acetylator status in patients with acute alcohol related pancreatitis appears to be significantly greater than in the normal population.

A validation study is underway to confirm this finding, examining polymorphisms of the NAT2 gene in a new group of patients with acute alcohol related pancreatitis, in patients with chronic alcohol related pancreatitis and in those with separate alcohol related illnesses such as cirrhosis.

References

1. Braganza JM. Towards a novel treatment strategy for acute pancreatitis. 1. Reappraisal of the evidence on aetiogenesis. Digestion 2001; 63:69–91.
2. Smith CAD, Wadelius M, Gough AC, et al. A simplified assay for the arylamine N acetyltransferase 2 polymorphism validated by phenotyping with isoniazid. J Med Genet 1997; 34:758–760.
3. Brockton N, Little J, Sharp L, et al. N acetyltransferase polymorphisms and colorectal cancer: a HuGE review. Amer J Epi 2000; 151 (9):846–861.
4. Smith CAD, Smith G, Wolf CR. Genetic polymorphisms in xenobiotic metabolism. Eur J of Cancer 1994; 30A (13):1921–1935.
5. Nordback IH, MacGowan S, Potter JJ, et al. The role of acetaldehyde in the pathogenesis of acute alcoholic pancreatitis. Ann Surg 1991; 214:671–8.
6. He ZJ, Ericksson P, Alho H, et al. Effects on endogenous acetaldehyde production by disulfiram and ethanol feeding on rat pancreas. J Gastrointest Surg 2001; 5:531–9.
7. Werner J, Saghir M, Warshaw AL, et al. Alcoholic pancreatitis in rats: injury from nonoxidative metabolites of ethanol. Am J Physiol Gastrointest Liver Physiol 2002; 283:G65–73.
8. Tsai K, Wang SS, Chen TS, et al. Oxidative stress: an important phenomenon with pathogenetic significance in the progression of acute pancreatitis. Gut 1998; 42:850–855.
9. Varga IS, Matkovics B, Hai DQ, et al. Lipid peroxidation and antioxidant system changes in acute L-Arginine pancreatitis in rats. Acta Physiologica Hungarica 1997; 85 (2):129–138.
10. Wallig MA. Xenobiotic metabolism, oxidant stress and chronic pancreatitis. Digestion 1998; 59 (Suppl 4):13–24.
11. Coskun T, Bozoklu S, Ozenc A, et al. Effect of hydrogen peroxide on permeability of the main pancreatic duct and morphology of the pancreas. Am J Surg 1998; 176:53–58.
12. Neuschwander-Tetri BA, Ferrell LD, Sukhabote RJ, et al. Glutathione monoethyl ester ameliorates caerulein-induced pancreatitis in the mouse. J Clin Invest 1992; 89:109–116.
13. Stenson WF, Lobos E, Wedner HJ. Glutathione depletion inhibits amylase release in guinea pig pancreatic acini. Am J Physiol 1983; 244:G273–G277.
14. Neuschwander-Tetri BA, Presti ME, Wells LD. Glutathione sythesis in the exocrine pancreas. Pancreas 1997; 14:342–349.
15. Bondy SC. Ethanol toxicity and oxidative stress. Toxicology letters 1992; 63:231–241.
16. Braganza JM, Schofield D, Snehalatha C, et al. Micronutrient antioxidant status in tropical compared with temperate-zone chronic pancreatitis. Scand J Gastroenterol 1993; 28:1098–1104.

17. Segal I, Gut A, Schofield D, et al. Micronutrient antioxidant status in black South Africans with chronic pancreatitis: opportunity for prophylaxis. Clinica Chimica Acta 1995; 239:71–79.
18. De las Heras Castano G, Garcia de la Paz A, Fernandez Forcelledo JL. Use of antioxidants to treat pain in chronic pancreatitis. Rev Enferm Dig 2000; 92:381–385.
19. Heaney AP, Sharer N, Rameh B, et al. Prevention of recurrent pancreatitis in familial lipoprotein lipase deficiency with high dose antioxidant therapy. J Endocrine Metab 1999; 84:1203–1205.
20. Demols A, Van Laethem JL, Quertinmont E, et al. N-acetylcysteine decreases severity of acute pancreatitis in mice. Pancreas 2000 Mar; 20 (2):161–9.
21. Kim H, Seo JY, Roh KH, et al. Suppression of NFkB activation and cytokine production by N acetylcysteine in pancreatic acinar cells. Free Radical Biology & Medicine 2000; 29:674–683.
22. Vaquero E, Gukovsky I, Zaninovic V, et al. Localised pancreatic NFκB activation and inflammatory response in taurocholate-induced pancreatitis. Am J Physiol Gastrointest Liver Physiol 2001; 280:G1197–G1208.
23. Lin JH, Levy G. Sulfate depletion after acetaminophen administration and replenishment by infusion of sodium sulfate or N acetylcysteine in rats. Biochem Pharmacol 1981; 30:2723–2725.
24. Golenhofen N, Heuner A, Schwegler JS, et al. Mercapturic acid formation in cultured opossum kidney cells. Ren Physiol Biochem 1995; 18 (4):191–197.
25. Okajima K, Inoue M, Morino Y, et al. Topological aspects of microsomal N acetyltransferase, an enzyme responsible for the acetylation of cysteine S-conjugates of xenobiotics. Eur J Biochem 1984; 142 (2):281–286.
26. Hein DW, Rustan TD, Martin WJ, et al. Acetylator genotype-dependant N acetylation of arylamines in vivo and in vitro by hepatic and extra hepatic organ cytosols of Syrian hamsters congenic at the polymorphic acetyltransferase locus. Arch Toxicol 1992; 66 (2):112–7.

27 Trypsin Activation and Inhibition in Pancreatitis

Markus M. Lerch, Manuel Ruthenbürger, Frank Ch. Mooren, Verena Hlouschek, Julia Mayerle, Peter Simon and F. Ulrich Weiss

Pancreatitis is a common disorder in which the passage of gallstones and the consumption of immoderate amounts of alcohol induce an inflammatory process. Recent studies involving animal and isolated cell models have elucidated many of the pathophysiological, cellular and molecular processes involved in the disease onset. More than a century ago it was proposed that pancreatic digestive enzymes are involved in the onset of pancreatitis and that the disease is essentially the result of an auto-digestion of the gland. Why and how digestive zymogens undergo activation, in spite of numerous protective mechanism, has been the topic of intense research efforts and debate. In this chapter we review the most recent progress in this enterprise and will specifically focus on mechanisms involved in gallstone-induced and hereditary pancreatitis.

Etiology and Pathogenesis of Pancreatitis

Pancreatitis is a common disease with an incidence of approximately 25/100 000 population per year. It differs from other inflammatory disorders in that infectious agents and autoimmune processes are considered exceedingly rare causes of the disease. The mild form of acute pancreatitis, which accounts for some 75% to 80% of cases has virtually no mortality and patients recover more or less spontaneously whereas the severe form is characterized by local and systemic complications, may lead to multi-organ failure and is burdened with a mortality rate of between 5 and 20 %. No specific treatment for pancreatitis is known today. The most common etiological factors are alcohol abuse and gallstone migration which, together, account for more than 80% of cases with acute pancreatitis in most Western countries. While the mechanisms involved in causing pancreatitis through alcohol consumption are still being explored and poorly understood much progress has been made in elucidating the role of gallstones in the pathophysiology of acute pancreatitis. We will therefore begin our review with some of the recent advances in understanding gallstone-induced pancreatitis.

Pathophysiology of Gallstone-induced Pancreatitis

Claude Bernard discovered in 1856[1] that bile is an agent that, when injected into the pancreatic duct of laboratory animals, can cause pancreatitis. Since that time many studies have been performed to elucidate the underlying mechanisms. While it is firmly established today that the initiation of pancreatitis requires the passage of a gallstone from the gallbladder through the biliary tract,[2] whereas gallstones that remain in the gallbladder will not cause pancreatitis, the various hypotheses that were proposed to explain this association are often contradictory. In 1901 Eugene Opie postulated that impairment of the pancreatic outflow due to obstruction of the pancreatic duct causes pancreatitis.[3] This initial 'duct obstruction hypothesis' was somewhat forgotten when Opie published his second 'common channel' hypothesis during the same year.[4] This later hypothesis predicts that an impacted gallstone at the papilla of Vater creates a communication between the pancreatic and the bile duct (the said 'common channel') through which bile flows into the pancreatic duct and thus causes pancreatitis.

Although Opie´s 'common channel' hypothesis seems rational from a mechanistic point of view and has become one of the most popular theories in the field, considerable experimental and clinical evidence is incompatible with its assumptions.[5,6] Anatomical studies have shown that the communication between the pancreatic duct and the common bile duct is much too short (<6 mm) to permit biliary reflux into the pancreatic duct,[7] and an impacted gallstone would most likely obstruct both the common bile duct and the pancreatic duct.[8] Even in the event of an existing anatomical communication pancreatic secretory pressure would still exceed biliary pressure and pancreatic juice would flow into the bile duct rather than bile into the pancreatic duct.[9,10] Late in the course of pancreatitis when necrosis is firmly established a biliopancreatic reflux due to a loss of barrier function in the damaged pancreatic duct may well explain the observation of a bile-stained necrotic pancreas at the time of surgery. This, however, should not be regarded as evidence for the assumption that reflux of bile into the pancreas is an initial triggering event for the disease onset. Experiments performed on the American opossum, an animal model that is anatomically well suited to test the common channel hypothesis, have revealed that neither a common channel, nor biliopancreatic reflux is required for the development of acute necrotizing pancreatitis.[6]

In order to overcome the inconsistencies of the 'common channel' hypothesis it was proposed that the passage of a gallstone could damage the duodenal sphincter in a manner that results in sphincter insufficiency. This, in turn, could permit duodenal content, including bile and activated pancreatic juice, to flow through the incompetent sphincter and into the pancreatic duct[11] thus inducing pancreatitis. While this hypothesis would, indeed, avoid most of the inconsistencies of Opie's 'common channel' hypothesis it was shown not to be applicable to the human situation in which sphincter stenosis, rather than sphincter insufficiency, results from the passage of a gallstone through the papilla and flow of pancreatic juice into the bile duct, rather than flow of duodenal content into the pancreas, is the consequence.[12] A final argument against the 'common channel' hypothesis is that the perfusion of bile through the pancreatic duct has been shown to be completely harmless[13] and only a potential influx of infected bile, which might occur after prolonged obstruction at the papilla when the pressure gradient between the pancreatic duct (higher) and the bile duct (lower) is reversed,[14,15] may represent an aggravating factor, as opposed to an initiating event, for the course of pancreatitis.

Taken together these data suggest that the initial pathophysiological events during the course of gallstone-induced pancreatitis affect acinar cells[16] and are triggered, in accordance with Opie's initial hypothesis, by obstruction or impairment of flow form the pancreatic duct.[17] A reflux of bile into the pancreatic duct – either through a common channel created by an impacted gallstone or through an incompetent spincter caused by the passage of a gallstone – is neither required nor likely to occur during the initial course of acute pancreatitis.

Cellular Events During Pancreatic Duct Obstruction

An animal model based on pancreatic duct obstruction in rodents was recently employed to investigate the cellular events involved in gallstone-induced pancreatitis.[18] In addition to a morphological and biochemical characterization of this experimental disease variety the intracellular calcium release in response to hormonal stimuli was investigated. Under physiological resting conditions most cell types, including the acinar cells of the exocrine pancreas, maintain a Ca^{2+}-gradient across the plasma membrane with low intracellular (nanomolar range) facing high extracellular (millimolar range) Ca^{2+}-concentrations. A rapid Ca^{2+}-release from intracellular stores in response to external and internal stimuli is used by many of these cells as a signaling mechanism that regulates such diverse biological events as growth and proliferation, locomotion and contraction, and the regulated secretion of exportable proteins. An impaired cellular capacity to maintain the Ca^{2+}-gradient across the plasma membrane has previously been identified as a common pathophysiological characteristic of vascular hypertension,[19,20] malignant tumor growth,[21,22] and cell damage in response to toxins.[23] It has also been observed in a secretagogue-induced model of acute pancreatitis.[24,25] Up to 6 h of pancreatic duct ligation in rats and mice, a condition that mimics the situation in human gallstone-induced pancreatitis, induced leukocytosis, hyperamylasemia, pancreatic edema and increased lung myeloperoxidase activity, all of which were not observed in bile duct-ligated controls.[18] It also led to a profound intracellular activation of pancreatic proteases such as trypsin, an event we will discuss in the next paragraph in more detail. In acinar cells of isolatd acini from these animals the resting $[Ca^{2+}]_i$ in isolated acini rose by 45% to 205±7 nmol, whereas the acetycholine- and cholecystokinin-stimulated calcium peaks as well as amylase secretion declined. However, neither the $[Ca^{2+}]_i$ signaling pattern nor the amylase output in response to the Ca^{2+}-ATPase inhibitor thapsigargin, nor the secretin-stimulated amylase release, were impaired by pancreatic duct ligation. On the single cell level pancreatic duct ligation reduced the percentage of cells in which a physiological secretagogue stimulation was followed by a physiological response (i.e. Ca^{2+}-oscillations) and increased the percentage of cells with a pathological response (i.e. peak-plateau or absent Ca^{2+}-signal). Moreover, it reduced the frequency and amplitude of Ca^{2+}-oscillation as well as the capacitative Ca^{2+}-influx in response to secretagogue stimulation.

To test whether these prominent changes in intra-acinar cell calcium signaling not only parallel pancreatic duct obstruction but are directly involved in the initiation of pancreatitis, animals were systemically treated with the intracellular calcium chelator BAPTA-AM. As a consequence, both the parameters of pancreatitis as well as the intrapancreatic trypsinogen activation induced by duct ligation were found to be significantly reduced. These experiments suggest that pancreatic duct obstruction, the critical event involved in gallstone-induced pancreatitis, rapidly changes the physiological response of the exocrine pancreas to a pathological Ca^{2+}-signaling pattern. This pathological Ca^{2+}-signaling is associated with premature digestive enzyme activation and the onset of pancreatitis – both of which can be prevented by administration of an intracellular calcium chelator. We set out below why we and others believe that alterations in calcium signaling and the premature activation of digestive proteases represent such critical events in the onset of pancreatitis.

Mechanisms of Pancreatic Autodigestion

The exocrine pancreas synthesizes and secretes more protein per cell than any other exocrine organ. Much of its protein secretion consists of digestive proenzymes, called zymogens that require proteolytic cleavage of an activation peptide by a protease. After entering the small intestine, the pancreatic zymogen trypsinogen is first processed to trypsin by the intestinal protease, enterokinase. Trypsin then proteolytically processes other pancreatic enzymes to their active forms. Under physiological conditions pancreatic proteases thus remain inactive during synthesis, intracellular transport, secretion from acinar cells, and transit through the pancreatic duct. They are activated only when reaching the lumen and brushborder of the small intestine. About a century ago, the pathologist Hans Chiari suggested that the pancreas of patients who had died during episodes of acute necrotizing pancreatitis "had succumbed to its own digestive properties," and he created the term "auto-digestion" to describe the underlying pathophysiological disease mechanism.[26] Since then, many attempts have been made to prove or disprove the role of premature, intracellular zymogen activation as an initial or an initiating event in the course of acute pancreatitis. Only recent advances in biochemical and molecular techniques have allowed investigators to address some of these questions conclusively.

Experimental Models for Intrapancreatic Protease Activation

Much of our current knowledge regarding the onset of pancreatitis was not gained from studies involving the human pancreas, or patients with pancreatitis, but came from animal and isolated cell models. There are several reasons why these models are being used: 1) The pancreas is a rather inaccessible organ due to its anatomical location in the retroperitoneal space. Biopsies of the human pancreas are difficult to obtain for ethical and medical reasons. 2) Patients who are admitted to the hospital with acute pancreatitis have already passed through the initial stages of the disease when the initial triggering events could have been studied. 3) The autodigestive process that characterizes this disease is a particularly significant impediment for investigations that attempt to address initiating pathophysiological events using autopsy or surgical specimens. The issue of premature protease activation has therefore been studied mostly in animal models of the disease.[27–29] These models can be experimentally controlled, are highly reproducible, and recapitulate many of the cellular events that are associated with the clinical disease.

Initial Cellular Site of Onset in Pancreatitis

The question where pancreatitis begins and through what mechanisms the disease is initiated has not been easily resolved. Early hypotheses were based on autopsy studies of patients who had died in the course of pancreatitis. One of these early theories based on human autopsy material suggested that peripancreatic fat necrosis represents the initial event from which all later alterations arise.[30] This hypothesis was attractive because it implicated pancreatic lipase as the culprit for pancreatic necrosis. Lipase is secreted from acinar cells in its active form and does not require activation by brushborder enterokinase. Another hypothesis suggested that periductular cells represented the site of initial damage and that the extravasation of pancreatic juice from the ductal system is responsible for initiating the disease onset.[31] Subsequent controlled studies performed in animal models that simulate the human disease have demonstrated that the acinar cell is the initial site of morphological damage.[16] The conclusion that pancreatitis begins in exocrine acinar cells, as opposed to some poorly defined extracellular space, is important because it represents a shift from earlier mechanistic and histopathological interpretations of the disease onset and it led to cell biological investigations of the underlying causes of pancreatitis. The concept of acinar cells as the primary site of the disease onset is also supported by recent clinical and genetic data[32,33] that are summarized below.

PathoPhysiological Importance of Digestive Protease Activation

Trypsinogen and other pancreatic proteases are synthesized by acinar cells as inactive proenzyme precursors and stored in membrane-confined zymogen granules. After activation in the small intestine, trypsin converts other pancreatic zymogens such as pro-elastase, pro-carboxypeptidase, or pro-phospholipase A2 to their active forms.[34] Although small amounts of trypsinogen are probably activated within the pancreatic acinar cell under physiological conditions, a number of protective mechanisms normally prevent cell damage from proteolytic activity. These protective intracellular mechanisms include: a) the presence of large amounts of pancreatic secretory trypsin inhibitor (PSTI), the product of the SPINK1 gene, b) an acidic pH within the distal secretory pathway, including the zymogen granule, which is below the optimum for most digestive proteases, and c) the presence of proteases that degrade other already active proteases. Theoretically a premature activation of large amounts of trypsinogen could overwhelm these protective mechanisms, lead to damage of the zymogen-confining membranes and the release of activated proteases into the cytosol. Moreover, the release of large amounts of calcium from zymogen granules into the cytosol might activate calcium-dependent proteases such as calpains which, in turn, could contribute to cell injury.

The suggestion that prematurely activated digestive enzymes play a central role in the pathogenesis of pancreatitis is based on the following observations: a) the activity of both pancreatic trypsin and elastase increases early in the course of experimental pancreatitis,[35,36] b) the activation peptides of trypsinogen and carboxypeptidase A_1 (CPA_1), which are cleaved from the respective proenzyme during the process of activation, are released into either the pancreatic tissue or the serum early in the course of acute pancreatitis,[34,37–41] c) pretreatment with gabexate mesilate, a serine protease inhibitor, reduces the incidence of ERCP-induced pancreatitis,[42,43] d) serine protease inhibitors reduce injury in experimental pancreatitis[44,45] and e) hereditary pancreatitis is often associated with various mutations in the cationic trypsinogen gene that could render trypsinogen either more prone to premature activation or may render active trypsin more resistant to degradation by other proteases.[46,47]

In clinical and experimental studies that investigated the time course of pancreatitis it was found that zymogen activation occurs very early in the disease course. One study that employed the caerulein model of acute pancreatitis reported a biphasic pattern of trypsin activity that reached an early peak after 1 h and a later second peak after several hours.[41] This observation is interesting because it suggests that more than one mechanism may be involved in the activation of pancreatic zymogens and the second peak may require the infiltration of inflammatory cells into the pancreas.[41] Taken together these observations represent compelling evidence that premature, intracellular zymogen activation plays a critical role in initiating acute pancreatitis.

Subcellular Site of Initial Protease Activation

One piece of information that would be critical for understanding the pathophysiological mechanisms involved in premature intrapancreatic protease activation would be the subcellular site where it begins. This question was addressed by three different approaches. Using a fluorogenic, cell permeant substrate specific for trypsin, confocal microscopy could clearly localize trypsinogen activation to the secretory compartment in acinar cell within minutes after supramaximal secretagogue stimulation, an *in vitro* situation that mimics a model of experimental pancreatitis.[48] When subcellular fractions containing different classes of secretory vesicles were subjected to density gradient centrifugation it was found that trypsinogen activation does not begin in mature zymogen granules but in membrane confined vesicles of lesser density that most likely correspond to immature condensing secretory vacuoles.[48] Experiments, in which antibodies directed against the activation peptide of trypsin (TAP) were used for ultrastructural immunocytochemistry electron microscopy, confirmed that the initial site of TAP generation and thus trypsinogen activation during experimental pancreatitis is, indeed, the secretory pathway. Again, within minutes of pancreatitis induction TAP was found in membrane confined secretory vesicles that were much less condensed than mature zymogen granules.[49] Taken together these data not only confirm that digestive protease activation begins within pancreatic acinar cells, as opposed to the pancreatic ducts or the interstitial space, but that mature zymogen granules in which digestive proteases are highly condensed are not necessarily the primary site of this activation. The first trypsin activity in acinar cells following a pathological stimulus is clearly detectable in membrane confined secretory vesicles in which trypsinogen, as well as lysosomal enzymes, are both physiologically present.

Clinical Role of Digestive Protease Activation

Recent studies involving patients have greatly contributed to understanding the role of zymogen activation in pancreatitis. In patients who underwent endoscopic retrograde cholangio-pancreatography (ERCP), the prophylactic administration of a small molecular weight protease inhibitor reduced the incidence of pancreatitis.[42,43] While protease inhibitors have not been found to be effective when used therapeutically in patients with clinically-established pancreatitis,[50] the result of the prophylactic study supports the conclusion that activation of pancreatic proteases is an inherent feature of the disease onset. Moreover, since reasonably specific antibodies have become available that detect the trypsinogen activation peptide (TAP) but do not cross react with either active trypsin or inactive trypsinogen,[51] the presence of TAP in serum and urine of patients with acute pancreatitis provides direct evidence for an activation of trypsinogen during pancreatitis. The amount of TAP released also appears to correlate with the disease severity.[52]

Evidence from Genetic Studies

A very different line of evidence comes from studies of the genetic changes in pancreatitis. Most patients in which pancreatitis was found in association with a genetic risk factor either carry point mutations in the cationic trypsinogen gene[32,53,54] or in the most abundant protease inhibitor PSTI (SPINK1).[55–57] The fact that the most common disease-associated mutations found in pancreatitis patients so far involve either a digestive zymogen or its intracellular inhibitor leads to two conclusions: a) pancreatitis in humans, just as in animal models, begins not only within the pancreas but the initiating events must affect exocrine acinar cells which synthesize and store the mutated proteins and, b) digestive protease activation is, after all, a critical event that not only parallels pancreatitis but is directly involved in its onset. Which role individual proteases have in the activation cascades that eventually lead to acinar cell damage and necrosis is, however, another matter. While trypsinogen clearly undergoes activation during pancreatitis and all reported protease mutations associated with pancreatitis (16 in all) exclusively affect trypsin, its ultimate role in the disease onset may be more complex than previously assumed.

Cathepsin B in Premature Digestive Protease Activation.

Several lines of evidence have suggested a possible role for the lysosomal cystein protease cathepsin B in the premature and intrapancreatic activation of digestive enzymes reviewed (in Refs. 58,59). Observations that would support such a role of cathepsin B include the following: a) cathepsin B can activate trypsinogen *in vitro*,[60,61] b) subcellular fractionation experiments using animal tissue from experimental pancreatitis models indicate that cathepsin B is redistributed from its lysosomal to a zymogen-granule enriched subcellular compartment,[62] and c) lysosomal enzymes such as cathepsin D have been reported to colocalize with digestive zymogens in membrane-confined organelles during the early course of experimental pancreatitis.[63] Although the cathepsin hypothesis appears attractive from a cell biological point of view and testable alternative hypotheses have not been proposed, it has received much criticism because the following experimental observations appear to be incompatible with its assumptions: a) a colocalization of cathepsins with digestive zymogens has not only been observed in the initial phase of acute pancreatitis but also under physiological control conditions and in secretory vesicles that are destined for regulated secretion from healthy pancreatic acinar cells,[64,65] b) a redistribution of cathepsin B into a zymogen-enriched subcellular compartment can be induced *in vivo* by experimental conditions that interfere with lysosomal sorting and are neither associated with, nor followed by, the development of acute pancreatitis,[66] c) the administration of potent lysosomal enzyme inhibitors *in vivo* does not prevent the onset of acute experimental pancreatitis,[67] d) both increases and decreases in the rate of intracelluar trypsinogen activation have been reported in experiments that used lysosomal enzyme inhibitors *in vitro*,[68,69] and e) even a protective role against a premature zymogen activation has been considered for cathepsin B.[70,71]

In view of the limited specificity and bioavailability of the available inhibitors for lysosomal hydrolases, the only remaining option to address the cathepsin hypothesis conclusively was therefore to generate cathepsin B deficient animals. When experimental pancreatitis in a strain of mice in which the cathepsin B gene had been deleted by targeted disruption was studied, the disease course was altered in a number of ways.[72] The most dramatic change in comparison to wild-type control animals, and also the most relevant in regard to the cathepsin hypothesis of acute pancreatitis, was a reduction in premature, intrapancreatic trypsinogen activation. In terms of substrate-defined trypsin activity, this reduction amounted to more than 80% over the course of 24 h. When the greater pancreatic trypsinogen content of cathepsin B knock-out animals was taken into account, less than 10% of the amount of trypsinogen detected in wild-type animals was activated during the course of pancreatitis in the cathepsin B-deficient animals. This observation alone can be regarded as the first direct experimental evidence for a critical role of cathepsin B in the intracellular events that determine premature digestive protease activation during the onset of acute pancreatitis.

Surprisingly, the decrease in trypsinogen activation was not paralleled by a dramatic prevention of pancreatic necrosis, and the systemic inflammatory response during pancreatitis was not affected at all. This observation and the fact that cathepsin B can activate pancreatic digestive zymogens other than trypsinogen[73] raises two important questions: a) whether trypsin activation itself, which is clearly cathepsin B-dependent, is directly involved in acinar cell damage and, b) whether a cathepsin B-induced activation of other digestive proteases ultimately causes the pancreatic necrosis for which trypsin is not the culprit. In order to study the role of cathepsin B in the human pancreas tissue specimens and pancreatic juice from patients with hereditary and sporadic pancreatitis were recently investigated. Cathepsin B was clearly shown to be abundantly present in the subcellular secretory compartment of the healthy human pancreas and in the pancreatic juice of controls and pancreatitis patients.[74] It was also found to be a potent activator of human trypsinogen. Its capacity to activate trypsinogen, however, was not affected by the most common trypsinogen mutations found in association with hereditary pancreatitis. While these data indicate that the onset of human pancreatitis may well involve mechanisms that depend on cathepsin B-induced protease activation the cause of hereditary pancreatitis cannot be easily reduced to an altered activation of mutant trypsinogen induced by cathepsin-B.

Role of Trypsin in Premature Digestive Protease Activation

The question of why structural changes in the cationic trypsinogen gene caused by germline mutations would lead to the onset of hereditary pancreatitis has been a matter of debate. Since trypsin is the oldest known digestive enzyme, because trypsin can activate multiple other digestive proteases in the gut, and because pancreatitis is regarded as a disease caused by proteolytic autodigestion of the pancreas it would be reasonable to assume that pancreatitis is caused by a trypsin-dependent protease cascade within the pancreas itself. If this hypothesis were correct the trypsinogen mutations that are found in association with hereditary pancreatitis could be predicted to confer a gain of enzymatic function,[32,33] meaning that mutant typsinogen would be more readily activated inside acinar cells or, alternatively, active trypsin would be less rapidly degraded inside acinar cells. Both events would lead to a prolonged or increased enzymatic action of trypsin within the cellular environment. In order to prove this hypothesis *in vitro* studies were performed that have analyzed the biochemistry of recombinant human trypsinogens into which pancreatitis-associated mutations were introduced. Some of these studies found, indeed, that either a facilitated trypsinogen autoactivation or an extended trypsin activity can result under defined experimental conditions.[75–77] Whether these *in vitro* conditions reflect the highly compartmentalized situation under which protease activation begins intracellularly and *in vivo*[78,79] is presently unknown, but the above studies would strongly be in favor of a gain of trypsin function as a consequence of defined mutations. A number of arguments, however, have been raised against the gain of trypsin function hypothesis of hereditary pancreatitis. Most hereditary disorders, including many autosomal dominant diseases, are associated with loss-of-function mutations that render a specific protein either defective or impair its intracellular processing and targeting.[80] Moreover, a total of 16 mutations in the cationic trypsinogen gene, scattered over the various regions of the molecule, have been reported to be associated with pancreatitis or hereditary pancreatitis. It is unlikely that such a great number of mutations located in entirely different regions of the PRSS1 gene would all have the same effect on trypsinogen and result in a gain of enzymatic function. A loss of enzymatic function *in vivo* would, accordingly, be a much simpler and consistent explanation for the pathophysiological role of hereditary pancreatitis mutations. This is especially true for the A16V mutation which affects the signal peptide cleavage site involved in the correct processing of trypsinogen.[81] This mutation would not be expected to have an effect on activation or catalytic activity of trypsin. The ultimate proof for the loss of function hypothesis would be a hereditary pancreatitis family in which a significant deletion in the cationic trypsinogen gene, preferably affecting the sequence that encodes the active site, would be found to segregate with the disease phenotype. This piece of evidence, however, is conspicuously missing so far.

In the absence of animal models in which human trypsinogen with a disease-relevant mutation has replaced the wild-type rodent trypsinogens – a daunting task because several genes and pseudogenes need to be exchanged – studies using isolated pancreatic acini and lobules are an alternative to study the role of trypsin in pancreatitis. In one study that used a specific, cell permeant and reversible trypsin inhibitor it was found that complete inhibition of trypsin activity does not prevent, not even reduce, the conversion of trypsinogen to trypsin.[82] A cell permeant cathepsin B inhibitor, on the other hand, prevented trypsin activation completely. In inhibitor wash-out experiments it was determined that, following hormone-induced trypsinogen activation in pancreatic acinar cells, 80% of the active trypsin is immediately and directly inactivated by trypsin itself. Taken together these experiments suggest that trypsin activity is neither required nor involved in trypsinogen activation, that trypsin does not autoactivate in living pancreatic acinar cell, and that its most prominent role is in autodegradation.[82] This, in turn, suggests that intracellular trypsin activity might have a role in the defense against other, potentially more harmful digestive proteases and that structural alterations that impair the function of trypsin in hereditary pancreatitis would eliminate a protective mechanism rather than generate a triggering event for pancreatitis.[83] Whether these experimental observations obtained from rodent pancreatic acini and lobules have any relevance to human hereditary pancreatitis is presently unknown because human cationic trypsinogen may have different characteristics in terms of its ability to autoactivate and to autodegrade *in vivo*.

Recently reported kindreds with hereditary pancreatitis that carry a novel R122C mutation[84–86] are very interesting in this context. The single nucleotide exchange in these families is located only one position upstream from the one found in the most common variety of hereditary pancreatitis and leads to an amino acid exchange at the same codon (R122C versus R122H). When recombinant protein was used for biochemical studies, the enterokinase-induced activation, the cathepsin B-induced activation, and the autoactivation of Cys-122 trypsinogen were found to be significantly reduced by 60–70% compared to the wild-type enzyme. A possible interpretation of these results would be that Cys-122 trypsinogen misfolds or forms mismatched disulfide bridges under intracellular *in vivo* conditions, both of which confer a dramatic loss of trypsin function that cannot be compensated for by increased autoactivation. If this scenario reflects, indeed, the *in vivo* conditions within the pancreas, it would represent the first direct evidence from a human study for a potential protective role of trypsin in pancreatitis.[84] The question of whether the gain of function hypothesis or the loss of function hypothesis correctly predicts the pathophysiology of hereditary pancreatitis can presently not be completely resolved, short of direct access to living human acini from carriers of PRSS1 mutations or a transgenic animal model into which the human PRSS1 mutations have been introduced. The data from rodent studies, however, suggest that the role of trypsin in the onset of pancreatitis may be more complex than previously assumed and that other proteases are more directly involved in the proteolytic damage during pancreatitis against which trypsin could represents a safeguard.[87]

Role of Calcium in Premature Pancreatic Protease Activation

Calcium is highly concentrated in zymogen granules and has a marked effect on the stability and activation kinetics of protease zymogens in pancreatic juice. Several factors, however, make it difficult to study a direct involvement of calcium in protease activation. First, cleavage of the activation peptide from the N-terminal end of trypsinogen can be catalyzed by enterokinase (enteropeptidase), by lysosomal enzymes such as cathepsin B,[61,62] and by trypsin itself. Furthermore, human trypsinogen, at least under *in vitro* conditions, can auto-activate.[88] To complicate matters further the auto-activation capacity of trypsin varies greatly between trypsin subtypes and among species.[88–90] Once active, trypsin can not only activate trypsinogen but can also degrade and inactivate trypsin, the predominant role of trypsin after intracellular activation within living acinar cells.[82] When a very small amount of active trypsin is added to a purified solution of inactive trypsinogen the substrate specific activity rapidly increases as trypsinogen is activated. After reaching a maximum activity, however, trypsin-induced trypsin degradation prevails and activity decreases. The role of calcium must be considered in the context of these factors. A number of elegant *in vitro* studies have shown that after trypsinogen activation, calcium stabilizes trypsin.[60,88–90] With regard to auto-activation and auto-degradation, calcium influences both events in a stabilizing manner and thus its presence significantly delays trypsin-induced trypsinogen activation as well as trypsin-induced trypsin-degradation, allowing trypsin activity to persist much longer once activation has occurred.

These *in vitro* mechanisms may be of clinical relevance in a situation where trypsinogen has been secreted from the pancreas but cannot flow freely from the pancreatic duct, e.g. in the event of an obstructing gallstone or tumor,[91] but they may not be applicable to the situation inside the acinar cell.

Ca^{2+} is also a critical intracellular second messenger for the regulated exocytosis of digestive enzymes from the apical pole of the acinar cell. Endocrine diseases that are associated with clinical hypercalcemia are known to predispose patients to develop pancreatitis[92] and those who develop pancreatitis after extracorporeal blood circulation for major cardiac surgery are thought to develop the disease because of an exposure to supraphysiological concentrations of calcium.[93] In animal experiments hypercalcemia was shown to either decrease the threshold level for the onset of pancreatitis or to induce morphological alterations equivalent to pancreatitis.[92,94] Moreover, in studies that have investigated the initial phase of experimental pancreatitis a progressive disruption of the intracellular Ca^{2+}-signaling was reported.[24] It has therefore been proposed that an elevation of acinar cytosolic free ionized calcium should be regarded as the most probable common denominator for the onset of various clinical varieties of acute or chronic pancreatitis.[95] Recent studies, in which the effect of a disruption of intracellular Ca^{2+}-signaling on premature protease activation in isolated acini was studied seem to confirm this hypothesis. Regardless of whether intracellular Ca^{2+}-stores were depleted by calcium-ATP-ase inhibition, withdrawal of extracellular Ca^{2+}, or complex formation with Ca^{2+}-chelators, intracellular protease activation in response to supramaximal hormone stimulation was greatly reduced or abolished[78,96]. However, increasing intracellular Ca^{2+}-concentrations with Ca^{2+}-ionophores or the Calcium ATPase inhibitor Thapsigargin did not induce premature protease activation. These experiments indicate that high intracellular Ca^{2+} concentrations are a requirement for premature protease activation but may not be sufficient to induce this process. While the requirement for calcium in protease activation is now undisputed some authors believe that elevated intracellular calcium in general, and regardless of its subcellular site and mechanism of release, is sufficient to trigger premature protease activation.[97] The latter view remains in conflict with trials that used other lines of evidence in addition to single cell measurements.[78,96] While all of the above studies used hormone-induced models of intra-acinar cell protease acitivation the most recent investigation could demonstrate that changes in intracellular calcium dynamics are also involved in the onset of pancreatitis in models that mimic the human disease.[18]

Conclusions

Recent advances in cell biological and molecular techniques have permitted the intracellular pathophysiology of pancreatitis to be addressed in a much more direct manner than was previously considered possible. Initial studies that have employed these techniques have delivered a number of surprising results that appear to be incompatible with long-standing dogmas and paradigms of pancreatic research. Some of these insights will lead to new and testable hypotheses that will bring us closer to understanding the pathogenesis of pancreatitis. Only progress in elucidating the intracellular and molecular mechanisms involved in the disease onset will permit the development of effective strategies for the prevention and cure of this debilitating disease.

References

1. Bernard C. Lecons de physiologie experimentale. Paris Bailliere 1856; 2:758.
2. Acosta JM, Ledesma CL. Gallstone migration as a cause of acute pancreatitis. N Engl J Med 1974; 290:484–487.
3. Opie E. The relation of cholelithiasis to disease of the pancreas and to fat necrosis. Johns Hopkins Hosp Bull 1901; 12:19–21.
4. Opie E. The etiology of acute hemorrhagic pancreatitis. John Hopkins Hosp Bull 1901; 12:182–188.
5. Neoptolemos JP. The theory of 'persisting' common bile duct stones in severe gallstone pancreatitis. Ann R Coll Surg Engl 1989; 71:326–331.
6. Lerch MM, Saluja AK, Runzi M, et al. Pancreatic duct obstruction triggers acute necrotizing pancreatitis in the opossum. Gastroenterology 1993; 104:853–861.
7. DiMagno EP, Shorter RG, Taylor WF, et al. Relationships between pancreaticobiliary ductal anatomy and pancreatic ductal and parenchymal histology. Cancer 1982; 49:361–368.
8. Mann FC, Giordano AS. The bile factor in pancreatitis. Arch Surg 1923; 6:1–30.
9. Carr-Locke DL, Gregg JA. Endoscopic manometry of pancreatic and biliary sphincter zones in man. Basal results in healthy volunteers. Dig Dis Sci 1981; 26:7–15.
10. Menguy RB, Hallenback GA, Bollmann JL, et al. Intradcutal pressures and sphincteric resistance in canine pancreatic and biliary ducts after various stimuli. Surg Gynecol Obstet 1958; 26:306–320.
11. McCutcheon AD. Reflux of duodenal contents in the pathogenesis of acute pancreatitis. Gut 1964; 5:260–265.
12. Hernandez CA, Lerch MM. Sphincter stenosis and gallstone migration through the biliary tract. Lancet 1993; 341:1371–3.
13. Robinson TM, Dunphy JE. Continuous perfusion of bile and protease activators through the pancreas. JAMA 1963; 183:530–533.
14. Arendt T, Nizze H, Monig H, et al. Biliary pancreatic reflux-induced acute pancreatitis–myth or possibility? Eur J Gastroenterol Hepatol 1999; 11:329–335.
15. Csendes A, Sepulveda A, Burdiles P, et al. Common bile duct pressure in patients with common bile duct stones with or without acute suppurative cholangitis. Arch Surg 1988; 123:697–699.
16. Lerch MM, Saluja AK, Dawra R, et al. Acute necrotizing pancreatitis in the opossum: earliest morphological changes involve acinar cells. Gastroenterology 1992; 103:205–213.
17. Lerch MM, Weidenbach H, Hernandez CA, et al. Pancreatic outflow obstruction as the critical event for human gall stone induced pancreatitis. Gut 1994; 35:1501–3.

18. Mooren FC, Hlouschek V, Finkes T, et al. Early changes in pancreatic acinar cell calcium signaling after pancreatic duct obstruction. J Biol Chem 2003; 8 [epub ahead of print] PMID: 12522141.
19. Blaustein MP. Physiological effects of endogenous ouabain: control of intracellular Ca2+ stores and cell responsiveness. Am J Physiol 1993; 264:C1367–1387.
20. Resnick L. The cellular ionic basis of hypertension and allied clinical conditions. Prog Cardiovasc Dis 1999; 42:1–22.
21. Poenie M, Alderton J, Tsien RY, et al. Changes of free calcium levels with stages of the cell division. Nature 1985; 315:147–149.
22. Alessandro R, Masiero L, Liotta LA, et al. The role of calcium in the regulation of invasion and angiogenesis. In Vivo 1996; 10:153–160.
23. Hameed A, Olsen KJ, Lee MK, et al. Cytolysis by Ca-permeable transmembrane channels. Pore formation causes extensive DNA degradation and cell lysis. J Exp Med 1989; 69:765–777.
24. Ward JB, Sutton R, Jenkins SA, et al. Progressive disruption of acinar cell calcium signaling is an early feature of cerulein-induced pancreatitis in mice. Gastroenterology 1996; 111:481–491.
25. Bragado MJ, San Roman JI, Gonzalez A, et al. Impairment of intracellular calcium homoeostasis in the exocrine pancreas after caerulein-induced acute pancreatitis in the rat. Clin Sci 1996; 91:365–369.
26. Chiari H. Über die Selbstverdauung des menschlichen Pankreas. Z Heilk 1896; 17:69–96.
27. Gorelick FS, Adler G, Kern HF. Cerulein-induced pancreatitis. In: The Pancreas: Biology, Pathobiology, and Disease, 1993; pp. 501–526, Go VLW, DiMagno EP, Gardner JD, et al. (ed.), Raven Press, New York.
28. Lerch MM, Adler G. Experimental pancreatitis. Curr Opinion Gastroenterology 1993; 9:752–759.
29. Lerch MM, Adler G. Experimental animal models of acute pancreatitis. Int J Pancreatol 1994; 15:159–170.
30. Kloppel G, Dreyer T, Willemer S, et al. Human acute pancreatitis: its pathogenesis in the light of immunocytochemical and ultrastructural findings in acinar cells. Virchows Arch A 1986; 409:791–803.
31. Foulis AK. Histological evidence of initiating factors in acute necrotizing pancreatitis in man. J Clin Path 1980; 33:1125–1131.
32. Whitcomb DC, Gorry MC, Preston RA, et al. Hereditary pancreatitis is caused by a mutation on the cationic trypsinogen gene. Nat Genet 1996; 14:141–145.
33. Whitcomb DC. Genes means pancreatitis. Gut 1999; 44:150.
34. Rinderknecht H. Activation of pancreatic zymogens. Normal activation, premature intrapancreatic activation, protective mechanisms against inappropriate activation. Dig Dis Sci 1986; 31:314–321.
35. Bialek R, Willemer S, Arnold R, et al. Evidence of intracellular activation of serine proteases in acute cerulein-induced pancreatitis in rats. Scand J Gastroenterol 1991; 26:190–196.
36. Luthen R, Niederau C, Grendell JH. Intrapancreatic zymogen activation and levels of ATP and glutathione during caerulein pancreatitis in rats. Am J Physiol 1995; 268:G592–G604.
37. Schmidt J, Fernandez-del Castillo C, Rattner DW, et al. Trypsinogen-activation peptides in experimental rat pancreatitis: prognostic implications and histopathologic correlates. Gastroenterology 1992; 103:1009–1016.
38. Appelros S, Thim L, Borgstorm A. Activation peptide of carboxypeptidase B in serum and urine in acute pancreatitis. Gut 1998; 42:97–102.
39. Gudgeon AM, Heath DI, Hurley P, et al. Trypsinogen activation peptides assay in the early prediction of severity of acute pancreatitis. Lancet 1990; 335:4–8.
40. Mithofer K, Fernandez-del Castillo C, Rattner D, et al. Subcellular kinetic of early typsinogen activation in acute rodent pancreatitis. Am J Physiol 1998; 274:G71–G79.
41. Gukovskaya AS, Vaquero E, Zaninovic V, et al. Neutrophils and NADPH oxidase mediate intrapancreatic trypsin activation in murine experimental acute pancreatitis. Gastroenterology 2002; 122:974–84.
42. Cavallini G, Tittobello A, Frulloni L, et al. Gabexate for the prevention of pancreatic damage related to endoscopic retrograde cholaniopancreatography. N Engl J Med 1996; 335:919–923.
43. Tympner F, Rosch W. Effect of secretin and gabexate-mesilate (synthetic protease inhibitor) on serum amylase level after ERCP. Z Gastroenterol 1982; 20:688–693.

44. Lasson A, Ohlsson K. Protease inhibitors in acute pancreatitis: correlation between biochemical changes and clinical course. Scand J Gastroenterol 1984; 19:779–786.
45. Niederau C, Grendell JH. Intracellular vacuoles in experimental acute pancreatitis in rats and mice are an acidified compartment. J Clin Invest 1988; 81:229–236.
46. Gorry MC, Gabbaizedeh D, Furey W, et al. Mutations in the cationic trypsinogen gene are associated with recurrent acute and chronic pancreatitis. Gastroenterology 1997; 113:1063–1068.
47. Varallyay E, Pal G, Patthy A, et al. Two mutations in rat trypsin confer resistance against autolysis. Biochem Biophys Res Commun 1998; 243:56–60.
48. Hofbauer B, Saluja AK, Lerch MM, et al. Intra-acinar cell activation of trypsinogen during caerulein-induced pancreatitis in rats. Am J Physiol 1998; 275:G352–62.
49. Krüger B, Lerch MM, Tessenow W. Direct detection of premature proteases activation in living pancreatic acinar cells. Lab Invest 1998; 78:763–764.
50. Büchler M, Malfertheiner P, Uhl W, et al. Gabexate mesilate in human acute pancreatitis. German Pancreatitis Study Group. Gastroenterology 1993; 104:1165–70.
51. Hurley PR, Cook A, Jehanli A, et al. Development of radioimmunoassays for free tetra-L-aspartyl-L-lysine trypsinogen activation peptides (TAP). J Immunol Methods 1988; 111:195–203.
52. Neoptolemos JP, Kemppainen EA, Mayer JM, et al. A multicentre study of early prediction of severity in acute pancreatitis by urinary trypsinogen activation peptide. Lancet 2000; 355:1955–1960.
53. Teich N, Mössner J, Keim V. Mutations of the cationic trypsinogen in hereditary pancreatitis. Hum Mutat 1998; 12:39–43.
54. Simon P, Weiss FU, Zimmer KP, et al. Spontaneous and sporadic trypsinogen mutations in idiopathic pancreatitis. JAMA 2002; 288:2122.
55. Witt H, Luck W, Hennies HC, et al. Mutations in the gene encoding the serine protease inhibitor, Kazal type 1 are associated with chronic pancreatitis. Nat Genet 2000; 25:213–216.
56. Pfützer RH, Barmada MM, Brunskill AP, et al. SPINK1/PSTI polymorphisms act as disease modifiers in familial and idiopathic chronic pancreatitis. Gastroenterology 2000; 119:615–623.
57. Threadgold J, Greenhalf W, Ellis I, et al. The N34S mutation of SPINK1 (PSTI) is associated with a familial pattern of idiopathic chronic pancreatitis but does not cause the disease. Gut 2002; 50:675–81.
58. Steer ML, Meldolesi J. The cell biology of experimental pancreatitis. N Engl J Med 1987; 316:144–50.
59. Gorelick F, Matovcik L. Lysosomal enzymes and pancreatitis. Gastroenterology 1995; 109:620–625.
60. Figarella C, Miszczuk-Jamska B, Barrett A. Possible lysosomal activation of pancreatic zymogens: activation of both human trypsinogens by cathepsin B and spontaneous acid activiation of human trypsinogen-1. Biol Chem Hoppe-Seyler 1988; 369:293–298.
61. Greenbaum LA, Hirshkowitz A. Endogenous cathepsin activaties trypsinogen in extracts of dog pancreas. Proc Soc Exp Biol Med 1961; 107:74–76.
62. Saluja A, Hashimoto S, Saluja M, et al. Subcellular redistribution of lysosomal enzymes during caerulein-induced pancreatitis. Am J Physiol 1987; 253:G508–G516.
63. Watanabe O, Baccino FM, Steer ML, et al. Supramaximal caerulein stimulation and ultrastructure of rat pancreatic acinar cell: early morphological changes during development of experimental pancreatitis. Am J Physiol 1984; 246:G457–G467.
64. Tooze J, Hollinshead M, Hensel G, et al. Regulated secretion of mature cathepsin B from rat exocrine pancreatic cells. Eur J Cell Biol 1991; 56:187–200.
65. Willemer S, Bialek R, Adler G. Localization of lysosomal and digestive enzymes in cytoplasmic vacuoles in caerulein-pancreatitis. Histochemistry 1990; 94:161–170.
66. Lerch MM, Saluja AK, Dawra R, et al. The effect of chloroquine administration on two experimental models of acute pancreatitis. Gastroenterology 1993; 104:1768–1779.
67. Steer ML, Saluja AK. Experimental acute pancreatitis: studies of the early events that lead to cell injury. In: The pancreas: Biology, Pathobiology, and Disease, 1993; pp. 489–500, Go VLW, DiMagno EP, Gardner JD, et al. (ed.) Raven Press, New York.
68. Leach SD, Modlin IM, Scheele GA, et al. Intracellular activation of digestive zymogens in rat pancreatic acini. Stimulation by high does of cholecystokinin. J Clin Invest 1991; 87:362–366.
69. Saluja AK, Donovan EA, Yamanaka K, et al. Cerulein-induced in vitro activation of trypsinogen in rat pancreatic acini is mediated by cathepsin B. Gastroenterology 1997; 113:304–310.

70. Gorelick FS, Modlin IM, Leach SD, et al. Intracellular proteolysis of pancreatic zymogens. Yale J Biol Med 1992; 65:407–420.
71. Klonowski-Stumpe H, Luthen R, Han B, et al. Inhibition of cathepsin B does not affect the intracellular activation of trypsinogen by cerulein hyperstimulation in isolated rat pancreatic acinar cells. Pancreas 1998; 16:96–101.
72. Halangk W, Lerch MM, Brandt-Nedelev B, et al. Role of cathepsin B in intracellular trypsinogen activation and the onset of acute pancreatitis. J Clin Invest 2000; 106:773–781.
73. Hakansson HO, Borgstrom A, Ohlsson K. Porcine pancreatic cationic pro-elastase. Studies on the activation, turnover and interaction with plasma proteinase inhibitors. Biol Chem Hoppe Seyler 1991; 372:465–72.
74. Kukor Z, Mayerle J, Kruger B, et al. Presence of cathepsin B in the human pancreatic secretory pathway and its role in trypsinogen activation during hereditary pancreatitis. J Biol Chem 2002; 277:21389–21396.
75. Teich N, Ockenga J, Hoffmeister A, et al. Chronic pancreatitis associated with an activation peptide mutation that facilitates trypsin activation. Gastroenterology 2000; 119:461–465.
76. Sahin-Tóth M, Tóth M. Gain-of-function mutations associated with hereditary pancreatitis enhance autoactivation of human cationic trypsinogen. Biochem Biophys Res Commun 2000; 278:286–289.
77. Sahin-Tóth M. Human cationic trypsinogen. Role of Asn-21 in zymogen activation and implications in hereditary pancreatitis. J Biol Chem 2000; 275:22750–22755.
78. Kruger B, Albrecht E, Lerch MM. The role of intracellular calcium signaling in premature protease activation and the onset of pancreatitis. Am J Pathol 2000; 157:43–50.
79. Kruger B, Weber IA, Albrecht E, et al. Effect of hyperthermia on premature intracellular trypsinogen activation in the exocrine pancreas. Biochem Biophys Res Comm 2001; 282:159–165.
80. Scriver CR. Mutation analysis in metabolic (and other genetic) disease: how soon, how useful. Eur J Pediatr 2000; 159:243–245.
81. Witt H, Luck W, Becker M. A signal peptide cleavage site mutation in the cationic trypsinogen gene is strongly associated with chronic pancreatitis. Gastroenterology 1999; 117:7–10.
82. Halangk W, Kruger B, Ruthenburger M, et al. Trypsin activity is not involved in premature, intrapancreatic trypsinogen activation. Am J Physiol Gastrointest Liver Physiol 2002; 282:G367–74.
83. Lerch MM, Gorelick FS. Trypsinogen activation in acute pancreatitis. Med Clin North Amer 2000; 84:549–563.
84. Simon P, Weiss FU, Sahin-Toth M, et al. Hereditary pancreatitis caused by a novel PRSS1 mutation (Arg-122 -> Cys) that alters autoactivation and autodegradation of cationic trypsinogen. J Biol Chem 2002; 277:5404–5410.
85. Le Marechal C, Chen JM, Quere I, et al. Discrimination of three mutational events that result in a disruption of the R122 primary autolysis site of the human cationic trypsinogen (PRSS1) by denaturing high performance liquid chromatography. BMC Genet 2001; 2:19.
86. Pfutzer R, Myers E, Applebaum-Shapiro S, et al. Novel cationic trypsinogen (PRSS1) N29T and R122C mutations cause autosomal dominant hereditary pancreatitis. Gut 2002; 50:271–2.
87. Ruthernbürger M, Krüger B, Halangk W, et al. Intracellular trypsinogen activation is not involved in acinar cell necrosis but may have a protective role. Pancreatology 2001; 1:176–177.
88. Kassell B, Kay J. Zymogens of proteolytic enzymes. Science 1973; 180:1022–1027.
89. Colomb E, Figarella C. Comparative studies on the mechanism of activation of the two human trypsinogens. Biochim Biophys Acta 1979; 571:343–51.
90. Colomb E, Figarella C, Guy O. The two human trypsinogens. Evidence of complex formation with basic pancreatic trypsin inhibitor-proteolytic activity. Biochim Biophys Acta 1979; 570:397–405.
91. Allan BJ, Tournut R, White TT. Intraductal activation of pancreatic zymogens behind a carcinoma of the pancreas. Gastroenterology 1973; 65:412–418.
92. Mithofer K, Fernandez-del Castillo C, Frick TW, et al. Acute hypercalcemia causes acute pancreatitis and ectopic trypsinogen activation in the rat. Gastroenterology 1995; 109:239–46.
93. Fernandez-del Castillo C, Harringer W, Warshaw AL, et al. Risk factors for pancreatic cellular injury after cardiopulmonary bypass. N Engl J Med 1991; 325:382–387.
94. Frick TW, Fernandez-del Castillo C, Bimmler D, et al. Elevated calcium and activation of trypsinogen in rat pancreatic acini. Gut 1997; 41:339–343.
95. Ward JB, Petersen OH, Jenkins SA, et al. Is an elevated concentration of acinar cytosolic free ionised calcium the trigger for acute pancreatitis? Lancet 1995; 346:1016–1019.

96. Saluja AK, Bhagat L, Lee HS, et al. Secretagogue-induced digestive enzyme activation and cell injury in rat pancreatic acini. Am J Physiol 1999; 276:G835–42.
97. Raraty M, Ward J, Erdemli G, et al. Calcium-dependent enzyme activation and vacuole formation in the apical granular region of pancreatic acinar cells. Proc Natl Acad Sci USA 2000; 97:13126–13131.

Part 4

Acute Pancreatitis

Selecting Severe Acute Pancreatitis for Trials and for Treatment

28 Selecting Patients for Trials and Treatment: Apache-II?

Mike Larvin

Acute pancreatitis continues to perplex clinicians as the most unpredictable acute digestive disease. In the absence of a specific treatment of universally acclaimed benefit, clinical management has accented the need for prompt identification of potentially life-threatening complications. This permits patients to be channelled towards the most appropriate supportive interventions. Although the Marseilles[1,2] and Cambridge[3] classifications defined severe attacks as those complicated by life-threatening (or fatal) organ–system failure or pancreatic collection, individual complications were not defined. A working agreement of what constitutes a life-threatening complication was reached at the Atlanta International symposium (Table 28.1).[4] It ensured that clinical trial groups could be compared across different geographical settings. The approach was confirmed at the Santorini conference of 1997,[5] but further refinements are likely as knowledge increases and the treatment of individual complications improves. Using these criteria, in most series 25–30% of attacks are classified as 'severe', and the remainder as 'mild'.

So *clinical severity* is defined from the occurrence of complications and overall outcome, and represents a 'gold-standard' for the evaluation of severity and prognosis. Accurate *severity assessment* is used to obtain more detailed information in order to quantify the severity of illness. But the actual situation is complex. Clinical progress and overall outcome depend on many factors, and they may be too crude as measures to assess the effectiveness of individual treatments. The initial biological insult in acute pancreatitis varies, as does an individual's response. The latter is modulated by genetic polymorphic idiosyncrasies, and by the deleterious effects of prior illness and existing co-morbidity on biological reserve. The level of care and attention given during the attack also affects outcome. In clinical trials, the measurement of *initial biological severity* of illness would be most useful at entry, in order to stratify entry and to provide an accurate baseline for comparisons of progress. Although the assessment of *host responses* is more useful in the fine-tuning of clinical management, it is also useful for assessing the effect of treatment.

The accuracy of a predictive test can be measured by various contingencies (Table 28.2). The proportion of severe and mild attacks correctly detected are known respectively as *sensitivity* and *specificity*. Good sensitivity ensures that high-risk patients are stratified to receive appropriate interventions and enter research studies, whilst high specificity excludes those at low-risk. Sensitivity and specificity are influenced by the *prevalence* of severe attacks. In a comprehensive review, prevalence in series assessing prognostic systems ranged from 14% to

Table 28.1. Atlanta International Symposium 1992: a clinically-based classification.[5]

MILD ACUTE PANCREATITIS
75% of attacks. Organ-system dysfunction minimal, recovery uneventful.
Pathology: mainly interstitial oedema. Fat necrosis may be present

SEVERE ACUTE PANCREATITIS
Complicated by life-threatening *systemic complications* or *pancreatic collections*:
Systemic complications:
- **Cardiovascular:** systolic blood pressure *<90 mmHg*
- **Respiratory:** arterial pO_2 *<8 kPa (60 mmHg)*
- **Renal:** creatinine *>177 mmol/L (2 mg/dl)* (after rehydration)
- **Coagulation:** platelets *<100,000/mm³*, or fibrinogen *<1g/L*, or fibrinogen degradation products *>80 mg/ml*
- **Metabolic:** hypocalcaemia *<1.87 mmol/L (7.5mg/dL)*
- **Gastro-intestinal:** haemorrhage *>500 ml/24 hours*
- **Multiple organ-system dysfunction:** ***Ranson*** *or* ***Glasgow*** *scores >2, or* ***APACHE-II*** *(Acute Physiology and Chronic Health Enquiry) score >7*

Pancreatic collections:
- **Pancreatic necrosis**: diffuse or focal area(s) of *non-viable pancreatic parenchyma*. Gangrenous, necrotic tissue may be surrounded by small amounts of inflammatory exudate or pus. Typically associated with peri-pancreatic fat necrosis. Acute fluid collections commonly co-exist. An inflammatory capsule beings to form only after 7 to 10 days
- **Pancreatic abscess**: well circumscribed *collection of pus*, usually in proximity to the pancreas, containing little or no necrotic tissue. Frequently loculated. Surrounded by mature, thickened wall. Occurs usually at least 4 weeks after onset of attack*
- **Acute pseudocyst**: collection of viscous, enzyme-rich, pancreatic juice enclosed by a mature wall of fibrous or granulation tissue. Occasionally contains small amounts of necrotic debris. Occur at least 4 weeks after onset of attack.[1] May communicate with an obstructed pancreatic duct. If infection is present–re-classify as pancreatic abscess

** if <4 weeks from onset, reclassify as* ***acute fluid collection*** *(sterile or infected)*

42%.[6] High sensitivity is harder to achieve than specificity for mild attacks, which are more numerous. Misclassification of severe attacks is more harmful than overtreatment of mild attacks, although the latter increases costs. Thus *receiver operating characteristic (ROC) curve* analysis, *overall accuracy* (the proportion of all attacks correctly predicted), and *significance testing* is less useful. Performance can be evaluated independently of prevalence by examining the accuracy of positive and negative predictions. For severe attacks this is the *positive predictive value* (PPV), and for mild the *negative predictive value* (NPV). A high PPV promotes confidence in clinical decisions or research stratification, whilst a high NPV reassures the continuation of simple management and exclusion from research and costly treatments. In the past, varying definitions of severity and of individual complications, disparities in analytical and reporting methods, varying case-mix and timing all hindered accurate comparison of prognostic methods. At the very least, claims for 'improved' prognosticators are difficult to measure if not set against internationally agreed standards such as the Atlanta and Santorini criteria.[4,5]

Clinical Assessment

Bedside clinical prognostic assessment is simple, rapid and repeatable, and is the usual *modus operandi* of good clinical practice. Studies of clinical assessment after

Table 28.2. Contingencies of prognostic systems

	Outcome MILD	Outcome SEVERE	*TOTAL*
Predicted MILD	A	B	C
Predicted SEVERE	D	E	F
TOTAL	G	H	I

SENSITIVITY (E/H)
The proportion of severe attacks correctly predicted

SPECIFICITY (A/G)
The proportion of mild attacks correctly predicted

POSITIVE PREDICTIVE VALUE or TRUE POSITIVE RATE (E/F)
The proportion of predicted severe attacks which proved to be severe

NEGATIVE PREDICTIVE VALUE or TRUE NEGATIVE RATE (A/C)
The proportion of predicted mild attacks which proved to be mild

OVERALL or PROGNOSTIC ACCURACY, or EFFICIENCY (A+E/I)
The proportion of all attacks in which outcome was correctly predicted

INACCURACY RATE (D+B/I)
The proportion of all attacks in which outcome was incorrectly predicted

24 or 48 h suggested that although it tends to offer poor sensitivity but excellent specificity, it is as accurate as multiple prognostic criteria after 48 h. However, a review of these studies pointed out that assessments were made by experienced clinicians, often in a research setting, and performance may be poorer in routine clinical practice.[7] Moreover, it is inherently subjective, dependent on the assessor's expertise and experience, and as such, therefore unsuitable for the objective demands of clinical trials.

'Traditional' Multiple Prognostic Criteria

A variety of predictive severity assessments, or *prognostic* systems, were developed in the 1960s and 1970s, in order to assist clinical management and facilitate clinical trials. Acknowledging the complexity of acute pancreatitis would suggest that no single prognostic criterion would suffice; an analysis of multiple factors by the late John Ranson in New York City led to the refinement of practical prognostic criteria.[8] A similar system was developed in parallel by Clem Imrie in Glasgow[9]. Both involved a mix of clinical and laboratory criteria measured during the first 48 h of hospitalisation. The Ranson system has been assessed in 12 published series. An analysis of series reporting a total of 1307 reported attacks (23% severe) yielded 75% sensitivity and 77% specificity (49% PPV, 91% NPV),[7] more sensitive but considerably less specific and with lower PPV than Ranson's index series. The Glasgow system is scored with a smaller number of criteria again using data from the first 48 h of hospitalisation. Analysis of the most recent modification evaluated in 12 published series,[7] involved 2122 attacks (24% severe), in which it offered 69% sensitivity and 84% specificity (57% PPV, 90% NPV). More sensitive, slightly less specific but with a considerably greater PPV than the initial retrospective analysis. Thus the Glasgow system appears slightly less sensitive but has greater specificity and PPV than the Ranson system. In practice, the Glasgow system is used wherever clinical laboratories have adopted *systeme internationale* (SI) unit reporting.

Despite their limitations, the Ranson and Glasgow criteria remain dominant as objective assessments of severity. They were incorporated in the Atlanta criteria for severity,[4] and despite the elapsed time which might be required to score 'positive', many national and international clinical guidelines recommend their use, including those published in the UK.[10] This appears to be principally an attempt to inspire clinical vigilance amongst less experienced clinicians, who manage the majority of patients. However, in the three decades since their development, requirements of the Ranson and Glasgow criteria by researchers has altered. Whilst they both offer a track record and a known level of accuracy, they have an inbuilt delay of up to 48 h, are cumbersome, do not work as well outwith their original case-mix, and provide only a 'one-off' overall prediction. A need for speed, more accuracy and ease of use led to refinements of the original systems, and a host of competitors of which none has endured.

Laboratory Criteria

Increased understanding of inflammatory responses underpinning organ-system failure has spawned a legion of laboratory based prognostic tests. A simple, speedy, cheap, reliable and repeatable laboratory test would form an ideal objective stratification system.

Acute Phase Response

The appearance of C-reactive protein (CRP) in plasma marks the acute phase host response to systemic inflammatory stimulation, and is routinely available in many hospitals. CRP rises significantly only after 48 hours, and various thresholds have been used from 80 mg/l to 210 mg/l. Disregarding these differences, an analysis of 584 attacks (38% severe) from nine published reports[7] reported 80% sensitivity and 76% specificity (67% PPV, 86% NPV). CRP has an accuracy and delay period similar to that of traditional prognostic systems, but offers the advantage of serial monitoring and thus may provide a useful barometer of progress.

Methaemalbuminaemia reflects haemoglobin degradation and was first reported as a useful prognostic indicator during the 1960s.[11] In an analysis of 94 attacks (24% severe) from two studies[7] methaemalbuminaemia provided only 22% sensitivity and 92% specificity (45% PPV, 78% NPV). Methaemalbuminaemia may not develop for 72 h, thus restricting its usefulness. Methaemalbumin also forms the basis for *body wall ecchymosis*. A study from Glasgow demonstrated a fourfold increased mortality,[12] and this, together with a delay of 48 to 72 h for the appearance of ecchymosis renders it useless for stratification in clinical trials.

Neurophil Activation

There is now overwhelming evidence that inflammatory changes mediate multiple organ-system failure, including the release of proteases from activated leukocytes. Phospholipase A_2 (PLA_2) degrades surfactant via lysolecithin production. Measurement of circulating immunoreactive PLA_2 parallels clinical severity, but phospholipase-A_2 activity provides better discrimination between mild and severe attacks. In three analysable publications of 295 attacks (37% severe),[7] elevated PLA_2 activity provided 56% sensitivity and 96% specificity (90% PPV, 79% NPV).

The peak in circulating polymorphonuclear (PMN) elastase appears to precede that of CRP. In an analysis of three studies of 394 attacks (30% severe),[7] elevated PMN elastase offered 88% sensitivity and 99% specificity (76% PPV, 95% NPV). PMN elastase appears superior to Ranson and Glasgow scores, PLA_2 activity and CRP.

Tumour necrosis factor (TNF), interleukins-1 and -6 are important mediators of the acute phase response, their appearance in the circulation should predate the acute phase response. In an analysis of three published studies of 107 attacks (44% severe), elevated interleukin-6 levels on day 1 or 2 provided 89% sensitivity and 85% specificity (82% PPV, 91% NPV), similar to CRP 24 h later.[7] Similarly, in 38 attacks (36% severe by Atlanta criteria),[7] initial interleukin-8 greater than 30 ng/l offered 100% sensitivity and 81% specificity (75% PPV, 100% NPV). Circulating TNF appears to be more evanescent and appears inferior to CRP although measurement of the TNF receptor may be more reliable.[13]

Trypsinogen activation peptide (TAP), a unique fragment cleaved on trypsinogen activation, detectable in urine by immunoassay, has been a prominent newcomer. In an initial UK study of 55 attacks (27% severe), initial urinary TAP exceeding 2 nmol/l provided a remarkable 80% sensitivity and 90% specificity (75% PPV, 92% NPV), superior to CRP and Glasgow scores at 48 h.[14] These findings were replicated in the USA, when 139 patients (40 severe attacks, 28%) studied within 48 h of symptom onset, the sensitivity for admission urinary TAP of 10 ng/ml or more was 100% and specificity 85%.[15] The negative predictive value was 100%. A recent large prospective European study involved 172 attacks (35 with severe disease, 20%).[16] Urinary TAP at 24 h after symptom onset provided sensitivity for TAP>35 nmol/l of 58%, specificity 73%, PPV 39% and NPV 86%. This compared well with CRP at 48 h, APACHE II >7, Ranson and Glasgow scores, TAP at 48 h showed improved discrimination. Carboxypeptidase activation perptide (CAPAP) also shows promise as a predictor of severity.

Computed Tomography

Dynamic computed tomographic and magnetic resonance imaging have also been used to 'stage' pancreatic inflammatory changes for prognosis. Initial studies focused on pancreatic swelling and extra-pancreatic inflammatory findings. The first CT grading system from New York applied five grades: A, normal; B, pancreatic swelling; C, peripancreatic fat abnormalities; D, single fluid collection; and E, multiple collections or gas.[17] The relationship to general morbidity was poor, even though CT grades correlated well with Ranson scores. In an analysis of three studies which formally analysed extra-pancreatic inflammatory changes, using differing, but comparable criteria,[7] in 315 attacks (37% severe), this offered 81% sensitivity and 75% specificity (66% PPV, 87% NPV). Non-ionic contrast agents and more rapid dynamic scanning in the late 1980s led to acceptance of CT for the diagnosis of pancreatic necrosis,[18–21] but few studies have investigated its prognostic role. The importance of pancreatic necrosis in prognosis was acknowledged by its incorporation within the revised New York grading system.[22] Applied in 88 attacks (25% had necrosis), a high CT severity index was associated with 92% morbidity and 17% mortality, and a low index with 2% morbidity and no mortality. Although both CT and magnetic resonance imaging provide morphological assessments of severity and prognosis, they represent an expensive, and not necessarily more accurate, alternative to existing prognosticators. Significant necrosis may occur without organ-system failure, leading to the aphorism 'treat the man, not the scan', and the converse is also true. A preoccupation with prognosis may detract from the most important function of imaging techniques, which remains primarily diagnostic, and to provide precise localisation, differentiation and management of pancreatic collections.

Critical Illness Scoring Systems

The Acute Physiology and Chronic Health Enquiry (APACHE) score was developed by the Intensive Care Research Group, George Washington University Medical Centre, Washington DC, USA to assess and monitor critically patients.[22] Simplifications were made in 1985, reducing from 35 to 14 criteria (Table 28.3),[23] and APACHE-II remains the most commonly evaluated scoring system in acute pancreatitis patients. Like Ranson and Glasgow scores, APACHE-II is also a multiple factor system, comprising pre-existing risk factors, vital signs and simple laboratory criteria. However, APACHE-II can be scored within minutes and repeated whenever required. Each parameter allows for up to four points for both high and low abnormal values, thus the range extends from zero to 72 points, and allows more accurate selection of cut-off levels when used for prognostic assessment. In an initial study of APACHE-II from Leeds of 290 attacks (20% severe), admission scores of 10 or more offered 63% sensitivity and 81% specificity (46% PPV, 90% NPV). By 24 hours scores greater than 10 provided better sensitivity at 71% with 91% specificity (67% PPV, 93% NPV), outperforming Ranson and Glasgow scores at 48 h.[24] These findings were largely confirmed by the Glasgow group.[25] Despite the different casemix, the performance of APACHE-II was remarkably similar in these studies, and in both no patient with a score exceeding 20 points survived. Preliminary results of a joint study of 719 attacks from Leeds and Glasgow provided comparable performance from both centres, and demonstrated that mortality rises sharply when 48 h scores rise from 10 to 12 points, and exceeds 90% for 24 points or more (Fig. 28.1).[26] APACHE-II appears to operate equally accurately in specialist centres in the United States,[27,28] the Netherlands,[29,30] and Spain.[31] Considering three fully analysable studies of 48 h APACHE-II scores in 627 attacks (20% severe), this provided 76% sensitivity and 84% specificity (54% PPV, 93% NPV).[7] The Atlanta criteria incorporated an APACHE-II score of eight points or moreas denoting a severe attack (Table 28.1).[4] Although APACHE-II appears to offer greater flexibility and speed than existing systems, it is essentially similar to the Ranson and Glasgow systems in that it measures systemic responses. However, it can do so repeatedly, and improved accuracy may result simply from an inherently greater score range from which bespoke cut-off levels may be selected. Nevertheless, APACHE-II remains cumbersome and more practical methods are required. APACHE-III was published in 1991,[32] with the introduction of greater score weights, complex scoring matrices, and new variables. Although diagnostic categories are provided for the calculation of risk in individual patients, these are only available for purchasers of a software package.

Table 28.3. Acute physiology and chronic health enquiry (APACHE-II) Score[23]

Parameter	Value range	Score	Parameter	Value range	Score
CORE TEMPERATURE	*0–29.9*	4	**PLASMA POTASSIUM**	*0–2.4*	4
°C	*30.0–31.9*	3	***mmol/L***	*2.5–2.9*	2
	32.0–33.9	2		*3.0–3.4*	1
	34.0–35.9	1		*3.5–5.4*	0
	36.0–38.4	0		*5.5–5.9*	1
	38.5–38.9	1		*6.0–6.9*	3
	39.0–40.9	3		7.0 or more	4
	41 or more	4			
			PLASMA CREATININE	*0–52*	2
PULSE RATE	*0–39*	4	***mmol/L***	*53–132*	0
per minute	*40–54*	3	*(double points for*	*133–176*	2
	55–69	2	*acute renal failure)*	*177–308*	3
	70–109	0		*309 or more*	4
	110–139	2			
	140–179	3	**ARTERIAL pH**	*0–7.14*	4
	180 or more	4		*7.15–7.24*	3
				7.25–7.32	2
MEAN BLOOD PRESSURE	*0–49*	4		*7.33–7.49*	0
mmHg	*50–69*	2		*7.50–7.59*	1
(2xsys.BP)+ dia.BP	*70–109*	0		*7.60–7.69*	3
3	*110–129*	2	or: *(if no blood gases)*	*7.7 or more*	4
	130–159	3	**VENOUS BICARBONATE**	*0–14.9*	4
	160 or more	4	***mmol/L***	*15.0–17.9*	3
				18.0–21.9	2
RESPIRATORY RATE	*0–5*	4		*22.0–31.9*	0
per minute	*6–9*	2		*32.0–40.9*	1
(omit if patient	*10–11*	1		*41.0–51.9*	3
is ventilated)	*12–24*	0		*52 or more*	4
	25–34	1			
	35–49	3	**ARTERIAL pO_2**	*0–7.32*	4
	50 or more	4	***kPa***	*7.33–8.12*	3
				8.13–9.33	1
WHITE CELL COUNT	*0–0.9*	4	or: *(if FiO_2>50%)*	*9.34 & over*	0
10^9/L	*1.0–2.9*	2	**ALVEOLAR/ARTERIAL**	*0–26.6*	0
	3.0–14.9	0	**pO_2 DIFFERENCE**	*26.7–46.6*	2
	15.0–19.9	1	kPa (p_A-p_aO_2)	*46.7–66.6*	3
	20.0–39.9	2		*66.7 & over*	4
	40 or more	4			
			AGE	*0–44*	0
HAEMATOCRIT	*0–19.9*	4	***years***	*45–54*	2
%	*20.0–29.9*	2		*55–64*	3
	30.0–45.9	0		*65–74*	5
	46.0–49.9	1		*75 or more*	6
	50.0–59.9	2			
	60 or more	4	**GLASGOW COMA SCORE**		
			(Score as 15 points minus actual score)		
PLASMA SODIUM	*0–110*	4			
mmol/L	*111–119*	3	CHRONIC HEALTH SCORE		
	120–129	2	Cardiac: *New York Heart Ass. Grade IV*		
	130–149	0	Respiratory: *minimal effort dyspnoea*		
	150–154	1	Hepatic *cirrhosis/portal hypertension*		
	155–159	2	Renal: *receiving dialysis.*		
	160–179	3	Immunodeficiency/suppression: *any cause*		
	180 or more	4	(If post-emerg.op 2 points; other 5 points)		

Weighted parameter scores are added, plus points for age, and chronic illness, depending on whether post-operative, to form the total. Unmeasured parameters are considered normal

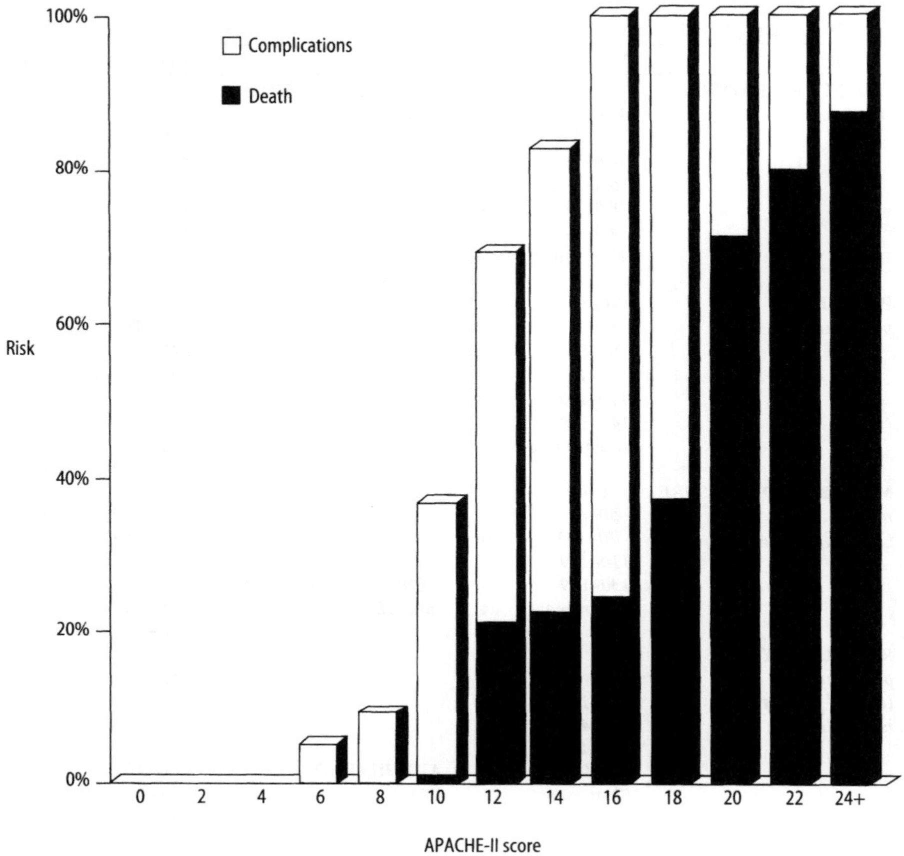

Figure 28.1. 48 h APACHE-II scores, morbidity and mortality.[26]

APACHE-II in Recent Clinical Trials

By the mid 1990s, Ranson,[33,34] Glasgow[34-38] and APACHE-II[39] scores, and dynamic CT criteria[40,41] had all been used to stratify patients entering clinical therapeutic trials. The first study in the UK to use APACHE-II as an entry-stratification was the multi-centre study of lexipafant in severe acute pancreatitis.[42] On the basis of data analysed from previous studies in Leeds and Glasgow, an APACHE-II cut-off score of greater than 6 was used which was predicted to achieve a 40% incidence of severe attacks. Some 290 patients were recruited from 87 hospitals. Some 57% of randomised patients experienced severe attacks, so the pre-trial modelling using APACHE-II scores was demonstrably effective in this study. However, patients could be randomised as late as 72 h after onset of symptoms, and this may explain why 44% already had established organ-system failure at entry and that there was no significant difference in attributable mortality between lexipafant (9.5%) and placebo (15.4%) therapy. A significantly lower mortality was demonstrated if patients were randomised less than 48 h after onset of symptoms, at 7.7% for lexipafant and 17.9% for placebo ($p = 0.03$).

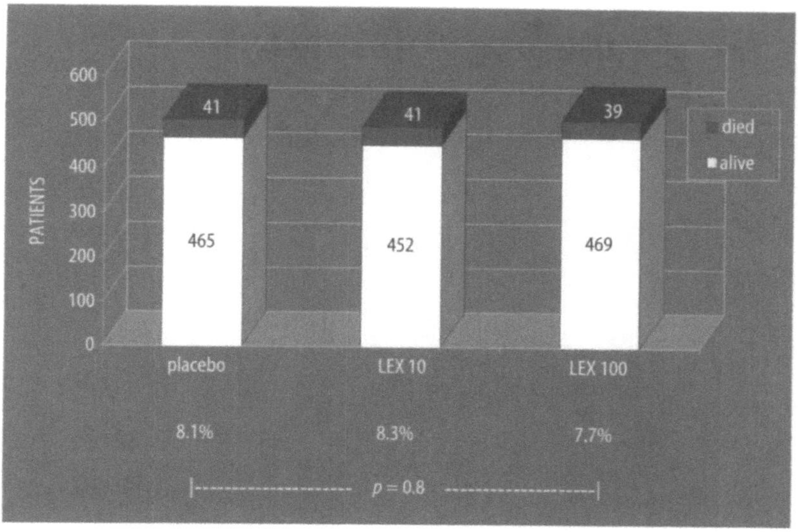

Figure 28.2. International Lexipafant study: All causes of 28 day mortality.[43]

Encouraged by this result, a further study of a two dose regimen of lexipafant therapy was undertaken in the USA, in which Europe later participated.[43] A total of 121 hospital units (83 US, 28 European) participated in the study which extended from January 1996 until January 1999. Some 1518 patients were randomised after entry stratification on the basis of an APACHE-II or 6 or more, making this the largest therapeutic trial in acute pancreatitis. The median APACHE-II was only 10.5 points and mortality was almost even at 8% across placebo and both treatment groups (Fig. 28.2).

Clearly, despite the use of data available from previous studies in the UK, APACHE-II score stratification with a cut-off of 6, or more, unexpectedly yielded an experience of severity lower than that generally expected in unstratified disease in previous UK trials and clinical series. Previous data from the UK suggested a steep rise in mortality when entry APACHE-II scores rise from 6 to 10 points. Would a higher cut-off have been more effective? Analysing this trial retrospectively by only including patients with scores of 8 or more would have left 80% in the study, with an overall mortality of 12%, rising to 15% with scores of 10 more. However, there were no significant differences between treatment and placebo groups at any cutoff level in this study. The variation in the performance of APACHE-III in this study with original trial data from the UK suggested the possibility of a lower mortality in the US, but there was no significant difference between US and European patients (Fig. 28.3). A diligent search has not uncovered any obvious reason for the poor stratification achieved, although it is perhaps notable that some 46% of centres randomised fewer than 10 patients each.

Conclusions

With regard to the needs of clinical trials, better *prognostic systems* are required for stratification as close as possible to the initial insult. Better systems for the

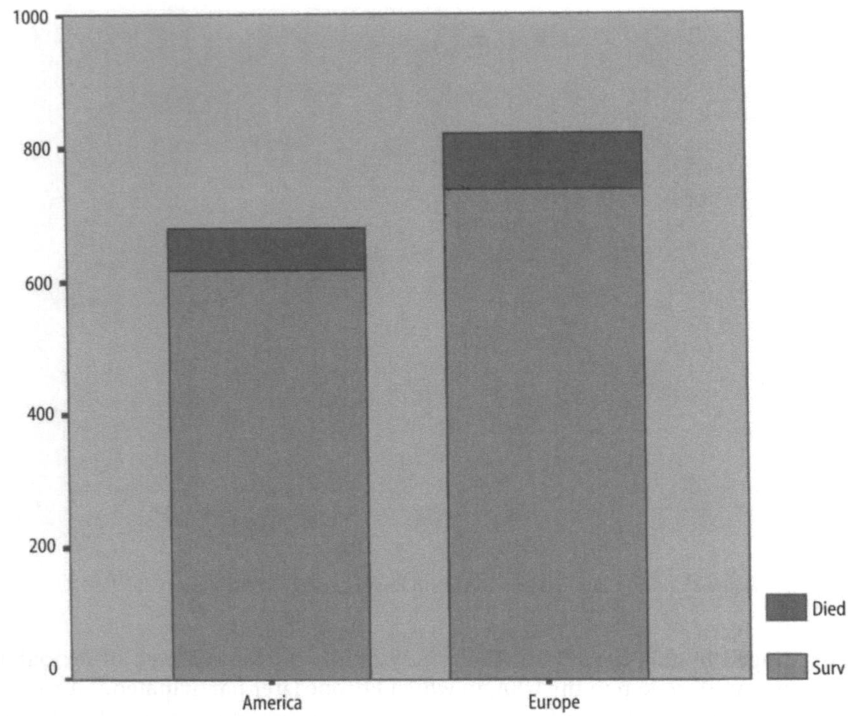

Figure 28.3. International Lexipafant study: outcome by continent.[42]

assessment of *host responses* to determine the effectiveness of therapy are also needed. Comparison of competing stratification systems has been marred by problems in evaluation, and this impedes any attempt at meta-analysis, but adoption of agreements achieved at Atlanta symposium may facilitate further progress. Should a specific treatment become available after successful evaluation, then efficient stratification systems will also prove necessary to enable appropriate therapeutic targeting.

Ranson, Glasgow and APACHE-II scores and CRP measurements are currently routinely available, and have become accepted as assessments of clinical severity and prognosis. APACHE-II and CRP offer additional serial monitoring capabilities.

APACHE-II has proved disappointing in a large scale clinical trial, and this recent experience suggest that like other currently available scoring systems, it is insufficiently rapid or accurate enough for confident use in further trials. Thought must now be applied to the newer contenders. Urinary activation peptides are promising in this regard. TAP provides an index of the initial biological severity of the attack by quantifying the degree of pancreatic protease activation. TAP is commercially available in the UK. It may also be useful to measure the activation peptide of carboxypeptidase-B (CAPAP) as an index of host inflammatory responses. One caveat for the future may be that advanced almost a decade ago by Heinrich Rindernecht, namely that genetic polymorphisms could condition host responses to acute pancreatitis, and thus largely determine outcome.[44] Evidence is now emerging to this effect, and such variations must be considered when geographically diverse populations are entered into therapeutic trials.

APACHE-II has been used successfully to stratify patients entering a clinical trial for septic shock,[45] as an outcome measure,[46] and to stratify outcome.[47,48] However, perhaps the ideal combination lies with a combination of APACHE-II and rapid diagnostics stick tests for the markers of severity, such as IL-5, which has been used to stratify entry to a clinical trial of an anti-TNF agent in severe sepsis.[49]

References

1. Sarles H. (Ed.) Pancreatitis. New York, Karger, 1965.
2. Singer MV, Gyr K, Sarles H. Revised classification of pancreatitis. Gastroenterology 1985; 89:683–685.
3. Sarner M, Cotton PB. Classification of pancreatitis. Gut 1984; 25:756–759.
4. Bradley EL. A clinically based classification system for acute pancreatitis. Summary of the International Symposium on Acute Pancreatitis, Atlanta, Sept. 11–13 1992. Arch Sur 1993; 128:586–590.
5. Dervenis C, Johnson CD, Bassi C, et al. Diagnosis, objective assessment of severity, and management of acute pancreatitis. Santorini consensus conference. Int J Pancreatol 1999; 25:195–210.
6. Steinberg WM. Predictors of severity of acute pancreatitis. Gastroenterology Clin of N Amer 1990; 19:849–861.
7. Larvin M. Chapter 46. Clinical assessment of severity (from Section V: Acute Pancreatitis). pp. 489–502. In: Beger HG, Warshaw AL, Carr-Locke DL, et al. (Editors). The Pancreas: A Clinical Textbook. Blackwell Scientific Publications, Oxford, 1998.
8. Ranson JHC, Rifkind KM, Roses DF, et al. Prognostic signs and the role of operative management in acute pancreatitis. Surg Gyn and Obst 1974; 139:69–81.
9. Imrie CW, Benjamin IS, Ferguson JC, et al. A single centre double blind trial of Trasylol therapy in primary acute pancreatitis. Br J Surg 1978; 65:337–341.
10. Anon. United Kingdom guidelines for the management of acute pancreatitis. British Society of Gastroenterology. Gut 1998; 42 (Suppl 2):S1–13.
11. Winstone NE. Methemalbumin in acute pancreatitis. Br J Surg 1965; 52:804–808.
12. Dickson AP, Imrie CW. The incidence and prognosis of body wall ecchymosis in acute pancreatitis. Surg, Gyne and Obst 1984; 159:343–347.
13. de Beaux AC, Goldie AS, Ross JA, et al. Serum concentrations of inflammatory mediators related to organ failure in patients with acute pancreatitis. Br J Surg 1996; 83: 349–53.
14. Gudgeon AM, Heath DI, Hurley P, et al. Trypsinogen activation peptides assay in the early prediction of severity of acute pancreatitis. Lancet 1990; 335:4–8.
15. Tenner S, Fernandez-del Castillo C, Warshaw A, et al. Urinary trypsinogen activation peptide (TAP) predicts severity in patients with acute pancreatitis. Int J Pancreatol 1997; 21:105–10.
16. Neoptolemos JP, Kemppainen EA, Mayer JM, et al. Early prediction of severity in acute pancreatitis by urinary trypsinogen activation peptide: a multicentre study. Lancet 2000; 355 (9219):1955–60.
17. Balthazar EJ, Ranson JH, Naidich DP, et al. Acute pancreatitis: prognostic value of CT. Radiology 1985; 156:767–772.
18. Larvin M, Chalmers AG, Robinson PJ, et al. Debridement and closed cavity irrigation for the treatment of pancreatic necrosis. Br J Surg 1989; 76:465–471.
19. Bradley EL, Murphy F, Ferguson C. Prediction of pancreatic necrosis by dynamic pancreatography. Ann Surg 1989; 210:495–503.
20. Larvin M, Chalmers AG, McMahon MJ. Dynamic contrast enhanced computed tomography: a precise technique for identifying and localising pancreatic necrosis. Br Med J 1990; 300:1425–1428.
21. Balthazar EJ, Robinson DL, Megibow AJ, et al. Acute pancreatitis: value of CT in establishing prognosis. Radiology 1990; 174:331–336.
22. Knaus WA, Zimmerman JE, Wagner DP, et al. APACHE: acute physiology and chronic health evaluation: a physiologically based classification system. Crit Care Med 1981; 9:591–597.
23. Knaus WA, Draper EA, Wagner DP, et al. APACHE-II: A severity of disease classification. Crit Care Med 1985; 13:818–829.

24. Larvin M, McMahon MJ. APACHE-II score for assessment and monitoring of acute pancreatitis. Lancet 1989; 2:201–205.
25. Wilson C, Heath DI, Imrie CW. Prediction of outcome in acute pancreatitis: a comparative study of APACHE II, clinical assessment and multiple factor scoring systems. Br J Surg 1990; 77:1260–1264.
26. Heath D, Alexander D, Wilson C, et al. Which complications of acute pancreatitis are most lethal. A prospective evaluation of 719 episodes. (Abstract). Gut 1995; 36:A478.
27. Stanten R, Frey CF. Comprehensive management of acute necrotizing pancreatitis and pancreatic abscess. Arc Surg 1990; 125:1269–74.
28. Banks PA. Predictors of severity in acute pancreatitis. Pancreas 1991; 6: Suppl 1: S7–12.
29. Tran DD, Cuesta MA. Evaluation of severity in patients with acute pancreatitis. Amer J Gastr 1992; 87:604–608.
30. Roumen RM, Schers TJ, de Boer HH, et al. Scoring systems for predicting outcome in acute hemorrhagic necrotizing pancreatitis. European J Surg 1992; 158:167–171.
31. Dominguez-Munoz JE, Carballo F, Garcia MJ, et al. Evaluation of the clinical usefulness of APACHE II and SAPS systems in the initial prognostic classification of acute pancreatitis: a multicenter study. Pancreas 1993; 8:682–686.
32. Knaus WA, Wagner DP, Draper EA, et al. The APACHE-III prognostic system. Risk prediction of hospital mortality for critically ill hospitalized adults. Chest 1991; 100:1619–1636.
33. Neoptolemos JP, Carr-Locke DL, London NJ, et al. Controlled trial of urgent endoscopic retrograde cholangiopancreatography and endoscopic sphincterotomy versus conservative treatment for acute pancreatitis due to gallstones. Lancet 1988; 2:979–983.
34. Leese T, Holliday M, Watkins M, et al. A multicentre controlled clinical trial of high-volume fresh frozen plasma therapy in prognostically severe acute pancreatitis. Ann of the Royal College of Surg of England 1991; 73:207–214.
35. Mayer AD, McMahon MJ, Corfield AP, et al. Controlled clinical trial of peritoneal lavage for the treatment of severe acute pancreatitis. New Eng J Med 1985; 312:399–404.
36. Kingsnorth AN, Galloway SW, Formela LJ. Randomized, double-blind phase II trial of Lexipafant, a platelet-activating factor antagonist, in human acute pancreatitis. Br J Surg 1995; 82:1414–1420.
37. Paran H, Neufeld D, Mayo A, et al. Preliminary report of a prospective randomized study of octreotide in the treatment of severe acute pancreatitis. J of the American College of Surg 1995; 181:121–124.
38. Luiten EJ, Hop WC, Lange JF, et al. Controlled clinical trial of selective decontamination for the treatment of severe acute pancreatitis. Anns Surg 1995; 222:57–65.
39. Pederzoli P, Bassi C, Falconi M, et al. Gabexate mesilate in the treatment of acute pancreatitis. Annali Italiani Di Chirurgia 1995; 66:191–195.
40. Leese T, Holliday M, Watkins M, et al. A multicentre controlled clinical trial of high-volume fresh frozen plasma therapy in prognostically severe acute pancreatitis. Ann of the Royal College of Surg Eng 1991; 73:207–214.
41. Luiten EJ, Hop WC, Lange JF, et al. Controlled clinical trial of selective decontamination for the treatment of severe acute pancreatitis. Ann Surg 1995; 222:57–65.
42. Johnson CD, Kingsnorth AN, Imrie CW, et al. Double blind, randomised, placebo controlled study of a platelet activating factor antagonist, lexipafant, in the treatment and prevention of organ failure in predicted severe acute pancreatitis. Gut 2001; 48:62–9.
43. Larvin M, Ammori B, McMahon MJ, et al. on behalf of the International Study Group on Acute Pancreatitis. A Double-Blind, Randomised, Placebo-Controlled Multi-Centre Trial to Evaluate Efficacy And Safety of Two Doses of Lexipafant in Acute Pancreatitis Therapy. Pancreatology 2001; 1:279.
44. Rinderknecht H. Genetic determinants of mortality in acute necrotizing pancreatitis. Intl J Panc 1994; 16:11–15.
45. Poeze M, Froon AH, Ramsay G, et al. Decreased organ failure in patients with severe SIRS and septic shock treated with the platelet-activating factor antagonist TCV-309: a prospective, multicenter, double-blind, randomized phase II trial. TCV-309 Septic Shock Study Group. Shock 2000; 14:421–8.
46. Shukla VK, Ojha AK, Pandey M, et al. Pentoxifylline in perforated peritonitis: results of a randomised, placebo controlled trial. Eur J Surg 2001; 167:622–4.
47. Abraham E, Reinhart K, Svoboda P, et al. Assessment of the safety of recombinant tissue factor pathway inhibitor in patients with severe sepsis: a multicenter, randomized, placebo-controlled, single-blind, dose escalation study. Crit Care Med 2001; 29:2081–9.

48. Lin MT, Kung SP, Yeh SL, et al. The effect of glutamine-supplemented total parenteral nutrition on nitrogen economy depends on severity of diseases in surgical patients. Clin Nutr 2002; 21:213–8.
49. Reinhart K, Menges T, Gardlund B, et al. Randomized, placebo-controlled trial of the anti-tumor necrosis factor antibody fragment afelimomab in hyper-inflammatory response during severe sepsis: The RAMSES Study. Crit Care Med 2001; 29:765–9.

29 Selecting Severe Cases of Acute Pancreatitis for Trials and for Treatment: Enzymes and Activation Peptides

Pauli A. Puolakkainen

Acute pancreatitis (AP) is a common disease with wide variation in severity. At present, there is no 'gold standard' for diagnosing AP nor assessing its severity. However, early identification of AP and especially detection of patients with a severe form of the disease is nowadays known to be of utmost importance.

Various digestive enzymes are produced by pancreatic acinar cells. Premature intrapancreatic activation of trypsinogen and other proenzymes leading to tissue damage and eventually to autodigestion of the pancreas is a crucial early event in the pathophysiology of AP. Therefore, enzyme and activation peptide-based assays would theoretically provide attractive means of detecting AP and assessing its severity.

In this chapter the current knowledge of measuring enzymes and activation peptides for selecting patients with severe AP for trials and for treatment is reviewed. To date, none of them alone provides sufficient predictive power to facilitate clinical decision-making.

Several factors are involved in determining the severity of an episode of acute pancreatitis. Patient related factors include age, co-morbidity and genetic factors. Disease related factors include etiology of AP, development of pancreatic necrosis and organ failure and infection of the necrosis as well as the treatment. All these should be taken into account when disease severity is estimated clinically and with enzyme assays. Further, the clinical use of an assay depends on the available treatment options. If we consider expensive treatment or intervention with significant side-effects, high PPV of a test is required to avoid unjustified procedures in patients with mild AP. In case of a safe treatment regimen, high NPV of a test is needed to enable provision of appropriate care to all patients suffering from severe AP.

Detection of Severe Acute Pancreatitis

At present, the clinical classification of AP is based on the internationally recognised Atlanta criteria.[1] In an emergency setting, the identification of severe AP remains problematic and several patients with severe disease are diagnosed only at autopsy.[2] It has been shown that patients with severe AP and delayed transfer to the intensive care unit have higher mortality than those admitted directly.[3] There is also evidence that early enteral feeding, prophylactic antiobiotics and emergency endoscopic sphincterotomy in patients with biliary AP are beneficial in severe

AP.[4–10] Early diagnosis of patients with severe AP would enable their immediate referral to a centre with facilities for maximal intensive care and specialists in endoscopic, radiological and surgical management of AP, and would also allow comparisons between centres participating in trials. Further, since new immunomodulatory therapies may have undesirable side effects, it is of utmost importance to accurately identify patients who will benefit from immunomodulation. On the other hand, it is important to recognize patients with mild AP to allow their treatment in lower-cost hospital beds.

One of the main problems with AP has been the lack of accurate early predictors of disease severity, including organ failure. On admission, clinical assessment of severity has been shown to be unreliable.[11] Contrast enhanced-computed tomography (CE-CT) has improved the assessment of the disease severity by accurately identifying areas of necrosis.[12,13] Magnetic resonance imaging is increasingly used for assessing the severity of AP with promising results.[14]

There are several clinico-biochemical scoring systems such as the Ranson and Glasgow criteria and APACHE II for the assessment of the severity of AP.[15,16] Due to their complexity, the multi-factorial systems are seldom routinely used in clinical practice.[17]

Much effort has been directed to developing a single, simple, rapid, affordable and reliable laboratory test for the severity assessment of an attack of AP. The severity of AP does not correlate with the level of serum amylase and lipase.[18] C-reactive protein (CRP) is the most commonly used laboratory test in the assessment of the severity of AP but it is useful only 48–72 h after the onset of the disease and is insensitive earlier.[19] However, in the follow-up during the course of the disease, CRP has proven to be useful.[20] The rapid test measuring procalcitonin has recently given encouraging results.[21] Estimation of plasma levels of cytokines are expensive and/or laborious and time-consuming to perform.

Enzymes in Detecting Patients with Severe Pancreatitis

In published studies enzymes and activation peptides have not been used alone in discriminating mild and severe AP, since none of them is ideal for this purpose. In combination with prognostic factors enzymes such as ribonuclease, chymotrypsin, elastase and pancreatic isoamylase have, however, been used for diagnosis but do not reliably detect severe disease. Phospholipase A_2 was originally suggested to provide a method for predicting severity of AP.[20] Later studies have revealed, however, that pancreatic group I phospholipase A_2 does not correlate with the severity of AP.[22,23] On the other hand, secretory, non-pancreatic group II phospholipase A_2, a general inflammatory parameter, has been shown to have pathophysiological importance in severe AP-associated SIRS.[24] Unfortunately, this assay is not suitable for use in the emergency setting.

Trypsin-based Laboratory Methods for Detection of Severe AP

Trypsinogen, a serine protease precursor is the main protease in human pancreatic fluid. The conversion of trypsinogen to active trypsin, a 24-kDA protease, is catalysed normally in the duodenum by intestinal enterokinase,[25] which releases a peptide called trypsinogen activation peptide (TAP).[19,26] Trypsin is the key enzyme for rapid activation of all the proenzymes, including its own proenzyme, trypsinogen. There are two major isoenzymes of trypsinogen: cationic trypsinogen-1 and anionic trypsinogen-2.[27] In the normal state only a minor proportion of the total trypsinogen production leaks into circulation.[28] When active trypsin reaches the circulation the major trypsin inhibitors, alpha-1-antitrypsin and alpha-2-macroglobulin, inactivate it.[29]

Immunoreactive Trypsin and Trypsinogen

There are laboratory methods based on the determination of pancreatic enzymes in serum and urine, which measure the intrinsic biological severity of organ damage by estimating the degree of the primary pancreatic proteolytic insult. Levels of immunoreactive trypsin reflect the leakage of unactivated proenzymes from injured acinar cells. The original assays for determination of immunoreactive trypsin preferentially measured cationic trypsinogen i.e. trypsinogen-1 and abnormal concentrations were considered strongly to suggest a diagnosis of pancreatitis.[31–32] Using specific antibodies for trypsinogen-1 and trypsinogen-2 it was found that in AP, the serum concentrations of trypsinogen-2 were increased 50-fold and those of trypsinogen-1 only 15-fold. The corresponding increase in immunoreactive trypsin was also only 15-fold.[32] Moreover, patients with AP excrete large amounts of trypsinogen-2 into urine within hours of the disease onset. Thus, quantitative trypsinogen-2 assay has been shown to be an useful marker for AP[32–34] and both urine and serum values correlate with the severity of the disease.[33–35] Unfortunately, the assay is technicallly demanding and cannot be used in clinical emergency setting.

Our research group has earlier introduced a rapid urinary trypsinogen-2 test strip for diagnosis of AP, which is based on the use of immunochromatography with monoclonal antibodies.[36] The trypsinogen-2 strip test can be performed rapidly in health care centres with limited laboratory facilities. A modified 5-min dipstick, actimPancreatitis® (Medix Biochemica, Kauniainen, Finland), has recently been developed with new antibodies to detect elevated levels of trypsinogen-2 in urine. The accuracy of the actimPancreatitis® test[37] proved to be very similar to that of the preliminary dipstick (sensitivity 96%, specificity 92%), which has been reported in a retrospective[36] and a prospective[38] study. Due to the very high sensitivity and negative predictive value (NPV)(90.6%) of the actimPancreatitis® test strip, AP can be excluded with high probability with a negative dipstick result. It, therefore, appears to be suitable as a screening test for AP in patients with acute abdominal pain. However, in a recent report by Pezzilli et al. the actimPancreatitis® test strip showed high specificity but low sensitivity in the diagnosis of AP.[39] In all the studies reported so far, the dipstick has detected all the severe cases of AP very accurately, which is important in clinical practice. The quantitative measurements of urinary trypsinogen-2 showed a good correlation with the test strip result (the kappa value 0.86), supporting the use of the simple and rapid dipstick.[37]

Trypsinogen-antiprotease-complexes and Antiproteases

Biochemical indicators of AP and its severity include the antiproteases and their complexes with trypsin. High serum concentrations of immunoreactive trypsin-alpha-1-antitrypsin complexes have been demonstrated in AP, and the levels on admission correlate with the severity of AP.[40] Our study group has measured trypsin-2 complexed with alpha-1-antitrypsin using a specific monoclonal antibody to trypsin-2 and a polyclonal antibody to alpha-1-antitrypsin.[34] In this study of 110 patients with AP and 66 patients with acute abdominal pain, trypsin-2-alpha-1-antitrypsin complex in serum had the largest AUC both in differentiating AP from control patients (0.995) and detecting mild AP from severe disease (0.82) as compared to CRP, amylase and trypsinogen-2 12 hours after admission.[34] The assay, however, is not suitable for use in emergecy setting. Recently, the ratio of trypsin-2-alpha-1-antitrypsin to trypsinogen-1 in serum was reported to be a promising new indicator for discriminating between biliary and alcohol-induced AP.[41] Serum alpha-2-macroglobulin concentrations are found to be significantly lower in complicated attacks of AP suggesting its excessive consumption.[42] Additionally, concentrations of complexed alpha-2-macroglobulin have been shown to increase in severe AP.[43] However, measurement of alpha-2-macroglobulin is not currently in clinical use partly due to complicated and time-consuming assay methods.

Activation Peptides in Detecting Patients with Severe Pancreatitis

Potentially useful activation peptides in selecting severe cases of acute pancreatitis include trypsinogen activation peptide (TAP), pancreatic phospholipase A2 activation peptide (PROP) and carboxypeptidase B activation peptide (CAPAP).

TAP

TAP is a highly conserved amino-terminal peptide relased during trypsinogen activation to trypsin. Immunoreactive TAP reflects the amount of pathological intrapancreatic trypsinogen activation irrespective whether the resulting trypsin is active or blocked by inhibitors.[44,45] Thus, it is a marker specifically related to the onset of AP.[26] Free TAP is liberated into the peritoneal cavity and circulation, after which, because of its small size, the peptide is rapidly cleared by kidneys and excreted into the urine.[45] However, the measurement of TAP in urine is not a useful diagnostic test for AP, since Gudgeon *et al.* reported that 30% of patients with AP had normal TAP values on admission.[26] Further, in an ERCP study, urinary TAP was not useful in predicting mild post-ERCP AP.[46] It has also been shown that the concentrations of urinary TAP do not vary according to the cause of the disease.[19]

In an animal model of AP TAP concentration in ascites, urine, plasma and pancreatic tissue has been shown to correlate well with the extent of pancreatic necrosis.[47] The urinary TAP/creatinine ratio correlates with the severity of the disease in humans.[48] Concentrations of TAP in urine have been shown to predict severe AP with a sensitivity of 100% and a specificity of 85% on admission to hospital within 48 h of the onset of symptoms in an American multicenter study.[49] In a recent European multicenter study, urinary TAP was shown to have a somewhat lower accuracy for the assessment of the severity of AP already 24 h after the onset of symptoms with a sensitivity of 58% and a specificity of 73% .[19] Thus, urinary TAP values correlate with the severity of AP at admission.[19,26,49] Clinically the most favourable feature of urinary TAP is the capability to differentiate between severe and mild disease during the very early phase of the disease, when other methods are not yet useful. Windsor considered its wider use justified since it is a single assay performed early in the attack with accuracy as good as that of other prognostic factors. However, the general accuracy of urinary TAP alone does not reach levels that are reliable for clinical decision-making and the currently available ELISA kit is not ideal in emergency setting. In plasma, TAP showed maximal accuracy for distinction between mild and severe disease within 6 hours of the admission with a sensitivity of 70% and specificity of 78%. Thereafter the prognostic accuracy declined rapidly and TAP values showed a very variable pattern possibly due to burst-like secretion.[50]

PROP

Heath et al measured prophospholipase A2 activation peptide concentration in patients with AP. Activation peptide–creatinine ratios were significantly greater in those with severe AP.[48] Previously increased PROP values have been reported in patients with severe trauma and acute lung injury.[51,52] In a multicentre study, the median maximum values of PROP at 48 h after the onset of symptoms were significantly elevated in patients with severe AP as compared to mild disease. The levels of PROP were related to overall disease severity but did not correlate with distant organ failure. PROP detected severe AP with sensitivity, specificity, NPV and PPV of 71%, 59%, 88% and 32%, respectively (Meyer, unpublished results). Thus, the accuracy of the test did not prove to be sufficient to allow clinical decision-making.

CAPAP

Released activation peptides of zymogens reflect free trypsin activity. Procarboxypeptidase B has an activation peptide, carboxypeptidase activation peptide (CAPAP), that is larger than other peptides released during proenzyme activation.[53] The large size makes it more stable and, thus, suitable for measurement in serum and urine, and now, radioimmunoassay has been developed for this peptide.[54] It has been reported that the levels of CAPAP in urine and serum correlate well with the severity of AP.[55] The AUC, representing the discriminatory power for severe disease, was 0.9422 when CAPAP concentration was measured in urine. However, the study included only 60 inconsecutive AP patients and only 12 of them had severe disease. Eight of the 60 AP patients (all with mild disease) had undetectable levels of CAPAP in urine. This suggests that measurement of CAPAP cannot be used as a diagnostic test for AP, since many mild cases would be missed. As for the accuracy of the CAPAP assay for the severity assessment of AP, further prospective clinical studies with sufficient number of patients are needed.

Conclusion

At present, no single biochemical marker is ideal for diagnosis and/or early prediction of severity of AP. Assays based on trypsin pathophysiology have brought interesting new alternatives for diagnostics and severity grading of AP. Urinary TAP can be measured relatively easily and has prognostic value especially in combination with CRP and could help the physician in clinical practice. Urinary CAPAP seems very promising as a prognostic marker but should be studied with a large consecutive series of AP patients before wider clinical use. Of non-enzyme predictors, CRP remains in wide clinical use and procalcitonin has given some promising results. It seems obvious that no enzyme or activation peptide alone provides sufficient predicitive power to facilitate clinical decision-making or justify selecting severe cases of AP for trials or treatment and a combination of tests may be needed to predict severe AP and its systemic complications when new therapies are planned. In the future, additional studies with a sufficient number of patients will be needed to find out the most accurate set of markers.

References

1. Bradley III E. A clinically based classification system for acute pancreatitis. Summary of the international symposium on acute pancreatitis, Atlanta, GA, September 11–13, 1992. Arch Surg 1993; 128:586–90.
2. Appelros S, Borgström A. Incidence, aetiology and mortality rate of acute pancreatitis over 10 years in a defined urban population in Sweden. Br J Surg 1999; 86:465–70.
3. De Beaux A, Palmer K, Carter D. Factors influencing morbidity and mortality in acute pancreatitis; an analysis of 279 cases. Gut 1995; 37:121–6.
4. Fan S, Lai E, Mok F, et al. Early treatment of acute biliary pancreatitis by endoscopic papillotomy. N Engl J Med 1993; 328:228–32.
5. Barie P. A critical review of antibiotic prophylaxis in severe acute pancreatitis. Am J Surg 1996; 172 (Suppl 6A):38–43.
6. Neoptolemos J, Carr-Locke D, London N, et al. Controlled trial of urgent endoscopic retrograde cholangiopancreatography and endoscopic sphincterotomy versus conservative treatment for acute pancreatitis due to gall stones. Lancet 1988; 2:980–3.
7. Sainio V, Kemppainen E, Puolakkainen P, et al. Early antibiotic treatment in acute necrotising pancreatitis. Lancet 1995; 346:663–667.
8. Nowak A, Marek T, Nowakowska-Dulawa E, et al. Biliary pancreatitis needs endoscopic retrograde cholangiopancreatography with endoscopic sphincterotomy for cure. Endoscopy 1998; 30:256–9.
9. Brivet F, Emilie D, Galanaud P. The Parisian Study Group on Acute Pancreatitis. Pro- and anti-inflammatory cytokines during acute severe pancreatitis: An early and sustained response, although unpredictive of death. Crit Care Med 1999; 27:749–55.
10. Kanwar S, Windsor A. Early enteral nutrition in acute pancreatitis. Nutrition 1999; 15:951–2.
11. Büchler M. Objectification of the severity of acute pancreatitis. Hepato-Gastroenterol 1991; 38:101–8.
12. Kivisaari L, Somer K, Strandertskjöld-Nordenstam C, et al. Early detection of acute fulminant pancreatitis by contrast-enhanced computed tomography. Scand J Gastroenterol 1983; 18:39–41.
13. Balthazar E, Robinson D, Megibow A, et al. Acute pancreatitis: value of CT in establishing prognosis. Radiology 1990; 174:331–6.
14. Ward J, Chalmers A, Guthrie A, et al. T2-weighted and dynamic enhanced MRI in acute pancreatitis: comparison with contrast enhanced CT. Clin Radiol 1997; 52:109–14.
15. Wilson C, Heath D, Imrie C. Prediction of outcome in acute pancreatitis: a comparative study of APACHE II, clinical assessment and multiple factor scoring systems. Br J Surg 1990; 77:1260–4.
16. Brisinda G, Maria G, Ferrante A, et al. Evaluation of prognostic factors in patients with acute pancreatitis. Hepato-Gastroenterol 1999; 46:1990–7.
17. Toh S, Phillips S, Johnson C. A prospective audit against management of acute pancreatitis in the south of England. Gut 2000; 46:239–43.
18. Kazmierczak S, Van Lente F, Hodges E. Diagnostic and prognostic utility of phospholipase A activity in patients with acute pancreatitis: Comparison with amylase and lipase. Clin Chem 1991; 37:356–60
19. Neoptolemos J, Kemppainen E, Mayer J, et al. Early prediction of severity in acute pancreatitis by urinary trypsinogen activation peptide: a multicentre study. Lancet 2000; 355:1955–60.

20. Puolakkainen P, Valtonen V, Paananen A, et al. C-reactive protein (CRP) and serum phospholipase A2 in the assessment of the severity of acute pancreatitis. Gut 1987; 28:764–71.
21. Kylänpää-Bäck ML, Takala E, Kemppainen E, et al. Procalcitonin strip test in early detection of severe acute pancreatitis. Br J Surg 2001; 88:222–7.
22. Kemppainen E, Hietaranta A, Puolakkainen P, et al. Bactericidal/permeability-increasing protein and group I and II phospholipase A2 during the induction phase of human acute pancreatitis. Pancreas 1999; 18:21–27.
23. Nevalainen T, Hietaranta A, Gronroos J. Phospholiase A2 in acute pancreatitis: new biochemical and pathological aspects. Hepatogastroenterology 1999; 46:2731–35.
24. Hietaranta A, Kemppainen E, Puolakkainen P, et al. Extracellular phospholipases A2 in relation to systemic inflammatory response syndrome (SIRS) and systemic complications in severe acute pancreatitis. Pancreas 1999; 4:385–91.
25. Kassel B, Kay J. Zymogens of proteolytic enzymes. Science 1973; 180:1022–7.
26. Gudgeon A, Heath D, Hurley P, et al. Trypsinogen activation peptides assay in the early prediction of severity of acute pancreatitis. Lancet 1990; 335:4–8.
27. Rinderknecht H, Geokas M. Anionic and cationic trypsinogens (trypsins) in mammalian pancreas. Enzyme 1973; 14:116–30.
28. Borgström A, Ohlsson K. Studies on the turnover of endogenous cathodal trypsinogen in man. Eur J Clin Invest 1978; 8:379–82.
29. Ohlsson K. Acute pancreatitis. Biochemical, pathophysiological and therapeutic aspects. Acta Gastroenterol Belg 1988; 51:3–12.
30. Brodrick J, Geokas M, Largman C, et al. Molecular forms of immunoreactive pancreatic cationic trypsin in pancreatitis sera. Am J Physiol 1979; 237:474–80.
31. Elias E, Redshaw M, Wood T. Diagnostic importance of changes in circulating concentrations of immunoreactive trypsin. Lancet 1977; 9:66–8.
32. Itkonen O, Koivunen E, Hurme M, et al. Time-resolved immunofluorometric assays for trypsinogen-1 and 2 in serum reveal preferential elevation of trypsinogen-2 in pancreatitis. J Lab Clin Med 1990; 115:712–8.
33. Hedström J, Leinonen J, Sainio V, et al. Time-resolved immunofluorometric assay of trypsin-2 complexed with alpha1-antitrypsin in serum. Clin Chem 1994; 40:1761–5.
34. Hedström J, Sainio V, Kemppainen E, et al. Serum complex of trypsin 2 and alpha-1-antitrypsin as diagnostic and prognostic marker of acute pancreatitis: clinical study in consecutive patients. BMJ 1996; 313:333–7.
35. Sainio V, Puolakkainen P, Kemppainen E, et al. Serum trypsinogen-2 in the prediction of outcome in acute necrotizing pancreatitis. Scand J Gastroent 1996; 31:818–824.
36. Hedström J, Korvuo A, Kenkimäki P, et al. Urinary trypsinogen-2 test strip for acute pancreatitis. Lancet 1996; 347:729–31.
37. Kylänpää-Bäck M-L, Kemppainen E, Puolakkainen P, et al. Reliable screening for acute pancreatitis with rapid urine trypsinogen-2 test strip. Br J Surg 2000; 87:49–52.
38. Kemppainen E, Hedström J, Puolakkainen P, et al. Rapid measurement of urinary trypsinogen-2 as a screening test for acute pancreatitis. N Engl J Med 1997; 336:1788–93. [AN: 9187069].
39. Pezzilli R, Morselli-Labate A, d'Alessandro A, et al. Time-course and clinical value of the urine trypsinogen-2 dipstick test in acute pancreatitis. Eur J Gastroenterol Hepatol 2001; 13:269–74.
40. Borgström A, Lasson A. Trypsin-alpha1-protease inhibitor complexes in serum and clinical course of acute pancreatitis. Scand J Gastroenterol 1984; 19:1119–22.
41. Andersen J, Hedström J, Kemppainen E, et al. The ratio of trypsin-2-alpha(1)-antitrypsin to trypsinogen-1 discriminate alcohol-induced acute pancreatitis. Clin Chem 2001; 47:231–6.
42. Mero M, Schröder R, Tenhunen R, et al. Serum phospholipase A2, immunoreactive trypsin, and trypsin inhibitors during human acute pancreatitis. Scand J Gastroenterol 1982; 17:413–6.
43. Banks R, Evans S, Alexander D, et al. Alpha2 macroglobulin state in acute pancreatitis. Raised values of alpha2 macroglobulin-protease complexes in severe and mild attacks. Gut 1991; 32:430–4.
44. Ohlsson K, Balldin G, Bohe M, et al. Pancreatic proteases and antiproteases in pancreatic disease; biochemical, pathophysiological and clinical aspects. Int J Pancreatol 1988; 3 (Suppl 1):67–78.
45. Hurley P, Cook A, Jehanli A, et al. Development of radioimmunoassays for free tetra-L-aspartyl-L-lysine trypsinogen activation peptides (TAP). J Immunol Methods 1988; 111:195–203.
46. Banks P, Carr-Locke D, Slivka A, et al. Urinary trypsinogen activation peptides (TAP) are not increased in mild ERCP-induced pancreatitis. Pancreas 1996; 12:294–7.
47. Fernandez del Castillo C, Schmidt J, Rattner D, et al. Generation and possible significance of trypsinogen activation peptides in experimental acute pancreatitis in the rat. Pancreas 1992; 7:263–70.

48. Heath D, Cruickshank A, Gudgeon A, et al. The relationship between pancreatic enzyme release and activation and the acute phase protein response in patients with acute pancreatitis. Pancreas 1995; 10:347–53.
49. Tenner S, Fernandez-del Castillo C, Warshaw A, et al. Urinary trypsinogen activation peptide (TAP) predicts severity in patients with acute pancreatitis. Int J Pancreatol 1997; 21:105–10.
50. Kemppainen E, Mayer J, Puolakkainen P, et al. The predictive value of plasma trypsinogen activation peptide (TAP) in acute pancreatitis. Br J Surg 2001; 88:679–80.
51. Fiennes AG, Gudgeon AM, Jehanli A, et al. Released phospholipase A2 activation peptides in the rapid early prediction of trauma outcome: a preliminary report. Injury 1991; 22:219–222.
52. Rae D, Porter J, Beechey Newman N, et al. Type 1 prophospholipase A2 propeptide in acute lung injury. Lancet 1994; 344:1472–73.
53. Burgos F, Salva M, Villegas V, et al. Analysis of the activation process of porcine procarboxypeptidase B and determination of the sequence of its activation segment. Biochemistry 1991; 30:4082–9.
54. Appelros S, Thim L, Borgström A. Activation peptide of carboxypeptidase B in serum and urine in acute pancreatitis. Gut 1998; 42:97–102.
55. Appelros S, Petersson U, Toh S, et al. Activation peptide of carboxypeptidase B and anionic trypsinogen as early predictors of the severity of acute pancreatitis. Br J Surg 2001; 88:216–21.

30 Selecting Severe Cases of Acute Pancreatitis on the Basis of Organ Failure

Clement W. Imrie

The assessment of patients for inclusion in prospective studies of potential new treatments in the management of acute pancreatitis requires early individual patient assessment with an accurate system. The delay necessary for either the Ranson[1,2] or the Glasgow[3,4] system to be completed causes problems. In 1985 the Glasgow prognostic system was successfully used in the prospective assessment of peritoneal lavage in the management of severe acute pancreatitis.[5] However, more recently the APACHE II[6–8] system has been used to predict severity and the Atlanta systems has been used to define severe outcome,[9] but neither of these has proved ideal.

Ocreotide Therapy

In the assessment of the efficacy of any new agent in the management of acute pancreatitis it is essential to focus on patients who have severe disease. To this end the prospective studies of octreotide therapy did achieve selection of a group with an appreciable mortality rate. Thus study from Glasgow in which intravenous octreotide was assessed against placebo in 50 patients in a double blind fashion had a 26% mortality rate.[10] In a similar fashion the 302 patients selected for the subcutaneous octreotide therapy study included 43 who died (14%).[11] Early clinical presentation and a minimum APACHE II score of 6 were taken as criteria for study entry.

Lexipafant Study

Earlier studies with the intention of assessing lexipafant against a placebo had a mortality ratein the region of 17%,[12,13] while the larger multicentre UK study published in 2001 had a 12.6% mortality in the 286 patients studied.[14] The latest lexipafant study which included patients from the United States, Scandinavia and Europe found an overall mortality rate of only 8% in the 1518 patients studied.[15] These patients were predicted to have severe acute pancreatitis on the basis that they had an admission APACHE-II score of 6 or more. This was the major criterion for entry to the study and clearly with a mortality rate at this level for those predicted to have severe acute pancreatitis, the selection criteria were 'too soft'.

Table 30.1. Methods of severity assessment of patients with acute pancreatitis

Early (< 3 h).	Later (36–60 h)
Age > 70 years	Ranson score (3 or greater)
Body Mass Index > 30 kg/m^2	Glasgow score (3 or greater)
Pleural effusion on CXR	Marshall score* (2 or greater)
Marshall score*	C-reactive protein
	(CRP > 150 mg/l)
CT necrosis > 30%	
APACHE II @ 8 or more	
APACHE – 0	

Scoring

I would submit that the problem is that the APACHE-II system as the single criterion for admission to studies has to have a much higher cut-off than 6 if we are to focus on a group of patients with more severe disease. Certainly a cut-off in the region of 8 or more at admission (as proposed in the Atlanta criteria) would select a more severely ill group of patients and would be a step in the right direction. Were one to include obesity as a factor as well then utilisation of the APACHE-O system suggested by Toh and Johnson[16] could also improve prediction of severity step in the right direction. Obesity alone where body mass index (BMI) exceeds 30 kg/m^2[17,18] and age of 70 or more[19] are important prognostic factors (Table 30.1).

In addition to evidence of systemic disturbances as shown by APACHE-II or APACHE-O, infarcted or ischaemic pancreas on early contrast enhanced computed tomography (CT) scan may also help predict a 'severe' attack of acute pancraetitis, but the exact importance of necrosis in relation to overall outcome is still in debate. Certainly this criterion was used in several antibiotic studies as the main reason for inclusion[20–22] but the yield of patients is small indeed and the performance of CT soon after admission is not clinically indicated for many patients in the United Kingdom.

A blood level of C-reactive protein greater than 150 mg/l is another objective marker of severe acute pancreatitis[23,24] and it is often considered that a value of either 150 mg/l (or better still 200 mg/l), indicates the severe form of disease. A problem does exist with the skew distribution of results for this marker so that a fair proportion of patients with clinically mild disease do reach this level of the acute phase marker, but are rarely clinically threatened by organ failure.

An alternative way of grading severity of disease by using a critical illness scoring system, such as that described by Marshall[25] (Table 30.2), has been shown by our group in Glasgow to focus on a small group of patients with a very high mortality rate, if a score of 2 or more is sustained for more than 36 h. In our series of 121 patients considered to have severe acute pancreatitis the mortality rate rose to a rather astonishing 55% in the small group of 20 patients with persistent organ failure.[26] It is therefore probable that if we switched to the utilisation of organ failure scores to grade disease severity and a patient continued to have a total Marshall score of 2 or more 48 h into illness this would indicate a higher risk of both mortality and major morbidity. The utilisation of such a scoring system to select patients should identify a small high risk group. In this way, new experimental therapies may be assessed with the prospect of a definite answer as to possible efficacy or otherwise being obtained with much smaller numbers of patients.

Table 30.2. Modified Marshall Score (excluding hepatic index)

Score	0	1	2	3	4
Systolic BP (mmHg)	>90	<90 Responds to fluid	<90 Poor IV fluid response	<90 (pH < 7.3)	<90 (Ph<7.2)
FiO2 / pO_2	>400	301–400	201–300	101–200	<101
Glasgow Coma Score	15	13–14	10–12	6–9	<6
Platelet count × 10^9/l	>120	81–120	51–80	21–50	<21
Creatinine µmol/l	<134	134–169	170–310	311–439	<439

FiO_2 = fraction of inspired oxygen: pO_2 = partial pressure of oxygen

Johnson[27] has verified that the use of this approach which was devised by Colin McKay[26] equally applies to the group of 286 patients with APACHE-II scores >6 who entered the UK Multicentre Study of Lexipafant as a possible therapy for severe acute pancreatitis (see Chapter 31).[27] The strength of such an assessment method using the Marshall score awaits prospective evaluation. If proof can be provided that this is the way ahead then both individual clinical assessment of patients and possible future therapeutic assessment of new treatments will both have a more accurate basis. This group of most severely ill patients will encompass only about 20% of those previously described as predicted severe acute pancreatitis.[26]

For the management of individual patients this dynamic assessment process will identify a small group of patients at very high risk who should all be assessed for intensive care or high dependency therapy. With regard to prospective therapeutic trials patients with a mortality of 50% can be assessed in numerically smaller studies if an improvement is taking place with any new therapy.

Further evidence to support the suggestions of Buter[26] and Johnson[27] came from Beger's group.[28] By retrospective assessment of their database back to 1982 Isenmann has shown that what they describe as early severe acute pancreatitis (ESAP) has a mortality of rate 42%. It must be emphasised that in the tertiary referral centre of Ulm this amounted to only 47 patients in 15 years, or 3 per year.[28] A multicentre study involving 6–10 European centres with a special interest in AP management could recruit 18–30 such patients per year. It is therefore a possible practical method of bringing to focus a new treatment approach in the most severely ill patients.

Isenmann *et al.* defined ESAP as the presence of organ failure at admission.[28] Their 47 patients came from a dataset of 158 patients graded as severe AP who were admitted within 72 h of onset of major symptoms. The extent of CT necrosis was greater than 50% of pancreatic volume in 34% of these 47 patients compared to 13% of the other 111 patients (p <0.0002). The mean APACHE-II score was also significantly different (16.6 *vs.* 9.9 p <0.0001).

Bank *et al*[29] have also discussed of the identification of the highest risk patients utilising organ failure. De Beaux *et al*[30] in 1995 drew attention to the higher mortality rate associated with organ failure. However, it is only with the recent publication by our own group that emphasis has been given to the dynamic nature of early organ failure[26] that a more accurate prospective use of this approach now beckons. It was certainly not appreciated at the time of the Atlanta conference in 1992[8] that the satisfaction of an organ failure criterion could be so frequently a transient phenomenon. In our own study approximately two thirds of the patients who recorded a Marshall score of 2 recovered quickly with supportive measures and had minimal morbidity and mortality rates. This contrasts starkly with the outcome of those who have persistent organ failure. It is this deteriorating organ score which is the herald of major problems.

Conclusion

In conclusion while certain new markers such as serum amyloid A hold promise to identify a higher risk group of patients, the most tangible measure of the highest risk patients at the present time is sustained organ dysfunction acknowledging that 45% of patients who exhibit such dysfunction do so from the time of admission. The dynamics of the process are crucially important and in all studies respiratory failure has been the dominant system failure. Abnormalities on the admission chest x-ray (especially pleural effusion) are indicative of severe disease[31] and in all multifactorial systems hypoxaemia is a crucial marker of respiratory compromise.

Nevertheless, future assessments of severity must take into account of the dynamic nature of organ failure, and, only those patients in whom organ failure persists for more than 48 h deserve to be categorised as severe acute pancreatitis.

References

1. Ranson HJC, Rifkind KM, Roses DF, et al. Prognostic signs and the role of operative management in acute pancreatitis. Surg Gynecol Obstet 1974; 139:69–81.
2. Ranson HJC. The timing of biliary surgery in acute pancreatitis. Ann Surg 1979; 189:654–662.
3. Imrie CW, Benjamin IS, McKay AJ, et al. A single centre double blind trial of Trasylol therapy in primary acute pancreatitis. Br J Surg 1978; 65:337–341.
4. Blamey SL, Imrie CW, O'Neill J, et al. Prognostic factors in acute pancreatitis. Gut 1984; 25:1340–1346.
5. Corfield AP, Cooper MJ, Williamson RCN, et al. Prediction of severity in acute pancreatitis: a prospective comparison of three prognostic indices. Lancet 1985/II; 403–406.
6. Knaus WA, Wagner DP, Draper EA, et al. APACHE II final form and national validation results of a severity of disease classification system. Crit Care Med 1984; 12:213–224.
7. Larvin M, McMahon MJ. APACHE II score for assessment and monitoring of acute pancreatitis. Lancet 1989/II; 201–205.
8. Wilson C, Heath DI, Imrie CW. Prediction of outcome in acute pancreatitis: a comparative study of APACHE II, clinical assessment and multiple factor scoring systems. Br J Surg 1990; 77:1260–1264.
9. Bradley EL. A clinically based classification system for acute pancreatitis. Arch Surg 1993; 128:586–590.
10. McKay CJ, Baxter J, Imrie CW. A randomised controlled trial of octreotide in the management of patients with acute pancreatitis. Int J Pancreatol 1997; 21:13–19.
11. Uhl W, Buchler MW, Malfertheiner P, et al. A randomised double blind multicentre trial of octreotide in moderate to severe acute pancreatitis. Gut 1999; 45:97–104.
12. Kingsnorth AN, Galloway SW, Formela J. Randomised double blind phase II trial of lexipafant, a platelet activating factor antagonist in human acute pancreatitis. Br J Surg 1995; 82:1414–1420.
13. McKay C, Curran F, Sharples C, et al. Prospective placebo controlled randomised trial of lexipafant in predicted severe acute pancreatitis. Br J Surg 1997; 84:1239–1243.
14. Johnson CD, Kingsnorth AN, Imrie CW, et al. Double blind, randomised placebo controlled study of a platelet activating factor antagonist, lexipafant, in the treatment and prevention of organ failure in predicted severe acute pancreatitis. Gut 2001; 48:62–69.
15. Larvin M, Ammori B, McMahon MJ, et al. A double blind randomised placebo controlled multicentre trial to evaluate the efficacy and safety of 2 doses of lexipafant in acute pancreatitis therapy. Pancreatology 2001; 1:279–280.

16. Toh SKC, Walters J, Johnson CD. APACHE- O. A new predictor of severity of acute pancreatitis. Gut 1996; 38:Supplement 1 (A35).
17. Lankisch PG, Schirren CA. Increased body weight as a prognostic parameter for complications in the course of acute pancreatitis. Pancreas 1990; 5:626–629.
18. Funnell IC, Bornmann PC, Weakley SP, et al. Br J Surg 1993; 80:484–486.
19. McKay CJ, Evans S, Sinclair M, et al. Br J Surg 1999; 86:1302–1036.
20. Pederzoli P, Bassi C, Vesentini S, et al. A randomised multicenter clinical trial of antibiotic prophylaxis of septic complications in acute necrotising pancreatitis with imipenem. Surg Gynecol Obstet 1993; 176:480–483.
21. Sainio V, Kemppainen E, Puolakkainen P, et al. Early antibiotic treatment in acute necrotising pancreatitis. Lancet 1995; 346:663–667.
22. Delcenserie R, Yzet T, Ducroix JP. Prophylactic antibiotics in treatment of severe acute alcoholic pancreatitis. Pancreas 1996; 13:198–201.
23. Puolakkainen P, Valtonen V, Paananen A, et al. C-reactive protein (CRP) and serum phospholipase A2 in the assessment of the severity of acute pancreatitis. Gut 1987; 28:764–771.
24. Wilson C, Heads A, Shenkin A, et al. C-reactive protein, antiproteases and complement factors as objective markers of severity in acute pancreatitis. Br J Surg 1989; 76:177–181.
25. Marshall JC, Cook DJ, Christou NV, et al. Multiple organ dysfunction score, a reliable descriptor of a complex clinical outcome. Crit Care Med 1995; 23:83–92.
26. Buter A, Imrie CW, Carter CR, et al. Dynamic nature of early organ dysfunction determines outcome in acute pancreatitis. Br J Surg 2002; 89:298–302.
27. Johnson CD. Transient organ failure is not a lethal complication of acute pancreatitis. Pancreas 2002; 25:435(A).
28. Isenmann R, Rao B, Beger HG. Early severe acute pancreatitis: characteristics of a new subgroup. Pancreas 2001; 22:272–278.
29. Bank S, Wise L, Gersten M. Risk factors in acute pancreatitis. Am J Gastroenterol 1983; 78:637–640.
30. de Beaux AC, Palmer KR, Carter CD. Factors influence morbidity and mortality in acute pancreatitis. Gut 1995; 37:121–126.
31. Talamini G, Bassi C, Falconi M, et al. Risk of Death from Acute Pancreatitis. Int J Pancreatol 1996; 19:15–24.

31 Individual Features Related to Severity in Acute Pancreatitis

Colin D. Johnson

Severe acute pancreatitis was defined at the Atlanta symposium[1] as an attack in which a complication occurs. Prediction of severity may be made at the start of the hospital admission, based on a variety of clinical, biochemical and radiological features. Scoring systems have been developed to describe groups of patients with high probability of severe pancreatitis, and these are often used to categorise individual patients as 'predicted mild' or 'predicted severe' pancreatitis. Such prediction for individuals, although widely accepted, strays beyond the original purpose of the scores used, and should be applied with caution, remembering that the overall accuracy of these predictions is rarely greater than 75%.

Early prediction of severity for individual patients with acute pancreatitis is important, to identify as soon as possible those patients who are most severely ill, and who will require aggressive management in the intensive care unit or high dependency area. Specific therapy targeted to those patients with severe disease, or predicted severe disease, is becoming a clinical reality. Such therapy should not be offered to patients with mild pancreatitis, who will recover without complications, and who may suffer complications of the treatment offered. For example, there is good evidence to support the use of endoscopic sphincterotomy in patients with gallstones and predicted severe pancreatitis[2;3] and growing evidence for the use of enteral nutrition in patients with severe disease of any cause.[4–8] Selection of these patients for treatment depends on early identification of those at risk of complications. Finally, it is helpful when reporting studies of patients with pancreatitis to characterise the group of patients by indicating the numbers who meet criteria of predicted severity at the outset.

Prediction of severity in acute pancreatitis has for many years relied on the pancreatitis specific score of Ranson[9] and the Glasgow score developed by Imrie.[10] These scores allow correct prediction of severity in about 75% of cases, and were designed primarily for the third purpose outlined above, that is to allow comparison of different groups of patients. For an individual patient the classification of 'mild' or 'severe' is not absolute, as 25% of predictions will be incorrect. Furthermore, the complete set of data for these scores is not available until 48 h after admission to hospital, whereas early therapy may be needed before that time.

The clinician must use all available information to detect patients who require general intensive care, and pancreatitis-specific therapies. It is not sufficient to rely on a single measurement or system, as no single test is always accurate. Therefore this chapter deals with the individual clinical and biochemical features that may be useful to identify patients with a high probability of developing a complication. Particular attention is given to those features which may be identified during the first 24 h after admission to hospital.

Clinical assessment is important from the outset, but the initial assessment, although specific, lacks sensitivity. By 48 h after admission, clinical assessment is as accurate as the Glasgow score.[11]

APACHE-II Score

This was developed as a general intensive care score of severe systemic illness,[12] but it performs well as an initial assessment of acute pancreatitis.[13] The data collected represent the degree of disturbance of systemic function, because the acute physiology component of the APACHE-II score is a measure of organ–system failure. For this reason, it correlates well with severity, as all patients with organ failure will have a high score, and by definition already have severe pancreatitis. In practice, the APACHE-II score within 24 h of admission is as good a predictor of severity as the Glasgow score at 48 h, and so it can be used for early assessment to identify patients who require intervention.[13]

An additional feature of the APACHE-II score is the range of values; this permits variation of the cut-off level for prediction of severity. A low cut-off will identify almost all patients with severe disease, a high cut-off is more specific, but less sensitive. For example using a score of >6 will identify a group of patients with 12% mortality and 62% severe disease[14]. The Atlanta criteria recommend a cut-off of >8; our unpublished data suggest that almost all patients who die have a score >8 and at this cutoff, the APACHE-II score has a sensitivity of 70% and specificity of 78%. In contrast, with a cutoff of >10, sensitivity falls to 56%, but specificity is 90% for severe disease.

Patient Characteristics

Several studies have shown the increased risk of complications with advancing age[9;10], and in patients who are obese (BMI >30)[9;15-18]. This information is available on admission, and should be used in all severity assessments. There is no specific age at which the risk of complications becomes suddenly greater, but it is the case that for patients with similar physiological and biochemical disturbances, the older the patient, the greater is the risk of complications.

In contrast, data on the relationship between obesity and severity of acute pancreatitis are inadequate to describe the effect of obesity on outcome, other than that obese patients are at greater risk of complications and death. Our unpublished data indicate that body mass index (BMI) is a predictor of complications in the same way as age, but most series include too few severely obese patients (BMI >40) to decide whether this extreme obesity poses a specially high risk. We have found that being overweight or obese progressively increases the risk of all complications, and obesity is associated with higher mortality (Fig. 31.1).

Aetiology of pancreatitis is not a predictive risk factor. Although some authors have reported increased risk in patients with gallstone pancreatitis, and after ERCP, large studies have not confirmed this.

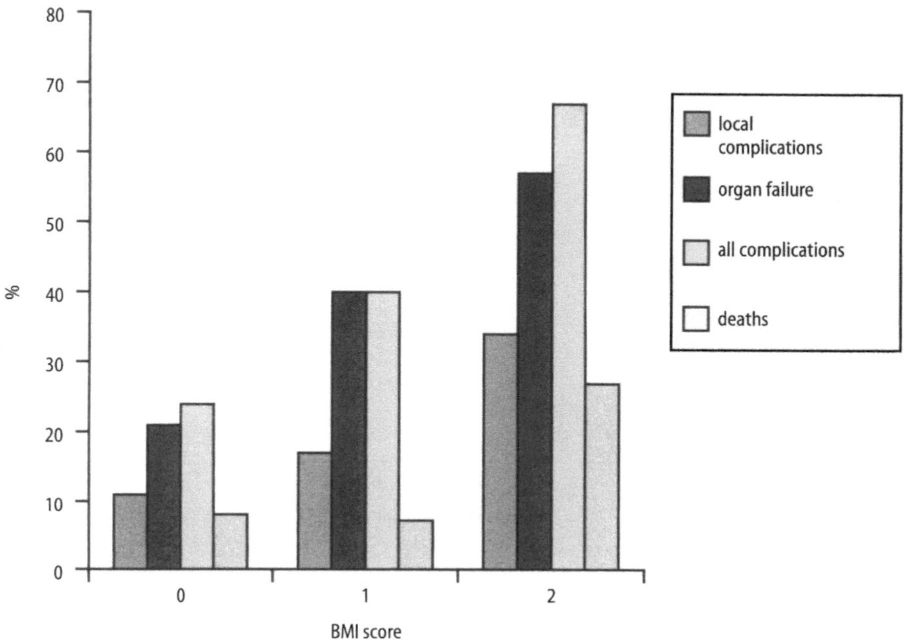

Figure 31.1. Percentage of 186 unselected patients with acute pancreatitis that developed complications, or died, related to body mass index (BMI): BMI score = 0 : normal; BMI score = 1 : overweight, ie BMI 26-30; BMI score = 2: obese, ie BMI >30. The association of complications and deaths with obesity was significant ($P < 0.01$, 2 df)

Inflammatory Markers

Plasma C-reactive protein (CRP) indicates an inflammatory response, and is elevated in severe pancreatitis. Values >150 mg/l are associated with a high risk of complications,[4] but these values are rarely achieved less than 48 h from the onset of symptoms, and peak values occur at about 96 h. CRP is specific, but not sensitive in the early stages of the disease. Nevertheless, a raised CRP is a reliable marker of severe disease.

Other markers of the inflammatory response become elevated before CRP. These were described in detail in a study of post-ERCP pancreatitis, which allowed the collection of samples during the very earliest stages of the disease[19]. IL8 and IL6 reliably correlate with severity, and neutrophil elastase is the earliest marker, which several authors have found to be accurate. However, assays of the cytokines are difficult, and at present are only suitable for use in research studies, with stored batches of samples. Neutrophil elastase has not fulfilled its earlier promise. None of these tests is currently available for clinical practice.

Other markers of the inflammatory response which show promise as predictors of severity include serum amyloid A (Fig. 31.2)[20;21] and procalcitonin (Fig. 31.3).[21;22] These acute phase proteins behave in a similar way to CRP, responding to changes in circulating cytokines, but it seems the response occurs earlier than with CRP.[20] Procalcitonin can now be applied in the clinical situation using a rapid test strip,[22] further evaluation of serum amyloid A is awaited with interest.

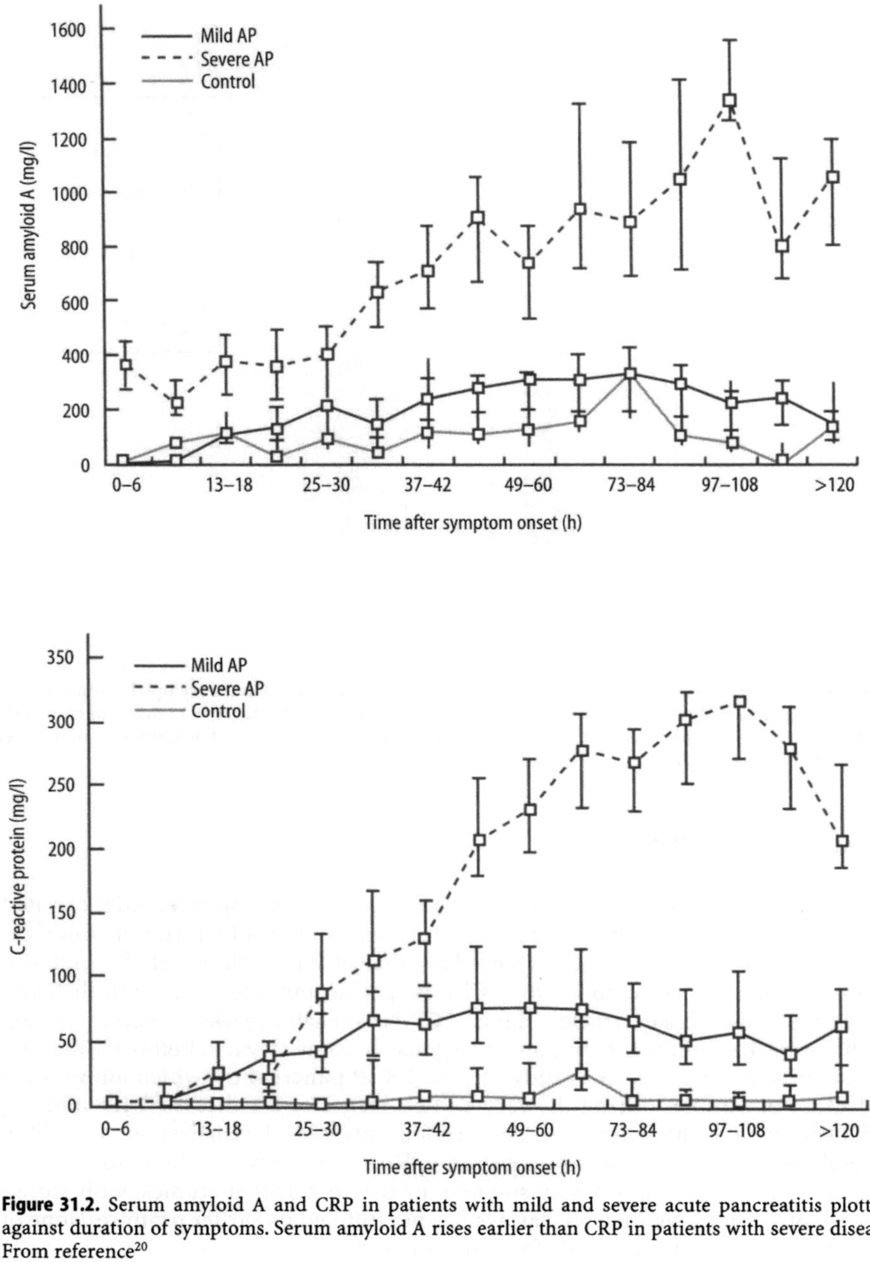

Figure 31.2. Serum amyloid A and CRP in patients with mild and severe acute pancreatitis plotted against duration of symptoms. Serum amyloid A rises earlier than CRP in patients with severe disease From reference[20]

Activation Peptides

It is now believed that activation of enzymes within the acinar cell is one of the earliest events in acute pancreatitis, possibly the major causative feature (see

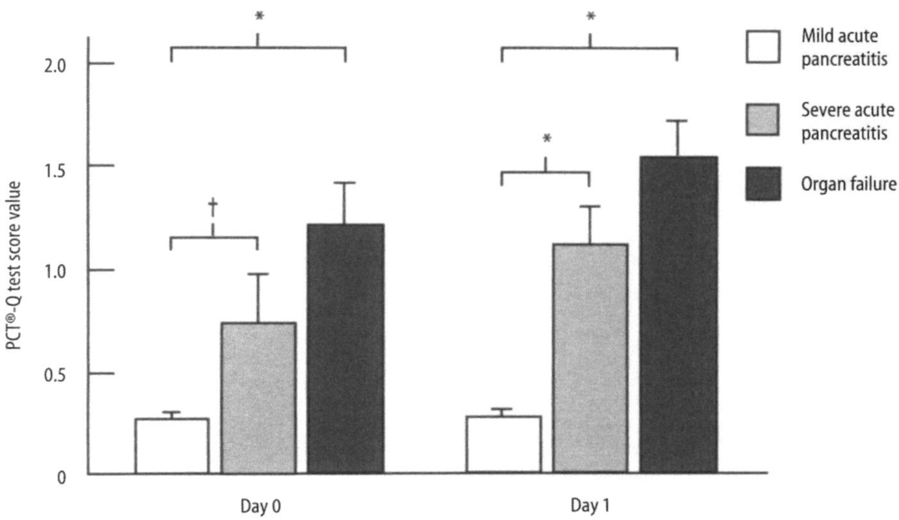

Figure 31.3. Procalcitonin test strip in the prediction of severity of acute pancreatitis. From reference[22]

Chapters 27 and 29). Activation peptides of pancreatic enzymes (trypsinogen activation peptide, TAP; carboxypeptidase activation peptide, CAPAP) are not normally present in the plasma, but are released in amounts that correspond to the extent of the pancreatic injury. Accordingly, both TAP and CAPAP are markers of severity, with the advantage that they are released from the pancreas at a very early stage in the disease. Because they are small molecules, they are filtered by the kidney, and best results for severity prediction are obtained from measurement of urine concentrations (Fig. 31.4)[23;24]. However, at present there is not a rapid assay for either of these peptides that could be used in clinical practice.

Morphological Changes

The chest radiograph gives useful information about severity: the presence of a pleural effusion is the most reliable sign associated with severe acute pancreatitis.[25]

Dynamic computed tomography (CT) within with the first four days in hospital is reported to identify patients with pancreatic necrosis, or extensive fluid collections.[24,26] Those patients have in effect severe disease, as the CT is showing the presence of a local complication, but they are also at high risk of systemic complications.

Concerns about the use of CT include the difficulty of transport to, and supervision of ill patients in, the radiology department during the examination, and the possible harmful effects of large doses of contrast agent, particularly if renal function is impaired. In addition, if no specific intervention is planned for patients with necrosis, there is little clinical benefit from early CT, and a substantial number of patients with apparently severe disease will settle and their symptoms resolve with no clinical feature to suggest extensive necrosis. For these reasons, many centres in

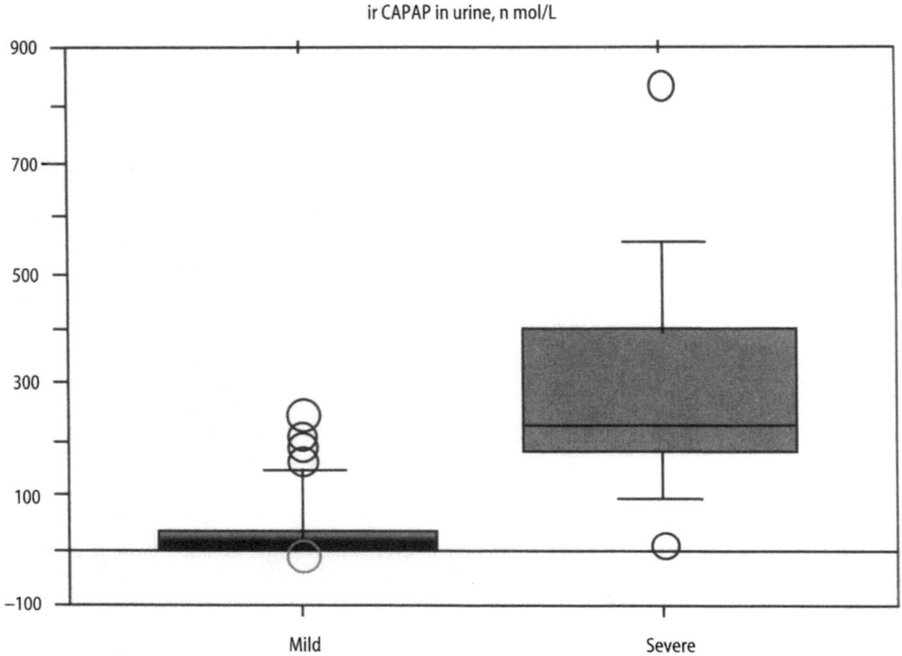

Figure 31.4. Urinary concentrations of ccarboxypeptidase activation peptide (CAPAP) in patients with mild and severe acute pancreatitis on admission to hospital. There is good separation between values in the two groups. Horizontal bars represent median values; boxes: interquartile range; error bars: range.

the UK delay CT until the end of the first week, and perform this examination only on those patients with signs of a continuing inflammatory response, or pain. At this stage, the detection of peripancreatic necrosis will prompt intervention such as fine needle aspiration to detect infection, or, when indicated, surgical debridement.

Integrated Risk Assessment

Can the clinician combine the findings of all these scores and tests to produce a reliable indicator of the risk that a complication will occur in an individual patient? If only one score or test is used, useful information will be lost. However, if a large number are used, and any one positive result is accepted as a positive prediction, sensitivity will be high, but specificity will be poor, and many patients will be wrongly classified as severe. Conversely, if the threshold is set for all or many tests to be positive before a prediction of severe disease is accepted, the predictions will be specific, but many patients with severe disease will not be included because they fail to reach the stringent threshold.

Combination of two independent features, such as the APACHE-II score, and the presence of obesity, can improve the prediction obtained with either alone[27]. The APACHE-O score, a simple addition of APACHE-II and an obesity score, has greater sensitivity and specificity than APACHE-II alone. At a cutoff of >8 for both

Table 31.1. Predictive values of APACHE-II and APACHE-O for prediction of severity in acute pancreatitis at a range of cutoff values. PPV: positive predictive value; NPV: negative predictive value

APACHE-II	Sensitivity	Specificity	PPV	NPV	Accuracy
>8	70	78	63	84	77
>9	68	84	71	81	80
>10	56	90	78	80	78
APACHE-O					
>8	89	79	67	94	82
>9	82	86	74	91	85
>10	69	90	80	85	82

scores, the APACHE-O had an overall accuracy of 85% for prediction of severe disease (**Table 31.1**). In making such combinations, it is important to ensure that the individual features independently predict severity, and that the combined judgement is more accurate than one or some of the features taken alone.

An alternative approach to the use of individual features in an empirical way is to combine them using a logistic equation to calculate a probability index (PI). This enables calculation of a probability of complications for an individual, based on that patient's own individual features. We have described such an approach in preliminary form[28]. While this approach is promising, development is limited by the need to collect large complete data sets in order to introduce new features. The advantage of the PI is that it makes clear the inherent uncertainty of prediction, which may be overlooked when predictions are into categories ('predicted mild' or 'predicted severe'). Further refinement of the PI will include the incorporation of other variables available during the first 24 hr in hospital, such as activation peptides, and the presence of pleural effusion.

Persistent Organ Failure

The Atlanta criteria[1] defined useful cut-offs for definition of organ failure, but recently these simple yes/no categories have been re-examined, with the appreciation that patients with acute pancreatitis follow a dynamic course, in which outcome depends not only on the presence of organ failure, but also on its timing, severity and duration. These will be affected by the patient's genetic makeup, the duration of symptoms before admission to hospital, and the effectiveness of early treatment. Approximately half the patients with organ failure recover rapidly, within 48 h. Other complications are rare in these patients.[29;30] Patients with persistent organ failure have a high mortality rate (30–50%).[1;29;30] Two studies with over 120 and nearly 300 patients with predicted severe acute pancreatitis showed very similar results: if organ failure is present for more than 48 h in the first week of the attack, the patient has a greater than 50% chance of a fatal outcome (**Table 31.2**). Conversely, even if organ failure is present, the patient is unlikely to die if the failure resolves within 48 h (see Chapter 30).

The importance of these observations lies in the possibility that patients with transient organ failure should perhaps be no longer regarded as having severe acute pancreatitis, as they will almost certainly have an uncomplicated recovery. The duration of organ failure is a feature that lies on the border between predictive feature, and marker of therapeutic response. Further work is required to determine

Table 31.2. Comparison of two UK studies

	OF in first week		Survived	Deaths
Glasgow[29]	None	68	65	2
	Resolved <48h	33	33	0
	Persistent >48h	20	9	11
UK study[30]				
(n=288)	none	114	111	3
	Resolved <48h	72	70	2
	Persistent >48h	102	67	35

whether organ failure and its resolution or otherwise is a marker of disease severity that depends on features of the patient or the illness not amenable to therapy, or whether in fact, aggressive early supportive therapy can alter the course of the disease.

Conclusions

In conclusion, individual features including a range of clinical and biochemical information give good prediction of severity in acute pancreatitis. Clinical information such as age, BMI, and chest X-ray can supplement the use of predictive scores, and best predictions will be made using combinations of markers. The ideal combinations remain to be determined.

The boundary between prediction and detection of severity is blurred, and perhaps should be removed altogether: patients with persistent organ failure, or CT evidence of local complications can be identified within 3 or 4 days in hospital, and clearly constitute a group that requires aggressive treatment.

References

1. Bradley EL, III. A clinically based classification system for acute pancreatitis. Summary of the International Symposium on Acute Pancreatitis, Atlanta, Ga, September 11 through 13, 1992. Arch Surg 1993; 128:586–90.
2. United Kingdom guidelines for the management of acute pancreatitis. British Society of Gastroenterology. Gut 1998; 42 (Suppl 2):S1–13.
3. Management of the biliary tract in acute necrotizing pancreatitis. J Gastrointest Surg 2001; 5:221–2.
4. Dervenis C, Johnson CD, Bassi C, et al. Diagnosis, objective assessment of severity, and management of acute pancreatitis. Santorini consensus conference. Int J Pancreatol 1999; 25:195–210.
5. Eatock FC, Brombacher GD, Steven A, et al. Nasogastric feeding in severe acute pancreatitis may be practical and safe. Int J Pancreatol 2000; 28:23–9.
6. Kalfarentzos F, Kehagias J, Mead N, et al. Enteral nutrition is superior to parenteral nutrition in severe acute pancreatitis: results of a randomized prospective trial. Br J Surg 1997; 84:1665–9.
7. Powell JJ, Murchison JT, Fearon KC, et al. Randomized controlled trial of the effect of early enteral nutrition on markers of the inflammatory response in predicted severe acute pancreatitis. Br J Surg 2000; 87:1375–81.
8. Windsor AC, Kanwar S, Li AG, et al. Compared with parenteral nutrition, enteral feeding attenuates the acute phase response and improves disease severity in acute pancreatitis. Gut 1998; 42:431–5.
9. Ranson JH, Rifkind KM, Roses DF, et al. Objective early identification of severe acute pancreatitis. Am J Gastroenterol 1974; 61:443–51.
10. Blamey SL, Imrie CW, O'Neill J, et al. Prognostic factors in acute pancreatitis. Gut 1984; 25:1340–6.

11. Corfield AP, Cooper MJ, Williamson RC, et al. Prediction of severity in acute pancreatitis: prospective comparison of three prognostic indices. Lancet 1985; 2:403–7.
12. Knaus WA, Draper EA, Wagner DP, et al. APACHE II: a severity of disease classification system. Crit Care Med 1985; 13:818–29.
13. Larvin M, McMahon MJ. APACHE-II score for assessment and monitoring of acute pancreatitis. Lancet 1989; 2:201–5.
14. Johnson CD, Kingsnorth AN, Imrie CW, et al. Double blind, randomised, placebo controlled study of a platelet activating factor antagonist, lexipafant, in the treatment and prevention of organ failure in predicted severe acute pancreatitis. Gut 2001; 48:62–9.
15. Funnell IC, Bornman PC, Weakley SP, et al. Obesity: an important prognostic factor in acute pancreatitis. Br J Surg 1993; 80:484–6.
16. Lankisch PG, Schirren CA. Increased body weight as a prognostic parameter for complications in the course of acute pancreatitis. Pancreas 1990; 5:626–9.
17. Porter KA, Banks PA. Obesity as a predictor of severity in acute pancreatitis. Int J Pancreatol 1991; 10:247–52.
18. Suazo-Barahona J, Carmona-Sanchez R, Robles-Diaz G, et al. Obesity: a risk factor for severe acute biliary and alcoholic pancreatitis. Am J Gastroenterol 1998; 93:1324–8.
19. Messmann H, Vogt W, Holstege A, et al. Post-ERP pancreatitis as a model for cytokine induced acute phase response in acute pancreatitis. Gut 1997; 40:80–5.
20. Mayer JM, Raraty M, Slavin J, et al. Serum amyloid A is a better early predictor of severity than C-reactive protein in acute pancreatitis. Br J Surg 2002; 89:163–71.
21. Pezzilli R, Melzi d'Eril GV, Morselli-Labate AM, et al. Serum amyloid A, procalcitonin, and C-reactive protein in early assessment of severity of acute pancreatitis. Dig Dis Sci 2000; 45:1072–8.
22. Kylanpaa-Back ML, Takala A, Kemppainen E, et al. Procalcitonin strip test in the early detection of severe acute pancreatitis. Br J Surg 2001; 88:222–7.
23. Appelros S, Petersson U, Toh S, et al. Activation peptide of carboxypeptidase B and anionic trypsinogen as early predictors of the severity of acute pancreatitis. Br J Surg 2001; 88:216–21.
24. Neoptolemos JP, Kemppainen EA, Mayer JM, et al. Early prediction of severity in acute pancreatitis by urinary trypsinogen activation peptide: a multicentre study. Lancet 2000; 355:1955–60.
25. Talamini G, Bassi C, Falconi M, et al. Risk of death from acute pancreatitis. Role of early, simple "routine" data. Int J Pancreatol 1996; 19:15–24.
26. Balthazar EJ, Robinson DL, Megibow AJ, et al. Acute pancreatitis: value of CT in establishing prognosis. Radiology 1990; 174:331–6.
27. Toh SKC, Walters J, Johnson CD. APACHE-O. A new predictor of severity in acute pancreatitis. Gut 1996; 38 (Suppl 1):A35.
28. Johnson CD, Phillips S, Toh S, et al. An individualised probability index for prediction of complications in acute pancreatitis. Gut 1998; 42 (Suppl 1):A10.
29. Buter A, Imrie CW, Carter CR, et al. Dynamic nature of early organ dysfunction determines outcome in acute pancreatitis. Br J Surg 2002; 89:298–302.
30. Johnson CD. Transient organ failure is not a lethal complication of acute pancreatitis. Pancreas 2002; 25:435.

Management of Necrosis in Acute Pancreatitis

32 Sterile Necrosis in Acute Necrotizing Pancreatitis: Current Concepts and Management Strategies

Shailesh Shrikhande, Helmut M. Friess, Jan Schmidt, Jens Werner, Waldemar Uhl and Markus W. Büchler

Acute necrotizing pancreatitis is possibly the most severe form of acute pancreatitis. While results have improved significantly in the past decade, acute necrotizing pancreatitis still carries a high morbidity and mortality. However, it is the infected necrosis of acute necrotizing pancreatitis that accounts for a major share of this high morbidity and mortality.[1] On the other hand, management of sterile necrosis has evolved considerably in recent years with improved results. This article discusses the current understanding of sterile necrosis and the approach to its management.

Diagnosis of Pancreatic Necrosis

Severe upper abdominal pain often radiating to the back and elevated serum amylase along with elevated serum lipase usually confirm the diagnosis of acute pancreatitis. However, the diagnosis of pancreatic necrosis is based on imaging findings or on serological markers (i.e. C-reactive protein levels).[2] Dynamic contrast enhanced computed tomography (CT) is the accepted gold standard for the diagnosis of pancreatic necrosis.[3,4] Focal or diffuse, well-marginated zones of non-enhanced pancreatic parenchyma that are larger than 3 cm or involve more than 30% of the area of the pancreas are considered as basic requisites for a CT diagnosis.[5] The contrast density, normally 50–150 Hounsfield units, fails to exceed 50 Hounsfield units in areas of necrosis after intravenous contrast medium injection.[5] However, it must be pointed out that while the overall sensitivity of CT in demonstrating parenchymal necrosis is more than 90%, one often encounters situations where the CT images and actual intraoperative findings are somewhat contradictory.

Sterile Necrosis

According to the Atlanta classification,[6,7] infected pancreatic necrosis has been defined as the appearance of bacteria in diffuse or focal areas of non-viable pancreatic parenchyma, associated with severe acute pancreatitis. Usually no areas

Table 32.1. Sensitivity of fine needle aspiration in detecting infection of sterile pancreatic necrosis

Author	Reference	Sensitivity / Specificity
Rau *et al.*, 1998	14	88% sensitivity 90% specificity
Büchler *et al.*, 2000	26	96% sensitivity

of pus collection are found. The appearance of bacteria is usually confirmed by fine needle aspiration. Thus sterile necrosis is pancreatic necrosis without proven pancreatic infection in a setting of acute necrotizing pancreatitis.

Pathology

Focal or diffuse areas of devitalized pancreatic parenchyma along with peripancreatic fat necrosis is evident. Microscopically, there is extensive interstitial fat necrosis with vessel damage and necrosis that affects acinar cells, islet cells and the pancreatic ductal system.[8–9] However, the distinction between a sterile and infected necrosis remains a clinical one and is not possible pathomorphologically.

The Role of Fine Needle Aspiration

Fine needle aspiration is useful in the early detection of infected pancreatic necrosis. It is the early detection of this condition that has a major impact on the further management and outcome in acute pancreatitis. Since clinical and laboratory findings can be often similar in patients with either sterile or infected necrosis),[10–12] this important differentiation is best made by a fine needle aspiration.[13] Fine needle aspiration can be performed either under CT[13] or under ultrasound guidance.[14] Ultrasonographically guided fine needle aspiration is a fast and reliable technique for the diagnosis of infected pancreatic necrosis. Since complication rates are very low, the procedure can be repeated at short intervals to improve the diagnostic accuracy. This technique has been recommended for all patients with necrotizing pancreatitis in whom a systemic inflammatory response syndrome persists beyond the first week after onset of symptoms[14] or when there is deterioration in the clinical situation. The technique is safe and accurate[4,13–18] and a positive result is an indication for surgical intervention without undue delay (Table 32.1).

In contrast, it has also been reported that percutaneous aspiration and drainage can often predispose to secondary infection of an originally sterile necrosis.[19]

Course of Sterile Necrosis

The data before routine antibiotic prophylaxis was used showed that 40–70% of all pancreatic necrosis ultimately became infected.[20–23] The incidence of infection tends to rise gradually with time after the onset of acute pancreatitis.[24] It has been observed that the highest incidence of infection is around three weeks after the initial attack of acute necrotizing pancreatitis.[24] Sterile necrosis that is treated with conservative intensive care treatment right from the onset of necrotizing pancreatitis runs a better course and many patients can be prevented from infection of the pancreatic necrosis and subsequent surgical intervention.

Pancreatic necrosis and organ failure are the principal determinants of severity in acute pancreatitis. However, it must be noted that not all cases of severe necrotizing pancreatitis, whether infected or sterile, develop organ failure.

Conservative Treatment of Sterile Pancreatic Necrosis

Between 15-20% of all acute pancreatitis patients develop severe necrotizing pancreatitis. In this subgroup, stratification according to infection status is crucial[15, 17, 18, 25]. Infection of pancreatic necrosis is currently the most important risk factor contributing to death in severe necrotizing pancreatitis and surgical necrosectomy along with debridement is the most widely accepted modality for management of infected pancreatic necrosis.[1,17,18,26] In contrast, the management of sterile necrosis even when associated with organ failure, is controversial and has evolved considerably in recent years.[26–28] Although necrosis confirms the presence of severe disease and the extent of the sterile necrotic tissue is proportional to the rate of organ failure,[29] sterile necrosis is primarily managed conservatively with antibiotics, nutritional support and active intensive care measures.

Role of Antibiotics

Conservative intensive care management of pancreatic necrosis primarily involves treatment with broad spectrum antibiotics. In 1991, Bradley *et al.* demonstrated that 11 patients with sterile necrosis were managed successfully without surgery[30] and attracted attention to the fact that a major treatment aim of acute necrotizing pancreatitis should be prevention of pancreatic infection. In 1992, our group undertook a study to evaluate pancreatic parenchymal penetration of various broad spectrum antibiotics. It was observed that imipenem, along with ciprofloxacin and ofloxacin, achieved high pancreatic tissue levels along with a high bactericidal activity against most of the organisms present in pancreatic infections.[31] There is now increasing evidence in the medical literature that antibiotic prophylaxis in the initial management of severe acute pancreatitis improves the overall outcome[32] and that the frequency of infection of pancreatic necrosis can be reduced by antibiotics. In a large study, Ho *et al.* demonstrated that intravenous antibiotic prophylaxis significantly reduced the incidence of pancreatic infection with a trend towards improved survival. In this analysis, patients with sterile necrosis had a mortality rate of 2% (2/97).[33] In another study, Rau *et al.* analyzed the clinical course and outcome of patients with sterile necrotizing pancreatitis treated surgically versus non-surgically. They observed that most patients with limited and sterile necrosis respond to intensive care treatment and that infected necrosis is best managed surgically.[34] Confirming these observations, our own group undertook a prospective single center trial to evaluate the role of non-surgical management including early antibiotic treatment with imipenem/cilastatin in patients with documented sterile necrosis. We observed a mortality rate of 1.8% (1/56) in patients with sterile necrosis managed without surgery.[26] Our findings were recently confirmed by a retrospective analysis of 99 patients

Table 32.2. Major series with conservative management of sterile pancreatic necrosis

Sr. No.	Author	Design	Ref	Number of Patients	Death rate
1	Bradley *et al.*, 1991	Prospective	30	11	0%
2	Rau *et al.*, 1995	Retrospective	34	65	6.2%
3	Ho *et al.*, 1997	Retrospective	33	97	2%
4	Büchler *et al.*, 2000	Prospective	26	56	1.8%
5	Ashley *et al.*, 2001	Retrospective	15	62	11%

with necrotizing pancreatitis in which patients with sterile necrosis could be successfully managed conservatively.[1] Considered together, all these results appear to suggest non-surgical management, including early antibiotic treatment, as the primary treatment approach in patients with sterile pancreatic necrosis (Table 32.2).

Indications for Surgery in Sterile Pancreatic Necrosis

Before considering the indications for intervention, whether endoscopic or surgical, in sterile pancreatic necrosis, it must be pointed out that the mortality rate in medically managed patients with extensive sterile pancreatic necrosis is approximately 10% and surgical intervention has not reduced this mortality rate.[3] Bearing this in mind, the principal indication for surgery should now be infection of an originally sterile pancreatic necrosis documented by fine needle aspiration. Other indications are sterile necrosis with persistent multiple organ failure and situations where sterile necrosis involves more than 50% of the pancreas. The latter two indications however, need to be individualized to the specific clinical situation.[26,36] An additional indication for surgery that deserves consideration is symptomatic (severe pain, gastric outlet obstruction etc) sterile pancreatic necrosis where the presence of infection is not the sole determinant of intervention.[37]

Timing of Surgical Intervention

In the last decade, the timing of surgical intervention for all forms of necrotizing pancreatitis has changed remarkably. Currently, it is accepted that surgical intervention should be as late as possible. The primary reason for this is that demarcation between viable and non-viable pancreatic tissue is better defined and this enables a more complete surgical necrosectomy and debridement that is also easier to perform.[38] For all practical purposes, the timing of surgical intervention is around three weeks after the initial attack of acute necrotizing pancreatitis.[38]

Surgical Techniques

The surgical principles and techniques for sterile pancreatic necrosis are essentially the same as those for infected necrosis. The aim for surgical intervention is local and adequate removal of the necrosis.[39] The commonly adopted techniques have been necrosectomy with closed continuous lavage,[20,40] repeated necrosectomies with planned relaparotomies[41] and necrosectomy with 'open packing'.[42]

These surgical strategies have enabled major centers to reduce mortality rates below 15%.[26,29] Other options such as pancreatic resections are now considered obsolete owing to their high rate of post-operative complications and the problems associated with exocrine and endocrine deficiency.[38] Peritoneal dialysis has also been shown to be ineffective because it has no effect on the inflammatory processes in the retroperitoneum.[38,43]

Non-surgical Interventions

Though interventional radiology techniques such as percutaneous placement of catheters under CT guidance have been introduced,[44–46] quite often operative drainage of undrained necrosis is still necessary. The formation of external fistulae is also a problem with percutaneous methods. Endoscopic treatment for pancreatic necrosis has been attempted with some success.[47] There is a belief that endoscopic interventions are less traumatic, reduce the incidence of external fistulae and possibly reduce hospital stay. On the other hand, there is a definite possibility of introducing infection and quite often complete and adequate drainage of necrosis, especially peripheral necrosis, is difficult to achieve. Thus sufficient data in favour of these treatment options is still lacking and surgery appears to be the current gold standard whenever intervention is contemplated in sterile pancreatic necrosis.

Conclusions

The outcome of acute necrotizing pancreatitis depends on the extent of necrosis, organ failure, and the development of infection in a previously sterile necrosis. While documented infection of pancreatic necrosis is a definite indication for surgery, current opinion supports conservative management of sterile necrosis. However, large, controlled, randomized trials are necessary to assess the role of different treatment approaches in the management of sterile pancreatic necrosis.

As things stand today, conservative management of sterile necrosis revolves around judicious use of intravenous antibiotics and nutritional support (enteral or parenteral) along with quality intensive care treatment. Surgical interventions in sterile necrosis, if at all considered necessary, should be carefully individualized to the specific situation.

References

1. Bradley EL III. Antibiotics in acute pancreatitis. Current status and future directions. Am J Surg 1989; 158:472–478.
2. Büchler M, Malfertheiner P, Schoetensack C, et al. Sensitivity of antiproteases, complement factors, and C-reactive protein in detecting pancreatic necrosis: Results of a prospective clinical study. Int J Pancreatol 1986; 1:227–235.
3. Clavein PA, Hauser H, Meyer P. Value of contrast enhanced CT in the early diagnosis and prognosis of acute pancreatitis: A prospective study of 202 patients. Am J Surg 1988; 155:457–466.
4. Staten R, Frey CF. Comprehensive management of acute necrotizing pancreatitis and pancreatic abscess. Arch Surg 1990; 125:1269–1275.

5. Balthazar EJ, Robinson DL, Megibow AJ. Acute pancreatitis: Value of CT in establishing prognosis. Radiology 1990; 174:331–336.
6. Bradley EL III. A clinically based classification system for acute pancreatitis. Arch Surg 1993; 128:586.
7. Frey CF, Reber HA. Clinically based classification system for acute pancreatitis. Pancreas 1993; 8:738.
8. Klöppel G, Von Gerkan R, Dreyer T. Pathomorphology of acute pancreatitis: Analysis of 367 autopsy cases and through surgical specimens. In: Gry KE, Singler MV, Sarles H, eds. Pancreatitis: Concepts and Classifications. Amsterdam, The Netherlands, Elsevier Science Publishers 1984; 29–35.
9. Bradley EL III. A natural history-based clinical classification system for acute pancreatitis. In: Büchler MW, Uhl W, Friess H, et al. eds. Acute Pancreatitis: Novel Concepts in Biology and Therapy. Berlin, Vienna, Blackwell Science, 1999; 181–192.
10. Block S, Maier W, Bittner R. Identification of pancreas necrosis in severe acute pancreatitis: Imaging procedures vs clinical staging. Gut 1986; 27:1035–1042.
11. Teerenhovi O. Fatal fulminant pancreatitis. Surg Res Comm 1988; 3:207–212.
12. Nordback I, Pessi T, Auvimen O. Determination of necrosis in necrotizing pancreatitis. Br J Surg 1985; 72:225–227.
13. Gerzof SG, Banks PA, Robbins AH, et al. Early diagnosis of pancreatic infection by CT-guided - aspiration. Gastroenterology 1987; 93:1315–1320.
14. Rau B, Pralle U, Mayer JM, et al. Role of ultrasonographically guided fine-needle aspiration cytology in the diagnosis of infected pancreatic necrosis. Br J Surg 1998; 85:179–184.
15. Ashley SW, Perez A, Pierce EA, et al. Necrotizing pancreatitis: contemporary analysis of 99 consecutive cases. Ann Surg 2001; 234:572–579.
16. Gloor B, Uhl W, Büchler MW. Changing concepts in the surgical management of acute pancreatitis. Baillieres Best Pract Res Clin Gastroenterol 1999; 13:303–315.
17. Gloor B, Muller CA, Worni M, et al. Late mortality in patients with severe acute pancreatitis. Br J Surg 2001; 88:975–979.
18. Gloor B, Muller CA, Worni M, et al. Pancreatic infection in severe pancreatitis: the role of fungus and multiresistant organisms. Arch Surg 2001; 136:592–596.
19. Paye F, Rotman N, Radier C, et al. Percutaneous aspiration for bacteriological studies in patients with necrotizing pancreatitis. Br J Surg 1998; 85:755–759.
20. Beger HG, Bittner R, Büchler M, et al. Necrosectomy and postoperative local lavage in necrotizing pancreatitis. Br J Surg 1988; 75:207–212.
21. Widdison Al, Karanjia ND. Pancreatic infection complicating acute pancreatitis. Br J Surg 1993; 80:148.
22. Bittner R, Block S, Büchler M, et al. Pancreatic Abscess and Infected Pancreatic Necrosis. Different Local Septic Complications in Acute Pancreatitis. Dig Dis Sci 1987; 32:1082.
23. Fedorak IJ, Ko TC, Djuricin G, et al. Secondary pancreatic infections: Are they distinct clinical entities? Surgery 1991; 161:19.
24. Beger HG, Bittner R, Block S, et al. Bacterial Contamination of Pancreatic necrosis – A Prospective Clinical Study. Gastroenterology 1986; 91:433.
25. Gloor B, Uhl W, Muller CA, et al. The role of surgery in the management of acute pancreatitis. Can J Gastroenterol 2000; 14 (Suppl D):136D–140D.
26. Büchler MW, Gloor B, Muller CA, et al. Acute necrotizing pancreatitis: treatment strategy according to the status of infection. Ann Surg 2000; 232:627–9.
27. Büchler M, Malfertheiner P, Uhl W, et al. Gabexate mesilate in human acute pancreatitis. German Pancreatitis Study Group. Gastroenterology. 1993; 104:1165–70.
28. Uhl W, Büchler MW, Malfertheiner P, et al. A randomised, double blind, multicentre trial of octreotide in moderate to severe acute pancreatitis. Gut 1999; 45:97–104.
29. Isenmann R, Rau B, Beger HG. Bacterial infection and extent of necrosis are determinants of organ failure in patients with acute necrotizing pancreatitis. Br J Surg 1999; 86:1020–1024.
30. Bradley EL 3rd, Allen K. A prospective longitudinal study of observation versus surgical intervention in the management of necrotizing pancreatitis. Am J Surg 1991; 161:19–25.
31. Büchler M, Malfertheiner P, Friess H, et al. Human pancreatic tissue concentration of bactericidal antibiotics. Gastroenterology 1992; 103:1902–1908.
32. Powell JJ, Miles R, Siriwardena AK. Antibiotic prophylaxis in the initial management of severe acute pancreatitis. Br J Surg 1998; 85:582–587.
33. Ho HS, Frey CF. The role of antibiotic prophylaxis in severe acute pancreatitis. Arch Surg 1997; 132:487–493.

34. Rau B, Pralle U, Uhl W, et al. Management of sterile necrosis in instances of severe acute pancreatitis. J Am Coll Surg 1995; 181:279–288.
35. Bradley EL III. Surgical indications and techniques in necrotizing pancreatitis. In: Bradley EL II ed. Acute Pancreatitis: diagnosis and therapy. Raven press, Ltd., New York, 1994; 105–117.
36. McFadden DW, Reber HA. Indications for surgery in severe acute pancreatitis. Int J Pancreatol 1994; 15:83–90.
37. Rattner DW, Legermate DA, Lee MJ, et al. Early surgical debridement of symptomatic pancreatic necrosis is beneficial irrespective of infection. Am J Surg 1992; 163:105–110.
38. Uhl W, Schrag HL, Büchler MW. Acute Pancreatitis: Necrosectomy and closed continuous lavage of the retroperitoneum. Dig Surg 1994; 11:245-251.
39. Hollender LF, Meyer C, Marrie A, et al. Role of surgery in the management of acute pancreatitis. World J Surg 1981; 5:361–368.
40. Beger HG, Krautzberger W, Bittner R, et al. Results of surgical treatment of necrotizing pancreatitis. World J Surg 1984; 9:972–979.
41. Sarr MH, Nagorney DM, Much P. Acute necrotizing pancreatitis: Management by planned, staged pancreatic necrosectomy/debridement and delayed primary wound closure over drains. Br J Surg 1991; 78:576–581.
42. Bradley EL III. Management of infected pancreatic necrosis by open drainage. Ann Surg 1987; 206:542–550.
43. Mayer AD, McMahon, Corfield AP, et al. Controlled clinical trial of peritoneal lavage for the treatment of severe acute pancreatitis. N Eng J Med 1985; 312:399–404.
44. Lee MJ, Rattner DW, Legemate DA, et al. Acute complicated pancreatitis: redefining the role of interventional radiology. Radiology 1992; 183:171–174.
45. Rotman N, Mathieu D, Anglade MC, et al. Failure of percutaneous drainage of pancreatic abscess complicating severe acute pancreatitis. Surg Gynecol Obstet 1992; 174:141–144.
46. Van Sonnenberg E, Wing VW, Casola G, et al. Temporizing effect of percutaneous drainage of complicated abscesses in critically ill patients. Am J Radiol 1984; 142:821–826.
47. Baron TH, Thaggard WG, Morgan DE, et al. Endoscopic therapy fpr organized pancreatic necrosis. Gastroenterology 1996; 111:755–765.

33 Management of Infected Pancreatic Necrosis

Ross Carter

Pancreatic necrosis occurs in 10–20% of patients presenting with acute pancreatitis.[1] Attitudes to the surgical approach to this have changed greatly in the last decade, and the role of surgical drainage is gradually evolving. Of those patients that die following an attack of severe acute pancreatitis, over half will succumb to overwhelming early organ dysfunction within the first week.[2] It is generally accepted that attempted pancreatic resection has little role in these patients,[3] and the only randomised trial was discontinued due to unacceptable mortality in the operative group.[4] Rarely, early surgical exploration may be required where the diagnosis is in doubt, or where bowel ischaemia or haemorrhage is suspected. For the majority however, despite the potential for continued deterioration and even death, the only appropriate treatment in the first week is maximal supportive care within an intensive care environment.

The role of surgical intervention in acute pancreatitis therefore lies in the management of local complications that develop during the evolution of the illness. Significant necrosis of either the pancreatic tissue or the surrounding adipose tissue does not in itself require treatment, as occasionally extensive necrosis may resolve without intervention,[5] although the extent of necrosis is related to the risk of developing complications.[6] The most frequent cause of death in patients with acute pancreatitis is multiple organ failure,[7] and recognition of the link between organ dysfunction and the outcome from surgical intervention has revolutionised the approach to the management of these patients in the last few years.[8]

Previously held dogma that development of infection demands urgent radical intervention[9] has been questioned. The overall mortality for radical debridement is between 20 and 30%, however various factors influence this, and mortality rates vary from less than 10%[10;11] to over 60%[9] in selected series from renowned units. Undoubtedly the results are better following intervention for sterile rather than infected necrosis,[12] minimal rather than extensive necrosis,[13] and drainage/debridement of a late pancreatic abscess containing necrosis rather than a true infected necrosis requiring debridement within the first 3–4 weeks of the illness.[14] The effect of differing referral patterns and patient co-morbidity must also be taken into account. Series have tended to report results of a single surgical approach applied to a moderately small and diverse cohort of acute pancreatitic patients. The results of these series have therefore often been more influenced by the selection criteria and clinical characteristics of the patients rather than the surgical technique employed. Surgeon preference has often been determined by either good, or bad, past experience, and no consensus has been achieved regarding a current 'gold standard'.

Indications for Intervention

The widespread use of contrast enhanced computed tomography (CT) has allowed the early identification of necrosis,[15] which develops within the first 3–4 days of the illness. Retro-peritoneal necrosis secondary to acute pancreatitis is not in itself and indication for surgery, as Bradley and his colleagues[1] have shown that even extensive necrosis can be adequately treated conservatively, at least initially. Secondary infection of pancreatic necrosis is most common in the second and third week[16] following disease onset, however broad-spectrum prophylactic antibiotics may delay this further.[17] There is undoubtedly a relationship between the extent of necrosis and the subsequent development of infection.[8] Once infection has occurred conservative management usually leads to escalating sepsis and death. Bacterial contamination of the necrotic material therefore traditionally mandated urgent and radical debridement for control of sepsis.[18]

Infection is usually heralded by an increase in the SIRS response or a secondary deterioration in organ failure scores. Bacteriological confirmation may be obtained by CT or ultrasound-guided FNA[18] of the pancreatic or peri-pancreatic area. Aspiration and culture of ascitic fluid leads to false negative aspirates and should be discouraged. Identification of gas within the retroperitoneum (Fig. 33.1) indicates infection without the need for FNA culture.[19] The confirmation of infection within the necrotic peri-pancreatic tissue should usually still be considered an indication for intervention, however the method chosen will be influenced by the

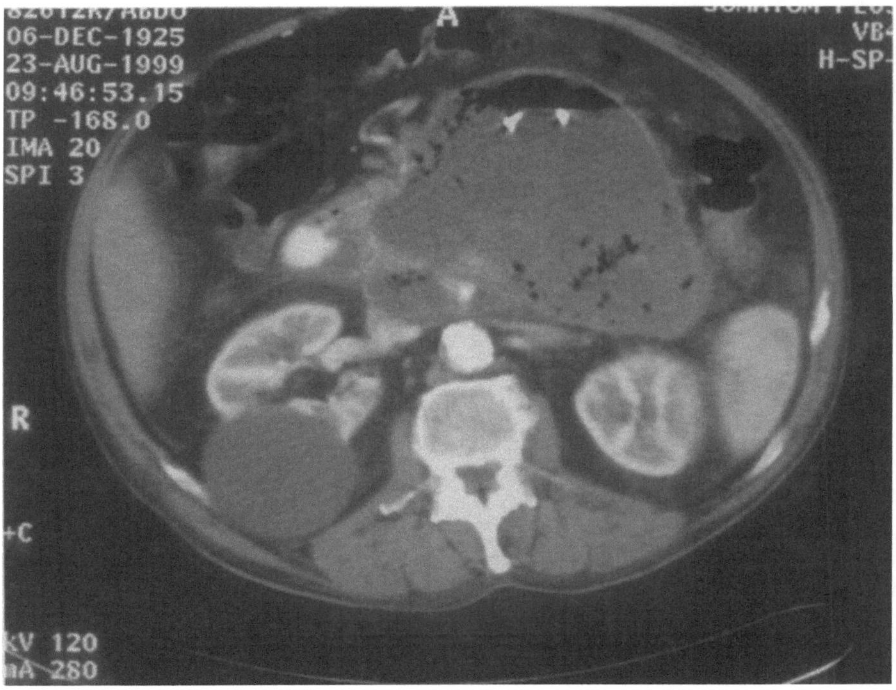

Figure 33.1. CT confirming extensive necrosis with retroperitoneal gas.

background condition of the patient. Aspiration may be repeated on a number of occasions should the culture be negative. Whilst occasionally sterile necrosis requires intervention, the lower mortality of late surgical drainage suggests that intervention in sterile necrosis should be delayed as long as possible.

Operative Techniques

Laparotomy, Retroperitoneal Exploration and Debridement

This is the most widely used approach to the management of infected necrosis. The process of blunt finger debridement of devitalized tissue evolved following recognition that attempts at formal pancreatic resection were associated with unacceptable mortality.[20;21] The technique has been further developed with particular reference to the management of the postoperative retroperitoneal bed. Skeletalisation of the coeliac and mesenteric vessels may occur with extensive necrosis (Fig. 33.2). The ease of debridement is dependent on the duration from onset of the acute pancreatitic episode, as the separation of necrotic and vital tissue is incomplete within the first few weeks of the illness. Debridement during this period results in increased oozing and often the need for packing for haemostasis. Some authors have argued that one advantage of antibiotic prophylaxis, is that while their use has often been shown not to influence the ultimate

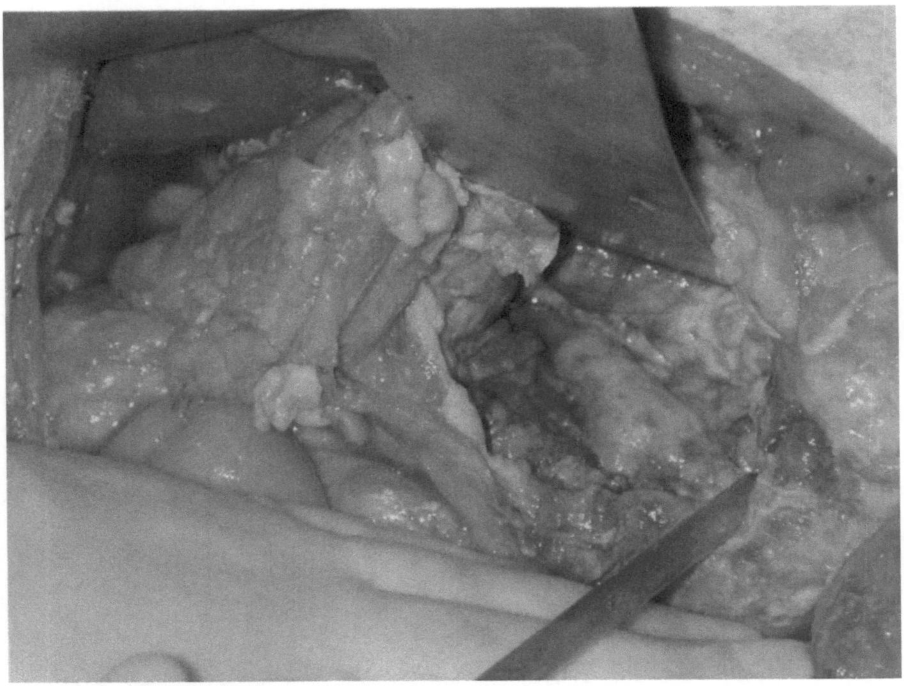

Figure 33.2. Exposed superior mesenteric vessels after debridement

need for intervention,[17] that intervention may be delayed by their use until a period when exploration is less hazardous.

Despite variations regarding the approach to the postoperative management of the retroperitoneum, the initial exploration and surgical technique has changed little in the last 25 years. Most specialists employ a rooftop-subcostal incision, however midline exposure is favoured by some. Following initial laparotomy, the lesser sac is opened either through the gastrocolic omentum or by lifting the omentum from the colon. Both colonic flexures are mobilised to expose the retroperitoneum, and allow access to the paracolic gutters particularly in patients with extensive 'horseshoe' necrosis. The peritoneum at the base of the lesser sac is usually opened and the necrosis is exposed during this mobilization, but occasionally the peritoneum may remain intact and require incision to gain access to the necrosis behind.

The necrotic material, usually of a soft putty consistency is teased from the underlying viable tissue by a blunt finger dissection technique. This often leaves some adherent devitalized tissue, however overzealous clearance can lead to bleeding from the raw surface that becomes difficult to control. The procedure usually includes a cholecystectomy with an operative cholangiogram. Occasionally the vascular integrity of the colon is questionable and an extended right hemicolectomy with terminal ileostomy may be required. Many authors recommend a feeding jejunostomy although recently we have preferred naso-enteric feeding as this avoids the risks of jejunostomy complications particularly when further surgical exploration may be required. There are several approaches to the management of the residual abscess cavity, the ultimate choice being determined by a combination of personal preference, operative findings and extent of residual necrosis.

With Drainage

Simple drainage, often with multiple retroperitoneal tube drains was the original approach to the postoperative management of the debrided pancreatic and peripancreatic bed. Warshaw has reported respectable mortality figures using this technique, although over 40% of the patients treated had pancreatic abscess rather than true infected necrosis.[22] Whilst mortality was less than with resective procedures, multiple second-look laparotomies were often required for residual sepsis. This led to the development of the packing or lavage techniques described below

With Open Packing

Bradley and his colleagues[23;24] have been the principal proponents of the open laparostomy technique, which was widely practiced in the 1980s as the treatment of choice. In this, at the conclusion of the debridement, the divided gastrocolic omentum is sutured to the wound edges leaving the wound open. The lesser sac is packed with lubricated cotton gauze, allowing planned re-explorations/wound dressings, every few days until granulation tissue forms. This approach has the advantage that subsequent explorations/dressings can be carried out under sedation in the ITU/HDU without recourse to further anaesthetics. The technique may be modified closing part of the wound leaving the left side open to allow access for

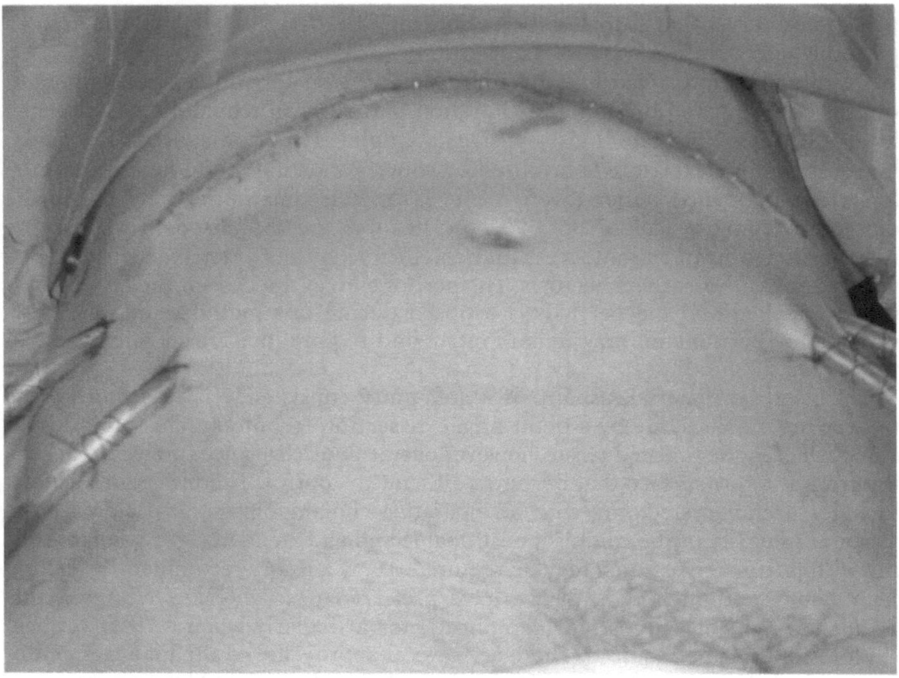

Figure 33.3. Multiple drains inserted for closed continuous postoperative lavage

gentle manual exploration. Enteric fistula and secondary haemorrhage are not uncommon, and the technique is rarely now performed as a first option. Fagniez[25] and his colleagues described a further modification with a lateral (retroperitoneal) approach utilizing a limited loin/subcostal incision, proceeding behind the colon for debridement of pancreatic and peripancreatic necrosis. The technique was however associated with major morbidity (enteric fistula 45%, haemorrhage 40%, and colonic necrosis 15%), and has not gained popularity.

With Closed Lavage

Radical debridement combined with postoperative closed lavage as described by Beger *et al.*[26], is now widely used for the management of infected pancreatic necrosis, the aim of the lavage being the continuous removal of devitalised necrotic material and bacteria. Having completed the debridement, the lesser sac is closed over multiple large diameter tube drains (Fig. 33.3). Continuous lavage is then commenced, our own preference being for peritoneal dialysis fluid (Dianil 7, Baxter Healthcare, potassium free, Iso-osmolar) warmed through a blood warmer and delivered at 500 ml/h. The lavage is continued, for around 3 to 4 weeks on average, until the return fluid is clear, and the patient has no residual signs of systemic sepsis. Re-exploration may still be required for residual sepsis, and for blocked or dislodged drains.

Personal Policy

Traditionally, authors have tended to report series whereby one technique has been used in isolation. In our experience, the extent of necrosis, the presence of a coagulopathy, haemorrhage, colonic ischaemia or fistula, and the condition of the patient all influence how we would manage the necrosectomy cavity. Our own preference, would be to create a closed retroperitoneal lavage system, however surgical packing and planned re-operation after 2–3 days is sometimes required in the presence of an intraoperative coagulopathy. We would them aim to create a closed lavage system, following correction of the coagulopathy, at the time of subsequent pack removal, rather than persevere with the laparostomy technique.

Delayed Management of Necrosis

It is well recognised that the mortality of necrosectomy related mainly to patients requiring surgical drainage or debridement within the first 4 weeks following the onset of acute pancreatitis. Drainage of a pancreatic abscess containing some pancreatic necrosis is comparatively risk free and the inclusion of these patients in reported series has led to difficulties in interpreting the literature. Our preferred option for patients with a well demarcated infected pseudocyst (abscess) is internal drainage usually into the stomach. A surgical cystgastrostomy (10 cm) allows adequate drainage in addition to removal of any necrotic material contained within and is usually associated with a rapid recovery. Our own current preference is to perform this laparoscopically combined with a cholecystectomy as definitive treatment of cholelithiasis. These patients should not be included in series reporting results of necrosectomy.

Significance of Organ Failure

It has recently been recognized that the mortality associated with surgery is intimately related to the presence or absence of organ failure.[7] The degree of this organ dysfunction is not directly related to the extent of pancreatic or peripancreatic necrosis, or even the presence of infection, although an association exists.[12] Background co-morbidity and genetic predisposition both play a significant role.[27] The precise mechanism of the initiation of organ dysfunction is unknown, however the absence of organ dysfunction in the preoperative patient is the single most accurate determinant of ultimate survival.

Whilst the indication for surgery has usually been the identification of bacteria on FNA, the outcome from intervention is very different in patients with, rather than without, organ dysfunction. Timing of intervention is particularly important when assessing results of intervention. Whilst the reported overall mortality in series may be 20–25%, the mortality in patients with infected necrosis and multiple organ (>3) failure may exceed 80–90%. Postoperative clinical deterioration in these patients is common, and many cannot withstand the aggressive surgical approach described above. For this reason many groups have recently been exploring a more conservative approach, trying minimally invasive techniques to minimise the effect of intervention on peri- and postoperative organ function.

Minimally Invasive Approaches to Infected Necrosis

CT or ultrasound-guided aspiration and drainage has revolutionised the management of many surgical conditions and complications. In the presence of pancreatic necrosis, simple aspiration and percutaneous drainage alone rarely result in resolution in that it does not address the solid component within the abscess, and should therefore be discouraged as sole treatment. Percutaneous drainage may however have a role as a temporising measure in the hope of finding a 'window of opportunity' in which to perform more definitive intervention. Freeny and his colleagues,[28] took this approach to its limits by combining aggressive CT guided percutaneous drainage, tract dilatation and continuous post drainage lavage, using a median of four drains per patient. They confirmed that using this technique pancreatic sepsis may resolve, however nearly 75% of the patients will subsequently require surgical intervention for residual sepsis or necrosis. The logistic demands on the radiological department of this approach have restricted its appeal, although other groups have reported series managed by primarily conservative means.[29;30]

The technique of endoscopic cystgastrostomy for pancreatic sepsis was first described by Baron *et al.*[31] and developments in endoscopic ultrasound have greatly facilitated the ease and safety of performing a transmural drainage.[32] Tract dilatation combined with naso-cyst lavage will adequately drain any fluid component however the residual necrotic material results in a significant failure rate in resolution. The same group subsequently reported[33] that extensive necrosis was a contraindication, and highlighted that drainage must be combined with some form of surgical removal of the necrotic material.

Laparoscopy has transformed many surgical procedures and has been shown to reduce the inflammatory stimulus resulting from surgery. Some laparoscopic specialists[34;35] have presented a small series of patients undergoing a laparoscopic necrosectomy, with encouraging results, however the surgical difficulty limits its universal application. In 2000, we described[36] our technique of percutaneous necrosectomy involving intra-operative dilatation of a percutaneous drain tract, and subsequent necrosectomy using a urological rigid rod lens system, usually from the left flank or right subcostal approach. To avoid contamination by bowel puncture, double contrast CT guided FNA is performed. Our preferred route is through the left fat plane between the spleen posteriorly and the colon anteriorly, although for right sided collections access can usually be obtained anterior to the duodenum, between colon and liver. The tract is first dilated using a balloon dilator, allowing insertion of a 34FG Amplatz sheath. Initial intermittent copious lavage and suction is performed until the irrigant clears sufficiently to see within the cavity. Devitalised tissue is easily identified and to can be removed by gentle traction in a piecemeal fashion (Fig. 33.4). Experience has suggested that overzealous attempts at cavity clearance are unnecessary and can lead to bleeding. An 8FG umbilical catheter sutured to a 28FG tube drain is then passed to the far end of the cavity to allow continuous post-operative lavage (500 ml/h Dianil 7). Planned second look procedures are then performed every 7–10 days, until the cavity is clean.

We have now treated over 40 patients using this technique; the major advantages appear to be the lack of the almost universal deterioration in organ function seen following an open approach, and therefore a significant reduction in the need for

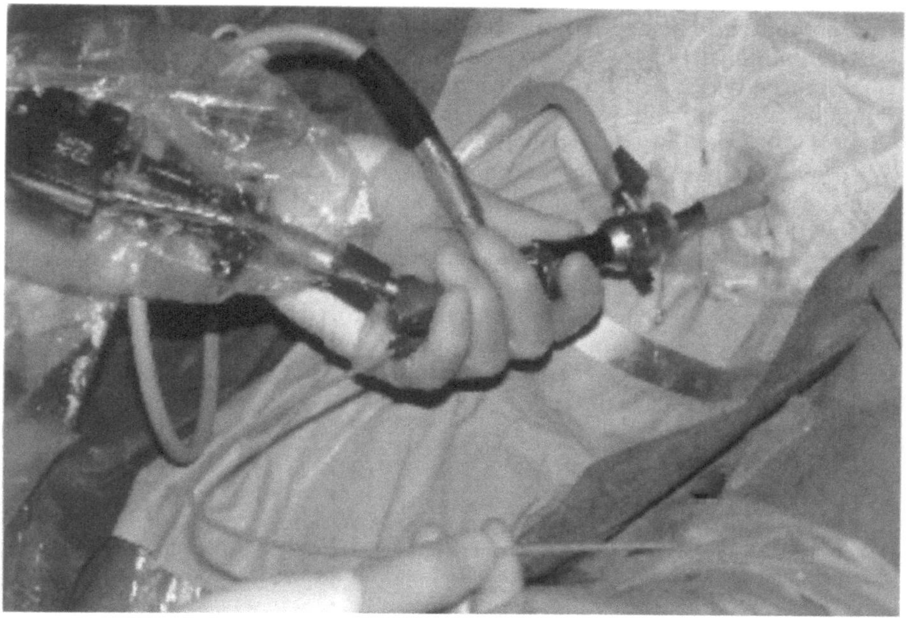

Figure 33.4. Percutaneous necrosectomy.

postoperative intensive care management. The preliminary results have been encouraging, however ongoing assessment of this approach continues.

Conclusion

Infected necrosis remains a major surgical challenge and the diversity of reported treatment strategies testifies to the lack of a universally agreed gold standard. Much of this controversy relates to the variability of clinical presentation, particularly of organ dysfunction, and the lack of uniformity in patient selection for procedures. Half of the patients who die as a result of severe acute pancreatitis do so within the first few days of the illness,[2] and may never reach a specialised unit, whilst others may not be considered fit for intervention. Background morbidity of patients within a series is difficult to determine and undoubtedly has a major influence on outcome. The potential effect of patient selection can be seen where overall mortality following surgery for infected necrosis has been reported[37] as being less than the mortality for all-comers, with or without necrosis, recruited to trials in patients with predicted severe pancreatitis.[38]

It is evident that no single treatment or technique is the answer. As these patients are relatively uncommon, most surgeons have adopted a favoured, but consistent, approach to infected necrosis. Within specialized units, it has become increasingly obvious that not all patients respond equally to a given surgical stimulus. As a generalisation, patients with infected necrosis but without significant organ dysfunction will do well regardless of the approach chosen, and in these an aggressive open debridement may be the most appropriate choice as it may hasten recovery. A patient with multiple organ dysfunction and sepsis however, may be more appropriately managed by a carefully timed percutaneous drain followed by a delayed minimally invasive or even open necrosectomy.

The mortality associated with open surgical exploration in a patient with multi-organ dysfunction and sepsis is unacceptable. Undoubtedly the severity of systemic sepsis and organ dysfunction can be down-staged by percutaneous or endoscopic drainage, however the improvement tends to be temporary unless drainage is maintained together with some means of addressing the solid component of these abscesses. Tract dilatation and minimally invasive necrosectomy achieves drainage, addresses the solid component, whilst minimizing the surgical insult to the patient, and may be the optimum approach in a carefully selected high-risk group of patients. It is only through improved timing of intervention and understanding of the disease process, combining various different techniques tailored to the specific requirements of an individual patient, that the mortality in the high-risk group may fall.

Acknowledgements

I would like to acknowledge the considerable contribution of my colleagues, Mr. Colin McKay, Professor Clem Imrie and the members of the West of Scotland Pancreatic Research Unit to this work.

References

1. Bradley III, Allen KA. Prospective longitudinal study of observation versus surgical intervention in the management of necrotizing pancreatitis. Amer J of Surg 1991; 161:19–25.
2. McKay CJ, Evans S, Sinclair M, et al. High early mortality rate from acute pancreatitis in Scotland, 1984–1995. Bri J of Surg 1999; 86:1302–1305.
3. Hartwig W, Maksan SM, Foitzik T, et al. Reduction in mortality with delayed surgical therapy of severe pancreatitis. J Gastrointest Surg 2002; 6:481–487.
4. Meir J, Luque-de Leon E, Castillo A, et al. Early versus late necrosectomy in severe necrotising pancreatitis. Am J Surg 1997; 173:71–75.
5. Bradley EL. Operative vs. Nonoperative therapy in necrotizing pancreatitis. Digestion 1999; 60 (Suppl 1):19–21.
6. Isenmann R, Rau B, Beger HG. Bacterial infection and extent of necrosis are determinants of organ failure in patients with acute necrotizing pancreatitis. Bri J of Surg 1999; 86:1020–1024.
7. Buter A, McKay CJ, Carter CR, et al. The time course of the development of organ failure in acute pancreatitis and its relationship to mortality. Digestion 1999; 60:371(abst).
8. Tenner S, Sica G, Hughes M, et al. Relationship of necrosis to organ failure in severe acute pancreatitis. Gastroenterology 1997; 113:899–903.
9. Rau B, Uhl W, Buchler MW, et al. Surgical treatment of infected necrosis. World J Surg 1997; 21:155–161.
10. Farkas G, Marton J, Mandi Y, et al. Progress in the management and treatment of infected pancreatic necrosis. Scand J Gastroenterol Suppl 1998; 228:31–37.
11. Fernandez-Del CC, Rattner DW, Makary MA, et al. Debridement and closed packing for the treatment of necrotizing pancreatitis. Ann Surg 1998; 228:676–684.
12. Isenmann R, Beger HG. Natural History of Acute Pancreatitis and the Role of Infection. Bailliere's Best Pract Clin Gastroenterol 1999; 13 (2):291–301.
13. Ashley SW, Perez A, Pierce EA, et al. Necrotizing pancreatitis: contemporary analysis of 99 consecutive cases. Ann Surg 2001; 234:572–579.
14. Tsiotos GG, Sarr MG. Management of fluid collections and necrosis in acute pancreatitis. Curr Gastroenterol Rep 1999; 1:139–144.
15. Balthazar EJ, Ranson JHC, Naidich DP, et al. Acute pancreatitis: prognostic value of CT. Radiology 1985; 156:767–772.

16. Beger HG, Bittner R, Block S, et al. Bacterial contamination of pancreatic necrosis. A prospective clinical study. Gastroenterology 1986; 91:433–438.
17. Slavin J, Neoptolemos JP. Antibiotic prophylaxis in severe acute pancreatitis – what are the facts? Langenbecks Arch Surg 2001; 386:155–159.
18. Rau B, Pralle U, Mayer JM, et al. Role of ultrasonographically guided fine-needle aspiration cytology in the diagnosis of infected pancreatic necrosis. Bri J of Surg 1998; 85:179–184.
19. Balthazar EJ, Robinson DL, Megibow AJ, et al. Acute pancreatitis: Value of CT in establishing prognosis. Radiology 1990; 174:331–336.
20. Alexander JH, Guerreri MT. Role of total pancreatectomy in the treatment of necrotising pancreatitis. World J of Surg 1981; 5:369–377.
21. Watts CT. Total pancreatectomy for fulminant pancreatitis. Lancet 1963; 2:384–389.
22. Warshaw AL, Jin G. Improved survival in 45 patients with pancreatic abscess. Ann Surg 1985; 202:408–415.
23. Bradley EL, III. A fifteen year experience with open drainage for infected pancreatic necrosis. Surg Gynaecol Obstet 1993; 177:215–222.
24. Bradley EL, III. Open packing in infected pancreatic necrosis. Digestive Surg 1997; 14:77–81.
25. Fagniez PL, Rotman N, Kracht M. Direct retroperitoneal approach to necrosis in severe acute pancreatitis. Br J Surg 1989; 76:264–267.
26. Beger HG, Buchler M, Bittner R, et al. Necrosectomy and postoperative local lavage in patients with necrotizing pancreatitis: Results of a prospective clinical trial. World J of Surg 1988; 12:255–262.
27. Buter A, Eskdale J, Gallagher G, et al. The IL-10. R3 microsatellite allele is associated with fulminant early organ dysfunction in acute pancreatitis. Pancreas 1999; 19:417 (abst).
28. Freeny PC, Hauptmann E, Althaus SJ, et al. Percutaneous CT-guided catheter drainage of infected acute necrotizing pancreatitis: Techniques and results. Amer J of Roentgenology 1998; 170:969–975.
29. Echenique AM, Sleeman D, Yrizarry J, et al. Percutaneous catheter-directed debridement of infected pancreatic necrosis: results in 20 patients. J Vasc Interv Radiol 1998; 9:565–571.
30. Lee MJ, Wittich GR, Mueller PR. Percutaneous intervention in acute pancreatitis. Radiographics 1998; 18:711–724.
31. Baron TH, Thaggard WG, Morgan DE, et al. Endoscopic therapy for organised pancreatic necrosis. Gastroenterology 1996; 111 (3):755–764.
32. Grzebieniak Z, Woyton M, Kielan W. Surgical and endoscopic treatment of pancreatic pseudocysts. Przegl Lek 2000; 57 (Suppl 5):50–52.
33. Morgan DE, Smith JK, Baron TH, et al. Pancreatic fluid collections prior to drainage: evaluation of MR imaging compared with CT and US. Radiology 1997; 203 (3):773–778.
34. Cuschieri A. Pancreatic necrosis: pathogenesis and endoscopic management. Semin Laparosc Surg 2002 Mar; 9 (1):54–63
35. Hamad GG, Broderick TJ. Laparoscopic pancreatic necrosectomy. J Laparoendosc Adv Surg Tech 2000; 10:115–118.
36. Carter CR, McKay CJ, Imrie CW. Percutaneous necrosectomy and sinus tract endoscopy in the management of infected pancreatic necrosis: An initial experience. Ann of Surg 2000; 232:175–180.
37. Farkas G, Marton J, Mandi Y, et al. Surgical strategy and management of infected pancreatic necrosis. Bri J of Surg 1996; 83:930–933.
38. Johnson CD, Kingsnorth AN, Imrie CW, et al. Double blind, randomised, placebo controlled study of a platelet activating factor antagonist, lexipafant, in the treatment and prevention of organ failure in predicted severe acute pancreatitis. Gut 2002; 48 (1):62–69.

34 Antibiotics in Acute Pancreatitis

Hans G. Beger and Rainer Isenman

The overwhelming majority of patients suffering from acute pancreatitis suffers from mild disease which responds to conservative treatment. Fatalities and complications are rare. The pathomorphological picture is characterized by interstitial oedema, and complete functional and morphological restitution of the gland is the rule.

Approximately 10 to 20 percent of the patients, however, develop severe disease which is characterized by the development of intra- or peripancreatic necrosis. Severe acute pancreatitis is associated with a considerable rate of organ failure and local complications. The majority of deaths due to the disease is observed in patients with pancreatic necrosis. Bacterial infection of pancreatic necrosis is found in 1–10% of all patients suffering from acute pancreatitis and in 40–70% of those with necrotizing pancreatitis.[1–4] It is defined as the presence of bacteria in diffuse or focal areas of non-viable pancreatic parenchyma. Infected necrosis is a phenomenon of the later phase of severe acute pancreatitis, becoming relevant during the second to third week after onset of the disease. Among all complications of severe pancreatitis, infected necrosis has the most striking impact on the patients course and prognosis.

Today, there is no doubt, that bacterial infection of pancreatic necrosis is the leading cause of death in patients with necrotizing pancreatitis. Mortality rates of 15–30% are commonly reported from patients with infected pancreatic necrosis. Most deaths in this entity are the sequel of ongoing sepsis and septic multiple organ failure.[1;5]

Infected Pancreatic Necrosis

Infected pancreatic necrosis has a well-defined bacterial spectrum (Table 34.1). In man, prospective data have been obtained from smears either performed during surgical necrosectomy[6;7] or by computed-tomography (CT)-guided fine needle aspiration.[8] In the majority of cases, pancreatic infection is monomicrobial. The bacterial spectrum of interest resembles an intestinal flora. It is dominated by gram-negative bacteria but also comprises gram-positive bacteria, anaerobes and fungi.

There is experimental evidence, that the bacteria originate from the gastrointestinal tract, as especially the colon contains the greatest variety and number of micro-organisms in the body. A number of different routes have been proposed by

Table 34.1. Bacterial spectrum of infected pancreatic necrosis. Data from 92 patients treated at the Department of General surgery, University of Ulm 1982–1997. Given are the numbers of isolated strains and their percentages

Enterococci	33 (20%)
E. coli	30 (18%)
Klebsiella spp.	16 (10%)
Staph. aureus	15 (9%)
Staph. epidermidis	9 (6%)
Bacteroides spp.	5 (3%)
Proteus spp.	4 (2%)
Pseudomonas spp.	3 (2%)
Other bacteria	26 (16%)
Candida spp.	22 (14%)
Isolated bacterial strain in total	**163**

which the organisms might reach the necrotic areas, including direct translocation, haematogenous or lymphatic spreading or infection via the pancreatic duct and the common bile duct.[9–12] The exact mechanisms still are a matter of debate and under experimental investigation.

Clinical Relevance of Infected Pancreatic Necrosis

Today, there is no doubt that bacterial infection of pancreatic necrosis is most important determinant of outcome for patients with severe acute pancreatitis. Analysis of the courses of 273 patients with necrotizing pancreatitis treated in our institution clearly showed, that bacterial infection of pancreatic necrosis is the most important risk factor predisposing for systemic organ failure and subsequent death (Table 34.2). Compared to sterile necrosis, the incidence of systemic complications is significantly higher in patients with pancreatic infection.[13] In addition, a considerable percentage of patients with severe acute pancreatitis can successfully be managed by conservative treatment as long as the necrosis remains sterile ,[14–16] but surgical necrosectomy is the standard treatment of infected pancreatic necrosis.[2–4;15;17] It therefore is one of the main principles of all diagnostic and therapeutic algorithms in severe acute pancreatitis to identify patients with infected necrosis.

Table 34.2. Factor predisposing for organ failure in necrotizing pancreatitis (From Ref. (13), with permission)

Variable		Odds ratio	95% confidence limits	
			Lower	Upper
Bacterial status	Infected vs. sterile necrosis	4.15	1.72	11.42
Extent of necrosis	30–50% vs. <30%	1.78	0.83	4.01
	>50% vs. 30–50%	4.84	1.39	22.65
Etiology	Biliary vs. alcohol	0.48	0.20	1.11
	Others vs. alcohol	1.49	0.62	3.90

Table 34.3. Value of CRP, Procalcitonin and IL-8 in the prediction of complications of acute pancreatitis (Data from Ref. (24), with permission)

Prediction of infected necrosis	Cut-off	Sensitivity	Specificity
PCT	>1.8 ng/ml	94%	90%
IL-8	>112 pg/ml	72%	75%
CRP	>300 mg/L	83%	78%
Prediction of multiorgan failure			
PCT	>1.8 ng/ml	86%	92%
IL-8	>140 pg/ml	79%	81%
CRP	>325 mg/L	71%	78%
Prediction of death			
PCT	>5.7 ng/ml	100%	92%
IL-8	>140 pg/ml	91%	79%
CRP	>325 mg/L	64%	72%

Identification of Infected Pancreatic Necrosis

The gold-standard for identification of infected pancreatic necrosis is the performance of ultrasound- or CT-guided fine needle aspiration with subsequent gram-staining of the aspirate.[18;19] These procedures can be performed with high sensitivity and specificity, but they are associated with all the disadvantages of invasive procedures. Therefore, the search has continued for laboratory markers which allow precise identification of pancreatic infection. Serum C-reactive protein, which is a standard marker for identification of pancreatic necrosis[20–23] is not reliable in the identification of infected necrosis. At the moment, there are number of inflammatory mediators under clinical investigation for this purpose. First investigations with serum procalcitonin revealed this peptide as a promising candidate and superior to other inflammatory markers for reliable identification of infected pancreatic necrosis[24] (Table 34.3). These first results could not be confirmed in other clinical trials,[25;26] but further well designed studies are on their way which will provide us with more information about this controversial topic.

Rationales for Antibiotics in Severe Acute Pancreatitis

When discussing the question of whether or not antibiotics should be given to patients with acute pancreatitis three points should be carefully distinguished:

1. Mild severe acute pancreatitis without evidence of pancreatic necrosis does not need treatment with antibiotic drugs. Septic complications are rare in this entity and restitution of the gland without further functional damage is the rule. With regard to the development of antibiotic resistance, patients suffering from oedematous pancreatitis should not receive antibiotic drugs.
2. In patients with infected pancreatic necrosis, antibiotic treatment is a substantial and mandatory part of the treatment regime. Antibiotics should be chosen according to bacterial resistance and continued as long as there is evidence of local or systemic infection. Antibiotic treatment alone, however, is not likely to cure pancreatic infection; surgical necrosectomy still is the gold standard in these patients. Treatment of infected necrosis by prolonged antibiotic applica-

tion without adequate surgical treatment currently is a question undergoing clinical investigation.[27] Our information concerning this topic is scarce and we have to await the results of future clinical trials to draw meaningful conclusions.

3. Antibiotic prophylaxis in severe acute pancreatitis currently is a challenging and controversial issue. Prophylaxis attempts to reduce septic complications in patients with pancreatic necrosis. This question has been a matter of several experimental and clinical studies during the past years. This problem will therefore be the main topic of this chapter.

Antibiotics in Acute Pancreatitis – The History

Whether or not to include antibiotics in the treatment protocol of acute pancreatitis has been under discussion for decades.[28–32] The rationale of antibiotic application has always been to reduce infectious complications of acute pancreatitis. Twenty-five years ago, the first clinical trials of antibiotic application were conducted in patients with mild acute pancreatitis. Meanwhile, our increasing knowledge has shown that septic complications are rare in this group of patients and it is not surprising that these earlier studies were not able to find any positive effect as antibiotics were given to patients with mild acute pancreatitis.[28] During the following years, considerable efforts were made to provide the scientific basis for further investigation in this field. The clinical relevance of bacterial infection in severe acute pancreatitis has been investigated[6–8] and the pharmacokinetics of antibiotics in the human pancreas have been carefully elaborated.[33–37] The basic studies were followed by a number of controlled clinical trials.[38–44] Today, several guidelines[45–47] and analysis of pooled data[48;49] have been published as evidence based recommendations for the use of antibiotics in severe acute pancreatitis.

Pharmacokinetics of Broad Spectrum Antibiotics in Human Pancreatic Tissue

Numerous antibiotics have been tested for their capability to penetrate into human pancreatic tissue, as tissue concentrations are regarded to be the 'gold standard' for antibiotic treatment protocols. Tissue concentrations of imipenem, ciprofloxacin and ofloxacin exceed the minimal inhibitory concentrations of most of the bacteria relevant in pancreatic infection, whereas others, especially the aminoglycosides tobramycin and netilmicin, did not penetrate into human pancreatic tissue.[33;34] From the pharmacokinetic point of view, these drugs can be regarded as candidates for the prevention of pancreatic infection and subsequent clinical trials have been conducted almost exclusively with one or a combination of these drugs.

Experimental Studies of Antibiotic Prophylaxis

Among the large number of experimental investigations using antibiotics in animal models of acute pancreatitis, only a few have had an adequate design that allows reliable conclusions for the clinical situation. Most of these studies were designed to investigate the pathogenetic pathways of pancreatic infection and do not allow any statements concerning the effects of antibiotic treatment on the course and outcome of the disease, as the observation period of surviving animals should be at least 2–3 weeks, which is long enough for development of late septic complications.[11;50–52]

Mithoefer and co-workers published one of the rare experimental series which can be regarded as a treatment study.[53] In rats, a model of necrotizing pancreatitis of defined and reproducible severity was used. Either systemic Ciprofloxacin or Imipenem was given over a period of seven days after initiation of pancreatitis and animals were observed over a period of time long enough to allow a statement concerning late septic complications of the disease. Pancreatic infection rate as well as mortality were assessed 21 days after induction of pancreatitis in comparison to a non-treated control group. The results of this study clearly indicate that prophylactic antibiotic application reduced both the incidence of septic complications of severe acute pancreatitis and mortality in this experimental setting. Interestingly, a significant difference was observed in the mortality of animals treated with the two different antibiotics. In this respect, treatment with Ciprofloxacin was superior to Imipenem treatment.

Clinical Studies

Systemic Antibiotics

Shortly after publication of the experimental and pharmacokinetic basis of antibiotic prophylaxis in necrotizing pancreatitis, the first clinical trials with an improved design were initiated (Table 34.4). In 1993, the first controlled clinical study was published by Pederzoli and co-workers[38] which fulfilled all the necessary standards. Antibiotic treatment was started early after onset of acute pancreatitis, only patients with proven pancreatic necrosis were enrolled, the study design was a controlled one and antibiotic drugs with favourable pancreatic tissue kinetics were chosen. In this multicenter, randomized trial, patients with necrotizing pancreatitis received either intravenous imipenem (41 patients, 3×0.5g/day) or no antibiotic treatment (33 patients). The authors observed a statistically significant reduction of both, pancreatic and non-pancreatic sepsis in the treatment group. No statistical difference, however, was found with regard to mortality (12.2 *vs* 7.3%) and the rate of multi-organ-failure as well as the need for surgical treatment between both groups. Besides the fact that the number of enrolled patients might have been too small to find differences in these parameters, this study included all the problems encountered in multicenter-studies. The indications for surgery as well as the standards of medical treatment might have differed between the six contributing hospitals.

A second controlled series focused on the use of intravenous cefuroxime (3×1.5 g/day) in acute necrotizing pancreatitis.[42] The antibiotic drug was chosen according to its antimicrobial activity, regardless of the limited information about the pharmacokinetic profile of cefuroxime in the human pancreas. Interestingly, Sainio and co-workers observed a significant reduction in the mortality of the antibiotic-treated patients. Furthermore, 23 of 30 patients primarily not treated with antibiotics had to receive antibiotic treatment due to evident or strongly

Table 34.4. Literature survey of the effect of prophylactic antibiotic treatment in necrotizing pancreatitis. (– = no difference, + = significant difference)

		Antibiotic agent(s)	Patients	Mortality	Pancreatic Infection
Systemic anitbiotics					
Pederzoli *et al.*(38)	1993	Imipenem	41	–	+
		None	33		
Sainio *et al.*(42)	1995	Cefuroxime	30	+	–
		None	30		
Delcenserie *et al.* (39)	1996	Ceftazidime+ Amikacin+ Metronidazole	11	–	–
		None	12		
Schwarz *et al.*(41)	1997	Ofloxacin+ Metronidazole	13	–	–*)
		None	13		
Bassi *et al.*(40)	1998	Imipenem	30	–	+
		Pefloxacin	30		
Nordback *et al.* (43)	2000	Imipenem (early)	25	–	+**)
		Imipenem (late)	33		
Selective decontamination					
Luiten *et al.*(44)	1995	Norfloxacin Colistin Amphotericin Cefotaxim	50	+	+
		None	52		

* significant decrease of APACHE II score in treatment group
** surgical debridement less frequent in treatment group

suspected bacterial infection after a mean time of 6.1 days, suggesting that antibiotic treatment might be of special importance during the first few days of the disease. Although these data provide strong support for antibiotic treatment in necrotizing pancreatitis, they are conflicting. Given the fact, that pancreatic infection is the leading cause of deaths in necrotizing pancreatitis, one would assume that a reduction in mortality is associated with a reduction in the incidence of pancreatic abscess or infected pancreatic necrosis, but this was not observed by the authors of the cefuroxime-study. In addition, deaths during the first days of pancreatitis were included in the analysis for mortality, although they were most unlikely to be caused by septic complications. If these fatalities were excluded from analysis, the difference would not be significant at a statistical level.

In a series of 26 patients with necrotizing pancreatitis, receiving either ofloxacin and metronidazol or no prophylactic antibiotic treatment, our group found a significant decrease of the APACHE-II score during the course of the disease in the group of patients treated with antibiotic prophylaxis).[41]

Bassi and co-workers have compared Imipenem (3×500 mg/day) and Pefloxacin (2×400 mg/day) in a controlled clinical trial in patients with necrosis of more than 50% of the glands parenchyma.[40] Interestingly, imipenem was superior to pefloxacin in reducing the rate of infected pancreatic necrosis. Most surprisingly, in the Pefloxacin group, the incidence of infected necrosis was comparable to the incidence observed in the control groups of other series, were the patients did not receive prophylactic antibiotics.[38;42] This study provides several interesting aspects: First, all patients of the Imipenem group that developed pancreatic infection despite antibiotic prophylaxis died during the later course of the disease. Second, infection with *Candida glabrata* was a frequent finding after Pefloxacin prophylaxis and associated with poor prognosis. According to our opinion, this later finding supports the position that fungal infection in necrotizing pancreatitis is associated with poor prognosis and can be regarded as sequel of prolonged prior antibiotic treatment

In a most recent series from Finland,[43] Imipenem prophylaxis was compared to Imipenem treatment in necrotizing pancreatitis. Patients received either Imipenem prophylaxis immediately after hospital admission or delayed treatment with Imipenem once the indications for surgical treatment of necrotizing pancreatitis (proven pancreatic infection or strongly suspected infection with ongoing SIRS) were fulfilled. Most interestingly, the clinical condition of nine patients of the delayed treatment group improved after initiation of Imipenem therapy; they recovered without surgical intervention. Nevertheless, all patients of the treatment group who underwent surgical necrosectomy died during the later course of the disease. This interesting series reminds us of the fact that proven pancreatic infection still remains an absolute indication for surgical treatment.

Based on the experience of the above mentioned randomized trials, the routine use of Imipenem has recently been advocated for all patients with necrotizing pancreatitis. Büchler and co-workers[15] have included prophylaxis with this antibiotic drug in their treatment protocol of patients with necrotizing pancreatitis. In their series of 86 patients, all receiving Imipenem prophylaxis, the rate of pancreatic infection was 34% with a mortality in infected necrosis of 24% compared to a mortality rate of 3.5% in the group of patients with sterile necrosis. Although the difference in mortality is tempting enough to propagate prophylactic antibiotics as a future standard in the treatment of severe acute pancreatitis, it should be noted, that the infection rate of the overall population does not differ from the rates of other series which did not use prophylactic antibiotics and the infection rates of the control group of previously published randomized trials. Infection rate with *Candida albicans* was 29% in this series, which again raises the question whether the general use of antibiotics carries the risk of fungal infection with subsequent poor prognosis.[54]

As a sequel of the limited number of patients included in randomized trials and their heterogeneous results, analyses of pooled data have tried to provide more substantial information about the outcome of patients receiving prophylactic antibiotics.[48;49] In fact, if all studies are taken together, there seems to be an effect of antibiotic prophylaxis with regard to a reduction in mortality[48;49] as well as to a reduction in the incidence of septic complications.[49]

Selective Decontamination of the Digestive Tract

The assumption, that the bacteria relevant in pancreatic infection originate from the digestive tract led to the idea of selective decontamination of the digestive tract (SDD) by oral application of non-absorbable antibiotics. SDD has been shown to reduce nosocomial infection in critically ill patients as well as to reduce mortality in subgroups of patients with increased risk of septic complications.[55–58] Animal models of severe pancreatitis showed a reduction of pancreatic infection by full-gut decontamination, giving further support to this theory.[50;59;60]

In a retrospective analysis, course and outcome of nine patients with necrotizing pancreatitis receiving SDD was compared to an earlier series of six similar patients without SDD.[61] All patients suffered from acute respiratory failure requiring mechanical ventilation. This study showed a reduction of the rate of infectious complications favouring SDD treatment but no differences in the mortality rate. Both series were relatively small and the time of enrolment was five years. Thus, these data can only be regarded as vague support of the theory that reduction of the intestinal bacterial flora is associated with improvements in the patients course.

Luiten and co-workers published the results of a randomized, controlled multicenter trial about SDD in severe acute pancreatitis.[44] Patients were randomized to receive either standard medical treatment without use of antibiotics or SDD consisting of oral colistin sulphate, norfloxacin and amphotericin in combination with systemic cefotaxime. The authors report a reduction of late mortality due to a significant reduction of the incidence of gram-negative pancreatic infection. Pancreatic infection occurred in nine of 50 patients in the SDD group (18%) compared to 20 of 52 patients of the control group (38%). Although overall mortality in this series is rather high (22% in the SDD group, 35% in the control group), these controlled data for the first time provide evidence for a beneficial role of SDD in patients with necrotizing pancreatitis.

Evidence-based Guidelines

Today there is much enthusiasm for treatment protocols based on the results of adequately powered, randomized trials. Therefore, it is not surprising that the treatment guidelines for acute pancreatitis of a number of medical associations include a more or less clear position on prophylactic antibiotics in severe acute pancreatitis is concerned (Table 34.5). In the authors' opinion, these guidelines should be regarded with some caution. First, they are not based on the results of double-blinded trials. Although it is frequently assumed that the clinical trials of prophylactic antibiotics were double-blind studies, this is not the case. None of them was blinded and this could be the source of some bias which arises as the investigator strongly expects a beneficial effect in the treatment arm. Second, not more than 150 patients were treated up to now under controlled conditions with prophylactic antibiotics.

Table 34.5. International guidelines for the treatment of acute pancreatitis that include statements concerning the use of prophylactic antibiotics, including levels of evidence (if given)

American College of Gastroenterology[47]	1997	It is reasonable to initiate antibiotic therapy in severe acute pancreatitis
British Society of Gastroenterology[45]	1998	There is some evidence to support the use of prophylactic antibiotics. Cefuroxime is a reasonable balance between efficacy and cost.
Santorini Consensus Conference[69]	1999	Prophylactic antibacterial treatment is strongly recommended in severe pancreatitis (Cat. A)
German guidelines*[46]	2000	Antibiotic prophylaxis is not generally recommended. Indications could be: necrotizing pancreatitis, severe acute pancreatitis (Cat B)

* Consensus of the German Society of Surgery (DGC), the German Society of Abdominal Surgery (DGVC) and the German Society for Disorders of the Digestive Tract (DGVS)

Nevertheless, these guidelines have contributed to a wide-spread use of antibiotics not only in severe, but also in mild acute pancreatitis. A questionnaire survey conducted in the United Kingdom and Ireland revealed that 88% of the respondents used prophylactic antibiotic therapy in acute pancreatitis. Interestingly, 24% of them prescribe antibiotics to all patients with acute pancreatitis[62] which means that a considerable percentage of patients receive antibiotics in cases where no positive effect can be expected.

Risks and Problems of Antibiotic Prophylaxis

Given the fact that prophylactic antibiotic application seems to reduce the rate of severe complications of necrotizing pancreatitis and subsequently appears to improve survival, it remains a very controversial issue to discuss the presumptive risks and problems of this topic. Nevertheless, evidence exists that prolonged antibiotic treatment may lead to a change in the spectrum of bacteria of pancreatic infection with emergence of staphylococci and other gram positive bacteria. This so-called bacterial shift has been observed in patients undergoing imipenem treatment[63] and seems to be of considerable clinical importance. Most interestingly, infection with multi-resistant organisms or bacteria resistant to antibiotics used for prophylaxis has been shown to be a significant risk factor for a fatal outcome.[64]

An additional aspect in this regard is the increasing incidence of *Candida* infections in patients with infected necrosis; this organism is frequently associated with poor prognosis[65–68] although the relevance of this observation is not undoubted.[64] Whether there is a link between *Candida* infection and prior antibiotic treatment is another point of investigation. It is the authors' experience that *Candida* infection in necrotizing pancreatitis is a sequel of prolonged prior antibiotic treatment and associated with a high rate of fatalities (Fig. 34.1). In our series of patients with infected pancreatic necrosis we found that patients positive for *Candida* had longer episodes of prior antibiotic treatment than patients without *Candida*. This difference was observed regardless whether *Candida* was the primary microbial pathogen or whether it was found secondary to infection with other bacteria.[66]

Conclusions

In summary, there are some data indicating that patients suffering from necrotizing pancreatitis may benefit from the application of prophylactic antibiotics. Although this is a very tempting approach and (at the moment) the only drug application which seems to influence the course of the disease in a positive manner, one should not rush to hasty conclusions. Too many questions remain unanswered in this field and our clinical experience with this topic is limited.

From the authors' point of view, an adequately-powered, randomized double-blinded trial is necessary to provide more of the necessary information. Such a multicenter trial is on the way in Germany using Ciprofloxacin + Metronidazol *vs.* placebo, and first results are to be expected in the course of 2002.

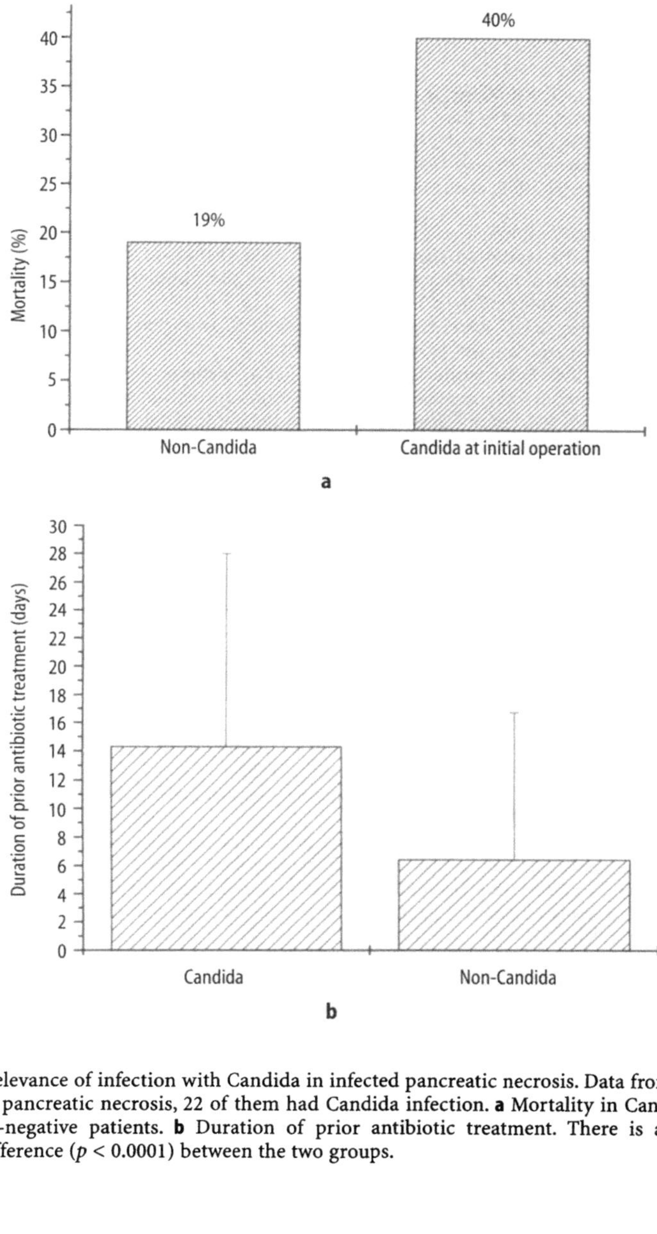

Figure 34.1. Relevance of infection with Candida in infected pancreatic necrosis. Data from 92 patients with infected pancreatic necrosis, 22 of them had Candida infection. **a** Mortality in Candida-positive and Candida-negative patients. **b** Duration of prior antibiotic treatment. There is a statistically significant difference ($p < 0.0001$) between the two groups.

References

1. Tsiotos GG, Luque-de Leon E, Sarr MG. Long-term outcome of necrotizing pancreatitis treated by necrosectomy. Br J Surg 1998; 85:1650–1653.
2. Fernandez Del-Castillo C, Rattner DW, Makary MA, et al. Debridement and closed packing for the treatment of necrotizing pancreatitis. Ann Surg 1998; 228:676–684.

3. Beger HG, Isenmann R. Surgical Management of Necrotizing Pancreatitis. Surg Clin North Am 1999; 79 (4):783–800.
4. Bradley ELI. A fifteen year experience with open drainage for infected pancreatic necrosis. Surg Gynecol Obstet 1993; 177:215–222.
5. Liu X-H, Kimura T, Ishikawa H, et al. Effects of Endothelin-1 on the Development of Hemorrhagic Pancreatitis in Rats. Scand J Gastroent 1995; 30:276–282.
6. Beger HG, Bittner R, Block S, et al. Bacterial Contamination of Pancreatic Necrosis – A Prospective Clinical Study. Gastroenterology 1986; 91:433–438.
7. Bassi C, Falconi M, Girelli R, et al. Microbiological findings in severe pancreatitis. Surg Res Comm 1989; 5:1–4.
8. Gerzof SG, Banks PA, Robbins AH, et al. Early Diagnosis of Pancreatic Infection by computed Tomography-Guided Aspiration. Gastroenterology 1987; 93:1315–1320.
9. Isenmann R, Beger HG. Role of Bacterial Translocation and Antibiotic Treatment in Necrotizing Pancreatitis. Pancreatology 2001; 1:79–89.
10. Widdison AL, Karanjia ND, Reber HA. Routes of spread of pathogens into the pancreas in a feline model of acute pancreatitis. Gut 1994; 35:1306–1310.
11. Foitzik T, Fernandez Del-Castillo C, Ferraro MJ, et al. Pathogenesis and Prevention of Early Pancreatic Infection in Experimental Acute Necrotizing Pancreatitis. Ann Surg 1995; 222:179–185.
12. Runkel NSF, Moody FG, Smith GS, et al. The role of the gut in the development of sepsis in acute pancreatitis. J Surg Res 1991; 51:18–23.
13. Isenmann R, Rau B, Beger HG. Bacterial infection and extent of necrosis are determinants of organ failure in patients with acute necrotizing pancreatitis. Br J Surg 1999; 86:1020–1024.
14. Rau B, Pralle U, Uhl W, et al. Management of Sterile Necrosis in Instances of severe acute Pancreatitis. J Am Coll Surg 1995; 181:279–288.
15. Büchler MW, Gloor B, Müller CA, et al. Acute necrotizing pancreatitis: Treatment strategy according to the status of infection. Ann Surg 2000; 232:619–626.
16. Bradley ELI, Allen K. A Prospective Longitudinal Study of Observation Versus Surgical Intervention in the Management of Necrotizing Pancreatitis. Am J Surg 1991; 161:19–25.
17. Tsiotos GG, Luque-de Leon E, Söreide JA, et al. Management of necrotizing pancreatitis by repeated operative necrosectomy using a zipper technique. Am J Surg 1998; 175:91–98.
18. Rau B, Pralle U, Mayer JM, et al. Role of ultrasonographically guided fine-needle aspiration cytology in the diagnosis of infected pancreatic necrosis. Br J Surg 1998; 85:179–184.
19. Paye F, Rotman N, Radier C, et al. Percutaneous aspiration for bacteriological studies in patients with necrotizing pancreatitis. Br J Surg 1998; 85:755–759.
20. Isenmann R, Büchler M, Uhl W, et al. Pancreatic necrosis: an early finding in severe acute pancreatitis. Pancreas 1993; 8:358–361.
21. Wilson C, Heads A, Shenkin A, et al. C-reactive protein, antiproteases and complement factors as objective markers of severity in acute pancreatitis. Br J Surg 1989; 76:177–181.
22. Büchler M, Malfertheiner P, Schoetensack C, et al. Sensitivity of antiproteases,complement factors and C-reactive protein in detecting pancreatic necrosis. Resúlts of a prospective clinical study. Int J Pancreatol 1986; 1:227–235.
23. Uhl W, Büchler M, Malfertheiner P, et al. PMN-Elastase in Comparison with CRP, Antiproteases and LDH as Indicators of Necrosis in Human Acute Pancreatitis. Pancreas 1991; 6 (3):253–259.
24. Rau B, Steinbach G, Gansauge F, et al. The potential role of procalcitonin and interleukin 8 in the prediction of infected necrosis in acute pancreatitis. Gut 1997; 41 (6):832–840.
25. Müller CA, Uhl W, Printzen G, et al. Role of procalcitonin and granulocyte colony stimulating factor in the early prediction of infected necrosis in severe acute pancreatitis. Gut 2000; 46:233–238.
26. Kylänpää-Bäck M-L, Takala A, Kemppainen E, et al. Procalcitonin, soluble interleukin-2 receptor, and soluble E-selectin in predicting the severity of acute pancreatitis. Crit Care Med 2001; 29:63–69.
27. Rünzi M, Layer P, Niebel W, et al. Konservative Therapie infizierter Nekrosen. Pancreas 1996; 13:455 (Abs.).
28. Cameron JL, Howes R, Zuidema GD. Antibiotic therapy in acute pancreatitis. Surg Clin North Am 1975; 55:1319–1324.
29. Bradley ELI. Antibiotics in Acute Pancreatitis. Current Status and Future Directions. Am J Surg 1989; 158:472–477.
30. Kim SL, Goldschmid S. Antibiotics in Acute Pancreatitis: The Debate Revisited. Am J Gastroenterol 1995; 90:666–667.
31. Kramer KM, Levy H. Prophylactic antibiotics for severe acute pancreatitis: The beginning of an era. Pharmacotherapy 1999; 19:592–602.

32. Powell JJ, Miles R, Siriwardena AK. Antibiotic prophylaxis in the initial management of severe acute pancreatitis. Br J Surg 1998; 85:582–587.
33. Büchler M, Malfertheiner P, Friess H, et al. Human Pancreatic Tissue Concentrations of Bactericidal Antibiotics. Gastroenterology 1992; 103:1902–1908.
34. Bassi C, Pederzoli P, Vesentini S, et al. Behaviour of Antibiotics during Human Necrotizing Pancreatitis. Antimicrob Agents Chemother 1994; 38 (4):830–836.
35. Roberts EA, Williams RJ. Ampicillin Concentrations in Pancreatic Fluid Bile Obtained at endoscopic Retrograde Cholangiopancreatography (ERCP). Scand J Gastroent 1979; 14:669–672.
36. Wallace JR, Cushing RD, Bawdon RE, et al. Assessment of Antimicrobial Penetrance into the pancreatic juice in humans. Surg Gynecol Obstet 1986; 162 (4):313–316.
37. Koch K, Drewelow B, Liebe S, et al. Die Pankreasgängigkeit von Antibiotika. Chirurg 1991; 62:317–322.
38. Pederzoli P, Bassi C, Vesentini S, et al. A Randomized Multicenter Clinical Trial of Antibiotic Prophylaxis of septic Complications in Acute Necrotizing Pancreatitis with Imipenem. Surg Gynecol Obstet 1993; 176:480–483.
39. Delcenserie R, Yzet T, Duccroix JP. Prophylactic Antibiotics in Treatment of Severe Acute Alcoholic Pancreatitis. Pancreas 1996; 13:198–201.
40. Bassi C, Falconi M, Talamini G, et al. Controlled clinical trial of pefloxacin versus imipenem in severe acute pancreatitis. Gastroenterology 1998; 115 (6):1513–1517.
41. Schwarz M, Isenmann R, Meyer H, et al. Antibiotika bei nekrotisierender Pankreatitis. Ergebnisse einer kontrollierten Studie. Dtsch med Wschr 1997; 122:356–361.
42. Sainio V, Kemppainen E, Puolakkainen P, et al. Early antibiotic treatment in acute necrotizing pancreatitis. Lancet 1995; 346:663–667.
43. Nordback I, Scand J, Saaristo R, et al. Early Treatment With Antibiotics Reduces the Need for Surgery in Acute Necrotizing Pancreatitis-A Single-Center Randomized Study. J Gastrointest Surg 2001; 5:113–120.
44. Luiten EJT, Hop WCJ, Lange JF, et al. Controlled Clinical Trial of Selective Decontamination for the Treatment of Severe Acute Pancreatitis. Ann Surg 1995; 222:57–65.
45. Glazer G, Mann D. United Kingdom guidelines for the management of acute pancreatitis. Gut 1998; 42 (Suppl 2):S1–S13.
46. Rünzi M, Layer P, Büchler MW, et al. Therapie der akuten Pankreatitis. Gemeinsame Leitlinien. Z Gastroenterol 2000; 38:571–580.
47. Banks PA. Practice guidelines in acute pancreatitis. Am J Gastroenterol 1997; 1997:377–382.
48. Golub R, Siddiqi F, Pohl D. Role of Antibiotics in Acute Pancreatitis: A Meta-Analysis. J Gastrointest Surg 1998; 2:496–502.
49. Sharma VK, Howden CW. Prophylactic antibiotic administration reduces sepsis and mortality in acute necrotizing pancreatitis: A meta-analysis. Pancreas 2001; 22:28–31.
50. Lange JF, van Gool J, Tytgat GNJ. The Protective Effect of a Reduction in Intestinal Flora on Mortality of Acute Haemorrhagic Pancreatitis in the Rat. Hepato-gastroenterol 1987; 34:28–30.
51. Widdison AL, Karanjia ND, Alvarez C, et al. Influence of Levamisole on Pancreatic Infection in Acute Pancreatitis. Am J Surg 1992; 163:100–104.
52. Isaji S, Suzuki M, Frey CF, et al. Role of Bacterial Infection in Diet-Induced Acute Pancreatitis in Mice. Int J Pancreatol 1992; 11:49–57.
53. Mithöfer K, Fernandez Del-Castillo C, Ferraro MJ, et al. Antibiotic Treatment Improves Survival in Experimental Acute Necrotizing Pancreatitis. Gastroenterology 1996; 110:232–240.
54. Warshaw AL. Pancreatic necrosis. To debride or not to debride – That is the question. Ann Surg 2000; 232:627–629.
55. Ramsay G, Van Saene HKF. Selective gut decontamination in intensive care and surgical practice: where are we? World J Surg 1998; 22:164–170.
56. Selective Decontamination of the Digestive Tract Trialists´ Collaborative Group. Meta-analysis of randomised controlled trials of selective decontamination of the digestive tract. Br Med J 1993; 307:525–532.
57. Stoutenbeek CP, Van Saene HKF, Miranda DR, et al. Nosocomial gram-negative pneumonie in critically ill patients. A 3-year experience with a novel therapeutic regimen. Intensive Care Med 1986; 419–423.
58. Van Saene HKF, Nunn AJ, Stoutenbeek CP. Selective decontamination of the digestive tract in intensive care patients. Br J Hosp Med 195; 54:558–561.
59. Marotta F, Geng TC, Wu CC, et al. Bacterial Translocation in the Course of Acute Pancreatitis: Beneficial Role of Nonabsorbable Antibiotics and Lactitol Enemas. Digestion 1996; 57:446–452.

60. Gianotti L, Munda R, Gennari R, et al. Effect of Different Regimens of Gut Decontamination on Bacterial Translocation and Mortality in Experimental Acute Pancreatitis. Eur J Surg 1995; 161:85–92.
61. McClelland P, Van Saene HKF, Murray A, et al. Prevention of bacterial infection and sepsis in acute severe pancreatitis. Ann Royal Surg Engl 1992; 74:329–334.
62. Powell JJ, Campbell E, Johnson CD, et al. Survey of antibiotic prophylaxix in acute pancreatitis in the UK and Ireland. Br J Surg 1999; 86:320–322.
63. Mai G, Gloor B, Uhl W, et al. Routine Antibiotic Prophylaxis in Necrotizing Pancreatitis Increased Gram-Positive Infections. Digestion 1999; 60:367.
64. Gloor B, Müller CA, Worni M, et al. Pancreatic infection in severe pancreatitis. The role of fungus and multiresistant organisms. Arch Surg 2001; 136:592–596.
65. Grewe M, Tsiotos GG, Luque-de Leon E, et al. Fungal infection in acute necrotizing pancreatitis. J Am Coll Surg 1999; 188:408–414.
66. Isenmann R, Schwarz M, Rau B, et al. Characteristics of infection with Candida species in patients with necrotizing pancreatitis. World J Surg 2001; in press.
67. Götzinger P, Wamser P, Barian M, et al. Candida infection of local necrosis in severe acute pancreatitis is associated with increased mortality. Shock 2000; 14:320–324.
68. Hoerauf A, Hammer ST, Müller-Myhsok B, et al. Intra-abdominal Candida infection during acute necrotizing pancreatitis has a high prevalance and is associated with increased mortality. Crit Care Med 1998; 26:2010–2015.
69. Dervenis C, Bassi C. Evidence-based assessment of severity and management of acute pancreatitis. Br J Surg 2000; 87:257–258.

Enteral Nutrition in Acute Pancreatitis

35 Enteral Nutrition in Acute Pancreatitis: Mucosal Barrier

Basil J. Ammori

The primary function of the intestinal mucosa is the digestion and absorption of nutrients. However, the mucosa also serves as an important mechanical barrier that helps to stop the bacteria within the lumen of the gut and their potentially harmful products such as endotoxin from gaining access to the deeper tissues and the blood stream. The gastrointestinal tract contains approximately 10^{12} total bacteria and 10^9 potentially pathogenic gram-negative 'enteric' bacteria, as well as potentially lethal amounts of endotoxin. The 'gut-barrier function' refers to the ability of the gastrointestinal tract to keep bacteria and endotoxin within its lumen, whilst allowing the absorption of nutrients.

Failure of the gut mucosal barrier has been implicated in the development of sepsis and multiple organ failure (MOF) in a wide spectrum of critical illnesses,[1-5] including severe acute pancreatitis.[6,7] Marshall and Meakins coined the terms 'undrained abscess'[4] and 'motor of MOF'[8] to describe the role of the gut in the pathogenesis.

The role of this chapter is to:

- Describe the clinical evidence that implicates the gut in the pathogenesis of severe attacks of acute pancreatitis
- Examine the available experimental evidence in man and in animals that demonstrates the derangement of the mucosal barrier in acute pancreatitis
- Discuss the underlying pathophysiological factors contributing to the derangement of the mucosal barrier
- Provide an overview of the potential avenues for preservation or restoration of the mucosal barrier, and discuss the role of enteral nutrition in detail.

The Role of the Gut in the Pathogenesis of Severe Acute Pancreatitis

There is convincing circumstantial clinical evidence that implicates the gut in the pathogenesis of severe attacks of acute pancreatitis in man.

Sepsis complicates approximately one-third of cases of necrotizing pancreatitis and accounts for the majority of late deaths in patients with severe acute pancreatitis [9-11]. Sepsis is usually associated with secondary infection of pancreatic or peripancreatic necrosis, which in the majority of patients is attributed to Gram-negative enteric organisms (Table 35.1).[9,12–16] This suggests a gastrointestinal origin, perhaps through 'bacterial translocation'; a process of migration of bacteria and bacterial fragments from the intestinal lumen to extraintestinal sites.[17] The possibility of translocation underscores a failure of gut-barrier function.

In a controlled clinical trial of selective digestive decontamination in patients with predicted severe acute pancreatitis,[18] intestinal colonization with Gram-negative bacteria preceded the development of pancreatic infections with micro-organisms of the same species, and significantly increased the risk of death.

However, limitations in investigation techniques due to technical and ethical reasons have so far limited our ability to prove the thesis of bacterial translocation in man. Indeed, using a polymerase chain reaction technique, Ammori and colleagues failed to detect the presence of bacterial nucleic acid in the peripheral blood of patients with severe acute pancreatitis.[19]

Derangement of the Mucosal Barrier in Acute Pancreatitis

However good evidence exists both in man and in animals to show that the gut mucosal barrier becomes deranged rather early in the course of acute pancreatitis.

Mucosal Barrier Dysfunction in Man

Two general methods have been used to assess the integrity of the gastrointestinal mucosal barrier in man: 1) A direct method that measures mucosal permeability to various hydrophilic compounds that may be divided into micromolecules (sugar probes such as lactulose) and micromolecules (such as polyethylene glycol 3350). 2) An indirect method that quantifies the extent of translocation of endotoxin, an important product of Gram-negative microorganisms that often originates from the gut,[20] and serves as a marker for the translocation of microbes

Studies that have evaluated the mucosal barrier function in patients with acute pancreatitis are scarce; their findings are summarised below:

Permeability probes. In a clinical study of 85 patients with acute pancreatitis, Ammori *et al*[21] demonstrated a significant increase in intestinal permeability to macromolecules (polyethylene glycol 3350) during severe attacks compared to patients with mild attacks and healthy controls. No change in intestinal permeability was evident in patients with mild acute pancreatitis. Changes in intestinal permeability occurred within 72 h of onset of severe disease and correlated strongly with clinical outcome, as permeability was significantly greater in patients who developed multiple organ failure (MOF) and/or died compared with the remainder of patients with severe disease.[21] The early changes in intestinal permeability predicted disease severity, development of sepsis, organ failure or death, and prolonged hospital stay (>10 days) as accurately as the Acute Physiology and Chronic Health Evaluation-II (APACHE-II)-scoring system and the peak values of serum C-reactive protein.[22]

In another clinical study of 23 patients with acute pancreatitis, Juvonen and colleagues[23] demonstrated significantly greater increases in intestinal permeability to micromolecules (sugar probes) in patients with severe attacks compared with mild attacks within 48 h of admission to hospital.

Table 35.1. Bacteria identified on cultures from infected pancreatic necrosis in humans

	Beger *et al.* [9]	Bittner *et al.* [12]	Fedorak *et al.* [13]	Bradley [14]	Farkas *et al.* [15]	Rau *et al.* [16]
No. of patients with ANP	114	152	N/A	N/A	N/A	286
Study period	1977–1982	1977–1984	1984–1991	1976–1993	1986–1993	1982–1995
Prophylactic antibiotics	No	No	N/A	N/A	No	N/A
No. of patients with infected ANP (%)	45 (40%)	56 (37%)	21	71	123	86 (30%)
Bacteriology: No. (%)						
E. coli	24 (53%)	(~50%)	5 (24%)	33 (46%)	16 (13%)	36 (44%)
Enterococcus species	16 (36%)	(~30%)	7 (33%)	14 (20%)	54 (44%)	23 (28%)
Pseudomonas aeruginosa	5 (11%)	(~10–20%)	3 (14%)	7 (10%)	46 (37%)	4 (5%)
Proteus species	5 (11%)	N/A	1 (5%)	N/A	N/A	3 (4%)
Klebsiella pneumoniae	3 (7%)	(~10–20%)	3 (14%)	10 (14%)	28 (23%)	13 (16%)
Anaerobes	5 (11%)	(8%)	2 (9%)	N/A	16 (13%)	7 (9%)
Streptococcus species	7 (16%)	N/A	3 (14%)	2 (3%)	43 (35%)	N/A
Staphylococcus species	5 (11%)	N/A	12 (57%)	1 (1%)	24 (20%)	12 (15%)
Candida species	3 (7%)	(5%)	4 (19%)	4 (6%)	21 (17%)	4 (5%)
Mortality (culture + vs. culture –)	37.8% vs. 8.7% 8.7%	32% vs. N/A	48% vs. N/A	14% vs. N/A	7% vs. N/A	N/A

ANP, acute necrotizing pancreatitis; N/A, not available

However, two other studies of intestinal permeability in patients with acute pancreatitis that employed the sugar probe lactulose found that intestinal permeability did not differ significantly between predicted severe and mild attacks.[24,25]

Endotoxin has been detected in the peripheral blood of a majority of patients with severe acute pancreatitis,[21,26,27] and at a significantly greater frequency[21,27] and larger magnitude[27] compared with mild attacks (Table 35.2).[21,26–29] Endotoxaemia has also been detected at a significantly greater frequency and concentration in non-survivors compared with survivors,[21,27] and in patients who developed MOF compared to those who did not.[21] Furthermore, a strong and significant correlation has been observed between the serum concentrations of endotoxin and the increases in intestinal permeability to macromolecules,[21] which attests to the gut origin of endotoxin. Other investigators, however, found no difference in the frequency of endotoxaemia between patients with predicted severe versus mild disease (Glasgow scores of ≥ 3).[26,29]

Antiendotoxin core antibodies bind to circulating endotoxin to form complexes that are subsequently eliminated from the circulation.[30] Unlike endotoxin, which is rather difficult to detect in blood due to its intermittent and transient appearance in the systemic circulation, antiendotoxin antibodies provide more stable evidence of systemic endotoxin exposure. Several investigators have shown that antiendotoxin antibodies become considerably depleted in patients with severe attacks of acute pancreatitis compared to mild,[21,29,31] which suggests a greater magnitude of systemic endotoxin translocation.

Mucosal Barrier Dysfunction in Animals

Unlike the situation in man, experimental studies in animal models of acute pancreatitis can provide direct evidence of bacterial, in addition to endotoxin, translocation across the mucosal barrier and provide clear evidence of gut barrier failure. Moreover, early changes in mucosal permeability can be clearly demonstrated. The evidence pertaining the animal studies is summarised below.

Bacterial translocation. Within hours of the induction of acute pancreatitis in animal models bacteria were detected in mesenteric lymph nodes and other extraintestinal sites such as the pancreas, liver, lungs and blood.[32–34] Several lines of evidence supported the thesis that these organisms originated from the gut. *Escherichia coli* was the most common organism isolated.[32–34] Using green fluorescent protein-transfected *E. coli* and intravital video microscopy, fluorescent bacteria were shown to translocate from the small bowel lumen into the pancreas[35] thus providing substantial experimental proof for the gut-origin-hypothesis of infectious complications in acute pancreatitis. In addition, the introduction of measures to reduce the colonic bacterial counts such as selective digestive decontamination,[36–39] colonic irrigation via a caecostomy[40] or retrograde enemas[41] significantly reduced bacterial translocation and reduced mortality in animal models of acute pancreatitis.

Permeability probes. In mice, Ryan *et al*[42] reported significant increases in intestinal permeability to macromolecules (polyethylene glycol 3350) within 24 h of induction of mild, moderate and severe acute pancreatitis, which correlated with disease severity.

Table 35.2. Endotoxaemia in patients with acute pancreatitis

Authors	Study population	No. of attacks (severe/mild)	No. of patients with endotoxaemia on admission		
			Severe	Mild	P value
Ammori *et al.* [21]	Acute pancreatitis	64 (22/42)	11	9	<0.02
Foulis *et al.* [26]	Acute pancreatitis	26 (8/18)	5	8	NS
Exley *et al.* [27]	Prognostically severe disease	38 (14/24)	12	7	0.002
Curley *et al.* [28]	Acute pancreatitis	29 (13/16)	2	2	NS
Windsor *et al.* [29]	Acute pancreatitis, non-consecutive series	33 (23/10)	10	3	NS

♣data represent median (interquartile range), ♠data represent mean (s.e.m.), N/A: data not available, NS: not significant

In another study, endotoxaemia was readily detected upon the induction of acute pancreatitis in animals, and was significantly reduced by colonic irrigation or the creation of caecostomy compared with controls.[40]

Pathogenesis of Gut-barrier Dysfunction

There are several important components to the physiological gut barrier (Table 35.3), and their derangement in acute pancreatitis is demonstrable in animals as well as in man. The pathophysiological factors that might lead to mucosal barrier dysfunction are listed in Table 35.4, and some of the most relevant factors are shown schematically in Figure 35.1.[43–47] We have recently reviewed this subject in a detail.[7] The role of nutritional factors affecting mucosal barrier functioning in man is as follows.

Intestinal abnormalities. Patients with acute necrotizing pancreatitis have an altered intestinal morphology and immunity with significant reduction in the height of villi and depletion of mucosal immune mast cells compared with healthy bowel.[48]

Disruption of the intestinal microbial ecology with significant increase in Gram-negative bacterial counts has been demonstrated in patients with acute pancreatitis.[18]

Of greater importance, perhaps, is the reduction in intestinal blood flow with mucosal ischaemia. Bonham *et al* demonstrated significantly lower gastric intramucosal pH within 48 h of admission in patients with predicted severe acute pancreatitis who required intensive care management compared with those who remained on the surgical ward, and in non-survivors compared with survivors.[49] Soong and colleagues reported significant correlations between intramucosal gastric pH and antiendotoxin antibodies.[31] These observations suggest intestinal ischaemia as an early event that contributes to the disruption of gut mucosal barrier and impacts the outcome of acute pancreatitis. Clinically overt intestinal ischaemia is known to occur in extreme cases and presents with colonic necrosis, fossilisation or stricture formation.[50,51] The pathophysiological factors that may contribute to mucosal ischaemia and reperfusion injury are listed in Table 35.5 [52–56].

Systemic immune modulators. Derangement of systemic immune function is known to occur in patients with acute pancreatitis. Significant alterations in lymphocyte surface marker antigen expression were demonstrated in man during the acute phase of severe attacks compared with mild attacks with reduced total

Table 35.3. Components of the gut-mucosal barrier

Local factors:
Immunological: Gut-associated lymphoid tissue, intra-epithelial lymphocytes, submucosal aggregates, Peyer's patches, mesenteric lymph nodes
Mechanical: Healthy enterocytes, tight junctions, cell turnover, normal intestinal motility
Chemical: Gastric acidity, salivary lysozyme, lactoferrin, mucus secretion, bile salts
Bacteriological: Aerobic and anaerobic micro-organisms
Systemic factors:
Circulatory lymphocytes
Hepatic Kupffer cells (gut-liver axis)

Table 35.4 Pathogenesis of gut barrier dysfunction

A. Local factors:
Disruption of mucosal epithelial integrity
Impaired mucosal immunity
Disruption of intestinal bacterial ecology
Mucosal ischaemia and reperfusion injury
B. Systemic factors:
Impaired systemic immunity
Systemic endotoxin exposure
Pro-inflammatory cytokines
Malnutrition and parenteral nutrition

T-lymphocyte (CD3), T-helper (CD4) and T-suppresser (CD8) cell numbers; abnormalities that were reversed during convalescence.[28,57] In contrast to mild attacks, severe pancreatitis is associated with impairment of systemic phagocytic function[58] with subsequent failure of systemic clearance of a_2 macroglobulin-protease complexes[59] as well as a decrease in delayed-type skin hypersensitivity.[60]

Endotoxin has also been shown to increase intestinal permeability and to promote bacterial translocation from the gastrointestinal tract. The intravenous administration of *E. coli* endotoxin to healthy humans resulted in a significant increase in intestinal permeability index (lactulose/mannitol urinary excretion ratio) within 2 h.[61]

In man, malnutrition impairs the gut-barrier function and increases mucosal permeability,[62] though it does not appear to induce villus atrophy.[63] In patients with severe acute pancreatitis, the associated hypermetabolic state may induce a

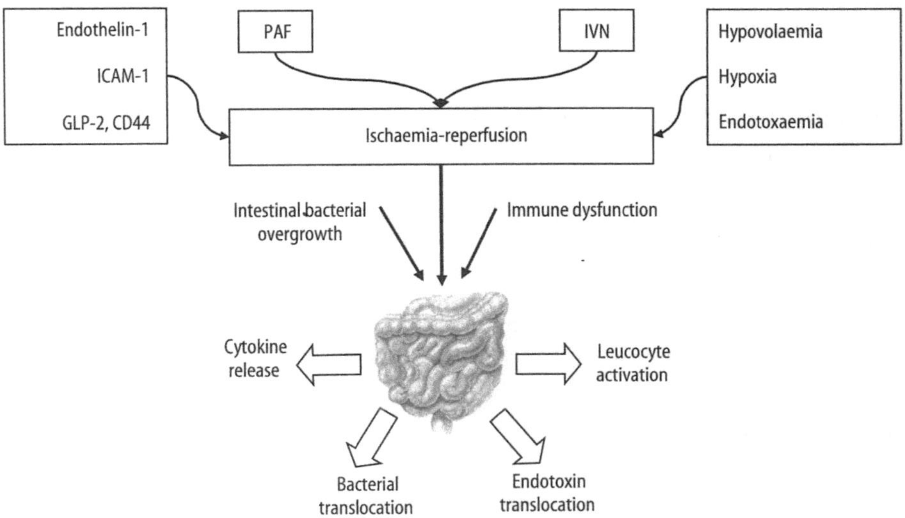

Figure 35.1. Diagram illustrating some of the important pathophysiological factors that promote mucosal barrier dysfunction. ICAM-1: inter-cellular adhesion molecule-1, GLP-2: glucagon-like peptide 2 [43,44], CD44: a trans-membrane glycoprotein involved in cell-cell and cell-matrix binding [45–47], PAF: platelet activating factor, IVN: intravenous nutrition

Table 35.5. Pathophysiological factors contributing to mucosal ischaemia and reperfusion injury in acute pancreatitis:

Systemic factors:
Hypovolaemia [52]
Hypoxia [53,54]
Systemic release of endothelin-1 [55]
Systemic release of intercellular adhesion molecule-1 (ICAM-1) [56]
Local factors:
Anatomical relationship between the superior mesenteric and middle colic arteries and the pancreas gland
Intra-abdominal hypertension and abdominal compartment syndrome

state of malnutrition[64] with its detrimental effects on intestinal mucosal morphology and function.

Although intravenous nutrition (IVN) is known to induce mucosal atrophy,[65] increase intestinal permeability,[65,66] impair mucosal immunity[67] and result in bacterial translocation in animals,[66,68] the deleterious impact of IVN on the mucosal barrier in man appears limited. Only a small decrease in intestinal villus height was observed after two weeks of IVN in man,[69] and more pronounced changes in intestinal mucosal morphology were observed only after a prolonged period (2–3 months) of IVN.[70] In patients with chronic pancreatitis, a greater extent of jejunal villous atrophy was observed in those parenterally fed compared to enterally nourished patients.[71] IVN, however, may impair systemic immunity, as healthy volunteers fed parenterally for 7 days had significantly lower levels of plasma C3a, lower absolute circulating neutrophil counts and reduced chemotaxis to leukotriene B4 compared with enterally fed controls.[72] The impact of IVN on mucosal morphological and functional integrity and systemic immunity in patients with acute pancreatitis in comparison with other forms of feeding has not been evaluated.

Measures to Preserve and/or Restore Gut Barrier Function

These may be divided into those that accept the thesis of translocation of endotoxin and bacteria across a defective intestinal barrier and respond by addressing these with systemic antibiotics or selective digestive decontamination, and measures that intend to restore the integrity of the mucosal barrier (Table 35.6).[24,73–90] We have reviewed these measures recently,[7] and concluded that enteral nutrition (EN) and in particular EN with immune-enhancing feeds (immunonutrition) is the most promising approach. The potential role of EN and enteral.

Enteral Nutrition

In animals, EN has been shown to preserve gastrointestinal mucosal mass,[91] reduce bacterial translocation,[92–94] and maintain systemic immune competence.[72] The jejunal administration of EN early in the course of experimental acute pancreatitis maintained immune responsiveness (CD4/CD8 ratio of T cells in spleen and peripheral blood) and gut mucosal integrity (mucosal thickness and villus height),

Table 35.6. Measures to counteract and restore the defective gut barrier

Measures to counteract gut barrier dysfunction:
Systemic antibiotics [73–76]
Selective digestive decontamination [77]
Probiotics [78]
Measures to restore gut barrier function:
Pharmacological manipulation:
Platelet activating factor antagonists [79]
Endothelin-1 receptor antagonism [80–82]
ICAM-1 monoclonal antibodies [83–85]
Probiotics [78]
Enteral nutrition [24,86–88]
Enteral immunonutrition [89,90]

and reduced bacterial and/or endotoxin translocation, though it did not improve outcome (mortality) compared with IVN.[94,95] Even when introduced at a low dose during IVN, EN proved beneficial and reduced bacterial translocation to mesenteric lymph nodes in an animal model.[93]

However, in a randomised controlled trial EN did not appear to have a beneficial effect on intestinal permeability after 3 days of administration in 13 patients with predicted severe attacks compared with conventional nil-by-mouth treatment in 14 patients.[24] The number of patients in this study, however, was small and the timing of the evaluation of outcome followed a rather short duration of feed delivery.

The clinical results of the randomised clinical trials of enteral nutrition in acute pancreatitis[24,86–88] are discussed in Chapter 37.

Enteral Immunonutrition

Enteral feeds with immune-enhancing ingredients such as glutamine, arginine, nucleotides and omega-3 fatty acids that modulate the host immune and inflammatory response have recently attracted considerable interest.[96] In severe rodent pancreatitis, supplementation of enteral feed with glutamine–an essential fuel for intestinal epithelial cells- improved colonic capillary blood flow, stabilized gut permeability, and reduced the numbers of secondary pancreatic infections and mortality rate.[89]

Perioperative immunonutrition in patients with intra-abdominal malignancies[90] and head and neck cancers[97] ameliorated the pro-inflammatory cytokine response and enhanced cell-mediated systemic immunity. When randomly compared with conventional enteral nutrition, enteral immunonutrition was associated with a significant reduction in bacteraemia, nasocomial infection and mortality rates of septic patients on the intensive care unit,[98] as well as requirements for ventilatory and intensive therapy and new organ failures in patients with adult respiratory distress syndrome.[99] However, conflicting evidence on the effect of enteral immunonutrition also exists that calls for caution in its administration in critically-ill patients.[96] The potential role of enteral immunonutrition in patients with predicted severe acute pancreatitis and its effect on mucosal barrier function are currently warrant future careful evaluation and study.

References

1. Carrico CJ, Meakins JL, Marshall JC, et al. Multiple-organ-failure syndrome. Arch Surg 1986; 121:196–208.
2. Border JR, Hassett J, LaDuca J, et al. Gut origin septic states in blunt trauma (ISS = 40) in the ICU. Ann Surg 1987; 206:427–445.
3. Deitch EA. Multiple organ failure. Pathophysiology and potential future therapy. Ann Surg 1992; 216:117–134.
4. Marshall JC, Christou NV, Meakins JL. The gastrointestinal tract. The 'undrained abscess' of multiple organ failure. Ann Surg 1993; 218:111–119.
5. Swank GM, Deitch EA. Role of the gut in multiple organ failure: Bacterial translocation and permeability changes. World J Surg 1996; 20:411–417.
6. Ammori BJ. Gut barrier dysfunction in patients with acute pancreatitis. J Hepatobiliary Pancreat Surg 2002; 9:411–412.
7. Ammori BJ. The role of the gut in the course of severe acute pancreatitis. Pancreas (in press).
8. Meakins JL, Marshall JC. The gastrointestinal tract: the "motor" of multiple organ failure. Arch Surg 1986; 121:197.
9. Beger HG, Bittner R, Block S, et al. Bacterial contamination of pancreatic necrosis - a prospective clinical study. Gastroenterology 1986; 91:433–438.
10. Bradley EL III, Allen K. A prospective longitudinal study of observation versus surgical intervention in the management of necrotizing pancreatitis. Am J Surg 1991; 161:19–24.
11. Gloor B, Muller CA, Worni M, et al. Pancreatic infection in severe pancreatitis: the role of fungus and multiresistant organisms. Arch Surg 2001; 136:592–596.
12. Bittner R, Block S, Buchler M, et al. Pancreatic abscess and infected pancreatic necrosis. Different local septic complications in acute pancreatitis. Dig Dis Sci 1987; 32:1082–1087.
13. Fedorak IJ, Ko TC, Djuricin G, et al. Secondary pancreatic infection: Are they distinct clinical entities? Surgery 1992; 112:824–831.
14. Bradley EL. A fifteen year experience with open drainage for infected pancreatic necrosis. Surg Gynecol Obstet 1993; 177:215–222.
15. Farkas G, Márton J, Mándi Y, et al. Surgical strategy and management of infected pancreatic necrosis. Br J Surg 1996; 83:930–933.
16. Rau B, Uhl W, Buchler MW, et al. Surgical treatment of infected necrosis. World J Surg 1997; 21:155–161.
17. Wolochow H, Hilderbrand GJ, Lamanna C. Translocation of microorganisms across the intestinal wall in rats: effect of microbial size and concentration. J Infect Dis 1966; 116:523–528.
18. Luiten EJ, Hop WC, Endtz HP, et al. Prognostic importance of gram-negative intestinal colonization preceding pancreatic infection in severe acute pancreatitis. Results of a controlled clinical trial of selective decontamination. Intensive Care Med 1998; 24:438–445.
19. Ammori BJ, Fitzgerald P, Hawkey P, et al. The early increase in intestinal permeability and systemic endotoxin exposure in patients with severe acute pancreatitis is not associated with systemic bacterial translocation: molecular investigation of microbial DNA in the blood. Pancreas 2003; 26:18–22.
20. Deitch EA, Xu D, Berg RD. Bacterial translocation from the gut impairs systemic immunity. Surgery 1991; 109:269–276.
21. Ammori BJ, Leeder PC, King RFGJ, et al. Early increase in intestinal permeability in patients with severe acute pancreatitis: correlation with endotoxemia, organ failure, and mortality. J Gastrointest Surg 1999; 3:252–262.
22. Ammori BJ. Importance of the early increase in intestinal permeability in critically ill patients. Eur J Surg (in press).
23. Juvonen PO, Alhava EM, Takala JA. Gut permeability in patients with acute pancreatitis. Scand J Gastroenterol 2000; 35:1314–1318.
24. Powell JJ, Murchison JT, Fearon KC, et al. Randomized controlled trial of the effect of early enteral nutrition on markers of the inflammatory response in predicted severe acute pancreatitis. Br J Surg 2000; 87:1375–1381.
25. McNaught CE, Woodcock NP, Mitchell CJ, et al. Gastric colonisation, intestinal permeability and septic morbidity in acute pancreatitis. Pancreatology 2002; 2:463–468.
26. Foulis AK, Murray WR, Galloway D, et al. Endotoxaemia and complement activation in acute pancreatitis in man. Gut 1982; 23:656–661.
27. Exley AR, Leese T, Holliday MP, et al. Endotoxaemia and serum tumour necrosis factor as prognostic markers in severe acute pancreatitis. Gut 1992; 33:1126–1128.

28. Curley PJ, McMahon MJ, Lancaster F, et al. Reduction in circulating levels of CD4-positive lymphocytes in acute pancreatitis: relationship to endotoxin, interleukin 6 and disease severity. Br J Surg 1993; 80:1312–1315.
29. Windsor JA, Fearon KC, Ross JA, et al. The role of serum endotoxin and antiendotoxin core antibody levels in predicting the development of multiple organ failure in acute pancreatitis. Br J Surg 1993; 80:1042–1046.
30. Barclay GR, Scott BB, Wright IH, et al. Changes in anti-endotoxin IgG antibody and endotoxaemia in three cases of Gram-negative septic shock. Circ Shock 1989; 29:93–106.
31. Soong CV, Lewis HG, Halliday MI, et al. Intramucosal acidosis and the inflammatory response in acute pancreatitis. Am J Gastroenterol 1999; 94:2423–2429.
32. Runkel NS, Moody FG, Smith GS, et al. The role of the gut in the development of sepsis in acute pancreatitis. J Surg Res 1991; 51:18–23.
33. Gianotti L, Munda R, Alexander JW. Pancreatitis-induced microbial translocation: a study of the mechanisms. Res Surg 1992; 4:87–91.
34. Tarpila E, Nystrom P-O, Franzen L, et al. Bacterial translocation during acute pancreatitis in rats. Eur J Surg 1993; 159:109–113.
35. Samel S, Lanig S, Lux A, et al. The gut origin of bacterial pancreatic infection during acute experimental pancreatitis in rats. Pancreatology 2002; 2:449–455.
36. Lange JF, van Gool J, Tytgat GN. The protective effect of a reduction in intestinal flora on mortality of acute haemorrhagic pancreatitis in the rat. Hepatogastroenterology 1987; 34:28–30.
37. Isaji S, Suzuki M, Frey CF, et al. Role of bacterial infection in diet-induced acute pancreatitis in mice. Int J Pancreatol 1992; 11:49–57.
38. Foitzik T, Fernandez-del Castillo C, Ferraro MJ, et al. Pathogenesis and prevention of early pancreatic infection in experimental acute necrotizing pancreatitis. Ann Surg 1995; 222:179–185.
39. Gianotti L, Munda R, Gennai R, et al. Effect of different regimens of gut decontamination on bacterial translocation and mortality in experimental acute pancreatitis. Eur J Surg 1995; 161:85–92.
40. Sulkowski U, Boin C, Brockmann J, et al. The influence of caecostomy and colonic irrigation on the pathophysiology and prognosis in acute experimental pancreatitis. Eur J Surg 1993; 159:287–291.
41. Marotta F, Geng TC, Wu CC, et al. Bacterial translocation in the course of acute pancreatitis: beneficial role of nonabsorbable antibiotics and lactitol enemas. Digestion 1996; 57:446–452.
42. Ryan CM, Schmidt J, Lewandrowski K, et al. Gut macromolecular permeability in pancreatitis correlates with severity of disease in rats. Gastroenterology 1993; 104:890–895.
43. Benjamin MA, McKay DM, Yang PC, et al. Glucagon-like peptide-2 enhances intestinal epithelial barrier function of both transcellular and paracellular pathways in the mouse. Gut 2000; 47:112–119.
44. Kouris GJ, Liu Q, Rossi H, et al. The effect of glucagon-like peptide 2 on intestinal permeability and bacterial translocation in acute necrotizing pancreatitis. Am J Surg 2001; 181:571–575.
45. Alho AM, Underhill CB. The hyaluronan receptor is preferentially expressed on proliferating epithelial cells. J Cell Biol 1989; 108:1557–1565.
46. Heel K, Blennerhassett L, Kong A-E, et al. Br J Surg 1998; 85:1086–1089.
47. Nagahama S, Korenaga D, Honda M, et al. Assessment of the intestinal permeability after a gastrectomy and the oral administration of anticancer drugs in rats: Nitric oxide release in response to gut injury. Surgery 2002; 131:S92–S97.
48. Ammori BJ, Cairns A, Dixon MF, et al. Altered intestinal morphology and immunity in patients with acute necrotizing pancreatitis. J Hepatobiliary Pancreat Surg 2002; 9:490–496.
49. Bonham MJD, Abu-Zidan FM, Simovic MO, et al. Gastric intramucosal pH predicts death in severe acute pancreatitis. Br J Surg 1997; 84:1670–1674.
50. Grodsinsky C, Ponka JL. The spectrum of colonic involvement in pancreatitis. Dis Colon Rectum 1978; 21:66–70.
51. Chaikhouni A, Regueyra FI, Stevens JR, et al. Colonic fistulization in pancreatitis: case report and literature review. Dis Colon Rectum 1980; 23:271–275.
52. Fiddian-Green RG. Studies in splanchnic ischemia and multiple organ failure. In: Marston A, Bukley GB, Fiddian-Green RG, et al. (eds). Splanchnic Ischemia and Multiple Organ Failure. London: Edward Arnold, 1989; pp. 349–363.
53. Ranson JHC, Roses DF, Fink SD. Early respiratory insufficiency in acute pancreatitis. Ann Surg 1972; 178:75–79.
54. Imrie CW, Ferguson JC, Murphy D, et al. Arterial hypoxia in acute pancreatitis. Br J Surg 1977; 64:185–188.
55. Eibl G, Hotz HG, Faulhaber J, et al. Effect of endothelin and endothelin receptor blockade on capillary permeability in experimental pancreatitis. Gut 2000; 46:390–394.

56. Kaufmann P, Tilz GP, Smolle KH, et al. Increased plasma concentrations of circulating intercellular adhesion molecule-1 (cICAM-1) in patients with necrotizing pancreatitis. Immunobiology 1996; 195:209–219.
57. Curley P, Nestor M, Collins K, et al. Decreased interleukin-2 production in murine acute pancreatitis: potential for immunomodulation. Gastroenterology 1996; 110:583–588.
58. Larvin M, Alexander DJ, Switala SF, et al. Impaired mononuclear phagocyte function in patients with severe acute pancreatitis; evidence from studies of plasma clearance of trypsin and monocyte phagocytosis. Dig Dis Sci 1993; 38:18–27.
59. Banks RE, Evans SW, Alexander D, et al. $Alpha_2$ macroglobulin state in acute pancreatitis. Raised values of a_2 macroglobulin-protease complexes in severe and mild attacks. Gut 1991; 32:430–434.
60. Garcia-Sabrido JL, Valdecantos E, Bastida E, et al. The anergic state as a predictor of pancreatic sepsis. Zentrabl Chir 1989; 114:114–120.
61. O'Dwyer ST, Michie HR, Ziegler TR, et al. A single dose of endotoxin increases intestinal permeability in healthy humans. Arch Surg 1988; 123:1459–1464.
62. Heyman M, Boudraa G, Sarrut S, et al. Macromolecular transport in jejunal mucosa of children with severe malnutrition: a quantitative study. J Pediatr Gastroenterol Nutr 1984; 3:357–633.
63. Reynolds JV, O'Farrelly C, Feighery C, et al. Impaired gut barrier function in malnourished patients. Br J Surg 1996; 83:1288–1291.
64. Sitzmann JV, Steinborn PA, Zinner MJ, et al. Total parenteral nutrition and alternate energy substrates in treatment of severe acute pancreatitis. Surg Gynecol Obstet 1989; 168:311–317.
65. Li J, Langkamp-Henken B, Suzuki K, et al. Glutamine prevents parenteral nutrition-induced increases in intestinal permeability. JPEN 1994; 18:303–307.
66. Illig KA, Ryan CK, Hardy DJ, et al. Total parenteral nutrition-induced changes in gut mucosal function: atrophy alone is not the issue. Surgery 1992; 112:631–637.
67. Alverdy J, Chi HS, Sheldon GF. The effect of parenteral nutrition on gastrointestinal immunity. Ann Surg 1985; 202:681–684.
68. Alverdy JC, Aoys E, Moss GS. Total parenteral nutrition promotes bacterial translocation from the gut. Surgery 1988; 104:185–190.
69. van der Hulst RR, van Kreel BK, von Meyenfeldt MF, et al. Glutamine and the preservation of gut integrity. Lancet 1993; 341:1363–1365.
70. Pironi L, Paganelli GM, Miglioli M, et al. Morphologic and cytoproliferative patterns of duodenal mucosa in two patients after long-term total parenteral nutrition: changes with oral refeeding and relation to intestinal resection. JPEN 1994; 18:351–354.
71. Groos S, Hunefeld G, Luciano L. Parenteral versus enteral nutrition: morphological changes in human adult intestinal mucosa. J Submicro Cytol Pathol 1996; 28:61–74.
72. Meyer J, Yurt RW, Duhaney R. Differential neutrophil activation before and after endotoxin infusion in enterally versus parenterally fed volunteers. Surg Gynecol Obstet 1988; 167:501–509.
73. Pederzoli P, Bassi C, Vesentini S, et al. A randomized multicenter clinical trial of antibiotic prophylaxis of septic complications in acute necrotizing pancreatitis with imipenem. Surg Gynecol Obstet 1993; 176:480–483.
74. Sainio V, Kemppaainen E, Puolakkainen P, et al. Early antibiotic treatment in acute necrotising pancreatitis. Lancet 1995; 346:663–667.
75. Delcenserie R, Yzet T, Ducroix JP. Prophylactic antibiotics in treatment of severe acute alcoholic pancreatitis. Pancreas 1996; 13:198–201.
76. Schwarz M, Isenmann R, Meyer H, et al. Antibiotic use in necrotizing pancreatitis. Results of a controlled study. Dtsch Med Wochenschr 1997; 122:356–361.
77. Luiten EJT, Hop WCJ, Lange JF, et al. Controlled clinical trial of selective decontamination for the treatment of severe acute pancreatitis. Ann Surg 1995; 222:57–65.
78. Mangiante G, Canepari P, Colucci G, et al. A probiotic as an antagonist of bacterial translocation in experimental pancreatitis. Chir Ital 1999; 51:221–226.
79. Andersson R, Wang X, Sun Z, et al. Effect of a platelet-activating factor antagonist on pancreatitis-associated gut barrier dysfunction in rats. Pancreas 1998; 17:107–119.
80. Foitzik T, Eibl G, Hotz HG, et al. Endothelin receptor blockade in severe acute pancreatitis leads to systemic enhancement of microcirculation, stabilization of capillary permeability, and improved survival rates. Surgery 2000; 128:399–407.
81. Eibl G, Hotz HG, Faulhaber J, et al. Effect of endothelin and endothelin receptor blockade on capillary permeability in experimental pancreatitis. Gut 2000; 46:390–394.
82. Foitzik T, Faulhaber J, Hotz HG, et al. Endothelin mediates local and systemic disease sequelae in severe experimental pancreatitis. Pancreas 2001; 22:248–254.
83. Werner J, Z'graggen K, Fernandez-del Castillo C, et al. Specific therapy for local and systemic complications of acute pancreatitis with monoclonal antibodies against ICAM-1. Ann Surg 1999; 229:834–840.

84. Foitzik T, Eibl G, Buhr HJ. Therapy for microcirculatory disorders in severe acute pancreatitis: comparison of delayed therapy with ICAM-1 antibodies and a specific endothelin A receptor antagonist. J Gastrointest Surg 2000; 4:240–246.
85. Inoue S, Nakao A, Kishimoto W, et al. LFA-1 (CD11a/CD18) and ICAM-1 (CD54) antibodies attenuate superoxide anion release from polymorphonuclear leukocytes in rats with experimental acute pancreatitis. Pancreas 1996; 12:183–188.
86. McClave SA, Greene LM, Snider HL, et al. Comparison of the safety of early enteral vs parenteral nutrition in mild acute pancreatitis. JPEN 1997; 21:14–20.
87. Windsor ACJ, Kanwar S, Li AGK, et al. Compared with parenteral nutrition, enteral feeding attenuates the acute phase response and improves disease severity in acute pancreatitis. Gut 1998; 42:431–435.
88. Kalfarentzos F, Kehagias J, Mead N, et al. Enteral nutrition is superior to parenteral nutrition in severe acute pancreatitis: results of a randomized prospective trial. Br J Surg 1997; 84:1665–1669.
89. Foitzik T, Kruschewski M, Kroesen AJ, et al. Does glutamine reduce bacterial translocation? A study in two animal models with impaired gut barrier. Int J Colorectal Dis 1999; 14:143–149.
90. Gianotti L, Braga M, Fortis C, et al. A prospective, randomized clinical trial on perioperative feeding with an arginine-, omega-3 fatty acid-, and RNA-enriched enteral diet: effect on host response and nutritional status. JPEN 1999; 23:314–20.
91. Levine GN, Derin JJ, Steiger E, et al. Role of oral intake and maintainence of gut mass and disaccharide activity. Gastroenterology 1974; 67:975–982.
92. Saito H, Trocki O, Alexander JW, et al. The effect of route of nutrient administration on the nutritional state, catabolic hormone secretion, and gut mucosal integrity after burn injury. JPEN 1987; 11:1–7.
93. Sax HC, Illig KA, Ryan CK, et al. Low-dose enteral feeding is beneficial during total parenteral nutrition. Am J Surg 1996; 171:587–590.
94. Qin H, Su Z, Hu L, et al. Effect of early intrajejunal nutrition on pancreatic pathological features and gut barrier function in dogs with acute pancreatitis. Clin Nutr 2002; 21:469–473.
95. Kotani J, Usami M, Nomura H, et al. Enteral nutrition prevents bacterial translocation but does not improve survival during acute pancreatitis. Arch Surg 1999; 134:287–292.
96. Suchner U, Kuhn KS, Furst P. The scientific basis of immunonutrition. Proc Nutr Soc 2000; 59:553–563.
97. Riso S, Aluffi P, Brugnani M, et al. Postoperative enteral immunonutrition in head and neck cancer patients. Clin Nutr 2000; 19:407–412.
98. Galban C, Montejo JC, Mesejo A, et al. An immune-enhancing enteral diet reduces mortality rate and episodes of bacteremia in septic intensive care unit patients. Crit Care Med 2000; 28:643–648.
99. Gadek JE, DeMichele SJ, Karlstad MD, et al. Effect of enteral feeding with eicosapentaenoic acid, gamma-linolenic acid, and antioxidants in patients with acute respiratory distress syndrome. Enteral Nutrition in ARDS Study Group. Crit Care Med 1999; 27:1409–1420.

36 Early Enteral Nutrition and Markers of the Inflammatory Response in Severe Acute Pancreatitis

James Powell and Ajith Siriwardena

Until recently conventional management of acute pancreatitis included an initial period of fasting in an attempt to reduce the systemic effects of acute pancreatitis. This management strategy was adopted because it was believed that the systemic effects of acute pancreatitis were a consequence of the circulation of activated pancreatic enzymes; therefore a 'nil-by-mouth' regime was thought to limit pancreatic stimulation, thereby leading to reduced pancreatic enzyme secretion. However, it is now thought that following the initial pancreatic acinar cell injury, disease extension is the result of a systemic inflammatory response involving a complex interaction between leukocytes, vascular endothelium and the effects of both of pro and anti-inflammatory cytokines.[1–3] Although it is still thought that aberrant pancreatic exocrine secretion initiates acute pancreatitis, the maintenance of the systemic inflammatory response is thought to be independent of further pancreatic exocrine secretion. Consequently, manoeuvres directed at reducing pancreatic exocrine secretion following onset of acute pancreatitis are not likely to be associated with improvements in disease outcome. Therefore, fasting in acute pancreatitis may not have the desired effect of reducing disease severity. In fact, evidence derived from the study of other conditions in which the systemic inflammatory response mediates outcome has suggested that loss of enteral nutrition may be detrimental to outcome.[4–7] Given this, an initial randomised controlled trial was undertaken which demonstrated that the provision of enteral nutrition in patients with mild/moderate acute pancreatitis was both feasible and safe.[8] Subsequently, three further randomised controlled trials have been published which have evaluated the efficacy and benefits of early enteral nutrition in patients with severe acute pancreatitis.[9–11] The findings of these three studies are the focus of this chapter.

Direct Comparison of Trials

Trial Design

In order to allocate appropriate weighting to the findings of the studies derived from Patras,[9] Leeds[10] and Edinburgh,[11] an appreciation of the variations between the studies in terms of trial design and execution is helpful. Table 36.1 demon-

Table 36.1. Study design of three recent randomised controlled trials of early enteral nutrition in predicted severe acute pancreatitis

	Patras[9]	Leeds[10]	Edinburgh[11]
Inclusion criteria	<48 h from admission; Glasgow ≥3 + APACHE ≥8.	< 48 h from admission; Glasgow ≥3.	<72 h disease onset; Glasgow ≥3 and/or APACHE II ≥7.
Groups	EN vs TPN	EN vs TPN	EN vs No supplemen tal feeding
Enteral nutrition	Reabilan® HN (Roussel) 1 litre contains 58 g protein, 52 g fat, 158 g carbohydrate providing 5583 kJ	Osmolite® (Abbott) 1 litre contains 40 g protein, 34 g fat, 136 g carbohydrate providing 4240 kJ	Jevity® (Abbott) 1 litre contains 40 g protein, 35 g fat, 148 g carbohydrate, 11g dietary fibre providing 4410 kJ
Rate of feeding	Started at 25 ml/h and increased by 25 ml/h every 4 h until target.	Started at 30 ml/h and increased until target.	Started at 25 ml/h and increased by 25 ml/h daily until target.
Parenteral nutrition	Kabi regimen 1 providing 9.4g N & 7.52 non-protein mJ in 2500 ml/24 h.	Kabi regimen 1 providing 9.4g N & 7.52 non-protein mJ in 2500ml/24 h.	Nil standard
Route of feeding	Nasojejunal	Nasojejunal	Nasojejunal
Method of tube placement	Radiological	Radiological	Radiological
Planned duration of study	Until discharge from ITU	Artificial nutritional support until day 7	Until introduction of normal diet or day 10 whichever is first
Outcome measure	Morbidity and mortality	Modulation of the inflammatory response	Modulation of the inflammatory response

strates the characteristics of each of these studies, while Table 36.2 outlines the patient demographics.

Trial Outcome

Table 36.3 outlines the principal results of the three studies.

Discussion

Of the three published trials, the studies from Leeds and Edinburgh are comparable. In these two trials the outcome measures established allowed evaluation of the effects of enteral nutrition on the inflammatory response in acute pancreatitis. In contrast, with its study design and longer follow up, the trial from Patras provides important insights into the benefits of enteral nutrition upon morbidity and mortality. It should also be noted that in contrast to the Edinburgh and Leeds trials which included a group of patients with end-of-episode mild acute pancreatitis the trial from Patras only recruited patients with severe acute pancreatitis.

Table 36.2. Patient characteristics in three recent randomised controlled trials of early enteral nutrition in predicted severe acute pancreatitis. Results are expressed as either median or mean depending on the method of reporting for each study

	Patras[9] Enteral	Control	Leeds[10] Enteral	Control	Edinburgh[11] Enteral	Control
Number of patients	18	20	16	18	13	14
Sex of patients	8M : 10F	7M : 13F	7m : 9F	7m : 11F	5M:8F	9M:5F
Age	Mean 63	Mean 63	Median 63	Median 63	Median 64	Median 52
Duration of symptoms (hours)	Mean 41	Mean 43	–	–	Median 31	Median 27
Aetiology						
Gallstone	14	16	9	14	7	3
Alcohol	3	2	2	2	4	7
Other	1	2	5	2	2	4
Glasgow score	Mean 4	Mean 5	Median 2	Median 2	Median 4	Median 4
Admission APACHE II score	Mean 12.7	Mean 11.8	Median 8	Median 10	Median 10	Median 12
Serum C-reactive protein (mg/l)	Mean 290	Mean 335	Median 156	Median 125	Median 144	Median 212
End of episode severe as defined by Atlanta	18	20	6	7	7	9
Days in study/artificial nutritional support	Mean 35	Mean 33	7	7	Median 5	Median 6

The studies from Leeds and Edinburgh provide conflicting results as to the efficacy of enteral nutrition in modulating the inflammatory response in acute pancreatitis. The results from Leeds suggested that the provision of enteral nutrition ameliorated the inflammatory response and may have reduced intestinal bacterial translocation. In contrast, the results from Edinburgh suggested that the provision of enteral nutrition has no effect on markers of the inflammatory response or on organ dysfunction, and may have had a deleterious effect on intestinal function. The differences in the reported results between the two studies may arise for several reasons.

Firstly and perhaps most importantly in the Edinburgh study a median of $1.8\,J \times 10^6$/day was delivered constituting a median of 21% of daily calorific requirement. In contrast, approximately 65% of non-protein calories were delivered over the study period during the Leeds trial. The difference in the provision of enteral nutrition between the two groups may be partly explained by the high rate of tube dislodgement in the Edinburgh trial and differences in the rate at which feeding was increased up to the calculated target, but differences in the disease severity of patients in the two studies may also have been a factor. The patient population in the Leeds study had lower serum C-reactive protein concentrations and multiple factor prognostic scores than patients included in the Edinburgh study. The greater number of patients in the Leeds study with mild acute pancreatitis suggests that the majority of patients had minimal ileus and therefore maximal rates of feeding could be achieved without difficulty. In a popu-

Table 36.3. Main study results in three recent randomised controlled trials of early enteral nutrition in predicted severe acute pancreatitis

	Main study results
Patras[9]	Significant reduction in total complications following the introduction of enteral nutrition
	Significant reduction in septic complications following the introduction of enteral nutrition
	Reduction in expenditure with the use of enteral nutrition
Leeds[10]	Significant reduction in serum CRP concentrations at day 7 when compared to admission following introduction of enteral nutrition
	Significant reduction in APACHE II score at day 7 when compared to admission following introduction of enteral nutrition
	Reduction in incidence of the systemic inflammatory response following introduction of enteral nutrition
	Significant rise in serum IgM anti-endotoxin core antibody at day 7 when compared to admission following introduction of parenteral nutrition
	Significant fall in anti-oxidant capacity at day 7 when compared to admission following introduction of enteral nutrition
Edinburgh[11]	Introduction of enteral nutrition did not affect the inflammatory response
	Introduction of enteral nutrition did not affect organ dysfunction
	Significant deterioration in intestinal permeability on day 4 when compared to admission following the introduction of enteral nutrition

lation of patients with more severe disease, ileus is an appreciable problem, indeed in the Edinburgh trial feed volumes had to be limited because of intestinal ileus in almost 25% of patients. With this in mind it is interesting to note that in the initial trial of enteral nutrition in acute pancreatitis, although 71% of nutritional requirements were delivered during the total study period, only 30% of nutritional requirements could be provided during the first four study days.[8] However, although ileus would appear to be a significant problem during the first few days of an episode of acute pancreatitis, the trial from Patras would suggest that it is possible to establish effective enteral nutrition in the majority of patients with severe acute pancreatitis. Over a period of 35 days, 74% of calorific requirements were delivered through enteral nutrition; unfortunately from the results reported it is not possible to determine what quantity could be delivered in the first few days.

It is not clear whether delivery of full caloric requirements by enteral nutrition is required to obtain benefit. It has been postulated that so-called minimal enteral nutrition is able to provide enough luminal nutrition to maintain intestinal function thereby limiting the effects mediated by the intestinal tract in the systemic inflammatory response syndrome. Experimental studies have demonstrated that minimal enteral nutrition maintains intestinal mass but does not necessarily affect intestinal tract immune function.[12,13] However, the addition of minimal enteral nutrition to parenteral nutrition in neonates requiring surgery is associated with an improvement in systemic immune function.[14] The results of the Edinburgh trial in which only 21% of nutritional requirements were met suggests that minimal enteral nutrition does not modify the inflammatory response in patients with acute pancreatitis.

Another major difference between the Edinburgh and Leeds trials is the use of parenteral nutrition.[15–17] In line with published guidelines, patients in the Edinburgh study did not receive parenteral nutrition from admission. In contrast, patients in the parenteral nutrition group in the Leeds trial received nutritional support from admission. Parenteral nutrition was therefore given to patients with mild disease, a group of patients that do not require routine artificial nutritional supplementation. More significantly however, in the Leeds trial a nil-by-mouth regime was maintained in the group receiving parenteral nutrition until the seventh study day irrespective of the clinical condition, therefore a group of patients remained fasted despite clinical resolution of the disease. The delivery of parenteral nutrition to patients with mild disease and abstinence until the seventh day may account for the some of the observed differences between the Leeds and Edinburgh trials. Fong and colleagues[18] have demonstrated that bowel rest and the institution of parenteral nutrition in normal volunteers is associated with an increased inflammatory response following a stimulus, whilst Welsh and colleagues[19] have reported that malnourished patients have an impairment of intestinal function and increased markers of the acute phase response. Therefore observed differences between patients receiving parenteral or enteral nutrition may not arise from a modulation of the disease process but may in fact be a direct consequence of the treatment modality.

Another reason for the failure to observe any effect on the inflammatory response in the Edinburgh trial may be a consequence of the earlier sampling on day 4 in contrast to day 7 in the Leeds trial. Measurement of the inflammatory response at day 4 may reflect the level of pancreatic inflammation and may be marginally influenced by the effects of bacterial translocation. Therefore by day 4 the effects of enteral nutrition may not yet be apparent.

Although surrogate markers such as C-reactive protein and organ dysfunction scores were used in both the Edinburgh and Leeds trials, benefits in these measure are not necessarily sufficient to mandate a change in management. Of more importance are outcome measures such as mortality and major complications. Therefore the results from Patras demonstrating a reduction in total and septic complications from the use of enteral nutrition in patients with severe acute pancreatitis are exciting, especially as this trial consisted of patients with severe acute pancreatitis in a intensive care setting. However, the ascribed benefits need to be confirmed in a larger study.

In summary, the published studies demonstrate that enteral nutrition is feasible in patients with prognostically severe acute pancreatitis. Moreover it would appear, that contrary to earlier hypotheses of the pathogenesis of severe acute pancreatitis, early enteral nutrition does not exacerbate organ dysfunction. However from the published data it is not clear whether early enteral nutrition ameliorates the inflammatory response although it may reduce overall morbidity and mortality.

References

1. Kingsnorth A. Role of cytokines and their inhibitors in acute pancreatitis. Gut 1997; 40:1–4.
2. Norman J. The role of cytokines in the pathogenesis of acute pancreatitis. Am J Surg 1998; 175:76–83.
3. Powell JJ, Fearon KCH, Siriwardena AK. Current concepts of the pathophysiology and treatment of severe acute pancreatitis. British Journal of Intensive Care 2000; 10:51–59.
4. Moore FA, Feliciano DV, Andrassy RJ, et al. Early enteral feeding, compared with parenteral, reduces postoperative septic complications. The results of a meta-analysis. Ann Surg 1992; 216:172–83.

5. Hadfield RJ, Sinclair DG, Houldsworth PE, et al. Effects of enteral and parenteral nutrition on gut mucosal permeability in the critically ill. Am J Respir Crit Care Med 1995; 152:1545–8.
6. Heys SD, Walker LG, Smith I, et al. Enteral nutritional supplementation with key nutrients in patients with critical illness and cancer: a meta-analysis of randomized controlled clinical trials. Ann Surg 1999; 229:467–77.
7. Beale RJ, Bryg DJ, Bihari DJ. Immunonutrition in the critically ill: a systematic review of clinical outcome. Crit Care Med 1999; 27:2799–805.
8. McClave SA, Greene LM, Snider HL, et al. Comparison of the safety of early enteral vs parenteral nutrition in mild acute pancreatitis. JPEN J Parenter Enteral Nutr 1997; 21:14–20.
9. Kalfarentzos F, Kehagias J, Mead N, et al. Enteral nutrition is superior to parenteral nutrition in severe acute pancreatitis: results of a randomized prospective trial. Br J Surg 1997; 84:1665–9.
10. Windsor AC, Kanwar S, Li AG, et al. Compared with parenteral nutrition, enteral feeding attenuates the acute phase response and improves disease severity in acute pancreatitis. Gut 1998; 42:431–5.
11. Powell JJ, Murchison JT, Fearon KC, et al. Randomized controlled trial of the effect of early enteral nutrition on markers of the inflammatory response in predicted severe acute pancreatitis. Br J Surg 2000; 87:1375–81.
12. Heel KA, Kong SE, McCauley RD, et al. The effect of minimum luminal nutrition on mucosal cellularity and immunity of the gut. J Gastroenterol Hepatol 1998; 13:1015–9.
13. McCauley RD, Heel KA, Christiansen KJ, et al. The effect of minimum luminal nutrition on bacterial translocation and atrophy of the jejunum during parenteral nutrition. J Gastroenterol Hepatol 1996; 11:65–70.
14. Okada Y, Klein N, van Saene HK, et al. Small volumes of enteral feedings normalise immune function in infants receiving parenteral nutrition. J Pediatr Surg 1998; 33:16–9.
15. Glazer G, Mann DV. United Kingdom guidelines for the management of acute pancreatitis. Gut 1998; 42:S1–S13.
16. Banks PA. Practice guidelines in acute pancreatitis. Am J Gastroenterol 1997; 92:377–86.
17. Dervenis C, Johnson CD, Bassi C, et al. Diagnosis, objective assessment of severity, and management of acute pancreatitis. Santorini consensus conference. Int J Pancreatol 1999; 25:195–210.
18. Fong YM, Marano MA, Barber A, et al. Total parenteral nutrition and bowel rest modify the metabolic response to endotoxin in humans. Ann Surg 1989; 210:449–56; discussion 456–7.
19. Welsh FK, Farmery SM, MacLennan K, et al. Gut barrier function in malnourished patients. Gut 1998; 42:396–401.

37 Enteral Nutrition in Acute Pancreatitis: Clinical Outcome

Christos Dervenis

Acute pancreatitis is a disease with a wide spectrum of clinical courses, ranging from the mild form with minimum morbidity and almost zero mortality, to a severe form with a high percentage of complications and a high risk for a lethal outcome.[1,2]

Severe acute pancreatitis is characterized by extensive necrosis of pancreatic parenchyma and local and systemic complications such as SIRS and organ dysfunction and failure. It represents a typical model of septic syndrome due to failure of the gut barrier to keep endogenous bacteria toxins and antigens away from the portal and systemic circulation.[3]

One of the main therapeutic aims in severe acute pancreatitis is to maintain the gut integrity to prevent bacteria and endotoxin translocation and at the same time to influence or even strengthen the immune system of the intestine. [4,5,6]

Metabolic and Nutritional Consequences in Severe Acute Pancreatitis –the Role of the Gut

Independently of the different proposed mechanisms for the pathogenesis of acute pancreatitis there is a common pattern that leads to the clinical course of the disease. This pathway involves activation of trypsinogen to trypsin and then a cascade activation of various enzymes is started, leading to autodigestion of the gland itself and of the peri-pancreatic tissues. At the same time liberation of acute phase reactants results in a haemodynamic response similar to that seen in sepsis syndrome (increased cardiac output, decreased peripheral resistance and increased oxygen consumption). This is accompanied by alterations in the metabolism of carbohydrates, proteins and lipids.

In parallel a hypermetabolic state develops, leading to an excessive negative nitrogen balance because of increased energy requirements and protein catabolism. This negative nitrogen balance together with starvation result in a rapid loss of lean body mass, which adversely affects host defences and immune competence.[7]

Malnutrition in acute pancreatitis is related to the severity of the disease and is the cause cause. Patients, for example, with alcoholic acute pancreatitis may be malnourished before the onset of the disease.

Although SIRS is the main cause of death in the early period of acute pancreatitis, sepsis due to contamination of pancreatic necrosis seems to be responsible for the late mortality. There are several routes of infection, but bacterial translocation through the gut wall is the main proposed mechanism for necrosis contamination.[8]

The gut acts as a physiological barrier against bacteria and endotoxins, and represents also the largest immune organ of the body. Secretory IgA, produced in the so-called gut associated lymphoid tissue, prevents bacterial and viral adherence to the mucosa.[9]

In summary, maintenance of the gut integrity is of a high priority in severe acute pancreatitis to prevent pancreatic necrosis contamination and preserve its immune function.

The Role of Enteral Feeding

Nutritional support in severe acute pancreatitis aims to reverse negative nitrogen balance and to protect gut barrier function and therefore prevent secondary pancreatic (super)infection.

For many years it has been suggested that by correcting malnutrition mortality and morbidity rates will decrease. In a relative study, among 73 patients, 50% of them with severe acute pancreatitis, who received early total parenteral nutrition (TPN), those in persistently negative nitrogen balance had significantly increased mortality.[10] Not in agreement with this a randomized controlled study was published by Sax et al[11] in late 80's comparing TPN with conventional therapy and found no advantage for TPN. In addition to these findings more complications related to catheter sepsis was found in TPN group. The problem with this study is that they included mostly patients with mild disease. A question still exists. Does providing parenteral nutritional support, compared to no nutritional therapy, makes a significant difference in clinical outcome? More trials are needed, as no strong level 1 information, regarding the role of parenteral nutritional support in pancreatitis, exists.

Despite these findings concerning the role of TPN in severe acute pancreatitis more recently attention has been given to the possible role of the enteral route of delivering the necessary calories and nutrients. The rationale behind the concept of enteral feeding is that there is at least some evidence that is important in restoring the gut-mucosal barrier and might prevent morphological changes in the intestine associated with starvation. Lack of nutrients in the gut lumen leads to loss of mucosal integrity as result of a decrease of mucosal thickness.[12] Enteral feeding also can reverse the reduction in villus height which occurred after TPN. In an experimental model rats with pancreatitis were infused with Ringer lactate solution for 48 hours followed by parenteral or enteral nutrition until day 7. Results showed lower endotoxin levels, higher villus height and T-cells levels in animals received enteral nutrition comparing with those received TPN.[5]

In theory, enteral nutrition could play an important role in the treatment of severe acute pancreatitis as it probably prevents sepsis and immune failure.

The Role of Pancreas Rest[11]

For many years to put the pancreas 'at rest' in acute pancreatitis was considered as the best medical practice and the cornerstone of therapeutic manipulations. The rational behind this practice was the concept that by withholding all enteral feeding, even water, the production of the proteolytic enzymes from the pancreas could be prevented and therefore the pancreatic inflammation could be facilitated.[13]

Exocrine pancreatic secretion can be divided in three phases: cephalic, gastric and intestinal.[14] However, the pattern of the pancreatic secretion is not so simple. For example although in the early postprandial phase, during the maximal endogenous stimulation, carbohydrates infused to the duodenum increases amylase secretion, in the late postprandial phase nutrients in the ileum inhibit pancreatic enzyme secretion.[15] These observations may explain the variations of human pancreatic secretion observed during the controlled experimental studies.

Although the pancreatic secretions, both the enzymes and bicarbonate, are linked with the digestion of food, the clinical significance of this was never shown. Moreover, there is evidence that after administration of enteral nutrition in patients with acute pancreatitis, an exacerbation of pancreatic inflammation was not observed. This is probably due to the fact that pancreatic exocrine secretion is severely reduced early after the onset of acute pancreatitis and cholecystokinin stimulated secretion is abolished at the time of maximal histological damage to the pancreas.

As there is no evidence that putting the pancreas 'at rest' has any clinical benefit this theory is very strongly challenged nowadays.[16]

Does Enteral Nutrition Affect Outcome in Acute Pancreatitis?

Since the mid 1980s there has been some evidence from critically ill patients, especially those with severe injury, showing that by giving very early enteral nutrition (EN), could alter favourably the outcome. Moore and co-workers[17] studied 32 patients with severe trauma and compared early EN with no nutritional intervention. They found statistically significant difference in septic morbidity (9% *vs.* 29%).

Although there are theoretical advantages and some experimental evidence that enteral feeding could affect outcome in severe acute pancreatitis, there are difficulties to prove its clinical effectiveness.

There are a number of trials proving that at least, to deliver nutrients through the intestine is safe, well tolerated and does not aggravate the disease in any case.

Two randomised studies have been published comparing enteral feeding with TPN. Kalfarentzos and co-workers[18] studied 38 patients, all with severe acute pancreatitis who were randomised into two groups (EN vs. TPN). They found a significant reduction in total, including septic, complications in the enteral feeding group. The cost of EN was one third that of TPN and they suggested the preferable use on EN in all patients with severe disease. The second study was from UK,[19] evaluating the 34 patients randomised also in two groups but they included patients with moderate and severe disease. Patients who received enteral feeding fared better after 7 days with respect to APACHE II score and C-reactive protein (CRP) levels compared with the TPN group. They also reported that serum IgM endotoxin core antibodies increased in the TPN group and remained unchanged in the EN group, and the total antioxidant capacity was less in the former group. They concluded that patients who received enteral nutrition were exposed to less endotoxin. Probably this was related to preserved host defence.

Recently, another randomised controlled trial was published by a Scottish group[20] (see Chapter 36). This group studied the effect of early enteral nutrition, compared with no nutritional support, on markers of the inflammatory response in predicted severe acute pancreatitis. Serum interleukin 6, tumor necrosis factor receptor I and CRP were used as inflammatory markers. Despite previous findings the authors found that early enteral nutrition did not ameliorate the inflammatory response in patients with severe acute pancreatitis compared with no nutritional intervention.

Finally, a randomised study is under way by our group, trying to identify the role of early enteral nutrition in severe acute pancreatitis compared with standard TPN in reducing the need for surgery in patients with predicted severe acute pancreatitis. We reported preliminary results recently (23 patients) where we showed that early enteral nutrition seems to reduce surgical interventions by reducing the incidence of sepsis (9% vs. 33%).[21]

As mentioned earlier, many believe that delivery of the enteral regimen proximal into the GI tract will cause stimulation of the exocrine pancreatic secretion, through CCK release, and in the case of acute pancreatitis, exacerbation of the inflammatory process. This was supported by animal and human studies, where the pancreatic secretion was higher when the nutrients were delivered either into the stomach or the duodenum compared with intra-jujenal route. However, the situation is different in acute pancreatitis where it known that secretion is suppressed. Although the current practice is to use naso-jejunal tubes, placed endoscopically or under radiographic screening, the Glasgow group[22] showed that nasogastric feeding is usually possible in severe acute pancreatitis. They reported that this practice is safe and well tolerated in most patients without any sign of clinical or biochemical deterioration.

Another question that should be answered is the possible role of the immune-enhanced enteral diets in severe acute pancreatitis.[23] There are a number of reports, mainly in severely injured patients, dealing with this aspect. A meta-analysis[xxiv] included 1009 patients from 11 trials showed that immune-modulated regiments resulted in a significant reduction of infectious complications and length of hospital stay, but with no effect on survival. Only one study was dealing with the use of glutamine in acute pancreatitis, as a supplement in the standard TPN. They found that glutamine improve leukocyte activity and reduce proinflammatory cytokine release in acute pancreatitis. No conclusions can be drawn from these studies, but as it seems possible, that immuno-enriched diets could play a role. Further trials are needed to clarify this issue.

Conclusions

At present there is no definite evidence that artificial nutritional support either total parenteral or enteral, alters outcome in most patients with acute pancreatitis, unless malnutrition is also a problem. Diagnosis of acute pancreatitis is not itself an indication for instituting artificial nutrition. Patients predicted to have severe acute pancreatitis may benefit from EN.

Enteral nutrition support is safe, well tolerated and does not stimulate the pancreas compared with parenteral feeding, and therefore should be used preferably in the treatment or prevention of malnutrition and probably immunosupression and infection, in patients with acute pancreatitis.

Finally, larger, well conducted trials, which recruit only patients with severe acute pancreatitis and stratify them for disease severity, nutritional status and etiology of pancreatitis before randomization, are needed before any conclusive statement on the benefits of nutritional support on outcome can be made.

References

1. Wycoll DL. The management of severe acute necrotizing pancreatitis: An evidence based review of the literature. Intensive Care Med 1999; 25:146–156.
2. Dervenis C, Johnson CD, Bassi C, et al. Diagnosis, objective assessment of severity and management of acute pancreatitis: Santorini consensus conference. Int J Pancreatol 1999; 25:195–210.
3. Saluja AK, Steer M. Pathophysiology of pancreatitis. Role of cytokines and other mediators of inflammation. Digestion 1999; 60 (Suppl 1):27–33.
4. Beger H, Bittner R, Block S, et al. Bacterial contamination of pancreatic necrosis. Gastroenterology 1986; 91:433–438.
5. Kotani J, Usami M, Nomura H. Enteral nutrition prevents bacterial translocation but does not improve survival in acute pancreatitis. Arch Surg 1999; 134:287–292.
6. Sigurdsson GH. Is translocation of bacteria and endotoxin from the gastrointestinal tract a source of sepsis in critically ill patients? Acta Anaesthesiol Scand 1995; 39:11–19.
7. Scolapio JS, Mahli-Chowla N, Ukleja A. Nutrition supplementation in patients with acute and chronic pancreatitis. Gastroenterol Clin N Am 1999; 28:695–707.
8. Schwarz M, Buchler M, Thomsen J, et al. Pancreatic infection in acute pancreatitis: a frequent finding. Digestion 1993; 54:A 119.
9. Underdown BJ, Schiff JM. Immunoglobulin A: Strategic defence initiative at the mucosal surface. Annu Rev Immunol 1986; 4:389–417.
10. Sitzmann J, Steinborn P, Zinner M, et al. Total parenteral nutrition and alternate energy substrates in treatment of severe acute pancreatitis. Surg Gynecon Obstet 1989; 168:311–317.
11. Sax H, Warner B, Talamini M, et al. Early total parenteral nutrition in acute pancreatitis: lack of beneficial effects. Am J Surg 1987; 153:117–124.
12. Johnson C, Kudsk K. Nutrition and intestinal mucosal immunity. Clin Nutr 1999; 18:337–344.
13. Wyncoll D. The management of severe acute necrotizing pancreatitis: An evidence-based review of the literature. Intensive Care Med 1999; 25:146–156.
14. Karamitsios N, Saltzman J. Enteral nutrition in acute pancreatitis. Nutr Rev 1997; 55:279–281.
15. Cassim M, Allardyce D. Pancreatic secretion in response to jejunal feeding of elemental diet. Ann Surg 1974; 180:228–231.
16. Lobo D, Memon M, Allison S, et al. Evolution of nutritional support in acute pancreatitis. Br J Surg 2000; 87:695–707.
17. Moore F, Moore E, Kudsk K, et al. Clinical benefits of an immune enhancing diets for early post-injury feeding. J Trauma 1994; 37:607–615.
18. Kalfarentzos F, Kehagias J, Mead N, et al. Enteral nutrition is superior to parenteral nutrition in severe acute pancreatitis: results of a randomised prospective trial. Br J Surg 1997; 83:349–353.
19. Windsor A, Kanwar S, Li A, et al. Compared with parenteral nutrition, enteral feeding attenuates the acute phase response and improves disease severity in acute pancreatitis. Gut 1998; 42:431–435.
20. Powell J J, et al. Randomized controlled trial of the effect of early enteral nutrition on markers of the inflammatory response in predicted severe acute pancreatitis. Br J Surg 2000; 87:1357–1381.
21. Paraskeva C, Smailis D, Priovolos A, et al. Early enteral nutrition reduces the need for surgery in Severe Acute Pancreatitis. Pancreatology 2001; 1 (4):372.
22. Eatock F, Brombacher G, Steven A, et al. Nasogastric feeding in severe acute pancreatitis may be practical and safe. Int J Pancreatol 2000; 28:25–31.
23. Early enteral nutrition in severe acute pancreatitis: a way of providing nutrients, gut barrier protection, immunomodulation or all of them? Scand J Gastroenterol 2001; 5:449–458.
24. Heys S, Walker L, Smith I, et al. Enteral nutritional supplementation with key nutrients in patients with critical illness and cancer. Ann Surg 1999; 229:467–477.

Part 5
Symptom Relief in Pancreatic Disease

38 Measurement of Symptoms and Quality of Life in Pancreatic Disease

Deborah Fitzsimmons and Colin D. Johnson

Assessment of quality of life (QoL) is now firmly established as an important endpoint in our evaluation of new treatments and interventions. An ever-increasing number of trials and studies report QoL as an outcome, in patients with non-malignant and malignant chronic diseases of the pancreas. The emergence of this approach to pancreatic disease has been an important move forward where there has been previously little consideration of the impact of these diseases and their treatment from the patients' perspective.

The Importance of Symptom and QoL Measurement in Pancreatic Disease

There is now established consensus of the need and demand in obtaining information about the quality of life of patients with pancreatic disease.[1–3] This can be attributed to two essential reasons. First, despite much progress, the vast majority of our patients will receive an intervention with palliative intent only. Second, within the context of limited survival for many of our patients, there is an increasing need and demand to consider the quality of this survival on the patients' health and general wellbeing. This is of particular importance when there is no significant survival advantage between two treatments. With the focus on more appropriate goals such as symptom relief and improvements on QoL, clinicians can then focus on what can be realistically achieved for their patients, and evaluate the effect of interventions using appropriate measures.

Approaches to Measuring Symptoms and QoL in Patients with Pancreatic Disease

Measurements of *quantity of life*, usually described in terms such as survival are a familiar concept to the clinician. These have been used widely, can be assessed objectively and direct comparisons can be made across individuals, groups or populations. However, measurements of *quality of life* has introduced a new and often, confusing area of health outcome measurement.[4]

With regard to health, the emphasis has been to develop appropriate methods to assess health-related quality of life, that is those aspects of quality of life that are most influenced by disease and treatment.[5] Within oncology, the predominant focus has been on assessing on physical functioning, disease symptoms, treatment side-effects and psychological well-being within the context of clinical trials.[6] Typically, assessment systems used comprise of psychometrically robust instruments that are either generic (capture broad areas of health related QoL relevant to all patients e.g. SF-36,[7] disease-specific (covers areas of QoL relevant to specific group of patients e.g. EORTC QLQ-C30 in cancer patients)[5] or dimension specific (focus on one domain of QoL e.g. Hospital Anxiety and Depression Score for psychological morbidity).[8]

Despite a plethora of instruments available to the clinician, there is no single assessment system available that can capture all relevant domains of patients' QoL.[6] In order to produce valid and reliable instruments that are able to capture the most important and relevant QoL issues of concern for patients for pancreatic disease, we have previously documented the development of a pancreatic cancer specific module, the EORTC QLQ-PAN26 to supplement the core EORTC cancer module, the EORTC QLQ-C30.[9] In this preliminary work, we highlighted the disparity and confusion in QoL assessment in pancreatic disease.[10] We will now review recent studies that have purported to measure QoL in patients with pancreatic disease.

Review of Recent Published Studies

From reviewing the evidence published since 1998, it appears that although progress has been made, there are still inconsistencies in the methods and approach to QoL assessment (see Table 38.1). Some studies have used validated instruments such as the EORTC QLQ-C30.[11] However, there are still many trials that appear to have given scant regard to the basic concepts underpinning QoL, using measures such as Clinical Benefit Response[12] or performance status as indicators of a patients' QoL. As Hoffman and Glimelius[13] conclude from their head to head evaluation of the CBR to the QLQ-C30, although the CBR is a better marker for clinical benefit than performance status or objective response, it is not sufficient at looking at the wider impact on a patient's QoL. In their evaluation of various treatments on patients' QoL and survival, Kokoska et al[14] conclude that QoL measurements do not support palliative pancreatic cancer treatments. Clearly, one of the methodological limitations of this study is that they used an inappropriate measure (Karnofsky performance status) as an indicator of QoL, albeit that they report that performance status was 'self reported' rather than measured by the clinician.

We also see little reference to any pancreatic cancer specific QoL instrument used in such trials. However, two international research programmes, have produced pancreatic specific QoL assessment systems. In parallel to the development of the EORTC QLQ-PAN26, the FACT-PA has been developed.[15] This has been recently updated by the FACIT-HEP, a validated measure for all hepato-pancreato- biliary malignancies.[16] Both assessment systems are currently incorporated into a range of clinical trials and academic studies. Table 38.2 summarises the content of the disease-specific QoL issues in these two instruments. It is anticipated that subsequent reporting of these instruments in large multi-centre studies will contribute valuable information on the optimum methods of assessing symptoms and QoL in patients with pancreatic disease.

Personal Experience of Measuring Symptoms and QoL in Patients with Pancreatic Disease

Pancreatic Cancer

As part of the on-going development of the EORTC QLQ-PAN26, we have provisionally assessed the reliability and validity of the EORTC QLQ-C30 and QLQ-PAN26 in pancreatic cancer patients in the UK. Patients were recruited from two sources, based on primary treatment intention. Group A consisted of 20 patients undergoing surgical resection. Eleven men and nine women were recruited with a median age of 64 (44–79) years and a median Karnofksy score of 90 (70–100). Group B consisted of 30 patients with inoperable disease receiving gemcitabine. Nineteen men and 11 women were recruited with a median age of 61.5 (39–78) years and a Karnofsky score of 80 (60–100). Assessment of QoL was undertaken before their treatment/ surgery and at one and three months afterwards.

All patients completed the QoL instruments in the presence of a research nurse, who was available to answer any queries on the QoL data. The majority of patients (90%) completed the QoL instruments themselves, and median time of completion was 9 minutes (5–25 minutes). The other patients (10%) completed the QoL instruments as part of a structured interview undertaken by the nurse. At baseline, there was 5% missing items within the instruments. This was mainly due to the non-completion of items related to information and support from health professionals.

As expected, the percentage of patients reporting symptoms associated with presentation and diagnosis (such as jaundice and pain) was higher at baseline but reduced at one and three months. This treatment reflects the effect of reducing these disease symptoms (see Table 38.3). Other symptoms synonymous with advancing disease (such as weight loss and ascites) rose at three months compared to baseline scores.

The internal consistency as measured by Cronbach's alpha coefficient of >0.70[17] was met on the majority of the multi-item scales on the QLQ-C30 and proposed scales of the QLQ-PAN26. Only the hepatic symptom scale in the QLQ-PAN26 consistently showed a low coefficient value of <0.35 at all time points.

In order to test construct validity, patients were differentiated at baseline (pre-treatment) scores based on performance status (Karnofsky score <80 versus 80+), treatment intention (surgery versus chemotherapy) and age (<70 years versus 70+ years), using one-way ANOVA on selected multi-item scales of the EORTC QLQ-C30 and QLQ-PAN26 (Emotional functioning, Global Health/ QoL., Pain, Fatigue, Pancreatic Pain, Digestive, Jaundice and Burden of Treatment). Significant difference was expected when patients were differentiated by performance status in the physical functioning and symptom scales. No significant difference would be expected at baseline based on treatment intention and age due to the generic scope of the module. Statistical significance was accepted at $p < 0.05$. Significant difference was seen in the jaundice scale when treatment groups were compared. This may be due to the presence of jaundice seen in some patients with a resectable

Table 38.1. Selection of recent studies (1998–2001) purporting to assess quality of life in pancreatic cancer

Author and year	Study population	Study design	QoL measure used	Main findings
Ekstom *et al.* 1998[23]	31 patients with advanced pancreatic and biliary cancer	Phase II study of single dose etoposide	EORTC QLQ-C30 CBR	QoL gains seen in some patients (19–29%)
Ferry *et al.* 200024	31 patients with advanced disease	Phase II trial of 5 lipooxygenase inhibitor	Not specified	QoL was maintained during therapy
Glimer-Hill *et al.* 2001[25]	9 inoperable patients with uncontrolled pain	Retrospective series of intrath ecal morphine using implanted infusion pumps	Pain visual analogue scale and level of activity	All patients reported good to excellent relief of pain
Hoffman and Glimelius 1998[13]	151 patients with gastrointestinal cancer, 53 with pancreatic cancer	Retrospective review of CBR versus QoL scores (EORTC QLQ-C30) from two trials of chemotherapy versus BSC	CBR EORTC QLQ-C30	CBR overestimated beneficial effects of chemotherapy CBR neglects impact of other symptoms on QoL CBR did show same differences between the two groups as QoL CBR limited as an indicator of QoL
Klapdor *et al.* 1999[26]	28 patients with advanced disease	Prospective study of mitomycin C with gemcitabine	Clinical benefit	75% of patients reported a clinical benefit compared to those receiving gemcitabine alone
Kokoska *et al.* 1998[14]	781 patients undergoing various treatments	Retrospective evaluation	QoL index based on self reported Karnosfky status	Performances scores not higher in treated patients QoL measurements do not support resection for patients with lymph node involvement
Glimelius *et al.* 1998[27]	100 patients with GI cancers including pancreatic cancer with low haemoglobin	RCT of low dose etpoetin beta versus high dose	EORTC QLQ-C30	QoL parameters showed improvements with correspon-ding increase in haemoglobin levels but was also linked to underlying malignancy
Maurer *et al.* 1998[28]	12 patients with non-resectable disease	Phase II study of a celiac axis infusion of mitoxantrone, 5-FU and folinic acid, and cisplatin	Symptom response and WHO toxicity scores	Nine patients experienced temporary relief of pain following treatment. 4 events of grade III

				toxicity and 10 events of grade II toxicity related to leucopenia and diarrhoea and vomiting
McLeod 1999[29]	25 patients post-Whipples procedure	Retrospective study of QoL, nutritional status and GI hormone profile <6 months post treatment compared to a control patients	Sickness Impact Profile GI QoL index Utility analysis	No/ minimal impairment in general well being and GI function Mean utility score of 0.98 suggesting near normal wellbeing QoL determined as excellent in these patients
Pietrabissa *et al.* 2000[30]	25 patients with unresectable disease	Consecutive series of patients undergoing thorascopic splanchnicectomy	Nottingham Health Profile	Significant improvement in each area of the NHP seen after thorascopic splanchnicetomy
Rauch *et al.* 2001[31]	Chemotherapy naïve patients with advanced disease	Phase II trial of gemcitabine in combination with continuous 5 Fu	Clinical benefit response	Overall clinical benefit effect with improved performance status in 39% of patients and reduction in pain in 65% of patients
Stehlin *et al.* 1999[32]	60 patients with advanced disease	Phase II study of oral nitrocampothecin	Not stated	
Wenger *et al.* 1999[33]	Patients with recurrent pancreatic cancer after resection	Prospective study of octreotide and tamoxifen	EORTC QLQ-C30	Treated patients suffered less from fatigue, nausea, appetite loss and pain compared to controls.

Table 38.2. Content of the disease specific QoL issues in the FACT-Pa and QLQ-PAN26

Common items	Abdominal swelling, back pain, digestion of food, changes in bowel habit, physical appearance, constipation, diarrhoea, nausea, lack of energy, weight loss, sexuality, fear of future health, burden of treatment
Additional items in the QLQ-PAN26 not covered in FACT-Pa	Jaundice, pruritus, indigestion, loss of muscle strength, flatulence, dry mouth, position related pain, night time pain, abdominal pain, communication and support from health care professionals
Additional items in the FACT-Pa not covered in QLQ-C30/ QLQ-PAN26	Meeting needs of family, feeling ill, family support, family acceptance of illness, family communication, closeness to main partner, coping with illness, maintaining hope, illness acceptance, enjoyment of life

Table 38.3. Percentage of patients reporting mean scores > 50 (moderate-severe)

Scale/Item	Baseline	Month 1	Month 3
Pancreatic pain	20	11	8
Digestive	15	6	12
Jaundice and pruritus	15	4	4
Body image	24	11	32
Ascites	28	6	15
Taste changes	15	15	24
Indigestion	11	12	24
Flatulence	20	9	24
Weight loss	19	15	28
Muscle strength	19	15	20
Burden of treatment	6	32	36
Dry mouth	3	18	24
Fear of future	23	41	36

tumour whereas patients treated with gemcitabine had had this jaundice relieved previously. When performance status was compared, statistical difference was seen in the digestive pancreatic pain and global QoL scales. There were no significant differences in patients stratified by age. This lack of statistical significance may be, in part, due to the similarities at diagnosis of these groups based on age, sex and performance status.

Chronic Pancreatitis

We have recently assessed the feasibility of the EORTC QLQ-C30 and QLQ-PAN26 in measuring the QoL of patients with chronic pancreatitis. The similarity of symptoms and treatments for pancreatic cancer and chronic pancreatitis has prompted interest in the application of this QoL assessment system in chronic pancreatitis. Sixty-five patients with chronic pancreatitis from four centres (Southampton; Cape Town, South Africa; Magdeburg, Germany; and Verona, Italy) were recruited. Sixty-three patients were able to self complete the instruments in a median time of 9 minutes (6–20 min). Content validity of the instrument was high with only issues related to alcohol dependency noted as a significant omission. All scales apart from the hepatic symptom scales met standards for internal consistency with an Alpha Coefficient Score of >0.70. With regard to construct validity, statistical difference was met in all scales of the EORTC QLQ-C30 and all symptoms scales and sexual functioning scale in the EORTC QLQ-PAN26 when comparisons made between good and poor Karnofsky performance status (80+ versus >80) and between those with a requirement for opioid analgesia, but there were no significant differences seen in any scale between patients who had had previous surgical or medical treatment.

The results of this present study suggest the EORTC QLQ-C30/PAN26 is a suitable measure for the cross-cultural assessment of HRQoL in chronic pancreatitis patients. There is an obvious benefit of simplicity in the use of a single assessment system to assess health related QoL in all patients with both malignant and non-malignant chronic pancreatic disease.

Recommendations for Incorporating QoL into Clinical Studies of Pancreatic Disease

Symptom and QoL assessment demands the same rigorous consideration as any other part of designing a clinical study and should not be an afterthought. Improvements in survival, disease free survival or response rates to therapy should still be considered the most important endpoints,[18] and there is debate as to whether QoL should only be used as an endpoint within a phase II trial. However, QoL can provide essential information on the patients' well being, which can supplement the more traditional clinical and laboratory indicators of illness, and incorporation into Phase III studies can allow important information to be gathered about the instruments' reliability and validity.

There are now a series of well-conducted reviews, which gives structured guidance to the clinician and researcher with regard to incorporating QoL assessment into clinical studies (for examples see Refs. 6 and 19). Attention should be given to the justification of using QoL as an endpoint, the evidence on which to select an appropriate assessment tool (including the validity, reliability, responsiveness to change and appropriateness of the instrument), the timing of QoL assessments, and the approaches taken to data collection and management, and the analysis of QoL data.

One of the issues that remain contentious for clinicians is the interpretation of QoL scores, particularly with the lack of a 'gold standard' within which to compare scores from a QoL instrument, and disparity in approaches taken to assess QoL. Current work is being undertaken to optimise current methods of QoL assessment such as the collection of reference data, development of statistical approaches such as Item Response Methods[20] and development of more individualised approaches to QoL assessment such as the SEIQOL.[21]

Incorporating QoL Assessment into Clinical Decision Making

One of the most important areas for future development is the clinical usefulness of QoL assessment. At present, there is little standardised or comprehensive method of evaluating the consequences of our care and treatment on the psychosocial wellbeing of the patient in the clinical setting. Several potential uses have been identified for QoL measures within this area.[22] These include prioritising problems, facilitating communication, screening for potential problems, identifying patient preferences, monitoring responses to treatment and education.

There are several hurdles to overcome in using QoL assessments within this context. At present, there are no reported studies that have considered this within pancreatic disease. It cannot be assumed that instruments that have been developed for use in clinical trials can be transferred directly to clinical practice. First, there is little evidence about the appropriateness of QoL instruments in specific patient groups, e.g. ethnic differences, the elderly or those at the terminal stages of their disease. Second, there is lack of consensus of the optimum method of presenting QoL scores within the clinical setting. Much of the interpretation of QoL scores is at group or population level. However, it is difficult to determine at present when a QoL score is of clinical significance for an individual patient, for example at what score a particular QoL score should be considered severe? Little work has been undertaken in the majority of QoL instruments. Third, the timing of assessments also requires careful consideration, so that a careful trade off can be made in obtaining comprehensive data about a patient's QoL, but not overburdening the patient with too many instruments to complete. The high attrition rate of QoL assessment is one of the most difficult hurdles to overcome in current clinical trials.

Once such systems have been developed for use in individual patient management, the next question is what should be done with this information. There is a lack of evidence to support the benefit of QoL assessment in facilitating decision making between clinician and patient.[22] A number of ethical dilemmas may be raised, as there may be the expectation that once QoL can be assessed, the clinician will be able to influence it. The application of QoL assessments into clinical practice is now highlighted as one of the priorities within the field of QoL research.

Conclusion

Pancreatic disease and its treatment affect all aspects of a patient's health-related QoL. Significant progress in measuring symptoms and QoL in the patient with pancreatic disease has been made in the past decade. However, there is still disparity of approaches taken to the measurement of these patient-based outcomes in recent reported studies. An international programme of research has resulted in the development of a single assessment system to assess health related QoL in all patients with both malignant and non-malignant chronic pancreatic disease in clinical studies. Further work is now required in developing or adapting QoL measures for use in clinical practice.

References

1. Alexandre JH, Bouillot JL. Quality of life assessment in pancreatic surgery. Theoretical Surgery 1992; 7:18–20.
2. Lionetto R, Puglises V, Bruzzi P, et al. No standard treatment is available for advanced pancreatic cancer. Eur J Cancer 1995; 31A:882–887.
3. Rothenberg ML, Abbruzzese JL, Moore M, et al. A rationale for expanding the endpoints for clinical trials in advanced pancreatic carcinoma. Cancer 1996; 78:627–632.

4. Cohen SR, Mount BM, MacDonald N. Defining quality of life. Eur J Cancer 1996; 32A:753–754.
5. Aaronson NK, Meyerowitz BE, Bard M, et al. Quality of life research in oncology. Past achievements and future priorities. Cancer 1991; 1 (3):839–843.
6. Bowling A. Measuring Health: A Review of Quality of Life Measurement Scales. Milton Keynes: Open University Press, 1991.
7. Ware JE, Snow K, Kosinski M, et al. SF-36. Health Survey. Manual and Interpretation guide USA Medical Outcomes Trust, 1993.
8. Zigmond A, Snaith RP. The hospital anxiety and depression scale. Acta Psychiatrica Scandinavia 1983; 67:361–370.
9. Fitzsimmons D, Johnson CD, George S, et al. Development of a disease specific quality of life (QoL) questionnaire module to supplement the EORTC core cancer QoL questionnaire, the QLQ-C30 in patients with pancreatic cancer. Eur J Cancer 1999; 35:939–41.
10. Fitzsimmons D, Johnson CD. Quality of Life after Treatment for Pancreatic Cancer. Lagenbeck's Archives of Surgery 1998; 383: 2:145–151.
11. Aaronson NK, Ahmedzai S, Bergman B, et al. The European Organization for Research and Treatment of Cancer QLQ-C30: a quality of life instrument for use in international clinical trials in oncology. J Natal Cancer Institute 1993; 85:365–376.
12. Burris HA, Moore MJ, Anderson J, et al. Improvements in survival and clinical benefit with gemcitabine as first line therapy for patients with advanced pancreas cancer: a randomised trial. J Clin Oncol 1997; 15:2403–2413.
13. Hoffman K, Glimelius B. Evaluation of clinical benefit of chemotherapy in patients with upper gastrointestinal cancer. Acta Oncol 1998; 37:651–9.
14. Kokoska ER, Stapleton DR, Virgo KS, et al. Quality of life measurements do not support palliative pancreatic cancer treatments Int J Oncol 1998; 13:1323–9.
15. Cella DF. Personal Communication September 28th 1999. Centre on Outcomes, Research and Education, Illinois, USA.
16. Cella DF. Personal Communication April 2000 Centre on Outcomes, Research and Education, Illinois, USA.
17. Streiner DL, Norman GR. Health Measurement Scales. A Practical Guide to Their Development and Use. Second Edition 1995 Oxford Medical Publications: Oxford.
18. de Haes J, Curran D, Young T, et al. Quality of life evaluation in oncological clinical trials-the EORTC model. Eur J Cancer 2000; 36:821–5.
19. Fitzpatrick R, Davey C, Buxton MJ, et al. Evaluating Patient-Based Outcome Measures for Use in Clinical Trials. Health Technology Assessment 1998; 2:14.
20. Fayers P, Grovenvold M, et al. Personal Communication. April 2000 EORTC Study Group Meeting. London.
21. O'Boyle CA, McGee HM, Hickey A, et al. The schedule for the evaluation of individual quality of life (SEIQoL): administration manual. Dublin: Royal College of Surgeons in Ireland, 1993.
22. Higginson IJ, Carr AJ. Measuring quality of life: Using quality of life measures in the clinical setting Br Med J 2001; 322:1297–1300.
23. Ekstrom K, Hoffman K, Linne T, et al. Single-dose etoposide in advanced pancreatic and biliary cancer, a phase II study. Oncol Rep 1998; 5:931–4.
24. Ferry DR, Deakin M, Baddeley J, et al. A phase II study of the 5-lipoxygenase inhibitor, CV6504 in advanced pancreatic cancer: correlation of clinical data with pharmokinetic and pharmodynamic endpoints. Ann Oncol 11:1165–70.
25. Gilmer-Hill HS, Boggan JE, Smith, et al. Intrathecal morphine delivered via subcutaneous pump for intractable pain in pancreatic cancer. Surg Neurol 1999; 51:6–11.
26. Klapdor R, Suetter E, Lang-Polckow EM, et al. Locoregional/systemic chemotherapy of locally advanced/metasized pancreatic cancer with a combination of mitomycin-C and gemcitabine and simultaneous follow-up by imaging methods and tumour markers. Anticancer Res 1999; 19:2459–69.
27. Glimelius B, Linne T, Hoffman K, et al. Epoetin beta in the treatment of anaemia in patients with advanced gastrointestinal cancer. J Clin Oncol 1998; 16:434–40.
28. Maurer CA, Borner MM, Lauffer J, et al. Celiac axis infusion chemotherapy in advanced non-resectable pancreatic cancer. Int J Pancreatol 1998; 23:181–6.
29. McLeod RS. Quality of life, nutritional status and gastrointestinal hormone profile following the Whipple procedure. Ann Oncol 1999; 10 (Suppl 4):481–4.
30. Pietrabissa A, Vistoli F, Carobbi A. Thorascopic splanchnicectomy for pain relief in unresectable pancreatic cancer. Arch Surg 2000; 135:332–5.
31. Rauch DP, Maurer CA, Aebi S, et al. Activity of gemcitabine and continuous infusion fluorouracil advanced pancreatic cancer. Oncology 2001; 60:43–8.

32. Stehlin JS, Giovanella BC, Natelson EA, et al. A study of 9-nitrocamptothecin (RFS-2000) in patients with advanced pancreatic cancer. Int J Oncol 1999; 14:821–831.
33. Wenger FA, Jacobi CA, Siderow A, et al. Hormone therapy of postoperative recurrent pancreatic carcinoma with octreotide and tamoxifen. Chirurg 1999; 70:694–9.

39 Mechanism of Nociception in Chronic Pancreatitis

Pierluigi Di Sebastiano and Fabio F. di Mola

Pain represents the leading symptom of chronic pancreatitis (chronic pancreatitis) and is usually so intense and long-lasting that the follow-up care of patients may be difficult and frustrating. In approximately 75% of cases, chronic pancreatitis presents with recurrent or continuous deep and gnawing abdominal pain, characteristically situated in the upper abdomen to the left of the midline passing round or through to the back.[1–2]

The pathophysiology of pain in chronic pancreatitis is incompletely understood and perhaps multifactorial: several hypotheses have been proposed including pancreatic and extrapancreatic mechanisms. In addition, the presence of different hypotheses to explain the genesis of pain in chronic pancreatitis directly reflects on the difficulty of pain treatment and subsequent relief in these patients.[2–3]

Earlier pain hypotheses include the increased intraductal and intraparenchymal pressure, as measured preoperatively or intra-operatively, or post-prandial pancreatic hyperstimulation caused by decreased enzyme secretion and the insufficient functioning of the so-called 'negative feedback mechanism'. These mechanisms are now often questioned as reliable explanations of abdominal pain in patients with chronic pancreatitis. The intrapancreatic ductal pressure might be related to the pancreatic secretion itself and to the presence of an obstruction in the pancreatic duct.[4] Several conditions that influence these two parameters are able to modulate pain intensity and frequency in patients with chronic pancreatitis.[5–6] In fact, many investigators have related the origin of pain to the increased pressure in pancreatic ducts and tissue.[7] The ductal hypertension hypothesis as an explanation for pain in chronic pancreatitis is derived from observations that decompression of a dilated pancreatic duct or pseudocyst frequently relieves pain in chronic pancreatitis patients.[8] However, after pancreatic duct drainage many chronic pancreatitis patients continue to experience unchanged pain postoperatively, or their pain recurs at a later time following duct drainage operations, suggesting that additional mechanisms are also involved in the pathogenesis of pain in this condition.[9–12]

Recent concepts have focused on the possible involvement of the nervous system in chronic pain and the inflammatory process in chronic pancreatitis. Supporting this fascinating hypothesis, Keith *et al.*[13] initiated that neural and perineural alterations might be important in the pathogenesis of pain in chronic pancreatitis. They demonstrated that pain severity correlated with the duration of alcohol consumption, pancreatic calcification and more interestingly with the percentage of eosinophils number in the perineural infiltrate, but not with duct dilatation.

The subsequent study[14] was the pioneer in this field that first demonstrated an increase both in number and diameter of pancreatic nerve fibres in the course of chronic pancreatitis compared to normal pancreas. In tissue specimens of patients suffering from chronic pancreatitis, foci of inflammatory cells were often found surrounding pancreatic nerves, which in electron-microscopic analysis exhibit a damaged perineurium and invasion with eosinophile granulocytes. These abnormalities might allow free access to inflammatory mediators or active pancreatic enzymes in the nerve bundles, thus generating and sustaining the inflammatory response and pain generation. The changed pattern of intrinsic and possibly extrinsic innervation of the pancreas in chronic pancreatitis suggested that there could be also an up-regulation of the neuropeptides that usually populate these enlarged nerves. In fact, a further study showed[15] that the striking changes in the peptidergic innervation pattern in chronic pancreatitis concerned only these altered nerves. This pattern includes an intensification of the immunostaining for calcitonin gene-related peptide (CGRP), and substance P (SP) in numerous fibres contained in these nerves. Double fluorescence immunohistochemistry revealed a coexistence of SP and CGRP immunoreactive fibres. Because both of these peptides are generally regarded as pain transmitters, these findings provided evidence for a role of pancreatic nerves in the long-lasting pain syndrome in chronic pancreatitis.

Another interesting finding of these studies was the observation of a close spatial relationship between neuronal structures and immune cells in chronically inflamed pancreas that led to the concept of neuroimmune mechanisms in the pathogenesis of chronic pancreatitis and the accompanying abdominal pain.

Interestingly, in the subsequent reports,[16–17] the presence of growth-associated-protein-43 (GAP-43, an established marker of neuronal plasticity, was correlated positively with pain scores in patients with chronic pancreatitis. GAP-43 is a neuronal protein known to be involved in the development of axonal growth cones and presynaptic terminals, and the expression of GAP-43 is increased at mRNA and protein level after neuronal lesions. GAP-43 is widespread in the developing, and adult, central and peripheral nervous systems of the rat and is expressed in the hippocampus of rats and humans, regions which continually undergo synaptic remodeling and after nerve damage. In the chronically inflamed human pancreas, by enzymatic and double fluorescence immunohistochemistry, a significant re-expression of GAP-43 in the majority of pancreatic nerve fibres was demonstrated. These immunohistochemical findings correlated with clinical and pathological findings in patients with chronic pancreatitis, including the parenchyma-fibrosis ratio, the degree of perineural immune cell infiltration, exhibiting a strong relationship with individual pain scores. Furthermore, the infiltration of pancreatic nerves by immune cells was significantly correlated with the pain intensity, whereas pain scores did not correlate neither with the degree of pancreatic fibrosis nor with the duration of the disease (Table 39.1). It is clear that the demonstration of a direct relationship between the degree of perineural inflammation and pain as clinical symptom, strongly supports the hypothesis of a neuroimmunological interaction as an important, if not predominant, factor in pain generation in chronic pancreatitis. In addition, the lack of a relationship between the degree of pancreatic fibrosis and pain could contradict the common concept that fibrosis leads to increased intraductal pressure in chronic pancreatitis and thereby contributes to pain pathophysiology during chronic inflammation of the pancreas.

Table 39.1. Relationship between clinical and immunocytochemical findings in chronic pancreatitis (From Ref. 17.)

	Infiltration score	Intensity of pain	Degree of fibrosis	GAP43-ir neurons	GAP43-ir nerve fibres
Infiltration score		$p < 0.01$			
Intensity of pain			$p < 0.05$	$p < 0.05$	$p < 0.05$
GAP43-ir	$p < 0.05$				
Duration of disease		$p < 0.09$		$p < 0.05$	$p < 0.05$

However, we have to remember also the mechanisms that contribute to the enlargement of pancreatic nerves. A recent study[18] analyzed the expression of nerve growth factor (NGF) and its high affinity receptor (TrkA) in patients suffering from chronic pancreatitis. NGF belongs to the neurotrophin family and plays a role in neuroblast proliferation and neuronal maturation, affecting neuronal phenotype and maintaining neuronal survival. NGF signaling is mediated via binding to a high and a low affinity receptor. The high affinity receptor is called TrkA, and signaling is transmitted via an internal tyrosine-kinase domain. p-75, the low affinity receptor of NGF, belongs to the G-protein receptor family and plays a minor role in signal transduction. TrkA is present in dorsal root and peripheral ganglia cells of primary sensory nerves, and is involved in signal transduction of noxious stimuli and tissue injury. Inflammation results in an elevation of NGF levels in different diseases. Interestingly, NGF may itself have cytokine-like functions; it can modify mast-cell, macrophage and B-cell functions, but may also activate TrkA located on sensory and sympathetic nerve fibres innervating the site of inflammation, thus modulating neuro-immune interactions. In chronic pancreatitis tissue samples NGF and TrkA mRNA expression were markedly increased and enhanced NGF mRNA expression was present in metaplastic ductal cells, in degenerating acinar cells, and in acinar cells dedifferentiating into tubular structures. TrkA mRNA was intensely present in the perineurium. Further, enhanced NGF and TrkA mRNA signals were also present in intrapancreatic ganglia cells in chronic pancreatitis samples. Analysis of the molecular findings with clinical parameters revealed a significant relation between NGF mRNA levels and pancreatic fibrosis and acinar cell damage and between TrkA mRNA and pain intensity thus indicating that the NGF/TrkA pathway is activated in chronic pancreatitis. It also appears that this activation might influence nerve growth and the pain syndrome most probably by modulating the sensitivity of NGF-independent primary sensory neurons, by increasing channel and receptor expression. Another mechanism by which NGF might influence pain is the regulation of transcription and the synthesis of SP and CGRP as well as through the release of histamine. In fact, the neuropeptide SP is the tachykinin mainly involved in neural transmission of sensory information, smooth muscle contraction, nociception, sexual behaviour and possibly wound healing and tissue regeneration.[19] SP has wide ranging functional effects, not only in the central and peripheral nervous systems, but also in the so-called cross-talk between nerves and the immune system by acting through its specific receptor, named neurokinin 1 (NK-1r). Interestingly, in a recent report Shrikhande *et al.*[20] demonstrated the significant correlation between NK-1r and the clinical-pathological findings in chronic pancreatitis patients. In this study quantitative PCR was used to determine the NK-1r mRNA expression levels, *in situ* hybridization and immunohistochemistry were used to localize expression sites of NK-1r mRNA and protein, respectively. In chronic pancreatitis samples, NK-1r mRNA expression and protein were localized mainly in the nerves, ganglia, blood vessels, inflammatory cells and occasionally in fibroblasts. Once again there was a significant relationship between NK-1r mRNA levels and intensity, frequency and duration of pain in chronic pancreatitis patients, but not with the degree of tissue inflammation. The expression of NK-1r in inflammatory cells and blood vessels also points to an interaction of immunoreactive SP nerves, inflammatory cells and blood vessels, and further supports the existence of a neuroimmune interaction that probably influences the pain syndrome and chronic inflammatory changes of chronic pancreatitis. Indeed, mechanisms that are involved in the interaction between inflammatory cells, nerves and ganglia – the neuroimmune cross-talk – are not yet fully clarified. Different cytokines have been shown to interact with SP in various paradigms for pain and inflammation. Interleukin-1 and SP were shown to increase synergistically the proliferation of a fibroblast cell line, and SP directly stimulates the release of interleukin-8 (IL-8) from macrophages. Inasmuch as IL-8 release also generates hyperalgesia by stimulation of post-ganglionic sympathetic neurons, these observations strongly suggest that neuropeptides and cytokines might be involved in the pathophysiology of inflammatory disorders and might contribute to the ongoing inflammation and destruction of the exocrine pancreas in chronic pancreatitis. In fact, in chronic pancreatitis tissue samples from patients with chronic pancreatitis a significant increase of IL-8 mRNA was found.[21] It was mainly present in macrophages surrounding the enlarged pancreatic nerves, but also in the remaining acinar cells of the exocrine parenchyma and often in the metaplastic ductal cells. This was associated with a positive correlation between the inflammatory score and the presence of ductal metaplasia in chronic pancreatitis tissue samples and IL-8 mRNA level of expression.

The pro-inflammatory cytokine IL-8 is a well-known a-chemokine involved in leukocyte recruitment and activation and it is representative of a family of factors. The reported findings in the literature on interaction of substance P and IL-8, in combination with what is reported in chronic pancreatitis, lead us to hypothesize that the increased mRNA expression of IL-8 in chronic pancreatitis could be in part mediated by substance P, released from sensory pancreatic nerves. This speculation is supported by considering that the major source of IL-8 is especially in those inflammatory cells present around the enlarged nerves in the so-called inflammatory foci. Thus, the induction of IL-8 in immune cells by SP might contribute to the amplification of the inflammatory process in chronic pancreatitis. In addition, the presence of IL-8 in the remaining exocrine pancreatic parenchyma, suggest the fascinating hypothesis of an intrinsic maintenance of the inflammatory response after the first damage to the pancreatic gland, thus sustaining disease progression and evolution.

Currently there exist we have recorded several hypotheses on pain pathophysiology in chronic pancreatitis. Indeed we have to admit that the data available on possible mechanisms of pain generation in chronic pancreatitis, implicate the involvement of neuropeptides released from enteric and sensory afferent neurons and their functional interactions with inflammatory cells in the pathogenesis of both pain generation and chronic inflammation of the pancreas. Taken together, the present data provides evidence for neuroimmune cross-talk in the pathogenesis of pain and inflammation in chronic pancreatitis. Although further studies are needed to clarify this interaction.

References

1. Beger HG, Büchler M, Malfertheiner P, eds. Standards in pancreatic surgery. New York: Springer-Verlag 1993; 41–46.
2. Wharshaw AL, Banks PA, Fernanfez-Del Castillo C. AGA Technical review: treatment of pain in chronic pancreatitis. Gastroenterology 1998; 115:765–776.
3. Beger HG, Krautzberger W, Bittner R, et al. Duodenum-preserving resection of the head of the pancreas in patients with severe chronic pancreatitis. Surgery 1985; 97:467–473.
4. Bradley EL 3d. Pancreatic duct pressure in chronic pancreatitis. Am J Surg 1982; 144:313–316.
5. Ebbehoj N. Pancreatic tissue fluid pressure and pain in chronic pancreatitis. Dan Med Bull 1992; 39:128–133.
6. Ebbehoj N, Borly L, Bulow J, et al. Pancreatic tissue fluid pressure in chronic pancreatitis. Relation to pain, morphology, and function. Scand J Gastroenterol 1990; 25:1046–1051.
7. Manes G, Buchler M, Pieramico O, et al. Is increased pancreatic pressure related to pain in chronic pancreatitis? Int J Pancreatol 1994; 15:113–117.
8. Ebbehoj N, Borly L, Madsen P, et al. Pancreatic tissue fluid pressure during drainage operations for chronic pancreatitis. Scand J Gastroenterol 1990; 25:1041–1045.
9. Kloppel G. Pathology of chronic pancreatitis and pancreatic pain. Acta Chir Scand 1990; 156:261–265.
10. Di Sebastiano P, Friess H, di Mola FF, et al. Mechanisms of pain in chronic pancreatitis. Ann Ital Chir 2000; 71:11–16.
11. Malfertheiner P, Buchler M, Stanescu A, et al. Pancreatic morphology and function in relationship to pain in chronic pancreatitis. Int J Pancreatol 1987; 2:59–66.
12. Ihse I, Borch K, Larsson J. Chronic pancreatitis: results of operations for relief of pain. World J Surg 1990; 14:53–58.
13. Keith RG, Keshavjee SH, Kerenyi NR. Neuropathology of chronic pancreatitis in humans. Can J Surg 1985; 28:207–211.
14. Bockman DE, Buchler M, Malfertheiner P, et al. Analysis of nerves in chronic pancreatitis. Gastroenterology 1988; 94:1459–1469.
15. Buchler M, Weihe E, Friess H, et al. Changes in peptidergic innervation in chronic pancreatitis. Pancreas 1992; 7:183–192.
16. Fink T, Di Sebastiano P, Büchler M, et al. Growth associated protein-43 and protein gene product 9.5 innervation in human pancreas: changes in chronic pancreatitis. Neuroscience 1994; 63:249–266.
17. Di Sebastiano P, Fink T, Weihe E, et al. Immune cell infiltration and growth-associated protein 43 expression correlate with pain in chronic pancreatitis. Gastroenterology 1997; 112:1648–1655.
18. Friess H, Zhu ZW, di Mola FF, et al. Nerve growth factor and its high affinity receptor in chronic pancreatitis. Ann Surg 1999; 230:615–624.
19. Di Sebastiano P, Weihe E, di Mola FF, et al. Neuroimmune appendicitis. Lancet 1999; 7; 354:461–466.
20. Shrikande S, Friess H, di Mola FF, et al. NK-1 receptor gene expression is related to pain in chronic pancreatitis. Pain 2001; 91:209–217.
21. Di Sebastiano P, di Mola FF, Di Febbo C, et al. Expression of Interleukin-8 (IL-8) and Substance P in human chronic pancreatitis. Gut 2000; 47:423–428.

40 Bilateral Thoracoscopic Splanchnicectomy in the Management of Pain in Patients with Chronic Pancreatitis

Jan B.M.J. Jansen, H.C.J.L.Buscher, R. van Dongen, R.P. Bleichrodt and H. van Goor

In this chapter we demonstrates that five years after bilateral thoracoscopic splanchnicectomy, pain relief is obtained in about 40% of patients with chronic pancreatitis. Although these results are considerably less than those reported by other operative techniques, such as resection of an inflammatory mass in the head of the pancreas or pancreatic duct drainage according to Partington–Rochelle, bilateral thoracoscopic splanchnicectomy may have a place in the management of pain in patients with chronic pancreatitis for several reasons: First, the operative procedure is simple, has acceptable side effects and a very low mortality rate, especially when compared to the other operative techniques applied for pain relief in chronic pancreatitis. The procedure also requires considerably less operation time and hospital stay. Second, we have followed up our patients for a median time of five years, while most papers on operative techniques for pain relief in chronic pancreatitis reported shorter follow up, whereby success rates of other operative techniques may also drop. Third, bilateral thoracoscopic splanchnicectomy is applicable to chronic pancreatitis patients without an inflammatory mass or without a dilated pancreatic duct and so may be used in patients who do not have indications for more traditional pancreatic procedures.

In about 80% of cases, chronic pancreatitis is complicated by pain.[1] In the early stages of the disease, pain is often present in episodes alternating with pain free periods (type A pain), whereas in the later stages of the disease, pain is often present continuously (type B pain). Pain in chronic pancreatitis is often so intense that patients become dependent on opiates. The pathophysiology of pain in chronic pancreatitis is not well understood. Many therapies for pain relief are based on decompression of the pancreatic duct, like the operation according to Partington–Rochelle, and stenting of the pancreatic duct, since ductal hypertension is believed to cause pain in chronic pancreatitis.[2–6] However in chronic pancreatitis patients without pain, ductal pressure is also found to be increased.[7] More recent data on the pathophysiology of pain in chronic pancreatitis has pointed to abnormalities in nerve sheets with increased concentrations of neuropeptides, such as substance-P and calcitonin gene related peptide.[8] It is believed that a considerable part of pain sensation is conducted through autonomic nerve fibers of the sympathetic nervous system assembling in the celiac ganglion and subsequently running into the splanchnic nerves.[9] This motivated us to attack these splanchnic nerves surgically in chronic pancreatitis patients in an attempt to manage type B pain.

Patients and Methods

From 1995 to 2000, 44 patients (26 men, 18 women) with chronic pancreatitis underwent bilateral thoracoscopic splanchnicectomy (TS). The mean age of the patients was 41 (range 15–63) years. The diagnosis chronic pancreatitis was based on conventional criteria.[10] At the time of operation, no pseudocysts were demonstrable in any patients. Twenty-one patients had neither a pancreatic mass in the head of the pancreas, nor a dilated pancreatic duct. In four patients the diameter of the main pancreatic duct was > 4 mm, and five patients had an enlarged (> 4 cm) pancreatic head on CT. Pancreatic surgery was performed previously in 21 patients. In five of these patients a duodenum preserving resection of the head of the pancreas (Beger operation) was performed, in three patients a Partington–Rochelle procedure was performed, while the remaining nine patients had a resection of the tail of the pancreas for pseudocyst. Papilloplasty (three), biliodigestive bypass (two) and pseudocyst drainage (three) had been performed in the remaining patients. Endoscopic drainage of the pancreatic duct by means of a plastic stent, in an attempt to decrease pain, had been performed in eight patients. Two patients had undergone neurolytic coeliac plexus blockade unsuccessfully.

The median interval between the onset of pancreatitis and bilateral thoracoscopic splanchnicectomy was 4.6 (range 1.4–14.8) years. In 24 patients alcohol consumption was considered to be the cause of pancreatitis, in four patients a pancreas divisum was found, four patients had hereditary pancreatitis, and in two patients trauma was considered to be the cause of pancreatitis. In ten patients the cause of pancreatitis was unknown. Thirty-four patients were referred from other hospitals.

Data on pain and pain medication were collected prospectively during regular outpatient visits before and after splanchnicectomy. Pain was scored on visual analogue scales (VAS; zero: no pain, 10: intractable pain). Use of medication was noted and divided into three groups: (1) no medication, or intermittent pain medication, (2) acetaminophen (paracetamol)or non-steroidal anti-inflammatory drugs (NSAIDs) and, (3) opioids. Failure of treatment was defined as persistence of pain needing additional therapy after operation or recurrence of pain necessitating the same or increased amounts of analgesics compared with the pre-operative situation. Pain scores were compared by Wilcoxon's signed rank sum test. Differences were considered of statistical significance when p was <0.05. Pain relief was analysed by the life-table method. Endpoints of follow up were failure of treatment, death or end-of-observation period.

The surgical procedure and early results have been described previously.[11]

Results

The median follow up was 5.1 (range 3.2–8.0) years. Twenty-two patients were followed up for five years or more. The median pre-operative VAS-score was

8.5 (range 7–10). Thirty-six patients required opioids pre-operatively. Median duration of opioid use was 38 (range 6–84) months.

Splanchnicectomy was technically successful in 40 patients, four patients had severe pleural adhesions on one or both sides due to pulmonary complications of acute necrotizing pancreatitis or after surgery. Transient pain lasting for 1–3 days related to cannula insertion was experienced by almost all patients. Three patients had intercostal neuralgia persisting for a longer period of time. Pre-operative aspiration of gastric contents occurred in one patient. In two patients pneumotharax required drainage. One patient had a wound infection and one patient had pneumonia. No deaths occurred. Median hospital stay was four (range 1–10) days. Despite pain related to cannula insertion, all patients reported significant pain relief immediately after surgery. Pain recurred within 6 months in 11 patients, and in another six between 6 and 12 months.

There were 19 patients with long-term failure. Re-administration of opiates was necessary in these patients at 15 (range 2–55) months after surgery. Nine patients required NSAID's for pain control, while 16 patients were free of pain. The VAS score of patients free of pain was 1.6 (range 0–3.1). The mean VAS-score of patients taking opiates or NSAIDs was 4.2 (range 1.1–8.6). Nine patients under went pancreatic surgery after TS (one distal pancreatectomy, four Partington–Rochelle procedures, Bour beger opeartions).Three patients died. One died from gastric cancer one year after thoracoscopic splanchnectomy: this patient had only mild epigastric discomfort at nine months follow-up, compared to severe pain before operation. One patient died from pulmonary insufficiency three years after TS. This patient still required opiates for pain relief due to chronic pancreatitis. One patient died from complications of excessive alcohol abuse. There was no difference in failure rate between the nine patients with a dilated duct or a pancreatic mass and the 21 patients without these features. Sixteen of the 44 patients (36%) remained pain free after TS during the entire follow-up period. The median follow-up period of these 16 patients was 6.2 (range 3.8-7.7) years. Two of these patients developed exocrine and endocrine insufficiency during follow up. Seven of these 16 patients had undergone pancreatic surgery before TS (four distal pancreatectomies, three Beger procedures).

Seven patients were operated on their pancreas after TS (three Beger resections, three operations according to Partington–Rochelle and one distal pancreatectomy). Only two of these seven patients ultimately became independent of opioids.

Pain medication, before, at 6 months and at 5 years after operation is shown in Table 40.1.

Fig. 40.1 shows the cumulative probability of pain reduction after splanchnicectomy. Most failures occured within the first year after surgery. The probablity of pain relief five years after splanchnicectomy is approximately 40 %.

Discussion

This study demonstrates that shortly after bilateral thoracoscopic splanchnicectomy, pain relief is obtained in about 70% of chronic pancreatitis patients with continuous, type B, pain. However, when time elapses, failure rates of pain relief by this technique increases. Five years after bilateral thoracoscopic splanchnicectomy, the success rate has dropped to approximately 40%. This is far less than the results

Table 40.1. Pain medication before, at 6 months and at five years after bilateral thoracoscopic splanchnicectomy

	Before (n=44)	6 months (n=44)	5 (3.2–8.0) years (n=29)
Opiods	36	2	19
NSAID's and acetaminophen	8	10	9
No pain medication	0	22	16

reported by other operative techniques, such as resection of an inflammatory mass in the head of the pancreas or pancreatic duct drainage techniques.[12–14] Despite this considerably lower success rate in the long run, bilateral thoracoscopic splanchnicectomy may have a place in the management of pain in patients with chronic pancreatitis for several reasons: First, the operative procedure is simple and has acceptable side effects and no associated deaths, especially when compared to the other operative techniques applied for pain relief in chronic pancreatitis. The procedure also requires considerably less operation time and hospital stay. Second, we have followed up our patients for a median time of five years, while most papers on operative techniques for pain relief in chronic pancreatitis which report high success rates, have reported shorter follow up. Thus it might be that the success rate of these operations may also drop when time elapses. Third, TS is also applicable to chronic pancreatitis patients without an inflammatory mass or without a dilated pancreatic duct and finally, the majority of patients included in this study were referred to us from other clinics. This may have introduced bias in favour of more severe cases. This is also illustrated by the high number of patients that had pancreatic surgery or endoscopic drainage procedures

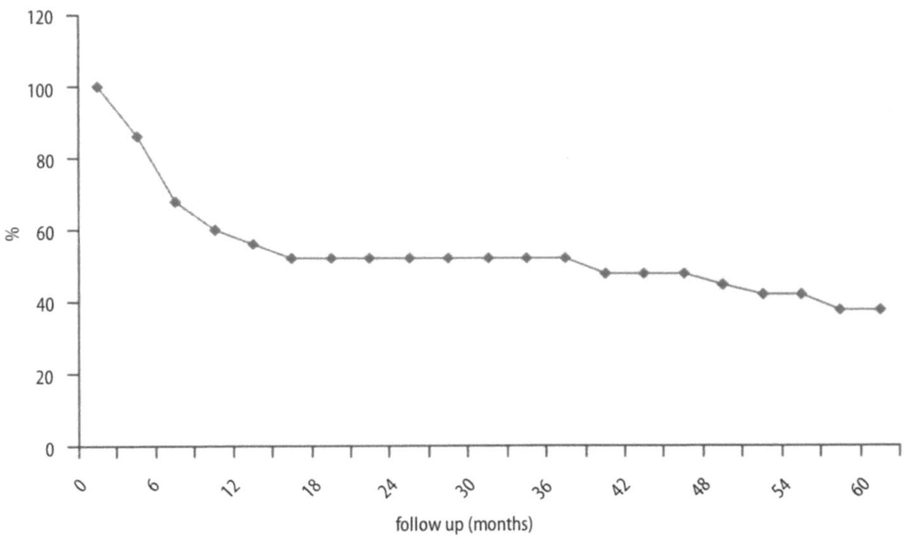

Figure 40.1. The cumulative probability of pain reduction after splanchnicectomy is depicted. Most failures occured within the first year after surgery. The probablity of pain relief five years after splanchnicectomy is approximately 40 %.

before TS and by the low success rate of traditional pancreatic surgery performed in seven patients that failed to respond adequately to TS.

During follow up, 60% of the patients had recurrent pain requiring daily administration of analgesics. There may be several explanations for pain recurrence. First, sympathetic nerves that are not cut during TS, may have taken over nociceptive transmission of pancreatic impulses. Second, parasympathetic innervation via the vagus nerve may carry pain signals from the pancreas. Based on this assumption, some authors advocate vagotomy in addition to splanchnicectomy.[15] The benefit of an additional vagotomy, however, has not clearly been demonstrated. Third patient selection as mentioned earlier may also have adversely influenced the outcome of this study. Despite this, we found the results of our study encouraging enough to advocate a randomised controlled trial to compare TS with conventional pancreatic surgery for pain relief in chronic pancreatitis.

References

1. Ammann RW, Akovbiantz A, Largiader F, et al. Course and outcome of chronic pancreatitis. Gastroenterology 1984; 86:820–8.
2. Bradley EL. Pancreatic duct pressure in chronic pancreatitis. Am J Surg 1982; 144:313–6.
3. Jalleh RP, Aslam M, Williamson RC. Pancreatic tissue and ductal pressures in chronic pancreatitis. Br J Surg 1991; 78:1235–7.
4. Okazaki K, Yamamoto Y, Kagiyama S, et al. Pressure of papillary sphincter zone and pancreatic main duct in patients with alcoholic and idiopathic chronic pancreatitis. Int J Pancreatol 1988; 3:457–68.
5. Raddai HM, Geenen JE, Hogan WJ, et al. Pressure measurements from biliary and pancreatic segments of sphincter of Oddi: comparison between patients with functional abdominal pain, biliary, or pancreatic disease. Dig Dis Sci 1991; 36:71–4.
6. Karanjia ND, Singh SM, Widdison AL, et al. Pancreatic ductal and interstitial pressures in cats with chronic pancreatitis. Dig Dis Sci 1992; 37:268–73.
7. Ebbehoj N, Borly L, Buelow J, et al. Pancreatic tissue fluid pressure in chronic pancreatitis: relation to pain, morphology and function. Scand J Gastroenterol 1990; 25:1046–51.
8. Buechler M, Weihe E, Friess H, et al. Changes in peptidergic innervation in chronic pancrewatitis. Pancreas 1992; 7:183–92.
9. Mayer EA, Gebhart GF. Basic and clinical aspects of visceral hyperalgesia. Gastroenterology 1994; 107:271–93.
10. Imrie CW, Menezes N, Carter CR. Diagnosis of chronic pancreatitis and newer aspects of pain control. Digestion 1999; 60 (Suppl):111–3.
11. Buescher HCJL, Jansen JBMJ, van Dongen R, et al. Long-term results of bilateral thoracoscopic splanchnicectomy in patients with chronic pancreatitis. Br J Surg 2002; 89:158–62.
12. Beger HG, Buechler M, Bittner RR, et al. Duodenum-preserving resection of the head of the pancreas in severe chronic pancreatitis: early and late results. Ann Surg 1989; 209:273–8.
13. Sato T, Noto N, Matsuno S, et al. Follow-up results of surgical treatment for chronic pancreatitis: present status in Japan. Am J Surg 1981; 142:317–27.
14. Lankisch PG. Prognosis of chronic pancreatitis. In: The Pancreas vol 1. Edited by Hans G. Beger et al. Blackwell Science 1998; pp. 740–47.
15. Stone HH, Chauvin EJ. Pancreatic denervation for pain relief in chronic alcohol associated pancreatitis. Br J Surg 1990; 77:303–5.

41 Nerve Pathways for Pain

Dale E. Bockman

Pain is a common symptom in diseases of the exocrine pancreas. It may be severe. If it is longstanding and is not amenable to alleviation by drugs, attempts are made to interrupt the neural pathways that lead from the pancreas to central terminals where the pain is perceived.

Mechanisms of Pain

If only one kind of stimulus acted on pancreatic nerve endings to initiate a nerve impulse, if one nerve conducted the impulse to the central nervous system, if only one pathway conducted the information within the central nervous system to only one central area for the interpretation of pain, and if none of these changed with time, alleviation of pain in patients with pancreatic disease would not be so difficult.

Alleviation of pain is, however, difficult because of multiple ways for it to be generated, the likelihood of multiple peripheral and central pathways, and not least because of our incomplete understanding. "Pain is not a passive consequence of the transfer of a defined peripheral input to a pain center in the cortex, but an active process generated partly in the periphery and partly within the CNS by multiple plastic changes that together determine the gain of the system.".[1]

The Plasticity of the Nervous System

Plasticity is present in the nervous system at the systematic, cellular and molecular levels.[2] Investigators provide evidence of changes in the nervous system variously described as synaptic plasticity, neuronal plasticity, functional plasticity, supraspinal plasticity and central neural plasticity. There may be profound changes in primary sensory neurons throughout the life of an organism and these changes account for clinically relevant alterations of pain perception.[3] Modification of the pain system involves an increase in constitutively expressed genes as well as induction of novel genes, including substance P.[1] Both receptors and transmitters are modified in dorsal horn neurons.

Neurons may change not only their function and chemical profile, but also their structure. Peripheral nerve injury results in a redistribution of the central terminals of myelinated afferents.[4] Remodeling within the central nervous system causes the physical pathogenesis of chronic pain. In chronic pain the cortical and subcortical processing of nociceptive input is modified. Reorganization in the primary somatosensory cortex is an example of neuronal plasticity induced by chronic pain.[5]

The afferent input generated by injury and intense noxious stimuli triggers an increased excitability of nociceptive neurons in the spinal cord. With severe, long lasting pain perception there develops an increased sensibility of the spinal cord, a progression known as action potential windup.

Generation of Pain in the Pancreas

The afferent nerves of the pancreas normally are 'silent'. That is, the normal functions proceed without perception. Reflex activity for secretion and vascular control is carried out with participation by the central nervous system without coming to consciousness.

Pain is evoked by excess stimulation. The manner in which pain is generated has been described as nociceptive pain, in which there is direct activation of pain receptors in response to tissue injury, usually with inflammation, and neuropathic pain. Nociceptive pain is initiated in various ways. Noxious substances such as the multitude of biologically active substances that might permeate the interstitial space in acute pancreatitis might reasonably be expected to stimulate afferent nerve endings. Unusual duct distention might initiate action potentials by stretching nerves. Edema and inhibition of blood flow could lead to anoxia and pH outside the normal range, initiating impulses carried by pancreatic nerves.

Neuropathic pain results from direct injury to nerves. For example, pancreatic adenocarcinoma seems to have an affinity to nerves.[6] As the cancer cells proliferate, they commonly approach and continue along a pancreatic nerve. The cancer cells may replace the perineurium and invade the nerve proper, distorting and damaging nerve fibers.

A less obvious process by which pancreatic nerves are damaged is through chronic inflammation. It has been demonstrated in patients with chronic pancreatitis that foci of chronic inflammatory cells frequently are found in association with nerves. The perineurium, which normally separates the interior of the nerve from the outside, providing a specialized microenvironment, is breached.[7] The result is a damaged nerve in which the nerve fibers are subjected to the many biologically active substances of the outside environment, and possible continuous stimulation.

Chronically injured nerves transmit a substantial abnormal impulse barrage known as ectopic discharges. Spontaneous discharges originate not only at the nerve injury but also at the soma of dorsal root ganglion neurons.[8] Both allodynia (pain due to a stimulus that normally is innocuous) and hyperalgesia (increased response to a stimulus that normally is painful) appear during inflammation and neuropathy.

Treatment of Pain

The surgical therapies available to treat chronic pain include pancreatic duct drainage, pancreatectomy, or severance of the neural pathways through which the impulses are thought to be conducted, such as truncal vagotomy, splanchnicectomy, or destruction of the celiac plexus.[9–11]

Nerves Associated with the Pancreas

Four sets of peripheral nerves have terminals in and around the pancreas: splanchnic, vagus, spinal, and phrenic. Consideration of pain pathways from the pancreas has focused almost exclusively on the splanchnic nerves.

Splanchnic Nerves

Afferent fibers in the splanchnic nerves begin as free nerve endings in the pancreas. As they progress toward the outside of the pancreas they wind with other fibers along the periphery of blood vessels. Close to the origin of the celiac and superior mesenteric arteries from the aorta, the afferent fibers run through the celiac plexus without synapse. The splanchnic nerves traverse from abdominal to thoracic cavities, where their segments branch off one by one to join dorsal root ganglia segmentally. The cell bodies of the splanchnic nerves lie in the dorsal root ganglia. Centrally directed fibers then join the spinal cord.

Interrupting the discharges in the splanchnic nerves has found considerable success in relieving chronic pain resulting from chronic pancreatitis and pancreatic cancer. Injection of alcohol into the region of the celiac plexus frequently improves or eliminates pain, at least for a time. Surgical interruption of the splanchnic nerves has also proven effective.

Splanchnic nerve section has been accomplished in different ways. At times only the left splanchnic nerve is divided. At other times, bilateral section is performed. Earlier approaches tended to cut the nerves in the abdominal region, although some surgeons cut above the diaphragm. Thoracoscopic surgery has been used more recently to identify and interrupt the splanchnic nerves or their segmental connections as they approach the sympathetic chain and has proved a relatively efficient approach.[12] Le Pimpec Barthes *et al.*[13] performed thoracoscopic splanchnicectomy on 20 patients. Pain was reported totally relieved in 10/11unilateral operations, 2/5 unilateral with associated vagotomy, and 4/4 bilateral.

Stone and Chauvin[10] treated patients with pain from chronic pancreatitis with left transthoracic splanchnicectomy with concomitant bilateral truncal vagotomy. Each patient experienced almost immediate pain relief. Five had return of pain, only in the right epigastrium. These five underwent right transthoracic splanchnicectomy, after which four noted complete and apparently permanent disappearance of pain.[10]

All of these approaches have proved effective in many patients. None has provided complete relief to all patients. The latter observation would seem to bring into question the extent of our understanding of pancreas-generated pain. More specifically, it brings into question the possibility of additional pathways for pancreatic pain.

There is little direct evidence for the participation of the vagus, spinal, and/or phrenic nerves in the transmission of pancreatic pain. However, given the uncertainty raised by the inability to relieve chronic pancreatic pain in all patients all of the time, it would seem reasonable to explore the possibility that nerves other than the splanchnics are involved. A first approach would be to determine if there is evidence that the afferent fibers in these nerves carry information interpreted as pain.

Vagus Nerve

Afferent fibers of the vagus nerve begin in the connective tissue of the pancreas, pass along the outside of arteries with other nerve fibers, traverse the celiac plexus without synapse, then progress cranially to their cell bodies located in the nodose or jugular nuclei. Centrally directed fibers then join the brainstem.

There is good evidence for a role of vagal afferents in nociception.[14] Facial pain is perceived by patients with lung cancer, the transmission presumably traveling through the vagus.[15] Facial pain as a symptom of lung cancer is presumed to be due to local invasion of the vagus nerve,[16] a process similar to that described for neuropathic pain generated in the pancreas. Pain resulting from hiatal hernia, angina, or myocardial infarction apparently may result in part from stimulation of the vagus.[17-19] Direct electrical stimulation of the vagus nerve, as a treatment for epilepsy, has led to severe pharyngeal pain.[20]

Hoyes *et al.*[21] studied afferent axons of neurons whose cell bodies were located in the nodose ganglion of the vagus nerve. These axons had terminals that resembled those which have been defined as pain afferents in ureter, cornea, and lung. Traub *et al.*[22] determined that noxious visceral input is carried via vagal afferent fibers when they found that distention of the stomach induced c-Fos in the nucleus of the solitary tract.

Bon *et al.* [23,24] have suggested that the dorsal vagal complex, where upper gastrointestinal vagal reflexes are integrated, could be the main hindbrain visceral pain center. They indicate that the fact that the dorsal vagal complex is the only hindbrain region to be differentially and maximally driven by visceral inflammatory inputs and whose activity coincided with that of the spinal cord makes it the best candidate for being the structure where both pain-related autonomic reflexes and visceral pain sensation are initially generated.

Other Nerves

The segmental spinal nerves supply the body wall and the parietal peritoneum. The pancreas is retroperitoneal, therefore it is situated close to some of the terminal branches of spinal nerves.

The phrenic nerves originate from the third and fourth cervical nerves. The terminal branches of the phrenic nerves pass through the diaphragm and are distributed on the abdominal surface to supply the diaphragm muscle and sensory fibers to the peritoneum. A branch communicates with the phrenic plexus, which in turn communicates with the celiac plexus.

Segawa *et al.*[25] have indicated that nociceptive neural information during upper abdominal surgery is conveyed by the sensory fibers included in the thoracic and lumbar spinal nerves that innervate the abdominal wall and the intra-abdominal viscera, and by the phrenic nerves that innervate the diaphragm.

Aida *et al.* (1999)[26] have suggested that in operations involving laparotomy (such as gastrectomy), viscero-peritoneal nociception is involved in postsurgical pain because the abdominal viscera and peritoneum are innervated by the vagus and/or phrenic nerves and by the spinal nerves. This suggests involvement of the brainstem and cervical spinal cord via the vagus and phrenic nerves.

Although the spinal and phrenic nerves may not be considered primary for the conduction of pancreatic pain, it remains possible that in time they may be incorporated into a complex of nerves providing discharges that converge in the central nervous system. It is likely that these nerves respond when pathological changes extend beyond the boundaries of the pancreas.

The likelihood that nerves in addition to the splanchnics are involved in pancreatic pain is shown by the observations of Bradley *et al.*[27] who showed that patients with somatic pain, predicted by differential epidural analgesia, were not helped by splanchnicectomy. In these cases the pain information may have been carried in part through the spinal nerves.

Central Pathways

Although it has been assumed that nociceptive signals arising from the viscera reached the brain via the spinothalamic tract, the primary ascending somatosensory pathway in the ventrolateral white matter of the spinal cord, evidence is accumulating that nociceptive information relayed to the thalamus is carried in the dorsal columns of the spinal cord. Ascending axons travel through the dorsal columns to synapse in the dorsal column nuclei. Neurons in the dorsal column nuclei in turn activate neurons in the contralateral ventral posterolateral nucleus of the thalamus through the medial lemniscus.[11]

Pain relief has been obtained in patients with unremitting lower abdominal and pelvic pain by interrupting tracts in the dorsal columns. The interruption was accomplished first by inserting a 16 gauge hypodermic needle 5 mm into the spinal cord immediately on each side of the midline.[28] The technique was altered to use a fine forceps which was inserted so the points were approximately 1 mm on either side of the midline, then closing the forceps to crush the axons.[29]

Animal studies support the presence of a 'pain pathway' through the dorsal columns, including modification of responses to upper abdominal pain by interrupting the pathway. Ascending visceral input from thoracic levels travels more laterally than that arising at sacral levels.

A dorsal column lesion at the cervical level in rats produced by a hypodermic needle significantly decreased responses of ventrobasal thalamic neurons and behavioral changes (writhing) in response to distension of the duodenum.[30]

Recent experimental studies demonstrate that nociceptive information about the pancreas is transmitted from the spinal cord through the dorsal columns.[11] Signals were recorded in the thalamus as bradykinin was applied to the pancreas through a cannula. Lesions of the dorsal column caused a decrease in electrical response in the thalamus, and a change in behavioral response to bradykinin.

How is it possible for unilateral splanchnicectomy to help some patients and not others? Similarly, why might bilateral splanchnicectomy not help some patients? The answer may lie in a process of summation of the discharges that arrive in a critical part of the brain. If numbers arriving through each of the pathways from the pancreas are insufficient to trigger what is interpreted as pain, the total arriving might be sufficient. In that case, interrupting one nerve might cause a decrease below the pain threshold. If, however, a nerve carrying sufficient discharges necessary to cause pain remained intact and other nerves were cut, pain might continue.

Additional observations about the possible contributions of different peripheral nerves, and about the central routes which may be taken to relay information from the pancreas, could help improve approaches to controlling chronic pancreatic pain.

References

1. Woolf CJ, Salter MW. Neuronal plasticity: Increasing the gain in pain. Science 2000; 288:1765–1768.
2. Zimmermann M, Herdegen T. Plasticity of the nervous system at the systematic, cellular and molecular levels: a mechanism of chronic pain and hyperalgesia. Prog Brain Res 1996; 110:233–259.
3. Koltzenburg M. The changing sensitivity in the life of the nociceptor. Pain 1999; 6:S93–102.
4. Woolf CJ, Shortland P, Coggeshall RE. Peripheral nerve injury triggers central sprouting of myelinated afferents. Nature 1992; 355:75–77.
5. Wiech K, Preissl H, Birbaumer N. Neural networks and pain processing. New insights from imaging techniques. [German] Anaesthesist 2001; 50:2–12.
6. Bockman DE, Büchler M, Beger HG. Interaction of pancreatic ductal adenocarcinoma with nerves leads to nerve damage. Gastroenterology 1994; 107:219–230.
7. Bockman DE, Büchler M, Malfertheiner P, et al. Analysis of nerves in chronic pancreatitis. Gastroenterology 1988; 94:1459–1469.
8. Kumazawa T. Primitivism and plasticity of pain–implications of polymodal receptors. Neurosci Res 1998; 32:9–31.
9. White TT, Lawinski M, Stacher G, et al. Treatment of pancreatitis by left splanchnicectomy and celiac ganglionectomy. Analysis of 146 cases. Am J Surg 1966; 112:95–99.
10. Stone HH, Chauvin EJ. Pancreatic denervation for pain relief in chronic alcohol associated pancreatitis. Brit J Surg 1990; 77:303–305.
11. Houghton AK, Wang CC, Westlund KN. Do nociceptive signals from the pancreas travel in the dorsal column? Pain 2001; 89:207–220.
12. Ihse I, Zoucas E, Gyllstedt E, et al. Bilateral thoracoscopic splanchnicectomy: effects on pancreatic pain and function. Ann Surg 1999; 230:785–790.
13. Le Pimpec Barthes F, Chapuis O, Riquet M, et al. Thoracoscopic splanchnicectomy for control of intractable pain in pancreatic cancer. Ann Thoracic Surg 1998; 65:810–813.
14. Berthoud H, Neuhuber WL. Functional and chemical anatomy of the afferent vagal system. Autonomic Neuroscience-Basic and Clinical 2000; 85:1–17.
15. Bindoff LA, Heseltine D. Unilateral facial pain in patients with lung cancer: a referred pain via the vagus? Lancet 1988; i:812–815.
16. Capobianco DJ. Facial pain as a symptom of nonmetastatic lung cancer. Headache 1995; 35:581–585.
17. Blau JN. Ear pain referred by the vagus. BMJ 1989; 299:1569–1570.
18. Meller ST, Gebhart GF. A critical review of the afferent pathways and the potential chemical mediators involved in cardiac pain. Neuroscience 1992; 48:501–524.
19. Rothwell PM. Angina and myocardial infarction presenting with pain confined to the ear. Postgrad Med J 1993; 69:300–301.
20. Duhaime AC, Melamed S, Clancy RR. Tonsillar pain mimicking glossopharyngeal neuralgia as a complication of vagus nerve stimulation: case report. Epilepsia 2000; 41:903–905.
21. Hoyes AD, Barber P, Jagessar H. Location in the nodose ganglion of the perikarya of neurons whose axons distribute in the epithelium of the rat trachea. J Anat 1982; 134:265–271.
22. Traub RJ, Sengupta JN, Gebhart GF. Differential c-fos expression in the nucleus of the solitary tract and spinal cord following noxious gastric distention in the rat. Neuroscience 1996; 74:873–884.
23. Bon K, Lanteri-Minet M, de Pommery J. Cyclophosphamide cystitis as a model of visceral pain in rats. A survey of hindbrain structures involved in visceroception and nociception using the expression of c-Fos an Krox-24 proteins. Exper Brain Res 1996; 108:404–416.

24. Bon K, Lanteri-Minet M, Michiels JF, et al. Cyclophosphamide cystitis as a model of visceral pain in rats: a c-fos and Krox-24 study at telencephalic levels, with a not on pituitary adenylate cyclase activating polypeptide (PACAP). Exper Brain Res 1998; 122:165–174.
25. Segawa H, Mori K, Kasai K, et al. The role of phrenic nerves in stress response in upper abdominal surgery. Anesth Analg 1996; 82:1215–1224.
26. Aida S, Baba H, Yamakura T, et al. The effectiveness of preemptive analgesia varies according to the type of surgery: a randomized, double-blind study. Anesth Analg 1999; 89:711–716.
27. Bradley EL 3rd, Reynhout JA, Peer GL. Thoracopic splanchnicectomy for "small duct" chronic pancreatitis: case selection by differential epidural analgesia. J Gastrointest Surg 1998; 2:88–94.
28. Nauta HJW, Hewitt E, Westlund KN, et al. Surgical interruption of a midline dorsal column visceral pain pathway. J Neurosurg 1997; 86:538–542.
29. Nauta HJW, Soukup VM, Fabian RH, et al. Punctate midline myelotomy for the relief of visceral cancer pain. J Neurosurg (Spine 2) 2000; 92:125–130.
30. Feng Y, Cui M, Al-Chaer ED, et al. Epigastric antinociception by cervical dorsal column lesions in rats. Anesthesiology 1998; 89:411–420.

42 Pain Management in Chronic Pancreatitis

Catherine Price

Universally it is stated that the pain of chronic pancreatitis is very difficult to treat. There are many differing issues that may make it so. This chapter explores some of these issues, looks at current United Kingdom practice and suggests some possible solutions.

In order to understand why chronic pancreatitis is difficult to treat, it may be just as important to look at the process of care as at the pathophysiological processes that are thought to occur in chronic pancreatitis. There have been tremendous advances in the understanding of the neurobiology of chronic pain in the past 10 years. Both the functioning of nociceptive pathways and how the brain deals with pain have been investigated. However, putting research into practice has been less spectacular and problems with developing coherent treatment packages are all too frequent.[1]

Pathophysiology of Pain in Chronic Pancreatitis

A highly complex set of changes may occur. Pain is multifactorial and patients may have greatly differing changes which may explain the variety of treatment responses. It is important to look at the state of the pancreas, its potential for pain generation and the state of the pain system after continued bombardment by noxious input. The pancreas becomes chronically inflamed and fibrosis occurs. Pain may occur because of persistent inflammation or because of obstruction of pancreatic ducts.[2] Locally increased pressure may occur with pseudocysts. Perineural scarring may also occur. Eventually the inflammation subsides and the pancreas is small and fibrosed. The mechanism of pain is multifactorial. There is increased intraductal pressure, interstitial hypertension, pancreatic ischaemia and neuronal inflammation.[3] The pathophysiology of chronic inflammation and pain generation in CP is not clear and is still under investigation. Substance P may itself have a role in further inflammation.[4]

Changes in the pain system may be profound. Normally the pain pathways are subject to modulation by peripheral and central mechanisms. However, during continued bombardment through inflammatory mediators, mechanical distension and possible nerve injury, the pain system undergoes peripheral and central sensitisation (Fig 42.1). Brain Derived Neurotrophic Factor has been found to be upregulated around pancreatic cells which may further contribute to the neuropathic pain in this condition.[5]

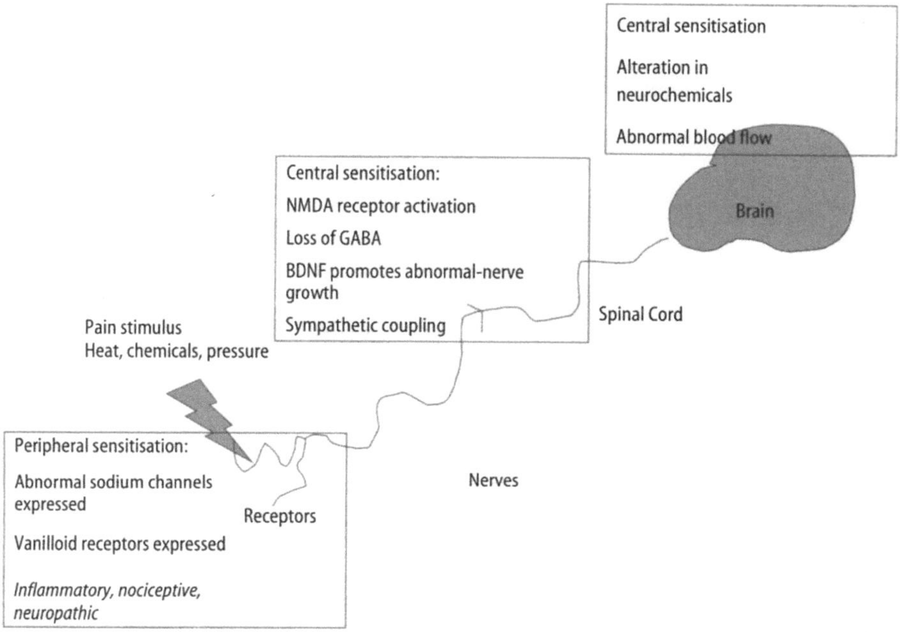

Figure 42.1. Some of the changes that occur in the central nervous system in chronic pain.

Voltage-gated sodium channels may be as important in visceral pain as they have been found to be in somatic pain. In inflammatory type pain, tetrado-toxin (TTX)-resistant sodium channels increase at the nociceptor. In nerve injury pain these channels decrease with an increase in TTX sensitive channels.

Visceral hyperalgesia is mediated centrally. Spinal cord neurons are increased in excitability. Perception of visceral stimuli depends on the temporal and spatial summation, there is considerable central plasticity of the threshold for the perception of visceral pain.[6] With continued bombardment of the central nervous system these thresholds decrease so that lack of descending modulation occurs.

Thus, through a process of peripheral and central sensitisation the pancreas may no longer be the cause of the pain itself. Instead the pain has become embedded within the nervous system. This leads to considerable confusion for both the patient and health care professional.

Psychology of Pancreatic Pain

Pain psychology in general looks at the way a person is thinking about their pain and how that influences their management of their pain. This approach then seeks to correct unhelpful biases in thinking by seeking alternative hypotheses that the patient can explore and arrive at a more helpful way of thinking about their pain. To take a dichotomous view of pain, that it is either physically based or psychologically based, creates an artificial distinction between mind and body which helps no-one, not least the patient.

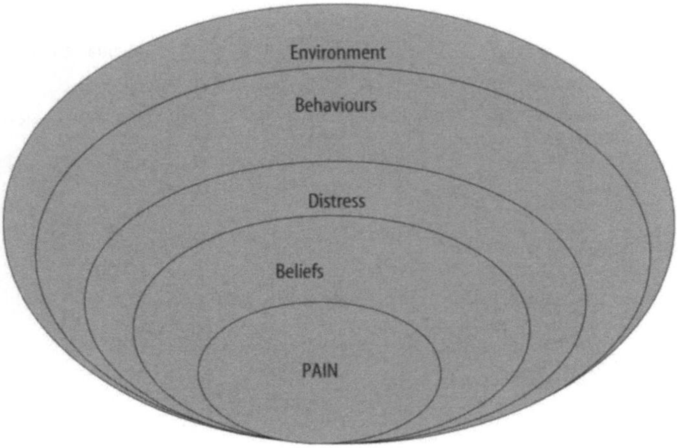

Figure 42.2. Biopsychosocial model of pain.

Pain is subject to behavioural, social learning, affective and cognitive factors (Fig. 42.2) in addition to the biomedical influences that caused the pain to begin with.[7] This is particularly so when the pain has gone on for some time. Emotional distress in pain patients may be due to a number of factors such as fear, inadequate or maladaptive support systems, iatrogenic complications, overuse of analgesics, inability to work, financial difficulties, prolonged litigation, disruption of usual activities and sleep disturbance. In addition the inability of medicine to adequately explain and provide evidence of a painful condition leads to the patient feeling disbelieved, compounding the distress already felt. Pain is such an aversive stimulus that the overriding desire to terminate pain is highly destructive. It can produce fear and ultimately depression and the lack of a will to live. Living with persistent pain requires considerable emotional resilience and external support.

In chronic pancreatitis there are additional problems. Often the only effective analgesics have been narcotics, the patient may have developed pancreatitis through alcohol dependency and there may be a pre-existing poor staff patient relationship.[8]

Addictive behaviour may be therefore common. If anxiety or depression is present this then compounds the problem, as does the use of placebos in a misguided attempt to wean the patient off analgesics. Addictive behaviour in chronic pain is difficult to diagnose as many of the DSM III-R criteria to meet this are physical and can equally be applied to the needs of someone with persistent pain.[9] Suicide attempts and self-injury behaviour are frequent.

Diagnosis

Diagnosis in chronic pain is along an axial diagnosis.[10] It is by site, aetiology, systems affected, pain intensity and possible mechanisms involved. In addition, factors that tend to maintain pain such as depression, anxiety, and deconditioning must be sought. Various standard questionnaires are available. The factors involved in pancreatitis may differ from one case to another. Multiple mechanisms may be involved such as interstitial hypertension, pancreatic ischaemia, nerve inflammation and increased ductal pressure may be involved.[11] It is important to delineate which factors are present in order to formulate a treatment plan for management of the pain.

Management

Approach to the Patient

In dealing with chronic pain one has to deal with both the cause (which may be the pain itself rather than any tissue fault) and its effects. The biopsychosocial model is the most heuristic for dealing with chronic pain problems.[12]

Management of chronic pancreatitis involves consideration of tissue-based generators of pain as well as traditional pain management interventions (Fig. 42.3). Antioxidants and low fat diet have been described.

Coeliac plexus blockade is popular in cancer pain although its efficacy in chronic pancreatitis is far from established.[11,13,14] Phenol blockade appears to offer no benefit over local anaesthetic blockade as pain returns due to central neuroplasticity. The advantages of blockade are that it offers temporary pain relief and thus time out from the pain. The disadvantages are that there may be serious complications due to the position of the coeliac ganglion near to major viscera and vessels and that a patient may become reliant on blockade as the sole method of dealing with pain rather than developing alternative coping strategies.

There appears to be little evidence to support the use of transcutaneous nerve stimulation and acupuncture.[15] In addition there is little information on the use of neuropathic pain medication.

Suggested Plan
Chronic pancreatitis
? Pain
Evidence that stricture present/inflammation
No Systemic upset
Pancreatitis
Disease management
Diet
Alcohol free
Surgery
Antioxidants
Pain flare-up
View as separate problem
Pain diagnosis
Pain effects
Flare-up plan

Figure 42.3. Suggested flow chart for management of pancreatitis pain.

Use of Opioids

Opioids are highly effective in chronic pancreatitis. However, the difficulties with their use are great including establishing appropriate use and building a degree of trust between the patient and health care professionals. Opioids may need careful review as the m and k receptors show considerable heterogeneity in their affinity for various opioids. It has been shown that opioid substitution may mean that either side-effects or effect are helped considerably.[16] The opioids used were morphine, oxycodone, methadone and transdermal fentanyl.

In managing patients on long term opioids who become highly distressed requiring hospital admission the following have been suggested:

- suicide risk should be evaluated
- the presence of any co-morbid psychiatric diseases should be established
- misconceptions of opiate analgesics among medical staff should be discussed
- poor staff–patient relationships should be managed aggressively
- factors causing a vicious cycle in pain control be identified

Above all the term addiction should be avoided.[8]

Dealing with Chronic Pain

General pain management principles should be applied. These include an explanation of chronic pain, difficulties in getting it to fit with a traditional biomedical perspective (in that there are no easily accessible investigations to confirm a diagnosis of chronic pain) and adoption of a self-management plan encouraged. Time-contingent analgesia should be instituted. General physical fitness combined with pacing (performance of a task in bite sized chunks) should be discussed. Flare up plans should be made which include distinguishing a flare-up of chronic pain from a flare–up of pancreatitis. This is hard when the principal symptom of both is pain, and nausea and vomiting may accompany both!

If secondary deconditioning is present and the patient is reluctant to engage in exercise then referral to physiotherapy is appropriate for graded exercise and stretch.

High distress and resistance to adoption of a self-management plan is best managed by interdisciplinary cognitive behavioural therapy or a pain management programme supervised by a clinical psychologist. Occasionally involvement of a psychiatrist is necessary for those at risk of self-harm.

Analysis of the National Chronic Pain Database reveals that pancreatitis accounts for only a small number of patients attending a pain clinic (74 of 12 000). There is a high fall off between assessment and re-visit. Very few patients are discharged. The majority of patients receive coeliac plexus blockade. The most common drug treatments are strong opioids and tricyclic analgesics. One third of patients undergo a pain management programme.

Overall, attendance at a pain clinic tends to improve physical measures and sleep, has little effect on psychological functioning, and pain intensity is unaltered. There appears to be substantial room for improvement. The outcomes for pain management programmes are not available. The small numbers coming into pain clinics make it hard to conduct any randomised controlled trials. Pain clinic methods might be better introduced at an earlier stage although this is often hard to implement.

The Future

The best form of treatment is multi-professional, where all parties have a good understanding of the disease and can plan interventions on a rational basis. Systems where a practitioner works in isolation are unlikely to be maximally effective. Crisis admissions should be recognised as often inevitable and should be planned for. The scope of investigations during those admissions should be clear. Rehabilitation should be encouraged at the outset in order to maximise quality of life for what is a difficult and often frustrating disease to manage.

References

1. Apte Minoti V, Keogh, Gregory W, et al. J Clin Gastroenterology October 1999; 29 (3):225–240.
2. Mergener K, Baillie J. Chronic Pancreatitis. Lancet 1997; 350:1379–1385.
3. Pitchumoni CS. Chronic pancreatitis: pathogenesis and management of pain. Gastroenterology 1999; 28; 2:109.
4. Di Sebastiano P, di Mola FF, Di Febbo C, et al. Expression of interleukin 8 (IL-8) and substance P in human chronic pancreatitis. Gut 2000; 47 (3):423–428.
5. Zhu ZW, Friess H, Wang L, et al. Brain Derived Neurotrophic Factor is upregulated and associated with pancreatitis. Dig Dis Sci 2001; 46; 8:1633–9.
6. Cervero F. Visceral hyperalgesia revisited. Lancet 2000; 356:1127–1128.
7. Gatchel RJ, Turk DC. Psychosocial Factors in Pain. Critical Perspectives. The Guilford Press, 1999.
8. Hung Ching-I, Liu Chia-Yih, Chen Ching-Yen, et al. Meperidine addiction or treatment frustration? General Hospital Psychiatry 2001; 23; 1:31–35.
9. Portenoy RJ. Opioid therapy in chronic non-malignant pain: a review of the critical issues. Pain and Symptom Management 1996; 11:203–17.
10. IASP taxonomy of terms. IASP press Seattle.
11. Pitchumoni CS. Chronic pancreatitis: pathogenesis and management of pain. Gastroenterol 1998; 27; 2:101–7.
12. Gatchel RJ. A biopsychosocial overview of pre-treatment screening of patients with pain. Clin J Pain 2001; 17:192–199.
13. Malfertheiner P, Dominguez-Munoz JE, Buchler MW. Chronic pancreatitis: management of pain. Digestion 1994; 55 (Suppl 1):29–34.
14. Vercauteren MP, Coppejans H, Adiaensen HA. Pancreatitis pain treatment: an overview. Acta Anaesthesiol Belg 1994; 45 (3):99–105.
15. Ballegaard S, Christophersen SJ, Dawids SG, et al. Acupuncture and transcutaneous nerve stimulation in the treatment of chronic pancreatitis. A randomised study. Scand J Gastroenterol 1985; 20:1249–54.
16. Quang-Cantagrel ND, Wallace MS, Magnuson SK. Opioid substitution to improve the effectiveness of chronic non cancer pain control: a chart review. Anaesth Analg 2000; 90:933–7.

43 Pancreatic Decompression in Chronic Pancreatitis

Claudio Bassi, Massimo Falconi, Roberto Salvia, Luca Casetti, Stefano Marcucci and Paolo Pederzoli

Chronic pancreatitis is a disease characterised by a dynamic course giving rise to fibrotic involution of the pancreatic parenchyma with a consequent progressive loss of both exocrine and endocrine function.

An excessive alcohol intake is universally accepted as being the most important risk factor for the onset of a pancreatic inflammatory process, though other factors, such as cigarette smoking and a high-fat diet also contribute to the aetiology of the disease along with organic and/or functional conditions which in some way chronically or recurrently obstruct the physiological outflow of the pancreas at the ampulla.[1]

Patients with chronic pancreatitis generally report a history of alcohol abuse and present recurrent abdominal pain that may develop into persistent pain associated with steatorrhoea, weight loss and diabetes. In some cases complications of adjacent organs are present as a result of the peripancreatic fibrosis itself or of the occurrence of pseudocysts which in turn give rise to the onset of jaundice and transit disorders.

The first approach to the patient with chronic pancreatitis is invariably medical and involves total abstention from alcohol consumption supported by pancreatic enzyme replacement therapy and the administration of analgesic drugs.

When the patient no longer responds to medical therapy, his or her condition becomes a matter for surgical care and this fact in itself implicitly signals the failure of medical therapy.

In the course of therapy, the endoscopist, in our opinion, plays an intermediate role. In view of the long clinical history of chronic pancreatitis, there is scope, in selected cases and in the context of a non-definitive temporary solution, for endoscopic and/or transcutaneous drainage of pseudocysts and for sphincterotomy with stenting of the main pancreatic duct. In chronic pancreatitis, we are against practice of indiscriminate stenting of the bile and pancreatic ducts.[2]

From an analysis of the literature[3,4] we find that from 30–60% of patients with chronic pancreatitis undergo surgical therapy in the course of their clinical history. The main indication for surgery is severe, disabling pain which no longer responds to drug therapy (pancreatic surgical target). There are also surgical indications relating to involvement of adjacent structures (extrapancreatic surgical targets) such as the presence of pancreatic pseudocysts, biliary or duodenal involvement, haemorrhage and the suspicion of pancreatic cancer. The presence of cystic dystrophy of the duodenal wall is, in our experience, also an indication for surgical treatment.[5]

The rationale underlying the decision to proceed with resective-type or anastomotic surgery depends primarily on the pancreatic and peripancreatic morphology and on the individual preference of the surgeon, based, in practical terms, on his personal convictions regarding the origin of the pancreatic pain in the course of the chronic disease. According to some surgeons[6] the pain stimulus due to the fibrosis can be eliminated only by removing pancreatic parenchyma, whereas others[7] believe that pancreatic decompression achieves the same result.

The aim of this chapter is to provide a retrospective assessment of our experience with anastomotic surgery in the treatment of chronic pancreatitis.

Surgical Patients and Procedures

Over the 10-year period from January 1989 to December 1999, 219 patients with chronic pancreatitis were submitted to surgery in our unit. Thirty-nine of these (17.8%) underwent resections and 180 (82.2 %) anastomotic procedures. This latter group constitutes our study population. In all cases, histology confirmed the diagnosis of chronic pancreatitis.

The 180 patients undergoing anastomotic surgery were 150 men and 30 women with a mean age of 39.6 ± 10.9 years, mean weight of 63.1 ± 11.1 kg, mean number of cigarettes smoked per day 20.1 ± 14.7 and mean daily alcohol intake 120.2 ± 104.5 g.

Table 43.1 summarises the preoperative morphological and clinical situations of these patients. In particular, 102 patients (56.6%) had pancreatic calcification and 155 patients (86.1%) dilation of Wirsung's duct. A pseudocyst was present in 61 patients (33.9%), while dilation of the bile ducts was present in 41 (22.7 %).

In our series, as can be clearly seen in Table 43.2, the main indication for surgical decompression was severe, disabling pain, followed by the presence of a 'symptomatic' pseudocyst and stenosis of the main bile duct. Table 43.3 schematically presents the main surgical procedures adopted in the series. In the context of anastomotic surgery, the most commonly performed operation up to 1997 was an extended pancreaticojejunostomy (at least 10 cm) according to Partington–Rochelle, to which, more recently, we have now added the Frey operation as a standard procedure. This surgical approach, however, is interpreted differently, in

Table 43.1. Preoperative features in 180 chronic pancreatitis patients who underwent a drainage procedure

	Number of patients	%
Calcification	102	56.6
Diabetes		
Type 1	17	9.4
Type 2	25	13.9
Wirsung dilatation (> 7 mm)	155	86.1
Pseudocyst	61	33.9
Main bile duct dilatation (> 5 mm)	41	22.7
Jaundice	16	8.9
Previous cholecystectomy	30	16.6
Biliary stones	19	10.5

Table 43.2. Indications for surgery in 180 patients with chronic pancreatitis

	Number of patients	%
Severe pain	124	68.8
Pseudocyst	20	11.1
Biliary complications	16	8.9
Suspicion of neoplasia	13	7.3
Other	7	3.9

Table 43.3. Surgical procedures adopted on 180 patients with chronic pancreatitis

	Number of patients	%
Pancreaticojejunostomy (Partington–Rochelle)	121	67.3
Pancreaticojejunostomy (Frey)	26	14.4
Cysto-pancrejejunostomy	18	10
Cystojejunostomy	15	8.3
Combined procedures		
Biliary by-pass	34	
Gastric by-pass	16	
Cholecystectomy	61	

that some surgeons class the Frey procedure as belonging to the resection group (it involves resection of a portion of the anterior wall of the head of the pancreas without transection of the gland at the portal axis level), while others interpret it as being a more strictly anastomotic procedure.[8,9]

Surgical Technique

The surgical technique we adopt involves complete exposure of the anterior surface of the pancreas after extensive opening of the gastrocolic ligament and a Kocher manoeuvre. This manoeuvre allows easy direct puncture of Wirsung's duct and the execution of intra-operative radiography of the duct so as to establish with precision the cranio-caudal extent of the ductal opening. We then lay open the main duct, removing any calculosis formations with resolution of the concomitant stenosis; we then proceed with the construction of the anastomosis on a Roux-en-Y loop.

As we have already stressed, it is extremely important to construct the largest possible anastomosis in order to drain the maximum possible amount of pancreatic parenchyma. In that sense, the Frey procedure, in addition to anastomosing the body-tail, makes it possible to retain all the head portion, removing a flap of tissue regarded as being the pace-maker site of the pain impulses.[7]

In the case of pseudocyst, we regard puncturing the pseudocyst along with contrast radiography as being of fundamental importance in order to detect the presence or otherwise of communication with the main duct. If there is no communication, our strategy consists in constructing a cystojejunostomy using the same intestinal loop in addition to the anastomosis with Wirsung's duct. If communication is detected, we proceed with the opening of both and the construction of a side-to-side anastomosis to the transmesocolic Roux-en-Y loop.

In patients suffering from chronic pancreatitis, the main bile duct is also of particular importance as it may be involved in the fibrotic processes even at an early stage. For this clinical reason, preoperative laboratory and radiographic investigations may modify the surgical timing. In the presence of stenosis of the terminal portion of the bile duct we construct a hepaticojejunostomy in preference to a choledocho-duodenostomy to prevent the onset of cholangitis-type phenomena facilitated by the lengthy natural history of the disease.

Results of Treatment

The postoperative course was uneventful in 148 patients (82.3%), while in 23 (12.7%) there were abdominal complications, in particular six pancreatic fistulas (26%), five bilio-pancreatic fistulas (21.7%), one biliary fistula (4.4 %) and one enteric fistula (4.4 %).

These complications did not entail any appreciable lengthening of the hospital stay. The perioperative mortality consisted of two deaths (1.1%), one related to a major coagulation deficit and the other resulting from haemorrhage due to rupture of a pseudoaneurysm of the gastroduodenal artery.

Long-term Outcome

During follow-up, the mean duration of which was 4.8 years (range: 13 months–11 years) there were 12 deaths due, respectively, to oesophageal cancer (one case), decompensated cirrhosis of the liver (two cases) pancreatic cancer (three cases, arising 2, 3.8 and 4.1 years after the anastomotic surgery), while in six cases we were unable to discover the cause of death. None of the patients in whom anastomoses were constructed subsequently underwent resection for persistence of pain symptoms.

Diabetes was present preoperatively in 23.3% of patients undergoing anastomotic surgery and this percentage subsequently rose to 37% during follow-up.

The incidence of pain recurrences showed a significant, progressive increase in the years preceding construction of the anastomosis (Fig. 43.1). In the postoperative period, 77.2 % of patients remained completely pain-free without any significant variations during the follow-up period.

As far as alcohol consumption is concerned, which was present in 84% of cases prior to anastomotic surgery, this was reduced in the postoperative period, but the percentage of patients who continued drinking (30%) remained fairly high. Body weight, which is an indirect indicator of nutritional status, showed a tendency to rise in the postoperative period with recovery of the weight lost preoperatively, when the 'feeding equals pain' equation prompted the patient to progressively reduce his or her consumption of a balanced calorie intake.

Conclusions

Chronic pancreatitis is a progressively developing disease that eventually leads to a state of severe physical debilitation with a progressive loss of acceptable quality of life, essentially as a result of the pain experienced.

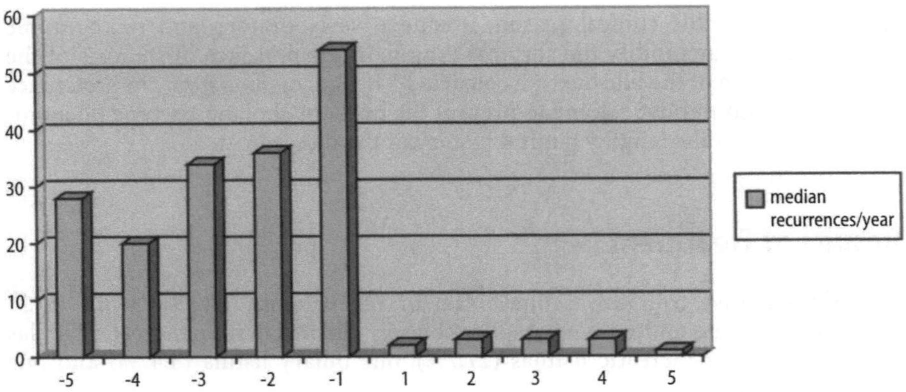

Figure 43.1. Symptomatic outcome in 180 chronic pancreatitis patients before and after surgery.

The role of the surgeon, when called upon to treat the patient, is aimed at enhancing the his or her quality of life by relieving the pain and preventing and/or treating the main complications.

The aetiopathogenesis of the pain is still unclear and the following hypotheses have been suggested:[10]

- intraductal hypertension with duodenal outflow obstruction;
- fibrotic involvement of the intrapancreatic nerve endings;
- concomitant neuritis;
- release of neurotransmitters by the inflamed pancreas.

As far as the type of surgical approach described here is concerned, the hypothesis that the pain is directly correlated with intraductal hypertension is borne out by the high percentage of patients undergoing surgical anastomosis who remain absolutely symptom-free after a lengthy follow-up period.[11]

We believe that these results are mainly related to the adoption of a surgical technique that involves the intra-operative identification of Wirsung's duct, the widest possible opening of the duct, complete removal, where possible, of any intraductual stones present, with resolution of the ductal stenosis and construction of the largest possible anastomosis.

One final consideration worthy of note is that anastomotic surgery presents a significantly lower operative risk and incidence of postoperative complications than resection procedures.[5,11] In our opinion, resection should be reserved for cases of pseudocyst of the pancreatic tail involving the splenic hilus with a haemorrhagic potential and for patients with suspected malignancies.

In conclusion, then, like others,[12] we believe that no single surgical technique is capable of constituting the gold standard in the treatment of chronic pancreatitis and its complications, but that the type of procedure adopted has to be identified on the basis of the individual patient's needs.

References

1. Talamini G, Bassi C, Falconi M, et al. Alcohol and smoking as risk factors in chronic pancreatitis and in pancreatic cancer. Dig Dis Sci 1999; 44:1303–1311.
2. Bassi C, Falconi M, Caldiron E, et al. To what extent is surgery superior to endoscopic therapy in the management of chronic pancreatitis? Ital J Gastroenterol 1998; 30:571–578.
3. Prinz RA. Surgical options in chronic pancreatitis. Int J Pancreatol 1993; 14:97–105.
4. Lankisch PG, Andersen-Sendberg A. Standards for the diagnosis of chronic pancreatitis and for the evaluation of treatment. Int J Pancreatol 1993; 14:205–212.
5. Falconi M, Valerio A, Caldiron E, et al. Changes in pancreatic resection for chronic pancreatitis over 28 years in a single institution. Br J Surg 2000; 87:428–433.
6. Backman DE. Pain in chronic pancreatitis: the role of nerves. Dig Surg 1996; 13:67–72.
7. Bradley EL III. Pancreatic duct pressure in chronic pancreatitis. Am J Surg 1982; 144:313–316.
8. Bell RH Jr. Surgical options in patients with chronic pancreatitis. Curr Gastroenterol Rep 2000; 2 (2):146–151.
9. Amikura K, Arai K, Kobari M, et al. Surgery for chronic pancreatitis extended pancreaticojejunostomy. Hepatogastroenterology 1997; 44:1547–1553.
10. Beglinger C. Pathophysiological events in chronic pancreatitis: the current concept. In: Malfertheiner P, Dominìnguez-Munoz JE, Sculz HU, et al., eds. Diagnostic Procedures in Pancreatic Disease, Springer 1996.
11. Bassi C, Falconi M, Caldiron E, et al. Surgical drainage and bypass. In: Izbicki JR, Binmoeller KF, Soehendra N, eds. Chronic Pancreatitis. Walter de Gruyter, Berlin, New York 1997.
12. Ho HS, Frey CF. Current approach to the surgical management of chronic pancreatitis. Gastroenterology 1997; 5 (2):128–36.

Index

Page numbers in **bold** represent tables, those in *italics* represent figures.

MIX
Papier aus verantwortungsvollen Quellen
Paper from responsible sources
FSC® C105338

If you have any concerns about our products,
you can contact us on
ProductSafety@springernature.com

In case Publisher is established outside the EU,
the EU authorized representative is:
Springer Nature Customer Service Center GmbH
Europaplatz 3, 69115 Heidelberg, Germany

Printed by Libri Plureos GmbH
in Hamburg, Germany